# The Pulmonary Circulation and Gas Exchange

*Edited by*

## Wiltz W. Wagner, Jr., Ph.D.

*VK Stoelting Professor of Anesthesiology*
*Professor of Physiology, Biophysics, and Pediatrics*
*Indiana University School of Medicine*
*Indianapolis, Indiana*

*and*

## E. Kenneth Weir, M.D.

*Professor of Medicine*
*Veterans Administration Medical Center*
*University of Minnesota School of Medicine*
*Minneapolis, Minnesota*

Futura Publishing Company, Inc
Armonk, NY

**Library of Congress Cataloging-in-Publication Data**

The Pulmonary circulation and gas exchange / edited by Wiltz W. Wagner, Jr. and E. Kenneth Weir.

    p. cm.

    Includes bibliographical references.

    ISBN 0-87993-572-3

    1. Pulmonary circulation—Biography. 2. Pulmonary circulation—History—20th century. I. Wagner, Wiltz W. Jr. II. Weir, E. Kenneth.

    [DNLM: 1. Pulmonary Circulation—physiology. 2. Pulmonary Gas Exchange—physiology. 3. Respiration. WF 600 P9807 1994]

QP107.P835 1994

612.2—dc20

DNLM/DLC

for Library of Congress

93-38017
CIP

Copyright 1994
Futura Publishing Company, Inc.

*Published by*
Futura Publishing Company, Inc.
135 Bedford Road
Armonk, New York 10504-0418

LC #: 93-38017
ISBN #: 0-87993-572-3

Printed in the United States of America.

This book is printed on acid-free paper.

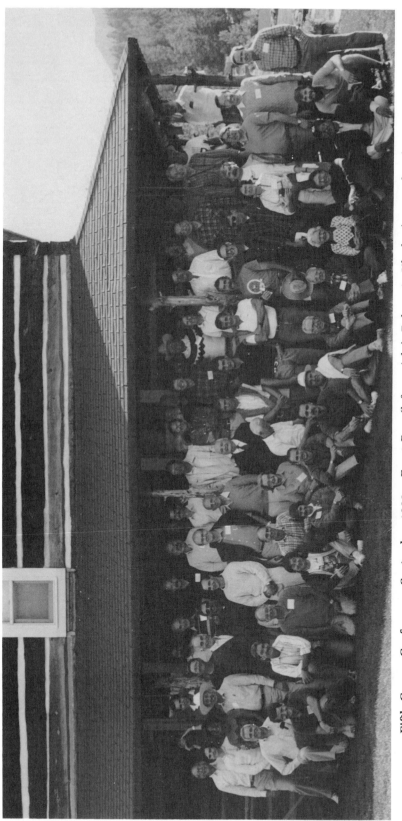

**Fifth Grover Conference, September 1992.** *Front Row* (left to right): Robert A. Klocke (on one knee), James R. Snapper, Mark N. Gillespie, Wiltz W. Wagner, Jr., Almas Aldechev, David J. Riley, Anne Clark, Gwenda R. Barer, Troy Stevens, Grant deJ. Lee (looking down), Tawfic S. Hakim, John N. Evans, Robert F. Grover, Norman C. Staub, Lynne M. Reid, J. Michael Kay, Michael R. T. Yen, Vaclav Hampl. *Middle Row:* Robert E. Forster II, Claire Doerschuk, J. Usha Raj, John B. West, Aubrey E. Taylor, Solbert Permutt, Christopher A. Dawson, Roy G. Brower, J. T. Sylvester, C. A. Wagenvoort, Donald Heath, S. Adnot, G. Simonneau, Phillipe Herve, Peter D. Wagner, John T. Reeves, David Badesch, Barbara O. Meyrick, Norbert Voelkel, A.N. Other, E. Kenneth Weir, Bertron M. Groves. *Back Row:* Albert L. Hyman (binoculars), Stephen Archer, Inder Anand, Peter Harris, Nicholas S. Hill, John A. Linehan, A.N. Other, Robert G. Presson, Stephen J. Lai-Fook, Robert L. Johnson, Jr., Ronald Capen, Leonard Latham, John Butler, Lorna Moore, Gregory J. Redding, Ewald R. Weibel, Y. C. Fung, Walker Long, K. Horsfield, John H. Newman, Thomas Jacobs.

# Preface

Scientific papers are inevitably highly polished, finely honed products that give few clues about the real process of science. In this book 21 pioneers in the wide fields of the pulmonary circulation and gas exchange write on their careers. To qualify from this elite group, they had to have worked on the pulmonary circulation and gas exchange for at least 25 years. Instead of the usual dry science, they were requested to write about how they got started, who influenced them, and what troubles they had; in other words to tell it like it was.

One theme that came out clearly was that this generation of scientists traveled widely to other centers and other countries to learn techniques, experimental methods, and the philosophy underlying scientific investigation. Travel of this kind was not unique to this group. Two prominent examples from generations past are Galen who went from Greece to the great museum in Alexandria to study the work of Herophilus and Erasistratus. Harvey studied in Padua and learned the concepts of Versalius, Columbo, and Fabricius. In the same manner, the authors of these chapters sought training in laboratories with international reputations; frequently they developed centers of excellence in their own careers that served to educate the next generation of investigators. Particular names and places recur throughout the narratives as sources of direction and inspiration. It is startling to realize how brief encounters may have determined the path of an illustrious career.

This volume provides a series of unique and fascinating autobiographies of the leaders in research on the pulmonary circulation and gas exchange. Their ability to persevere despite adversity should be an encouragement to all, whether scientist or not.

The editors gratefully acknowledge Cathy Kreyche and Linda Shaw who provided invaluable editorial expertise and James A. Will who provided some of the photographs of the contributors.

WILTZ W. WAGNER, JR.
E. KENNETH WEIR

# Introduction

In this volume the evolution of our current understanding of a number of areas of pulmonary function, both the physiology and the pathophysiology, are explained. The authors were specifically instructed to write in plain English and not to obfuscate the material with equations. This elite group of scientists succeeded brilliantly.

Subjects that are often difficult to understand such as the diffusion of gases are lucidly explained—not only the physiology of the subject, but the clinical areas when the gas exchange properties of the lung go awry. Contributions are made by: Robert E. Forster, M.D., Robert L. Johnson, M.D., Johannes Piiper, M.D.

How the pulmonary circulation is remodeled in disease is laid out by the scientists who did the original work. Their difficulties and disagreements are discussed in a way that leaves readers in a position to make up their own minds. Contributions are made by: Y. C. Fung, Ph.D., Donald Heath, D.Sc., M.D., Lynne Reid, M.D., Ph.D., C. A. Wagenvoort, M.D.

The fascinating area of high altitude physiology and medicine is described by the men and women who did the basic work. This area of research has always been interesting not only because of the inherent nature of the subject, but also because it serves as a good model for many lung diseases. Contributions are made by: Gwenda R. Barer, M.D., Robert F. Grover, M.D., Ph.D., Peter Harris, M.D., Ph.D.

The complex work on the relationships of pressure and flow in health and disease are explored. Pulmonary pharmacology, the anatomy of the pulmonary blood vessels, and alterations in the pulmonary circulation in relationship to respiration and in disease are all brought into sharp focus by the masters of these fields. Contributions are made by: John Butler, M.D., A. P. Fishman, M.D., Keith Horsfield, M.D., Albert L. Hyman, M.D., Grant deJ. Lee, M.D., Thomas C. Lloyd, M.D., Solbert Permutt, M.D., John T. Reeves, M.D., Norman C. Staub, M.D., Ewald R. Weibel, M.D., John B. West, M.D., Ph.D., D.Sc.

In addition to being a repository for considerable scientific information, the autobiographic details are filled with anecdotes that are sometimes amusing, sometimes touching, and always interesting.

WILTZ W. WAGNER, JR.
E. KENNETH WEIR

# Contents

Preface: Wiltz W. Wagner, Jr., Ph.D., and E. Kenneth Weir, M.D. . . . . . . . . . . . v
Introduction: Wiltz W. Wagner, Jr., Ph.D., and E. Kenneth Weir, M.D. . . . . . . . vii

1   Strength and Failure of Pulmonary Capillaries
     John B. West, M.D., Ph.D., D.Sc. . . . . . . . . . . . . . . . . . . . . . . . 1

2   Exploring the Structural Basis for Pulmonary Gas Exchange
     Ewald R. Weibel, M.D. . . . . . . . . . . . . . . . . . . . . . . . 19

3   Pulmonary Vascular Disease: A Joint Adventure
     C. A. Wagenvoort, M.D. . . . . . . . . . . . . . . . . . . . . . . . 47

4   Pulmonary Edema: Then and Now
     Norman C. Staub, M.D. . . . . . . . . . . . . . . . . . . . . . . . 59

5   Structural Remodeling of the Pulmonary Vasculature by Environmental
     Change and Disease
     Lynne M. Reid, M.D. . . . . . . . . . . . . . . . . . . . . . . . 77

6   A Personal View of Neonatal Pulmonary Hypertension
     John T. Reeves, M.D. . . . . . . . . . . . . . . . . . . . . . . . 111

7   Search for Diffusion Limitation in Pulmonary Gas Exchange
     Johannes Piiper, M.D. . . . . . . . . . . . . . . . . . . . . . . . 125

8   Pulmonary Mechanics and the Pulmonary Blood Vessels
     Solbert Permutt, M.D. . . . . . . . . . . . . . . . . . . . . . . . 147

9   Encounters with the Pulmonary Circulation
     Thomas C. Lloyd, M.D. . . . . . . . . . . . . . . . . . . . . . . . 167

10   My Studies of the Lung Microcirculation
     Grant de J. Lee, M.D. . . . . . . . . . . . . . . . . . . . . . . . 189

11   Adventures in Gas Exchange
     Robert L. Johnson, M.D. . . . . . . . . . . . . . . . . . . . . . . . 221

12   An Approach to the Study of the Pulmonary Circulation
     Albert L. Hyman, M.D. . . . . . . . . . . . . . . . . . . . . . . . 235

13   The Pulmonary Vascular Tree Seen as a Convergent Tree
     Keith Horsfield, M.D. . . . . . . . . . . . . . . . . . . . . . . . 253

14   Pulmonary Vascular Disease in Sheffield, the Andes, Tibet, and Tanzania
     Donald Heath, D.Sc., M.D., Ph.D. . . . . . . . . . . . . . . . . . . . . . . . 265

15  The Pulmonary Circulation of Some Domestic Animals at High
    Altitude: The Real Story
        Peter Harris, M.D., Ph.D. . . . . . . . . . . . . . . . . . . . . . 283

16  Pulmonary Hypertension: The Price of High Living
        Robert F. Grover, M.D., Ph.D. . . . . . . . . . . . . . . . . . . 317

17  Pressure, Flow, Stress, and Remodeling in the Pulmonary Vasculature
        Yuan-Cheng B. Fung, Ph.D. . . . . . . . . . . . . . . . . . . . 343

18  The Exotic Gases, CO, $O_2$, and $CO_2$
        Robert E. Forster, M.D. . . . . . . . . . . . . . . . . . . . . . 365

19  A Physician-Scientist's Tale
        Alfred P. Fishman, M.D. . . . . . . . . . . . . . . . . . . . . . 381

20  Reflections on the Waterfall in the Chest
        John Butler, M.D. . . . . . . . . . . . . . . . . . . . . . . . . 389

21  Acute and Chronic Lack of Oxygen: Consequences for the Lung and
    Carotid Body; A Journey with *Bacillus Investigationis,* the
    Curiosity Bug
        Gwenda R. Barer, M.D. . . . . . . . . . . . . . . . . . . . . . 403

# 1

# Strength and Failure of Pulmonary Capillaries

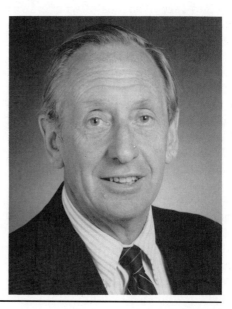

### John B. West, M.D., Ph.D., D.Sc.

*Professor of Medicine and Physiology, University of California, San Diego, La Jolla, California*

I was fortunate to attend a good school in Adelaide, Australia, and was greatly influenced by a Mr. Ray Smith, who taught physics and chemistry in the last three years of high school. He had an infectious enthusiasm and a wonderful clarity of exposition that had an important bearing on how I learned to write and talk about physiology. In my last couple of years at school my great love was high energy physics, and I probably would have gone into that area were it not for the fact that both my father and mother had medical backgrounds and that in the education system that I was brought up in it was necessary to elect your field of study by the age of 16 or 17.

I found medical school very tedious partly because the material was taught in a descriptive, nonanalytical manner. These were the days before full-time academic appointments in the clinical departments at Adelaide University. In particular, I was taught physiology very badly, and this probably set back my interest in the topic by about ten years. Most of my university friends were outside the medical school, and I spent a good deal of my time studying music and other humanities. As a result, I barely scraped through in my final year.

After the required year of residency, I left for England on the first available boat (this was before long distance air travel was feasible) and started to put down roots in London, a city I still regard as the most stimulating city in the world. Fortunately I had a link with someone at the Postgrad-

From: Wagner WW, Jr, Weir EK (eds): *The Pulmonary Circulation and Gas Exchange.* ©1994, Futura Publishing Co Inc, Armonk, NY.

uate Medical School, Hammersmith Hospital (later to become the Royal Postgraduate Medical School), and after a year or so I was accepted there as an intern. At this stage I had very little idea of what area of medicine to pursue except that, being interested in physical phenomena such as pressures and flows, I considered cardiology or pulmonary diseases. It happened that the Postgraduate Medical School was soon to embark on a new program in clinical pulmonary physiology, and Dr. Charles Fletcher suggested that I spend a year at the Pneumoconiosis Research Unit near Cardiff, learn some pulmonary physiology, and then return to Hammersmith. While I was at Cardiff, Julius Comroe's green-covered book, *The Lung,* appeared and I devoured every word. That exceptional book persuaded me that I had found my niche.

When I returned to Hammersmith, two new technical developments determined my research program. The first was that Kemp Fowler had just built the first mass spectrometer designed specifically for pulmonary research. We used it to study the alveolar gas composition both in expired gas[58,59,61] and during bronchoscopy by passing the sampling tube of the mass spectrometer down the old, rigid bronchoscope.[28,60] The procedure we developed at that time for determining the amount of ventilation-perfusion inequality in the lung from measurements of the respiratory exchange ratio in expired gas was exploited on Spacelab SLS-1 in June 1991, when we found, to our surprise, that there was considerable ventilation-perfusion inequality present during space flight.

The second technical development was that the first cyclotron specifically for medical research was just coming on line, and, among the exotic radioisotopes it produced, the most remarkable was oxygen-15, with a half life of only 2 min. Together with Phillip Hugh-Jones and others, I studied the patterns obtained when a patient inhaled a single breath of this gas and counters were placed over different regions of the lung.[14,15] To our utter astonishment, the rate at which the radioactive oxygen was removed from the apex of the normal upright lung was much less than that at the base.[56,57]

It is difficult now to realize that at that time there was no notion that the distribution of blood flow in the lung was uneven. Admittedly, in retrospect, some early measurements using bronchospirometry and small catheters passed into the bronchi were consistent with uneven blood flow. But the significance of these observations had not been fully appreciated, and therefore the demonstration using oxygen-15 of the striking regional differences of blood flow was enormously exciting. Subsequently we found that if we labeled carbon dioxide with the same radioisotope, the rates of removal were faster and easier to measure. Figure 1 shows one of the early tracings made using [15]O-labeled carbon dioxide in 1958. Much of my research over the subsequent 10 years was devoted to the factors responsible for the inequality of blood flow and ventilation in the lung and their effects on regional and overall gas exchange.

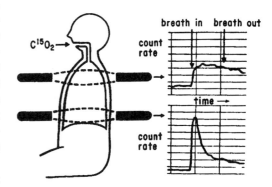

**Figure 1.** Early tracings obtained with [15]O-labeled carbon dioxide showing the striking difference in blood flow between the top and bottom of the upright lung. The subject took a single breath of the gas and held his breath for 15 s. Note the slow rate of removal of the gas at the apex of the lung compared with the pattern at the base of the lung.

I spent almost 15 years at the Postgraduate Medical School, with three interruptions. The first was to join Sir Edmund Hillary on a Himalayan high-altitude physiology expedition in 1960. This was followed by a year with Hermann Rahn in Buffalo and later a year at the NASA Ames Research Center at Moffett Field in California. I became interested in space physiology because I had spent a great deal of time thinking about the effects of gravity on the lung. While I was in California, the new medical school at the University of California, San Diego, was recruiting its first faculty members, and this seemed like a wonderful opportunity. It was, and I have spent the last 22 years very happily at UCSD. I have been away only for a period in 1981 during the American Medical Research Expedition to Everest.

I would now like to turn to the recent work on the strength and failure of pulmonary capillaries, carried out in collaboration with Dr. Odile Mathieu-Costello. It is well known that the blood-gas barrier is extremely thin. Indeed in the human lung, approximately half of the barrier has a thickness of only 0.2–0.4 μm.[20] However, the integrity of the blood-gas barrier must be maintained because otherwise plasma or even blood from the capillaries will leak into the alveolar spaces and interfere with gas exchange. Therefore the blood-gas barrier needs to be strong as well as thin. It is curious that physicians and physiologists have rarely asked the question: how strong is the blood-gas barrier?

We approached this problem by taking anesthetized rabbits, opening the chest, cannulating the pulmonary artery and left atrium, and perfusing the lung with the rabbit's own blood. After only 1 min of autologous blood perfusion, we washed the blood out with a saline/dextran mixture and followed with buffered glutaraldehyde to fix the lungs for electron microscopy. We used pulmonary arterial pressures of 20, 40, 60, and 80 cmH$_2$O. The pulmonary venous pressure

was always set 5 cmH$_2$O below the arterial pressure, and the alveolar pressure was 5 cmH$_2$O. Therefore the capillary transmural pressures were at 12.5, 32.5, 52.5, and 72.5 ± 2.5 cmH$_2$O.[52,64]

Two interesting findings emerged. The first was that at the high pressures the capillaries bulged into the alveolar spaces (Fig. 2). This was not surprising because Glazier and coworkers[22] had shown a similar appearance in an entirely different preparation, where dog lung capillaries had been rapidly frozen during perfusion with their own blood. In addition, a similar appearance was reported by Gil and coworkers[21] in rabbit lungs.

The second finding was more surprising. At capillary transmural pressures of 52.5 cmH$_2$O and above we saw ultrastructural damage to the blood-gas barrier, including disruption of the capillary endothelial cells, alveolar epithelial cells, and sometimes all layers of the barrier. An

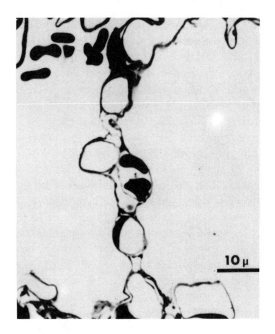

**Figure 2.** Photomicrograph of pulmonary capillaries of rabbit at a transpulmonary pressure of 52.5 cmH$_2$O. Note that the capillaries bulge into the alveolar spaces and that their average diameter is about 10 μm. (Reproduced with permission from reference 64.)

example is shown in Figure 3a, where the capillary endothelial layer shows disruption while its basement membrane remains intact, as does the basement membrane of the alveolar epithelial cell and the alveolar epithelium itself. Figure 3b shows another example. Here the alveolar epithelial lining is disrupted, and if you look carefully you can see that the capillary endothelial layer is also broken, with a red cell very close to the exposed endothelial basement membrane. A further example is shown in Figure 3c, where the alveolar epithelial layer is broken on one side of the capillary while the endothelial layer is disrupted on the other. Note the platelet apparently adhering to the exposed basement membrane. A final example is shown in Figure 3d, where all layers of the blood-gas barrier are broken and a red cell can be seen apparently moving out of the capillary lumen. Note also the appearance of "blebbing" in the alveolar epithelium near the break.

The breaks in the alveolar epithelial layer can also be seen very well by scanning electron microscopy. Here we had to be especially careful to avoid artifacts, and Figure 4a shows a normal appearance at a low capillary transmural pressure of 12.5 $cmH_2O$. The arrows point to junctions between adjacent type I alveolar epithelial cells. Figure 4b shows an example when the capillary pressure was raised to 52.5 $cmH_2O$. Several breaks can be seen. Interestingly, these generally occur at right angles to the longitudinal axis of the capillary.

Figure 5 shows the frequency of breaks in both the endothelial and epithelial layers. No breaks were seen in preparations, where the capillary transmural pressure was 12.5 $cmH_2O$. However, breaks were consistently seen when the pressure was raised to 52.5 $cmH_2O$ or above. A few breaks were seen at a transmural pressure of 32.5 $cmH_2O$, although most of these were in one preparation, which could have been abnormal.

The three principal forces acting on the capillary wall are shown in Figure 6. The first is the hoop or circumferential tension caused by the capillary transmural pressure acting across a curved surface and calculated from the Laplace relationship. At a capillary transmural pressure of 50 $cmH_2O$ (that is, at failure), the hoop tension is not particularly high, being about 25 dyn/cm (or 25 mN/m). The very small radius of curvature of the capillaries is an important factor in keeping this tension low. The second force is the surface tension of the alveolar lining layer. Because the capillaries bulge into the alveolar spaces at the high pressures (Fig. 2), we have argued that the surface tension will support the capillaries much as iron hoops support a barrel of beer. At normal lung volumes, the surface tension is believed to be 1–10 dyn/cm. It therefore represents a significant support to the bulging capillaries. At high lung volumes, where the surface tension might rise to 50 dyn/cm because of the behavior of surfactant, the support is predicted to be much greater. The third force is the longitudinal tension in the alveolar wall associated with lung inflation. This is probably very small at normal lung volumes but can rise to high levels at large lung volumes. We shall see later that the frequency of stress failure increases greatly at high lung volumes for the same capillary transmural pressure.

As indicated above, the hoop tension of the capillary wall at failure is relatively small. However, whether the wall gives way depends not on the tension but on the stress, that is, the tension divided by wall thickness. Figure 7 shows the calculation of wall stress for a capillary transmural pressure of 40 mmHg (= 54 $cmH_2O$), radius of curvature of 5 μm, and wall thickness of 0.3 μm. The calculated stress is $9 \times 10^5$ dyn/cm$^2$ (or $9 \times 10^4$ N/m$^2$, which is astonishingly high. Indeed this is approximately the same as the wall stress of the normal aorta, which is armored by substantial amounts of collagen and elastin. By contrast, the thin side of the

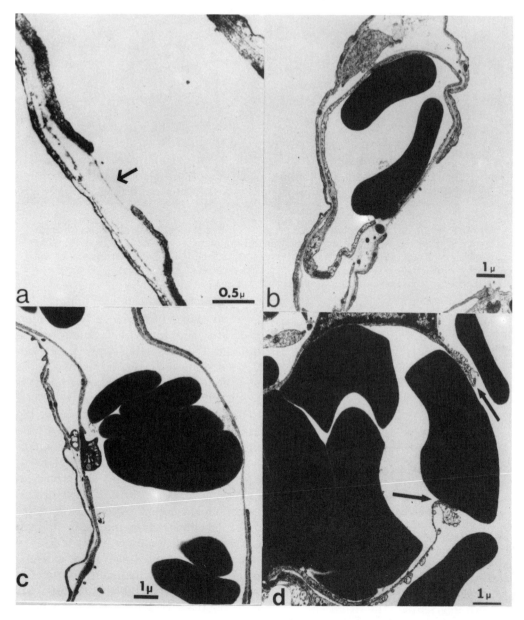

**Figure 3.** Electron micrographs showing stress failure in pulmonary capillaries. a. The capillary endothelium is disrupted, but the alveolar epithelium and the two basement membranes are intact. Capillary transmural pressure was 52.5 cmH$_2$O. b. Both the alveolar epithelium and capillary endothelium are disrupted, but the basement membrane is intact. Note the red blood cell closely applied to the exposed intact basement membrane. The capillary transmural pressure was 72.5 cmH$_2$O. c. The alveolar epithelial layer (right) and capillary endothelial layer (left) are disrupted. Note the platelet closely applied to the exposed basement membrane (left). The capillary transmural pressure was 52.5 cmH$_2$O. d. Disruption of all layers of the blood-gas barrier with red blood cell passing through the opening. Note "blebbing" of the alveolar epithelium. The capillary pressure was 72.5 cmH$_2$O. (a, b, c reproduced with permission from reference 64. d. reproduced with permission from reference 52.)

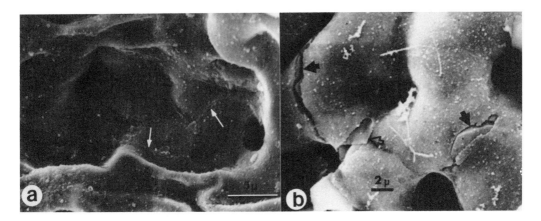

**Figure 4.** a. Scanning electron micrograph (SEM) showing normal appearance of alveolar epithelial cells at a capillary transmural pressure of 12.5 $cmH_2O$. b. SEM appearance at a capillary transmural pressure of 52.5 $cmH_2O$. Note disruptions of the alveolar epithelial cells with a flap of endothelium (open arrow) partly covering one break. (Reproduced with permission from reference 7.)

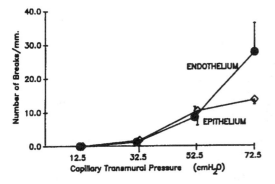

**Figure 5.** Number of breaks per mm of endothelial and epithelial boundary length plotted against capillary transmural pressure. Means ± SE. Very few breaks were seen at 32.5 $cmH_2O$, and the pressure had to be raised to 52.5 $cmH_2O$ before breaks were consistently seen. (Reproduced with permission from reference 52.)

blood-gas barrier has half of its thickness made up of endothelial and epithelial cell layers, which presumably contribute relatively little strength. What is remarkable is not that the capillaries fail at high pressures, but that they do not fail more often.

We have given a great deal of thought to what is responsible for the strength of the blood-gas barrier. Several pieces of evidence suggest that most of the strength can be attributed to the extracellular matrix. One piece of evidence is the pattern of failure commonly seen, which is illustrated in Figures 3a–c. Frequently the capillary endothelial layer and/or the alveolar epithelial cell layer breaks, but the basement membranes remain intact. This is not a universal finding, as shown by Figure 3d, but it is common and suggests that the strongest component of the blood-gas barrier is the extracellular matrix.

More evidence comes from the work of Welling and Grantham.[55] These investigators took isolated rabbit renal tubules, mounted them on a micropipette, and measured their diameter while increasing their transmural pressure. They were able to do this both with intact tubules and with tubules where the epithelium had been removed with detergent so that only the basement membrane remained. They found that the mechanical properties of the tubules in extension were the same, regardless of whether the epithelium was present. This ingenious experiment strongly suggested that the mechanical behavior of the isolated tubules was essentially determined by the extracellular matrix.

Further evidence comes from the work of Williamson et al.,[67] who showed

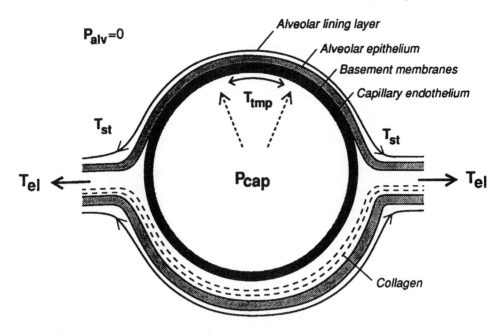

**Figure 6.** Diagram showing the three principal forces acting on the blood–gas barrier. These are the hoop or circumferential tension ($T_{tmp}$), surface tension of the alveolar lining layer ($T_{st}$), and longitudinal tension in the alveolar wall associated with lung inflation ($T_{el}$). (Reproduced with permission from reference 64.)

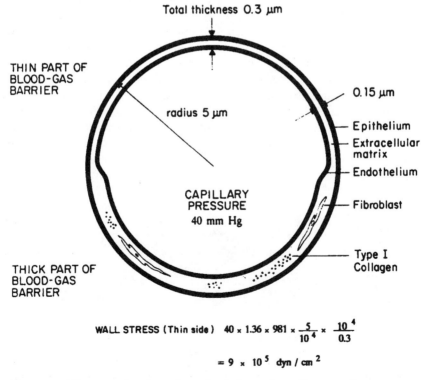

$$\text{WALL STRESS (Thin side)} \quad 40 \times 1.36 \times 981 \times \frac{5}{10^4} \times \frac{10^4}{0.3}$$

$$= 9 \times 10^5 \ \text{dyn / cm}^2$$

**Figure 7.** Diagram showing the calculation of capillary wall stress at a capillary transmural pressure of 40 mmHg. Radius of curvature is 5 μm and the thickness of the blood–gas barrier on the thin side is 0.3 μm.

that the width of the basement membrane in systemic capillaries down the human body from the abdomen to the calf increased along with the hydrostatic pressure. These authors were enterprising enough to show the same thing in the giraffe where the height is greatly increased! It is also well known that the basement membrane of pulmonary capillaries is thickened in patients with mitral stenosis who have a raised capillary pressure over months or years.[25,36] It has also been shown that the distensibility of systemic capillaries can be explained by the mechanical properties of basement membrane.[50] Finally, we know that glomerular capillaries, which normally maintain a hydrostatic gradient across them of about 40 mmHg, have a considerably thicker basement membrane than do pulmonary capillaries. All of these observations taken together strongly suggest that the extracellular matrix of pulmonary capillaries is responsible for most of their strength.

The extracellular matrix of the thin side of the blood-gas barrier is composed of the basement membranes of the two overlying cell layers, the capillary endothelium and alveolar epithelium. Alveolar wall basement membranes contain four main molecules: type IV collagen, which is believed to play a structural role; laminin, which is involved in linking the basement membrane with overlying cells; heparan sulfate proteoglycans, which

form a charge shield and probably affect capillary permeability; and entactin (or nidogen), which is thought to bind laminin and type IV collagen. The most likely candidate for the great strength of extracellular matrix is the type IV collagen, which has an interesting configuration.[51,69] The molecules are approximately 400 nm long, and two join at the C terminal end. Then four molecules join at the N terminal end to give a matrix configuration similar to chicken wire. This apparently combines great strength with porosity. Measurements show that the tensile strength of basement membranes approaches that of type I collagen.[18,55,64]

There is evidence that the type IV collagen is not uniformly distributed throughout the extracellular matrix. Vaccarro and Brody[53] have shown that the extracellular matrix has a central lamina densa with a lamina rara on either side (Fig. 8). In addition, antibodies to type IV collagen track the lamina densa as it is formed by the fusion of the basement membranes of the capillary endothelial and alveolar epithelial cells.[8] The lamina rara on either side of the lamina densa apparently predominantly contain molecules such as laminin, which link the type IV collagen to the overlying cells, and the heparan sulfate proteoglycans, which are responsible for the charge barrier. Thus the great strength of the thin part of the blood-gas barrier apparently comes from

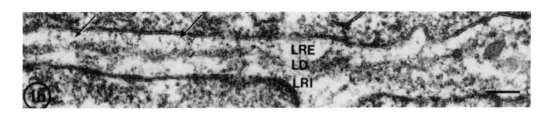

**Figure 8.** Ultrastructure of the thin part of the blood–gas barrier in rat. The alveolar epithelial cell is at the top and the capillary endothelial cell at the bottom. Note that the extracellular matrix has a central lamina densa (LD) with a lamina rara externa (LRE) and lamina rara interna (LRI) on each side. Most of the type IV collagen which is believed to be responsible for the strength of the blood-gas barrier is located in the lamina densa. Bar 0.1 μm. (Reproduced with permission from reference 53.)

an extremely thin layer of type IV collagen, only about 50-nm thick, which is sandwiched in the middle of the extracellular matrix.[62]

We have seen that in the rabbit lung, stress failure occurs at a capillary transmural pressure of about 52 cmH$_2$O, that is, about 40 mmHg. Is this such a high pressure that it is of little physiological or pathophysiological interest? The answer is no, because there is good evidence that in the human lung during maximal exercise the pulmonary capillary pressure rises above 30 mmHg. For example, Wagner et al.[54] exercised normal volunteers on a bicycle ergometer at an oxygen consumption of 3.7 L/m, that is, about 80% of their $\dot{V}O_2$ max. The mean pulmonary arterial pressure, measured with a Swan–Ganz catheter, was 37 mmHg, and the pulmonary arterial wedge pressure had a mean value of 21 mmHg. It is not known for certain where pulmonary capillary pressure lies in relation to arterial and venous pressure. However, Bhattacharya et al.[2] have shown by micropuncture that capillary pressure is about halfway between arterial and venous pressure, and Younes et al.[68] have obtained data suggesting that the capillary pressure is nearer to arterial pressure at high pulmonary blood flows. Therefore we can state that the capillary pressure at mid-lung is at least 29 mmHg. Because the bottom of the lung is some 10 cm below mid-lung, adding the hydrostatic gradient gives a capillary pressure there that exceeds 36 mmHg. Other studies on exercising normal subjects have provided similar data.[23,45]

Initially, we were very surprised to find that the capillary pressure during maximal exercise apparently rises to values close to those at which failure is seen. However, we now realize that this makes sense because of the dual role of the blood-gas barrier. Of course we cannot assume that stress failure occurs at the same pressures in the rabbit and human lung, and indeed we have recently obtained evidence in the dog lung that failure occurs at higher pressures than in the rabbit.

We can now summarize the events that occur as the pulmonary capillary pressure is gradually raised from low normal values to high values. Initially, as the Starling equilibrium is disturbed, fluid will move from the capillary lumen into the alveolar wall interstitium and possibly into the alveolar spaces. Nothing that we have said here goes against the Starling hypothesis. The result will be interstitial and perhaps alveolar edema. Then, as the pressure is raised to higher levels, we may see the phenomenon known as "pore stretching." This is somewhat controversial, but Pietra et al.[43] showed that when the pulmonary capillary pressure was increased, large tracer molecules such as hemoglobin moved between capillary endothelial cells into the interstitium of the alveolar wall. Finally, at even higher pressures, stress failure occurs with disruption of the capillary endothelial layer, alveolar epithelial layer, or sometimes all layers of the blood-gas barrier. The result will be a high permeability type of edema. Thus, as the capillary pressure is gradually raised from normal to high levels, the first stage is a low permeability, hydrostatic form of pulmonary edema, but this is later followed by a high permeability type of edema.

We can now turn to the pathophysiological conditions apparently associated with stress failure of pulmonary capillaries; these are listed in Table 1. The first group includes diseases in which an increased capillary pressure is associated with a high permeability type of pulmonary edema. Examples are neurogenic pulmonary edema, high altitude pulmonary edema, and possibly some cases of the adult respiratory distress syndrome.

There is strong evidence that neurogenic pulmonary edema is caused by stress failure of pulmonary capillaries. First, experimental models of this disease showed that both high pulmonary arterial

**Table 1**
Possible Conditions Involving Stress Failure

1. Increased pressure causing edema
   a. Neurogenic pulmonary edema
   b. High altitude pulmonary edema
   c. ? some cases of ARDS
2. Increased pressure causing hemorrhage
   a. EIPH in racehorses
   b. EIPH in greyhounds
   c. Bleeding in humans
3. Increased pressure causing edema and hemorrhage
   a. Chronic venous hypertension, e.g., mitral stenosis
4. Overinflation of lung
5. Abnormal extracellular matrix
   a. Goodpasture's syndrome
   b. Alpha-1 antitrypsin deficiency
   c. Emphysema

ARDS = adult respiratory distress syndrome;
EIPH = exercised-induced pulmonary hemorrhage.

and wedge pressures occur[47] and that these are associated with very high catecholamine levels in the blood. The exact mechanism by which this "sympathetic storm" causes elevated pulmonary vascular pressures is still debated, but it is probably acute left ventricular failure caused by systemic hypertension coupled with impaired myocardial relaxation. Next, Cameron and De showed that the edema is of the high permeability type with a large concentration of high molecular weight proteins and cells.[4] Finally, Minnear and his collaborators[38,39] showed ultrastructural damage to the blood-gas barrier that is essentially identical to the patterns that we have seen in the rabbit. They described both disruption of capillary endothelial cells[39] and breaks in alveolar epithelial cells,[38] although they did not recognize the mechanism. Thus the evidence that neurogenic pulmonary edema is caused by stress failure of pulmonary capillaries is extremely strong.

It is also probable that high-altitude pulmonary edema is caused by stress failure. First, it is now known that there is a strong association between the occurrence of high-altitude pulmonary edema and very high pulmonary arterial pressures caused by hypoxic pulmonary vasoconstriction.[30,41] Thus the edema presumably has a hydrostatic basis. However, recently Hackett et al.[24] and Schoene et al.[48] have shown that the alveolar edema is of the high permeability type with a large concentration of high molecular weight proteins and cells. Indeed one study showed that the protein concentration of the alveolar fluid in severe high-altitude pulmonary edema exceeded that in many cases of the adult respiratory distress syndrome.[48] Thus the problem is how to reconcile the occurrence of a high permeability type of edema with a presumed hydrostatic basis, which was what led us to begin this project on stress failure.

Other features of high-altitude pulmonary edema are also consistent with the stress failure mechanism. For example, postmortem studies often show vascular thrombi and fibrin clots in the lung.[1] These can be attributed to the exposed basement membranes caused by capillary endothelial cell distribution, which are highly reactive and cause adhesion of platelets, white cells, and red cells (Figures 3b and 3c). In addition, exercise at high altitude has been shown to be a provocative factor in high-altitude pulmonary edema.[27] It presumably acts by raising the pulmonary arterial pressure. The explanation of how hypoxic vasoconstriction can raise pulmonary capillary pressure is probably that given by Hultgren[29] some twenty years ago, that is, that the vasoconstriction is uneven, with the result that those capillaries not protected by arterial constriction see the high pressure. This would explain the patchy distribution of high-altitude pulmonary edema described both at autopsy and in chest radiographs.[31] Proof that stress failure of pulmonary capillaries is the mechanism of high-altitude pulmonary edema requires that the characteristic ultrastructural changes be demonstrated at autopsy, and this has not yet been done.

Some cases of the adult respiratory distress syndrome may have their origin in a transient large rise in pulmonary capillary pressure, which exposes endothelial basement membranes and leads to adhesion and activation of platelets and white blood cells. This could then initiate a biochemical cascade with the liberation of platelet activating factor, kallikrein, bradykinin, and other injurious substances. Such a sequence of events might occur in a patient who is involved in an automobile accident where the blood catecholamine levels are transiently greatly increased. This situation would be like an early subclinical type of neurogenic pulmonary edema.

The second category of conditions attributable to stress failure of pulmonary capillaries is where the increased pressure causes frank hemorrhage (Table 1). The best example of this is the remarkable condition of exercise-induced pulmonary hemorrhage, which is seen in thoroughbred racehorses. This is extremely common. Tracheobronchial washings carried out by bronchoscopy in thoroughbreds in training show that essentially 100% have evidence of alveolar bleeding,[65] although less than 5% of horses have epistaxis. The condition has apparently been recognized since Elizabethan times[37] and exercise-induced pulmonary hemorrhage is an enormous problem for thoroughbred veterinarians, but the cause has not been identified. We believe that there is strong evidence that the condition is caused by stress failure of pulmonary capillaries.

These horses develop enormously high pulmonary arterial pressures while galloping. Direct measurements made on a treadmill show that the mean pulmonary arterial pressures are 80–100 mmHg.[17] There are also reports of left ventricular end diastolic pressures in ponies exceeding 50 mmHg.[46] Therefore the pulmonary capillary pressures must be extremely high. Thoroughbreds have enormous maximal oxygen consumptions, of up to 180 ml/min/kg (compare the elite human athlete at 70–80 ml/min/kg). These high levels of aerobic activity are associated with very high cardiac outputs, which exceed 250 L/min.

Because these animals have been selectively bred for racing for over 400 years,[9] their cardiovascular systems have developed to the point that the pulmonary vascular pressures are so high that the capillaries fail because of the high wall stress. Exercise-induced pulmonary hemorrhage has also been described in racing greyhound dogs,[34] indicating that the condition is not confined to the thoroughbred but occurs in at least one other selectively bred, highly aerobic mammal. The fact that the pathological consequence is bleeding rather than the high permeability edema, which is seen both in neurogenic and high-altitude pulmonary edema, can be explained by the abrupt rise in pulmonary capillary pressure. There is evidence that exercise-induced pulmonary hemorrhage may occur in elite human athletes.[63]

Not everyone accepts that this is the mechanism for exercise-induced pulmonary hemorrhage. In an extensive autopsy study of horses with exercise-induced pulmonary hemorrhage, O'Callaghan et al.[40] concluded that the bleeding probably came from the bronchial circulation. Certainly enlarged bronchial vessels are seen at the sites of old bleeding, and these are associated with mild inflammatory changes of the small airways. However, it is likely that these changes constitute a reaction to the blood in the alveoli and small airways.

Another objection to the stress failure hypothesis is that the bleeding is chiefly seen in the dorsal-caudal regions of the lung. At first sight this suggests that the capillary hydrostatic pressure is not a major factor because one would expect the pressure to be greatest at the bottom of the lung. However, the important pressure for stress failure is the capillary transmural pressure, and it may well be that the alveolar pressure falls transiently to very low values in the dorsal-caudal region. We know that esophageal pressure falls by up to 30 mmHg during rapid inspiration during galloping,[17] and therefore substantial falls in alveolar pressure will occur at the same time. The dorsal-caudal regions of the lung are the furthest from the nares, and the changes in alveolar pressure are therefore likely to be particularly marked in these areas. In addition, these regions of the lung are close to the diaphragm, which has a very oblique orientation in the horse. Downward movements of the abdominal contents during galloping may cause large transient falls in alveolar pressure. Another factor may be the distended alveoli in the upper regions of the lung as a result of distortion of the lung by its weight. As we shall see below, stress failure of pulmonary capillaries is much increased at high lung volumes. We are presently collaborating with James Jones, John Pascoe, and Walter Tyler at the University of California, Davis, to obtain more data on this fascinating problem.

Chronic increases in pulmonary capillary pressure may give rise to a combination of pulmonary edema and hemorrhage. A good example is the patient with mitral stenosis (Table 1). Hemoptysis is a common symptom in severe disease, and autopsy studies have shown large amounts of hemosiderin in the lung. Pulmonary edema can also occur. An interesting ultrastructural feature is that type II alveolar epithelial cells are sometimes seen lining parts of the epithelium.[36] These may develop in response to damage to the type I epithelial cells as a result of stress failure (Figures 3b–3d). As pointed out earlier, marked thickening of the basement membrane is commonly seen in mitral stenosis, presumably in response to the chronically increased capillary pressure.[25,36]

Overinflation of the lung is an important contributing factor to stress failure of

pulmonary capillaries (Table 1). We have studied this in the anesthetized rabbit preparation by increasing the transpulmonary pressure from 5 to 20 $cmH_2O$ while keeping the capillary transmural pressure constant at 32.5 or 52.5 $cmH_2O$.[19] Figure 9 shows the striking increase in the number of breaks per mm cell boundary layer length for both endothelium and epithelium for a capillary transmural pressure of 32.5 $cmH_2O$. At this moderate capillary pressure there were almost no breaks in the endothelium or epithelium at a normal lung volume. However, when the transpulmonary pressure was increased to 20 $cmH_2O$ when the lung volume was close to total lung capacity, there was a large increase in the number of breaks. The differences were statistically significant at the

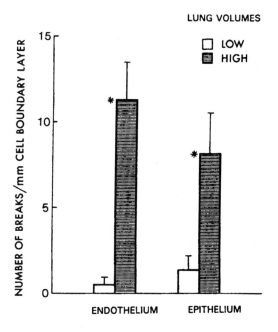

**Figure 9.** Effect of increasing lung volume on the frequency of stress failure. The transpulmonary pressure at the low lung volume was 5 $cmH_2O$ and 20 $cmH_2O$ at the high lung volume (that is, close to total lung capacity). In both instances, the capillary transmural pressure was 32.5 $cmH_2O$. Note the large increase in frequency of stress failure when the lung volume was increased. This provides a mechanism for the increased capillary permeability caused by overinflation.

5% level. A large increase in breaks was also seen when the capillary transmural pressure was kept at 52.5 cmH$_2$O and lung volume was increased.

These results provide a physiological mechanism for the increase in capillary permeability at high lung volumes that has been described by many investigators.[5,12,13,16,35,42] It is known that the increased permeability is due to the high lung volume rather than the high alveolar pressure because banding the chest prevents the increased permeability.[26] Ultrastructural evidence of damaged alveolar epithelium at high lung volumes has also been reported.[12,33]

As pointed out by others, this potential cause of damage to pulmonary capillaries at high states of lung inflation is particularly important in the intensive-care setting. It is often necessary to apply high airway pressures and substantial levels of positive end-expiratory pressure to obtain sufficiently high levels of PO$_2$ in the arterial blood. Often these diseased lungs have nonuniform mechanical properties, and it is difficult to avoid overexpanding some regions while preventing atelectasis in others. Barotrauma, as it is sometimes referred to, has emerged as one of the most challenging problems of intensive-care management.

This last group of conditions in which stress failure of pulmonary capillaries may play a role is when there is an abnormality of the extracellular matrix (Table 1). The first of these is Goodpasture's syndrome, where it has been shown that autoantibodies attack the NC1 globular domain of type IV collagen.[66] Because the type IV collagen apparently plays a critical role in maintaining the integrity of the blood-gas barrier, it is not surprising that bleeding occurs into the alveolar spaces. Donald et al. published ultrastructural evidence of breaches in the basement membrane in Goodpasture's syndrome.[11] As pointed out earlier, the glomerular capillaries are exposed to a high hydrostatic gradient of about 40 mmHg, and it is not surprising that damage to the basement membrane of these capillaries results in bleeding into the kidney.

It is also possible that stress failure of pulmonary capillaries is one of the earliest pathophysiological events in the development of the emphysema of alpha-1 antitrypsin deficiency. The basis for this disease is presumably an imbalance in the protease-antiprotease system as a result of the congenital lack of alpha-1 antitrypsin. Indeed many investigators believe that this imbalance is at the root of the more common types of emphysema, where the imbalance is associated with cigarette smoking.[32,49] It has been shown that neutrophil elastase attacks elastin in the alveolar wall, and it has been suggested that this is the initiating event in the breakdown of the wall. However, neutrophil elastase is known to cause degradation of type IV collagen,[44] and if this molecule plays the critical role in the integrity of the capillary wall that we have suggested, then the earliest destructive changes of emphysema may occur here. A possible scenario is stress failure of a pulmonary capillary at normal vascular pressures because of weakening of the wall, with the production of a small hole or fenestra.[3,6] That alveolar bleeding is not a feature of emphysema can be explained by the gradual development of the destructive changes over many years. Note, however, that pathologists have occasionally remarked on the presence of red blood cells on the alveolar surface in emphysema[3] and certainly alveolar hemorrhage is a prominent feature of animal models of emphysema produced by instilling neutrophil elastase into the lungs.[49]

Finally, I have emphasized those conditions in which the walls of the pulmonary capillaries fail because of exposure to high stresses or weakening of the walls by disease. However, it should not be concluded that the normal pulmonary blood-gas barrier is weak. On the contrary it is immensely strong. However, the lung has a basic bioengineering dilemma, as is shown in Figure 10. The blood-gas barrier must be extremely thin because gases pass through it by passive diffusion and the resistance that the barrier offers is proportional to its thickness (Fick's law). We know that the blood-gas barrier cannot afford to be any thicker because at maximal oxygen uptakes some elite human athletes show diffusion-limitation of oxygen transfer in the lung.[10,54] The extreme thinness of the barrier therefore confers a clear evolutionary advantage.

On the other hand, the blood-gas barrier needs to be extremely strong because it also forms the walls of the pulmonary capillaries, which are exposed to very high stresses when the pulmonary vascular pressures rise during maximal exercise. Indeed there is evidence that the capillary pressures during maximal exercise approach those at which stress failure occurs. In other words, the blood-gas barrier has evolved to be as thin as possible for maximum efficiency of gas exchange, with just enough strength to maintain its integrity under the most challenging conditions. Apparently in thoroughbred racehorses, which have been selectively bred for high aerobic levels over hundreds of years, the balance between the development of the cardiovascular system and the lung capillaries has been disturbed, and as a result all of these animals bleed into their lungs. It also follows that if the barrier is weakened by disease, alveolar

**Bioengineering dilemma of lung**

**Blood-gas barrier must be:**

**Extremely thin**

**Because: diffusion resistance ∝ thickness**

**Nevertheless: diffusion limitation at $VO_2$ max**

**Extremely strong**

**Because: wall stress ∝ capillary pressure**

**Nevertheless: close to failure at $VO_2$ max**

**Figure 10.** Basic bioengineering dilemma of the lung. The blood-gas barrier has to be both extremely thin and immensely strong.

edema or hemorrhage is inevitable. Stress failure in pulmonary capillaries is a hitherto overlooked factor of basic biological importance and a mechanism that apparently plays a role in many types of lung disease.

**Acknowledgments:** I am indebted to Odile Mathieu-Costello for her major contributions to the work described here on stress failure of pulmonary capillaries. I also acknowledge the collaboration of Michael L. Costello, Ann R. Elliot, Zhenxing Fu, Renato Prediletto, and Kiochi Tsukimoto. The work was supported by NIH Program Project HL17331-18.

# References

1. Arias-Stella, J., and H. Kruger. Pathology of high altitude pulmonary edema. *Arch. Pathol.* 76: 147–157, 1963.
2. Bhattacharya, J., S. Nanjo, and N. C. Staub. Micropuncture measurement of lung microvascular pressure during 5-HT infusion. *J. Appl. Physiol.* 52: 634–637, 1982.
3. Boren H. G. Alveolar fenestrae: Relationship to the pathology and pathogenesis of pulmonary emphysema. *Am. Rev. Respir. Dis.* 85: 328–344, 1962.
4. Cameron, G. R., and S. N. De. Experimental pulmonary edema of nervous origin. *J. Pathol. Bacteriol.* 61: 375–387, 1949.
5. Carlton, D. P., J. J. Cummings, R. G. Scheerer, F. R. Poulain, and R. D. Bland. Lung overexpansion increases pulmonary microvascular protein permeability in young lambs. *J. Appl. Physiol.* 69: 577–583, 1990.

6. Cosio, M. G., R. J., Shiner, M. Saetta, N.-S. Wang, M. King, H. Ghezzo, and E. Angus. Alveolar fenestrae in smokers: relationship with light microscopic and functional abnormalities. *Am. Rev. Respir. Dis.* 133: 126–131, 1986.

7. Costello M. L., O. Mathieu-Costello, and J. B. West. Stress failure of alveolar epithelial cells studied by scanning electron microscopy. *Am. Rev. Respir. Dis.* 145: 1446–1455, 1992.

8. Crouch, E. C., G. R. Martin, & J. S. Brody. Basement membranes. In: *The Lung: Scientific Foundations,* edited by R. G. Crystal and J. B. West. New York: Raven, 1991, p. 421–437.

9. Cunningham, P. The genetics of thoroughbred horses. *Scientific American* 264: 92–98, 1991.

10. Dempsey, J. A., P. G. Hanson, and K. S. Henderson. Exercise-induced alveolar hypoxemia in healthy human subjects at sea-level. *J. Physiol. (London)* 355: 161–175, 1984.

11. Donald, K. J., R. L. Edwards, and J. D. S. McEvoy. Alveolar capillary basement membrane lesions in Goodpasture's Syndrome and idiopathic pulmonary hemosiderosis. *Am. J. Med.* 59: 642–649, 1975.

12. Dreyfuss, D., G. Basset, P. Soler, and G. Saumon. Intermittent positive-pressure hyperventilation with high inflation pressures produces pulmonary microvascular injury in rats. *Am. Rev. Respir. Dis.* 132: 880–884, 1985.

13. Dreyfuss, D., and G. Saumon. Lung overinflation: physiologic and anatomical alterations leading to pulmonary edema. In: *Adult Respiratory Distress Syndrome,* edited by W. M. Zapol, and F. Lemaire. New York: M. Dekker, 1991, p. 433–449.

14. Dyson, N. A., P. Hugh-Jones, G. R. Newbery, J. D. Sinclair, and J. B. West. Studies of regional lung function using radioactive oxygen. *Br. Med. J.* 1: 231–238, 1960.

15. Dyson, N. A., P. Hugh-Jones, G. R. Newbery, and J. B. West. The preparation and use of oxygen-15 with particular reference to its value in the study of pulmonary malfunction. In: *The Second United Nations International Conference on the Peaceful Uses of Atomic Energy.* Geneva: United Nations, 1958.

16. Egan, E. A., R. M. Nelson, and R. E. Olver. Lung inflation and alveolar permeability to non-electrolytes in the adult sheep *in vivo. J. Physiol. (London)* 260: 409–424, 1976.

17. Erickson, B. K., H. H. Erickson, and J. R. Coffman. Pulmonary artery, aortic and oesophageal pressure changes during high intensity treadmill exercise in the horse: a possible relation to exercise-induced pulmonary hemorrhage. *Equine Vet. J.* (Suppl.) 9: 47–52, 1990.

18. Fisher, R. F., and J. Wakely. The elastic constants and ultrastructural organization of a basement membrane (lens capsule). *Proc. Roy. Soc. Lond. Ser. B* 193: 335–358, 1976.

19. Fu, Z., M. L. Costello, K. Tsukimoto, R. Prediletto, A. R. Elliott, O. Mathieu-Costello, and J. B. West. High lung volume increases stress failure in pulmonary capillaries. *J. Appl. Physiol.* 73: 123–133, 1992.

20. Gehr, P., M. Bachofen, and E. R. Weibel. The normal human lung: ultrastructure and morphometric estimation of diffusion capacity. *Respir. Physiol.* 32: 121–140, 1978.

21. Gil, J., H. Bachofen, P. Gehr, and E. R. Weibel. Alveolar volume-surface area relation in air- and saline-filled lungs fixed by vascular perfusion. *J. Appl. Physiol.* 47: 990–1001, 1979.

22. Glazier, J. B., J. M. B. Hughes, J. E. Maloney, and J. B. West. Measurements of capillary dimensions and blood volume in rapidly frozen lungs. *J. Appl. Physiol.* 26: 65–76, 1969.

23. Groves, B. M., J. T., Reeves, J. R. Sutton, P. D. Wagner, A. Cymerman, M. K. Malconian, P. B. Rock. P. M. Young, and C. S. Houston. Operation Everest II: elevated high-altitude pulmonary resistance unresponsive to oxygen. *J. Appl. Physiol.* 63: 521–530, 1987.

24. Hackett, P. H., J. Bertman, and G. Rodriguez. Pulmonary edema fluid protein in high-altitude pulmonary edema. *JAMA* 256: 36, 1986.

25. Haworth, S. G., S. M. Hall, and M. Patel. Peripheral pulmonary vascular and airway abnormalities in adolescents with rheumatic mitral stenosis. *Int. J. Cardiol.* 18: 405–416: 1988.

26. Hernandez, L. A., K. J. Peevy, A. A. Moise, and J. C. Parker. Chest wall restriction limits high airway pressure-induced lung injury in young rabbits. *J. Appl. Physiol.* 66: 2364–2368, 1989.

27. Houston, C. S. Acute pulmonary edema of high altitude. *N. Engl. J. Med.* 263: 478–480, 1960.

28. Hugh-Jones, P., and J. B. West. Detection of

bronchial and arterial obstruction by continuous gas analysis from individual lobes and segments of the lung. *Thorax* 15: 154–164, 1960.

29. Hultgren, H. N. High altitude pulmonary edema. In: *Biomedicine Problems in High Terrestrial Altitude,* edited by A. H. Hegnauer. New York: Springer, 1969, p. 131–141.

30. Hultgren, H. N., R. F. Grover, and L. H. Hartley. Abnormal circulatory responses to high altitude in subjects with a previous history of high-altitude pulmonary edema. *Circulation* 44: 759–770, 1971.

31. Hultgren, H. N., C. E. Lopez, E. Lundberg, and H. Miller. Physiologic studies of pulmonary edema at high altitude. *Circulation* 29: 393–408, 1964.

32. Janoff, A. Elastases and emphysema: current assessment of the protease-antiprotease hypothesis. *Am. Rev. Respir. Dis.* 132: 417–433, 1985.

33. John, E., M. McDevitt, W. Wilborn, and G. Cassady. Ultrastructure of the lung after ventilation. *Br. J. Exp. Path.* 63: 401–407, 1982.

34. King R. R, R. E. Raskin, and J. P. Rosbolt. Pulmonary hemorrhage in the racing greyhound dog. *Proceedings of the Eighth Annual Veterinary Medicine Forum, Am. Coll. Vet. Int. Med.,* Abstract no. 97, 1990.

35. Kolobow, T., M. P. Moretti, R. Fumagalli, D. Mascheroni, P. Prato, V. Chen, and M. Joris. Severe impairment in lung function induced by high peak airway pressure during mechanical ventilation. *Am. Rev. Respir. Dis.* 135: 312–315, 1987.

36. Lee, Y-S. Electron microscopic studies of the alveolar-capillary barrier in the patients of chronic pulmonary edema. *Jap. Circ. J.* 43: 945–954, 1979.

37. Markham, G. *Markham's Master-piece Revived: Containing All Knowledge Belonging to the Smith, Furrier, or Horse-Leach . . .,* London: Printed by Evan Tyler and Ralph Holt, 1681, Lib 2, p. 184.

38. Minnear, F. L., and R. S. Connell. Increased permeability of the capillary-alveolar barriers in neurogenic pulmonary edema (NPE). *Microvasc. Res.* 22: 345–366, 1981.

39. Minnear, F. L., C. Kite, L. A. Hill, and H. van der Zee. Endothelial injury and pulmonary congestion characterize neurogenic pulmonary edema in rabbits. *J. Appl. Physiol.* 63: 335–341, 1987.

40. O'Callaghan, M. W., J. R. Pascoe, W. S. Tyler, and D. K. Mason. Exercise-induced pulmonary hemorrhage in the horse: results of a detailed clinical, post-mortem and imaging study. V. Conclusions and implications. *Equine Vet. J.* 19: 428–434, 1987.

41. Oelz, O., M. Ritter, R. Jenni, M. Maggiorini, U. Waber, P. Vock, and P. Bärtsch. Nifedipine for high altitude pulmonary oedema. *Lancet* 2: 1241–1244, 1989.

42. Parker, J. C., M. I. Townsley, B. Rippe, A. E. Taylor, and J. Thigpen. Increased microvascular permeability in dog lungs due to high peak airway pressures. *J. Appl. Physiol.* 57: 1809–1816, 1984.

43. Pietra, G. G., J. P. Szidon, M. M. Leventhal, and A. P. Fishman. Hemoglobin as a tracer in hemodynamic pulmonary edema. *Science, (Washington, DC)* 166: 1643–1646, 1969.

44. Pipoly, D. J., and E. C. Crouch. Degradation of native type IV procollagen by human neutrophil elastase: implications for leukocyte-mediacted degradation of basement membranes. *Biochemistry* 26: 5748–5754, 1987.

45. Reeves, J. T., B. M. Groves, A. Cymerman, J. R. Sutton, P. D. Wagner, D. Turkevich, and C. S. Houston. Operation Everest II: cardiac filling pressures during cycle exercise at sea level. *Respir Physiol.* 80: 147–154, 1990.

46. Rugh, K. S., H. E. Garner, J. R. Miramonti, and D. G. Hatfield. Left ventricular function and haemodynamics in ponies during exercise and recovery. *Equine Vet. J.* 21: 39–44, 1989.

47. Sarnoff, S. J., E. Berglund, and L. C. Sarnoff. Neurohemodynamics of pulmonary edema. III. Estimated changes in pulmonary blood volume accompanying systemic vasoconstriction and vasodilation. *J. Appl. Physiol.* 5: 367–374, 1981.

48. Schoene R. B., P. H. Hackett, W. R. Henderson, E. H. Sage, M. Chow, R. C. Roach, W. J. Mills, and T. R. Martin. High-altitude pulmonary edema: characteristics of lung lavage fluid. *JAMA* 256: 63–69, 1986.

49. Snider, G. L., E. C. Lucey, and P. J. Stone. Animal models of emphysema. *Am. Rev. Respir. Dis.* 133: 149–169, 1986.

50. Swayne, G. T. G., L. H. Smaje, and D. H. Bergel. Distensibility of single capillaries and venules in the rat and frog mesentery. *Int. J. Microcirc* 8 *(Clin. Exp.)*: 25–42, 1989.

51. Timpl, R., H. Wiedemann, V. Van Delden, H. Furthmayr, and K. Kühn. A network model for the organization of type IV collagen molecules in basement membranes. *Eur. J. Biochem.* 120: 203–211, 1981.

52. Tsukimoto, K., O. Mathieu-Costello, R. Prediletto, A. R. Elliott, and J. B. West. Ultrastructural appearances of pulmonary capillaries at high transmural pressures. *J. Appl. Physiol.* 71: 573–582, 1991.

53. Vaccaro, C. A., and J. S. Brody. Structural features of alveolar wall basement membrane in the adult rat lung. *J. Cell Biol.* 91: 427–437, 1981.

54. Wagner, P. D., G. E. Gale, R. E. Moon, J. R. Torre-Bueno, B. W. Stolp, and H. A. Saltzman. Pulmonary gas exchange in humans exercising at sea level and simulated altitude. *J. Appl. Physiol.* 61: 260–270, 1986.

55. Welling, L. W., and J. J. Grantham. Physical properties of isolated perfused renal tubules and tubular basement membranes. *J. Clin. Invest.* 51: 1063–1075, 1972.

56. West, J. B., and C. T. Dollery. Distribution of blood flow and ventilation-perfusion ratio in the lung, measured with radioactive $CO_2$. *J. Appl. Physiol.* 15: 405–410, 1960.

57. West, J. B., C. T. Dollery, and P. Hugh-Jones. The use of radioactive carbon dioxide to measure regional blood flow in the lungs of patients with pulmonary disease. *J. Clin. Invest.* 40: 1–12, 1961.

58. West, J. B., K. T. Fowler, P. Hugh-Jones, and T. V. O'Donnell. Measurement of the ventilation-perfusion ratio inequality in the lung by the analysis of a single expirate. *Clin. Sci.* 16: 529–547, 1957.

59. West, J. B., K. T. Fowler, P. Hugh-Jones, and T. V. O'Donnell. The measurement of the inequality of ventilation and of perfusion in the lung by the analysis of single expirates. *Clin. Sci.* 16: 549–565, 1957.

60. West, J. B., and P. Hugh-Jones. Effect of bronchial and arterial constriction on alveolar gas concentrations in a lobe of the dog's lung. *J. Appl. Physiol.* 14: 743–752, 1959.

61. West, J. B., and P. Hugh-Jones. Experimental verification of the single breath tests of ventilatory and ventilation-perfusion ratio inequality. *Clin. Sci.* 18: 553–559, 1959.

62. West, J. B., and O. Mathieu-Costello. Strength of the pulmonary blood-gas barrier. *Respir. Physiol.* 88: 141–148, 1992.

63. West, J. B., O. Mathieu-Costello, and D. M. Geddes. Intrapulmonary hemorrhage caused by stress failure of pulmonary capillaries during exercise. (Abstract). *Am. Rev. Respir. Dis.* 143: A569, 1991.

64. West, J. B., K. Tsukimoto, O. Mathieu-Costello, and R. Prediletto. Stress failure in pulmonary capillaries. *J. Appl. Physiol.* 70: 1731–1742, 1991.

65. Whitwell, K. E., and T. R. C. Greet. Collection and evaluation of tracheobronchial washes in horse. *Equine Vet. J.* 16: 499–508, 1984.

66. Wieslander, J, and D. Heinegard. The involvement of type IV collagen in Goodpasture's Syndrome. *Ann. NY Acad. Sci.* 460: 363–374, 1985.

67. Williamson, J. R., N. J. Vogler, and C. Kilo. Regional variations in the width of the basement membrane of muscle capillaries in man and giraffe. *Am. J. Pathol.* 63: 359–370, 1971.

68. Younes, M., Z. Bshouty, and J. Ali. Longitudinal distribution of pulmonary vascular resistance with very high pulmonary blood flow. *J. Appl. Physiol.* 62: 344–358, 1987.

69. Yurchenco, P. D., and J. C. Schittny. Molecular architecture of basement membranes. *FASEB J.* 4: 1577–1590, 1990.

# 2

# Exploring the Structural Basis for Pulmonary Gas Exchange

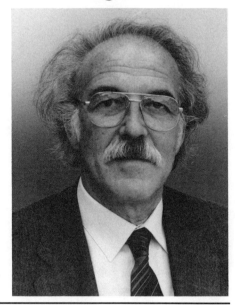

## Ewald R. Weibel, M.D.

*Professor and Chairman of Anatomy, University of Berne, Berne, Switzerland*

My story begins in the summer of 1959 when I joined, as a research fellow, the group of André F. Cournand and Dickinson W. Richards in the famous "C 6" Cardiopulmonary Laboratory of the Columbia University Division at Bellevue Hospital in New York City. This job had been offered to me in February of the same year following a seminar on the anatomy of collateral circulation to the lung that I gave at Bellevue on invitation by André Cournand. Relations between myself and Cournand had been strained, because a year before I had irritated Cournand—who had been awarded the Nobel prize in 1956 and clearly knew his worth—by taking a fellowship with Averill A. Liebow at Yale University instead of with him. I had written to Cournand from Switzerland in 1957

but never got an answer because, apparently, the U.S. Postal Service could not find this famous man in New York to deliver my letter. By the time I got a positive reply I had already committed myself to spending two years at Yale conducting experiments on the development of collateral circulation to the lung, a project in line with my previous research at the anatomy department in Zürich under the direction of Gian Töndury.

André Cournand was not a man to give up. Following my seminar he called me into the office of Dickinson W. Richards, Director of the First Medical Division, and bluntly said that I should leave Yale prematurely and come to work at Bellevue. Surprisingly, they offered me a substantial supplement to my modest fellowship,

From: Wagner WW, Jr, Weir EK (eds): *The Pulmonary Circulation and Gas Exchange.* ©1994, Futura Publishing Co Inc, Armonk, NY.

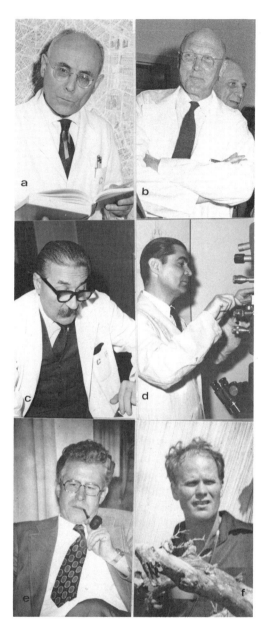

(a) André F. Cournand (1895–1989); (b) Dickinson W. Richards (1895–1973); (c) Domingo M. Gomez (1901–1978); (d) George E. Palade (1912); (e) Hans Bachofen (1938); (f) C. Richard Taylor (1939).

job—and, in turn, irritate Averill Liebow—was not the money but the task, for when I asked Cournand what he expected me to do, the reply was, "Do anything on the structure of the lung that is of interest for physiology." My mind was immediately made up because that was such a tremendous challenge. Back at Yale I worked frantically to complete my experiments and write a manuscript,[47] and, in preparation for my work in New York, developed a method for lung fixation by formalin steam that would be "more physiological" than conventional fixation.[64] Then I bundled my things and traveled with my wife through the United States on a camping trip in our 1951 Nash (purchased for $200). I took up my job at Bellevue after Labor Day 1959, ripped of my last penny.

Meanwhile, Domingo Gomez had arrived at the C 6 Laboratory. A Cuban refugee who had barely escaped with his life from Fidel Castro's revolution and reign of terror, he found refuge with his old friend Cournand. They had been acquainted in their young years in France and then again when Gomez had worked with Homer Smith at New York University. Afterwards Gomez returned to Cuba on invitation by the then-dictator Fulgencio Batista to create a Cuban Heart Institute, a project that never materialized. Gomez would prove to be the genius behind the work in which I was about to engage. A son of Cuban peasants, he had been sent by Batista to medical school in Paris, where he became a cardiologist and developed his extraordinary skills in mathematical reasoning. This training made him a biophysicist in the true sense of the word, one who would seek a rational explanation for life processes such as the circulation of blood,[21] the binding of $O_2$ to hemoglobin, and gas exchange in the lung—and later even for social problems in public health.

When I took on my new job I set up two laboratories, a small one in the pathology department to process specimens and serve as a link to morphology and one in

which was highly welcome because at Yale my wife and I lived in a shabby apartment without a bathroom and ate junk food like Chef Boyardee ravioli to make ends meet. But what really pushed me to take the

the C 6 Laboratory to serve as a link to physiology. My equipment was modest but adequate, and it was all brand new because the laboratory had not done any morphology. I had a microscope, a microtome, some glassware, and later on a calculator. I participated in some of the ongoing experiments and listened and talked to the many senior and junior physiologists bustling about the place. This gave me new perspectives but did not help me find a worthwhile morphological project "of interest for physiology." Cournand himself would be in and out of the place. It was his time of glory, when he was in great demand as a lecturer all over the world. And he certainly enjoyed it, as he later confessed in his autobiography.[10] He would come to the lab, stir up the crew, discuss all the projects, collect information and slides, and take off for the next lectures.

The first question that sent me on my track was put to me by Domingo Gomez who wanted to know how many alveoli there were in the human lung. The question was serious and pressing, for he needed the information to make calculations and predictions on gas exchange between air and blood. It also suggested the path for me to take: to provide sound quantitative information on the lung's structure because the customary meticulous anatomical descriptions would not be of sufficient interest for physiologists. But what we later came to call "morphometry" was not yet invented, so information was rare. When I searched the literature I found estimates of alveolar number to range from 66 to 725 million, not to mention even higher values. It was evident that I had to obtain my own estimate, but no method was available for counting such microscopic entities on histological sections. I found out only much later that such a method had indeed been worked out in 1925 by the Swedish mathematician Wicksell, but his paper[72] was too theoretical to be known among anatomists at that time.

So, as a first project, Domingo Gomez and I set out to develop a method for counting alveoli on sections. We analyzed theoretically the sectioning process, which presents, on sections, profiles of alveoli whose diameter would generally be smaller than that of the alveolus. The number of alveolar profiles counted on the unit area of microscopic sections, $N_A$ in contemporary symbolism, therefore depended not only on the number of alveoli in the unit volume, $N_V$, but also on their size. We devised a formula that would allow $N_V$ to be calculated from a count of $N_A$ and the estimation of the relative lung volume occupied by alveoli, $V_V$:

$$N_V = N_A^{3/2} / \beta \cdot V_V^{1/2} \qquad (1)$$

The method required an estimation of the shape factor $\beta$, which related alveolar volume and mean cross sectional area. We derived a "reasonable" set of values for $\beta$ for different geometric shapes and used linear integration to estimate relative alveolar volume. But we then wanted to verify the method on some model specimen of known composition. For that purpose we embedded a known number of peas and short segments of string beans into gelatin, cut the blocks with a sharp knife, and did the required measurements on the cut surfaces (Fig. 1): the method gave a correct result!

While we were doing this kitchen work in the laboratory next to the room where patients were being studied by cardiac catheterization, Cournand returned from one of his trips and stepped into the lab. He expressed utter consternation at our experimental object: "I did not hire you to study vegetable aspic," he told us, and walked out. We were evidently in trouble, but when we eventually submitted our method and the first estimates of alveolar number for the human lung obtained by a sound morphometric method to the *Journal of Applied Physiology*,[59] we included a photograph of our "vegetable

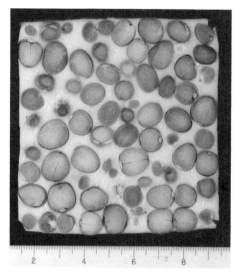

**Figure 1.** Cut surface of gelatine block containing peas used as models for spherical particles in testing particle counting method. (Reproduced with permission from reference 59.)

aspic" to support the method and got it published (Fig. 1). The number of alveoli we determined, about 300 million in an adult human lung, is still an accepted figure. Today we realize that our method is only approximate and not unbiased; better methods are now available,[11,41] but these improved methods have still not been used to estimate the number of alveoli in the human lung.

I soon found out that Domingo Gomez was not interested in the number of alveoli but merely wanted this number to calculate the lung's inner gas exchange surface. The question was whether this parameter could be measured directly. I then discovered that metallurgists were using a simple method for estimating interface area between grains in alloys, a method developed by the Russian metallurgist Saltikov in 1945.[36] It consists of drawing test lines on the section and counting the number of intersections they form with the surface trace. The intersection density per unit test line length, $I_L$, is directly proportional to the surface density in the unit tissue volume: $S_V = 2 \cdot I_L$. The application of this

method gave almost the same result as that obtained from the number of alveoli, but it was much easier to use and was free of assumptions about shape.

We then also needed to estimate the amount of capillary blood on the alveolar surface, which was difficult to do because the light microscope did not offer adequate resolution. I developed a rather cumbersome method based on a model of the capillary network and painstaking measurements of capillary segments obtained on en face images of alveolar septa. The calculations could be made only with a powerful digital computer, a huge machine that occupied a whole building but was less powerful than today's personal computer.

Two social events then occurred that had some significance for the future. The first helped give what we were doing a name. Domingo Gomez and I had usually described our enterprise as the study of the "architecture" of the human lung,[60] but that term was not satisfactory because it did not reflect the investigative process. One Sunday morning I woke up from a dream and the term "morphometry" surfaced. That afternoon I was invited to a barbecue at Dickinson Richards' home and immediately broke the news to him; he did not like it but later was the first to use the term in a lecture! The second event occurred a few weeks later, when Hans Elias, the anatomist from Chicago, visited me on his way home from Europe. I told him about "morphometry," and he informed me that he had himself just invented the term "stereology" to describe the methods of measuring three-dimensional structures on two-dimensional sections—precisely what we were doing—and had already founded the International Society for Stereology. This was a significant development because it would, over the next years, bring together morphologists from various disciplines to share methods of study that applied equally well to metals, rocks, lungs, or cells. We collaborated intensively over the years.[56]

After two years at the Cardiopulmonary Laboratory I had obtained as much information as I could with the methods and specimens I had available; the basic methods of morphometry were worked out, and a first data set "useful for physiology" was available. I collected and fixed five normal human lungs from victims of accidents or violence—of which there were plenty in New York at the time. I then studied the factors by which lung tissue shrinks on preparation for histology and estimated that, in the lung in vivo, the alveolar and capillary surface areas should be on the order of 75 m², and the capillary blood volume about 180 ml. Thus the most important parameters for estimating the effect of structure on pulmonary gas exchange were available (Table 1). When I presented these data to groups of established respiratory physiologists, my estimate of capillary volume particularly met with disbelief because the Roughton-Forster method gave a much lower value. But that is what I had found. I then soon came to realize that the estimates of gas exchange surface were probably too low because the light microscope did not allow the surface to be adequately resolved.[50]

I could of course have proceeded to collect more human lungs than the five I had fixed and could even have extended the studies into pathology. But this was made very difficult—to say it very politely—by some of my colleagues in the pathology department who did not appreciate my approach and its apparent success. Thus I found that the cadaver lungs that had been assigned to my study would almost invariably be damaged, "inadvertently" of course, by smaller or larger cuts, which then precluded their adequate fixation by the steam technique. So I decided to expand the approach in two directions: first, to study the morphometry of the airway tree and, second, to study the fine structure of the alveolar septum, its capillaries and the tissue barrier, by using the electron microscope to overcome the limits set by the resolving power of the light microscope.

## Studying the Human Airway Tree

The study of the airway tree was motivated by Domingo Gomez' interest in calculating the change of flow velocity of air as a breath of fresh air was drawn deep into the lung. He had predicted that there might be a critical point along the airways, owing to design, where flow velocity dropped so low that $O_2$ diffusion in the gas phase became the dominant means for ventilating alveoli, and he suspected that distortion of these critical airways was the

---

**Table 1**

Morphometric Data Describing the Human Pulmonary Gas Exchanger, as Originally Estimated by Light Microscopy in Weibel [48] and Subsequently by Improved Electron Microscopic Techniques by Gehr et al.[16]

|  | *1963* | *1978/87* |  |
| --- | --- | --- | --- |
| Age | 34–74 | 19–40 | years |
| Body mass | — | 74 ± 4 | kg |
| Alveolar surface area | 75 | 130 ± 12 | m² |
| Capillary surface area | 70 | 115 ± 12 | m² |
| Capillary blood volume | 180 | 194 ± 30 | ml |
| Tissue barrier thickness* | (0.46)# | 0.62 ± 0.04 | μm |
| Plasma barrier thickness* | — | 0.15 ± 0.01 | μm |

*Harmonic mean barrier thickness.
#estimated on rat lung

major disturbance in centrilobular emphysema.[22] Gomez and I began by setting up a model of the airway tree that we separated into conducting, transitory, and respiratory zones (Fig. 2). We assumed that dichotomous branching prevailed, which established a hierarchical order of the airways from the trachea to the terminal branches. This model also determined that the number of branches would double with each generation so that in generation $z$ it was $N(z) = 2^z$. The first task, then, was to estimate over how many generations the human airway tree branched to reach the terminal airways, the alveolar sacs. I used our new counting method to obtain the number of alveolar ducts and sacs in my five human lungs and found that it ranged from 12 to $16 \cdot 10^6$, from which we calculated that there must be, on average, about 23 generations of airway branching.[60]

The next task was to estimate the dimensions of airways, the diameter and length of the segments in relation to their position in the airway tree. For that purpose I borrowed one of the excellent plastic casts of the bronchial tree that Averill Liebow had produced while I was working with him at Yale. By painstaking measurement using a fine needle caliper, my devoted assistant Barbara Frank and I mapped the dimensions of well over 1,000 airways on a pedigree chart and then calculated the diameter and length ratios of paired daughter branches, the length-to-diameter ratio, and, finally, the distribution of lengths and diameters for each generation. We also compared the data obtained on the cast with in vivo bronchograms to check on whether our preparation faithfully represented the airway tree. Then, Domingo Gomez came into play when we went about to derive models of the human airway tree from all this information. We realized that the dichotomous airway branching was irregular but that it also revealed a basic progression in the airway dimensions from the trachea out to the peripheral airways. So we synthesized our data into two models: model "A," which reported the dimensions in relation to "regular dichotomy," where all branches in one generation had the same characteristic dimension, and model "B," which expanded the model to consider the irregularities of branching. Subsequently it turned out that model "A" was useful for many applications and is still widely used, whereas the more realistic model "B" was largely overlooked.

The main result of this analysis was that with each generation the average diameter of the airways decreased according

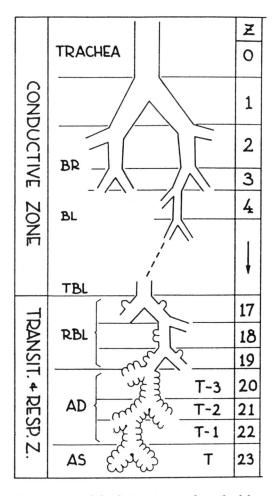

**Figure 2.** Model of airway tree described by generation *z* of dichotomous branching. (Reproduced with permission from reference 48.)

to an interesting law (Fig. 3). We found that conducting airways reduced their diameter by a factor of cube root of $1/2$, which led to the conclusion that the loss of energy due to frictional resistance in mass air flow was minimized in the conducting tree; in contrast, the peripheral transitory and respiratory airways retained a larger diameter, which we interpreted as favorable for diffusion of $O_2$ in the gas phase, as it must prevail at this level.[60] As a consequence, the total airway cross section increases dramatically along the tree and reaches about 1 m² in the most peripheral alveolar ducts. And, because the distance from one branch point to the next decreases from a few centimeters to less than 1 mm, the airways resemble a trumpet with a wide bell.

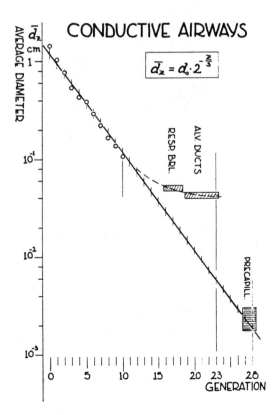

**Figure 3.** Average diameter of conductive airways, respiratory bronchioles, alveolar ducts, and precapillaries plotted against generations of dichotomous branching. (Reproduced with permission from reference 60.)

In recent years, I have reexamined the dimensional analysis of the peripheral airways using newer techniques, but this reexamination has largely confirmed the old data, except for a few details, which were refined.[23] Yet our model analysis has been challenged: first, by using an alternative way of ordering airways by "orders up" starting at the periphery[26] then by considering the airways as a fractal tree.[71] It still appears, however, that the simple model "A" is useful for many applications.

## Moving to a New Dimension

During my second year at Bellevue Hospital I realized that the light microscope did not allow the precise study of the pulmonary gas exchanger because the dimensions of the gas exchange barrier were at the limit of its resolving power. When discussing the progress of my work with Cournand and Richards, I said that I needed to learn electron microscopy to study the gas exchange barrier with adequate resolution. They asked me where I would like to do that, and I replied, without hesitation, that I would like to have George E. Palade at Rockefeller Institute as my mentor. Palade was one of the stars in the development of this then new technique, and I knew that he was interested in capillary endothelium. But he was also not easily accessible. That, however, was no problem for my famous mentors, and they quickly arranged for me to meet George Palade over lunch at Rockefeller, and he agreed to take me on. This move was facilitated by my appointment the year before as career investigator of the Health Research Council of the City of New York. This position allowed me to work anywhere in New York City, but it also created a problem: my salary was too high for Rockefeller, so I had to accept a pay cut to be admitted to Palade's lab. I also had to learn electron microscopy by working with one of his associates on a project on the spleen. This was more difficult to swallow because I found the project uninteresting and because I could not forget the lung. Although I had no problems abandoning collateral circulation when I moved to Bellevue, I was now completely hooked on morphometry of the lung. So I would sneakily also fix lung specimens along with the spleens of our experimental animals. Finally George Palade generously let me do what I wanted, although it was not in his line of interest.

At Rockefeller I had the unusual opportunity of joining a group that was at the forefront of the newly emerging field of cell biology. I was also completely ignorant of the new developments in molecular biology, but the environment at the institute was so stimulating that I made a special effort to get into the picture. This experience would have a great influence on the further development of my research interests, which henceforth always included some aspects of cell biology. Here, together with Domingo Gomez and Bruce W. Knight, a young mathematician at Rockefeller, I worked out methods for electron microscopic morphometry that allowed a precise analysis of the alveolar septum. I learned, for example, that the estimates of alveolar surface area I had obtained by light microscopy (Table 1) were probably underestimates.[50] We also developed methods for estimating the thickness of the air-blood barrier and realized that the conductance of the pulmonary gas exchanger was dependent on the harmonic mean of the tissue barrier rather than on its arithmetic mean, which estimates tissue mass[61]. The harmonic mean thickness is one third of the arithmetic mean, which is the result of alternating thin and thick parts of the barrier. The thick parts contain cells and fibers and hence serve a support function, whereas the thin parts act as the main gas exchanger between air and blood (Fig. 4).

At the end of this period I could write

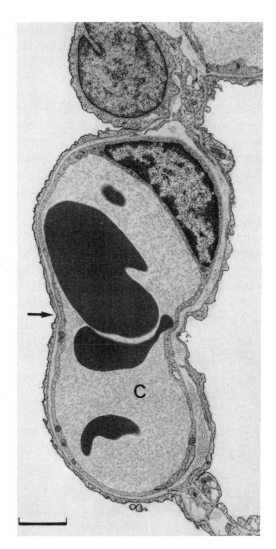

**Figure 4.** Electron micrograph of alveolar capillary (C). The alveolar epithelial surface (arrow) is exposed to the alveolar space. Scale marker: 2 μm.

my monograph *Morphometry of the Human Lung,*[48] which summarized the methods and results of nearly four years of research in two centers of excellence of biomedical research. I wrote this book because, on returning to Switzerland in 1963, I had to submit a thesis in view of my pending academic appointment. I do not think I would have written this book without this external pressure, but I certainly do not regret it. It concluded a fascinating period of apprenticeship with great masters, a period of freedom and stimulation that I would never experience again. This was made possible thanks to postdoctoral research fellowships, first from the Swiss Academy of Medical Sciences and then through an exchange arrangement between the U.S. National Institutes of Health and the Swiss National Science Foundation. When, in subsequent years, I served on the Swiss National Research Council as chairman of the Swiss Medical Research Council, I did all I could to promote the fellowship system because I believe it is important to allow promising young scientists first to be exposed to leading masters and then to give them freedom to pursue and develop their own ideas. This is how an investigator is made.

## Developing a Structural Model for Pulmonary Gas Exchange

One of the questions that had remained unsolved was how the morphometric information obtained could be used to establish a link with pulmonary physiology—in other words, how this information could be shown to be of interest to physiology. Maintaining contact with Domingo Gomez, I eventually worked out a model that allowed pulmonary diffusing capacity $DL_{O_2}$ to be calculated from morphometric data.[51] This was based on the classical model of Roughton and Forster[35] that broke $DL_{O_2}$ into two sequential components, the membrane-diffusing capacity $DM_{O_2}$ and the blood where the capillary volume $V_C$ and a chemical reaction velocity $\theta_{O_2}$ determined $O_2$ binding capacity:

$$1/DL_{O_2} = 1/DM_{O_2} + 1/\theta_{O_2} \cdot V_C \quad (2)$$

It is evident that $DM_{O_2}$ depends on the design of the barrier, on the area over which $O_2$ diffuses from the air into the blood, i.e., on the alveolar and capillary surface, and on the thickness of the tissue and plasma barriers. The model we had originally developed for the gas exchange barrier[61] suggested that the overall barrier thickness is to be estimated as the mean of reciprocal local thicknesses, i.e., as its harmonic mean. The morphometric model therefore comprised three serial conductances for tissue ($Dt_{O_2}$), plasma ($Dp_{O_2}$), and blood whose reciprocals had to be added:

$$1/DL_{O_2} = 1/Dt_{O_2} + 1/Dp_{O_2} + 1/\theta_{O_2} \cdot V_C \quad (3)$$

$Dt_{O_2}$ and $Dp_{O_2}$ were defined in terms of the corresponding surfaces and thicknesses.[51]

This method was first applied mostly to animal lungs because the measurements had to be obtained by electron microscopy. We had to await the availability of well-fixed human lungs before we could estimate the diffusing capacity of the human lung.[16] The current estimate based on the best available data (Table 1) suggests that the diffusing capacity of the human lung is about 200 $mlO_2 \cdot min^{-1} \cdot mmHg^{-1}$, a value that is about 10 times higher than the conventional physiological estimates obtained at rest. Is this a meaningful result? I believe so, for several reasons. First, if physiological $DL_{O_2}$ is estimated in the exercising individual, values up to 100 $mlO_2 \cdot min^{-1} \cdot mmHg^{-1}$ are reached; this indicates that the "capacity" of a functional system, i.e., its upper limit of performance, can be larger than what we measure physiologically. Second, it has now been shown repeatedly in animal experiments that morphometric $DL_{O_2}$ is a realistic estimate of functional capacity, which is, however, normally not completely utilized but includes a reserve that is exploited only in cases of very large $O_2$ demand, such as in top athletes, or in hypoxia.

By virtue of its structural design the lung is a very good gas exchanger, and the factors responsible for this are that (1) it maintains a very large surface, which is ventilated through the airways; (2) it keeps this surface loaded and perfused with a reasonable amount of blood, just one red cell layer thick; and (3) it maintains a very thin barrier of tissue as support for the capillaries. The problem is how this is achieved. Supporting a surface nearly the size of a tennis court by means of a tissue sheet 50 times thinner than a sheet of air mail stationery is no trivial matter. Mechanical problems must be addressed, and the question is to what extent they find their solution in properties of structural design.

## The Structural Basis of Lung Mechanics

Around 1960 much attention was devoted to surfactant as important in stabilizing the alveolar surface against surface tension effects. With the discovery by John Clements in 1962 that surfactant was a phospholipid, we could expect to see this material in electron micrographs because the lamellar bodies of type 2 cells from which surfactant presumably originated appeared made of pitch-black lamellae. After all, the fact that cellular membranes were so prominently visible resulted from fixation with osmium tetroxide, which became reduced on their phospholipid bilayer. But none of the electron micrographs of well-fixed lung tissue showed any traces of a phospholipid lining on the alveolar side (Fig. 4): the alveolar surface of the air-blood barrier was constituted of a bare cell membrane whose outer surface must be made of glycoproteins. But then, in studying the damage occurring in rat lungs poisoned with pure $O_2$, we noted that alveolar edema fluid contained a peculiar structure made of osmiophilic lamellae in a characteristic pattern that we called "tubular myelin."[31,66] Because small amounts of tubular myelin could also be found in normal lungs, we conjectured that this substance could be related

to surfactant. If that were so, then the absence of such a layer on the barrier surface could mean that our method of preparation did not retain it. Indeed, if the surfactant lining is fluid and loosely attached to the cell surface, then the instillation of fixative into the airways, the conventional procedure designed to preserve the content of the alveolar septum, would probably wash this lining off. The only hope to keep it in place would be to apply the fixative "from behind," that is through the capillary.

In the summer of 1967 I therefore fixed, together with Joan Gil, some rat lungs by perfusing a glutaraldehyde solution from the inferior vena cava through the pulmonary vasculature; the chest remained closed so that the lung was naturally air filled. On August 11, 1967, I looked at the first sections of one of these specimens and recorded the electron micrograph shown in Figure 5: it revealed an extracellular lining layer made of two parts, an amorphous hypophase topped by a strongly osmiophilic layer made of parallel lamellae strongly suggestive of a phospholipid nature. We repeated the experiment and confirmed the finding. We were convinced that we had demonstrated the existence of a duplex alveolar lining layer that was related to surfactant. I frantically wrote a paper, and by the end of the month it was submitted and rapidly accepted,[57] so I could finally go off for some holidays, which I had put off out of my excitement. The lining was not as perfect as we had expected it to be. So we improved the methods of fixation and preparation until what we saw fitted our concept of a continuous surface-active lining[19]: the hypophase-filled depressions in the alveolar epithelium thus smoothed the free surface, and the surface film was mostly smooth and made of a fine osmiophilic monolayer (Fig. 6). It was also associated with tubular myelin figures here and there.

The next question, evidently, was

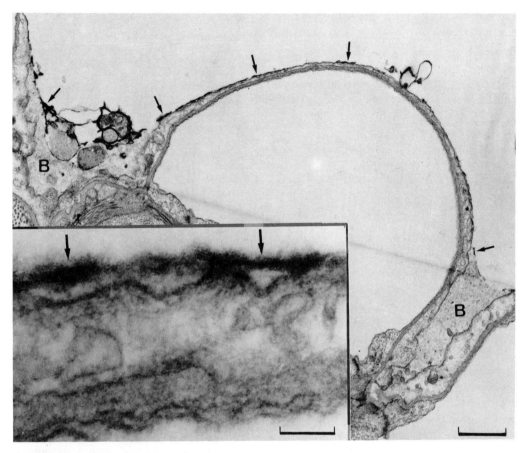

**Figure 5.** Electron micrographs of perfusion-fixed rat lung recorded on August 11, 1967, shows duplex lining layer with hypophase (B) and osmiophilic lamellae at surface (arrows), shown at higher magnification in inset. Scale markers: 1 µm, inset 0.1 µm. (Reproduced with permission from reference 57.)

whether this lining played a role in stabilizing the alveolar surface, i.e., whether we were really observing surfactant. We engaged in a series of experiments in which we attempted to fix lungs by vascular perfusion under various controlled inflation conditions, measuring the inflation pressure and then, on the micrographs, the mean surface curvature by a new stereological method developed by a metallurgist.[12] From this we described the structural changes associated with the pressure-volume hysteresis and even ventured to calculate the surface tension from the ratio of pressure to curvature: it appeared to fall, with deflation to values as low as

17 dyn/cm.[20] But these experiments were, from the point of view of lung mechanics, far from optimal. Real progress came when Hans Bachofen from the Pulmonary Division of our hospital, a disciple of Jack Hildebrandt, Leon Farhi, and Hermann Rahn, came to collaborate with us in a series of studies on structure-function relation of the lung's mechanical system.[2,18,37]

With better physiological experimentation, the demonstration of the lining layer and its disposition on the alveolar surface improved (Fig. 6), and it appeared that in the inflation range of normal breathing the surface tension must indeed

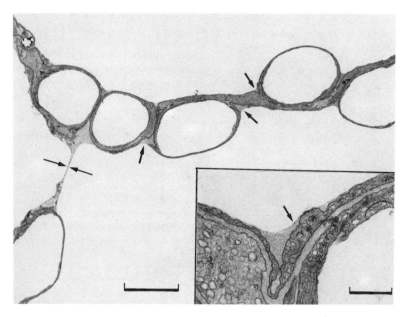

**Figure 6.** Demonstration of a smooth surface film by improved fixation method (arrows). The surface tension was very low as evidenced by bulging of capillaries and film of lining layer spanning interalveolar pore (paired arrows). Scale markers: 5 μm, inset 0.5 μm.

be very low. This allowed the capillaries to bulge somewhat toward the alveolar surface, with the result that the free alveolar surface was not much smaller than the tissue surface we had estimated by morphometry; accordingly, the existence of an extracellular lining layer reduced morphometric $DL_{O_2}$ by no more than 25%.[1]

Still the question remained of how important the surfactant lining is for stabilizing the gas exchange surface. Mead[34] had suggested that the tissue scaffold of lung parenchyma made adjacent alveoli "interdependent," which could prevent alveolar collapse. On the other hand, we had studied the connective tissue system of the lung and had come up with a model of a fiber continuum on which the capillary network was delicately supported within the alveolar septum, a continuum that extended, as axial fibers, from the hilum along the airway walls into the alveolar ducts and from there through the alveolar septa into the peripheral fibers that coursed through interlobular septa to the pleura.[58] Was this sufficient to support

the alveolar walls, or was surfactant needed? To answer this question Hans Bachofen compared normal lungs with air-inflated rabbit lungs depleted of surfactant by prior lavage with a detergent, fixing them by vascular perfusion at well-defined points of the pressure-volume curve.[2] Figure 7 compares specimens fixed at 60% of TLC on the deflation curve: in the air-filled normal lung the alveoli are patent pockets emanating from the alveolar duct, whereas in the surfactant-depleted lung the alveoli are collapsed. What is striking is that the free edges of the alveolar septa are stretched and pushed outward; the alveoli are therefore collapsed because the ring of strong connective tissue fibers that surrounds the alveolar mouths as the end part of the axial fiber tract cannot withstand the high surface tension generated at the margin of the alveolar septum if surfactant is missing. These studies brought enormous progress in our understanding of lung mechanics and its structural basis,[3,37] which finally allowed us to design a new model

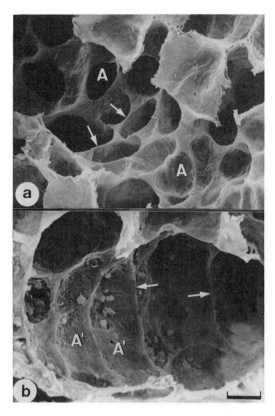

**Figure 7.** Scanning electron micrographs of normal air-filled (a) and surfactant-depleted (b) rabbit lungs fixed at 60% TLC on the deflation curve show alveoli to be open (A) in (a), collapsed (A′) in (b). The alveolar duct is widened in the surfactant-depleted lung, resulting in a stretching of the fiber strands around the alveolar mouths (arrows). Scale markers: 50 μm. (Reproduced with permission from reference 73.)

of alveolar or, rather, acinar mechanics that involves both the fiber continuum and a surfactant lining, as shown in Figure 8.[58,73]

This now establishes the link between lung mechanics and our attempts to characterize the pulmonary diffusing capacity from morphometric measurements. Mechanical factors are evidently important determinants of the configuration of the gas exchanger. The capillaries are supported on the fiber scaffold in such a way that one side of the barrier is very thin, made only of epithelial and endothelial

sheets (Fig. 4), whereas the other side contains a fiber tract. Capillary blood pressure tends to push the thin side out toward the alveolar space. This may be counteracted by surface tension, but surface tension appears low enough to allow some "crumpling" of the alveolar surface (Fig. 6), thus maintaining a large functional gas exchange surface. This may partially fail in high inflation, where surface tension is high, or under zone I or II conditions, where capillary pressure is low. In the range of physiological breathing it appears that at least 80% of morphometric $DL_{O_2}$ is available for gas exchange.[4]

## How Well Is the Lung Designed for Gas Exchange?

When, in 1970, I had set up a model for calculating $DL_{O_2}$ from morphometric data, we had in hand the means for attempting some quantitative studies on structure-function correlation in the lung. The Bohr equation sets $DL_{O_2}$ in relation to $O_2$ consumption:

$$\dot{V}_{O_2} = DL_{O_2} \cdot (PA_{O_2} - Pb_{O_2}) \qquad (4)$$

The first hypothesis suggested by this relation is that $DL_{O_2}$ should be matched to $\dot{V}_{O_2}$ if the lung is well designed as a gas exchanger. And, evidently, variations in ambient $P_{O_2}$ could also have an effect because they would affect the pressure head of the driving force, $PA_{O_2}$. So we engaged in three lines of research directed toward answering the question of whether $DL_{O_2}$ was matched to conditions of $O_2$ supply and consumption. Peter Burri, who had studied lung growth,[8] raised rats on the Jungfraujoch, our high alpine research station at 3,400 m altitude, and found them to develop a higher $DL_{O_2}$ than control rats raised in Berne.[7] We then discussed ways of modifying $O_2$ consumption. One day one of our medical students, Annemarie Geelhaar, returned from a shopping trip

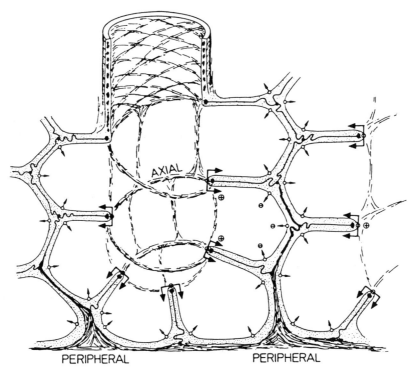

**Figure 8.** Model of the disposition of axial, septal, and peripheral fibers in an acinus showing the effect of surface force (arrows).

into town excited because she had discovered, in the window of a pet shop, the experimental animal we needed for that purpose: the Japanese waltzing mouse. We bought her some of these cute pets, which are continuously in motion, performing their waltz at a rate of nearly three turns per second. She measured their $\dot{V}_{O_2}$ and found that it was considerably higher than $\dot{V}_{O_2}$ in normal Swiss laboratory mice and that morphometric $DL_{O_2}$ was proportionally higher.[15] Of course, Japanese waltzing mice are genetically different from the Swiss mice, so this could not be interpreted as adaptation of the lung to increased $O_2$ demand by the body. But Peter Burri then succeeded in making artificial waltzing mice and found that they also had a larger diffusing capacity.[27] So it appeared that the size of the pulmonary gas exchanger was related to the $O_2$ needs of the body.

This suggested that we look for larger variations in $\dot{V}_{O_2}$ as they occur when body size varies. It is well known that $\dot{V}_{O_2}$ increases with body mass to the power 0.75,[32] which means that $\dot{V}_{O_2}$ of a mouse should be three times higher than that of a dog. Does $DL_{O_2}$ vary in parallel? Tenney and Remmers[45] had measured alveolar surface area in a large range of mammals, from shrew to whale, and found that it varied with $O_2$ consumption. Is this also true for $DL_{O_2}$? We began to collect animals of different size, from the dog of 30 kg down to mice; we even got a colony of the smallest mammal, the Etruscan shrew, which weighs no more than 2.5 g. Because of its small size this fascinating animal pushes its metabolism to extremes: we recorded an electrocardiogram and found the resting heart rate to be over 1,000 $min^{-1}$ and the respiration rate about 300 $min^{-1}$. Accordingly the metabolic rate per unit body mass was eight times greater in these shrews than in the rat.[55] The shrews also have an enormous demand for food: they consume about six times their own body weight in insects every day, and, as we now know, when they are short of food they go into torpor; we may have inadvertently killed several of our Etruscan shrews because we found them "dead" when they presumably were in torpor. In all these different species we measured the morphometric lung parameters required to calculate $DL_{O_2}$ and plotted these data against body mass and $\dot{V}_{O_2}$ (Fig. 9): it turned out that $DL_{O_2}$ was not proportional to $\dot{V}_{O_2}$ but increased nearly linearly with body mass.[52] On the other hand, free-living animals had a higher $DL_{O_2}$ than captive animals of the same size, which still suggested that $DL_{O_2}$ and $O_2$ needs could be related. I concluded that we were faced with an apparent paradox, with $DL_{O_2}$ related to $\dot{V}_{O_2}$ in one case, but not in the other.

I did not know what to do with these intriguing results. So when on a sabbatical in 1974 I spent some time at Yale with George Palade working on the endothelial granules we had discovered when I worked with him as a fellow.[62] I searched through the magnificent library at Yale Medical School for answers to my problem and fell upon a paper by one C. Richard Taylor, who had studied $\dot{V}_{O_2}$ in animals of different body mass. Measuring both resting and maximal $O_2$ consumption elicited by exercise, he concluded that the ratio of maximal to resting $\dot{V}_{O_2}$ was not constant but was highest in mid-size animals, such as dogs and lower in smaller and larger animals.[42] I had measured resting or average $\dot{V}_{O_2}$. When I superimposed Taylor's bell-shaped curve for $\dot{V}_{O_2}max/\dot{V}_{O_2}$ rest on my allometric plots of the relation between $\dot{V}_{O_2}$ and $DL_{O_2}$, I immediately jumped to the conclusion that $DL_{O_2}$ must be related to

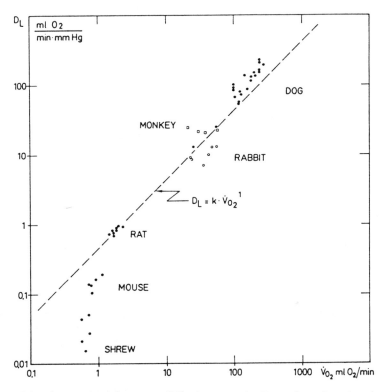

**Figure 9.** Morphometric pulmonary diffusing capacity $DL_{O_2}$ plotted against (average) $O_2$ consumption. (Reproduced with permission from reference 52.)

$\dot{V}_{O_2}$max, which, of course, made a lot of sense anyway: if the lung is designed well its gas exchange capacity must be matched to aerobic capacity or $\dot{V}_{O_2}$max rather than to any arbitrary measure of metabolic rate.

I located C. Richard Taylor at Harvard and called him by phone, explaining my problem and its possible solution to him. A few days later I was in Boston, and Dick Taylor and I had lunch at the Harvard Faculty Club, together with Tom MacMahon. We had never met before, not even heard about each other, but halfway into lunch we had already decided that we would launch a joint expedition to Kenya to collect a set of free-living wild mammals, covering a large range in body mass, for which we would measure $\dot{V}_{O_2}$max and $DL_{O_2}$—hopefully to support the hypothesis that $DL_{O_2}$ was related to $\dot{V}_{O_2}$max. This brief meeting triggered an extraordinary intense collaboration and close personal friendship and a refocusing of the research in both our labs on both sides of the Atlantic.

After our meeting, each of us wrote to his granting institution asking for a change in his research program and reallocation of funds, and we both got approval. Dick Taylor had worked in Kenya in 1969 and had good contacts, particularly with Geoffrey M. O. Maloiy, the professor of physiology and dean of the School of Veterinary Medicine at the University of Nairobi. He would offer us tremendous support, without which the study could not have been done. Dick had a treadmill built in Boston, large enough so that a small buffalo weighing half a ton could run on it. He shipped this heavy device to Kenya by sea, together with other equipment, and set it up at the Muguga field station outside Nairobi, where excellent facilities for housing animals existed as part of the East African Veterinary Research Organization. He took a sabbatical and in spring of 1977 went to Nairobi with a small group of young collaborators to work for 7 months.

For my part, I was unable to leave my job for a longer time, but I had a young zoologist, Peter Gehr, working with me who had done part of the morphometric studies on dog lungs as his thesis work. I dispatched him and my chief technician, Helgard Claassen, later also Odile Mathieu, to join Dick's group and eventually prepare the lung specimens for subsequent morphometric study in Berne. Our lab was set up in the Department of Veterinary Anatomy, then chaired by Wangari Muta Maathai, a beautiful and charming Kikuyu woman who helped us very generously in return for some lectures to her students. She would later get into political trouble but was just recently awarded the prestigious Africa Prize for her activities in the Green Belt Movement. She assigned some of her associates to work on our project, among them Deter Mwangi, who then spent a couple of years in Berne.

Using his many African contacts Dick had prepared our expedition well. But when he and the other members of the group arrived, an important political development occurred that nearly blocked our enterprise completely. The political powers had realized that tremendous damage was being done to African wildlife by ruthless commercial hunters, who nearly decimated the elephant population in amassing horrendous quantities of ivory. So the parliament of Kenya had passed a law that banned the capturing and hunting of wild animals, precisely what we had come for. A lot of diplomatic activity was necessary, particularly by Geoffrey Maloiy, until we could obtain permits and eventually get the animals we needed. But the whole enterprise retained a touch of illegality to the end, which, of course, only added to the excitement of this fascinating study. Indeed, one of the ministers told Dick that he could not protect him from being put into jail, but he promised to get him out fast! That was some consolation.

While this study on the relation of the

lung and maximal $O_2$ consumption was being set up in Nairobi, I acquired a new collaborator in Berne, Hans Hoppeler, who a few years before had done a remarkable thesis on the relation between muscle mitochondria and $\dot{V}_{O_2}$max in human athletes.[24] After completing medical school and a residency in surgery and obstetrics, he wanted to get back into research. When I went to Kenya to join the group for a few weeks I suggested that we expand the program to consider not only the lung as the supplier of $O_2$ to the body, but also the locomotor muscles as the chief $O_2$ consumers during maximal exercise. The study therefore became one of respiratory system physiology, more precisely on the design of the mammalian respiratory system in relation to function or its functional limits. The decision was rapidly made while we were all sitting under a tree behind the anatomy department on the Nairobi campus. We did not have much time for planning and thinking out detailed strategies because this was so new. What it required of my group was that, in addition to the lungs, samples from a variety of muscles had to be collected and fixed from all the animals, which would eventually be sacrificed after completion of the physiological studies. This was a tremendous additional load, and the working conditions were not optimal.

In Berne, I then reoriented my research program. Since my training period with George Palade at the Rockefeller Institute I had always maintained a research project in the field of cell biology in which we had explored the relation between cellular membranes and their enzymes in liver cells[6,40,68]; one project also dealt with cell damage in the lung.[5] In view of this new study I abandoned the liver cells and redirected the cell biology project to muscle and its mitochondria. The approach would be the same, namely, combing morphometric studies of cell composition with biochemical analyses in an integrated fashion, but the object was now the membrane system of muscle mitochondria instead of the endoplasmic reticulum of liver cells.[38,39] It also proved necessary to improve the stereological methods used to generate the extensive morphometric data that would now be needed. I had always maintained a personal interest in continuously developing this fascinating methodology with its beautiful mathematical appeal. This effort was greatly advanced by my friendship with Roger Miles, the eminent mathematician from Australia.[49,53,56,65] When Luis Cruz-Orive joined our group in 1976, we acquired an "in-house theoretician" who would continuously contribute to improving and updating our methods of sampling and measurement in this rapidly advancing field.[11,53]

The field study in Kenya lasted for 7 months, after which we had cratefulls of physiological data and tissue samples from lungs and 20 different muscles collected from over 20 different animals ranging in body size from 500 g to 250 kg. An important aspect of the study was that all the tissue samples had been obtained on the same animals that had been subjected to thorough physiological study. It took us over 3 years and involved some 20 investigators to analyze all this vast material. We finally produced nine papers, which we wanted to publish together in order to stress the systems physiology approach. We were fortunate to find in Pierre Dejours an editor of a renowned journal who was sympathetic to this idea; he eventually accepted the entire series for *Respiration Physiology*.[63] The papers had gone through an adequate peer review process, but Taylor got into some difficulties later with his granting agencies because some of them considered this "package of papers" as a non-peer-reviewed publication. The reason was that Pierre Dejours had generously named us "guest editors" for the issue of his journal in which our series was published, although he had personally handled the editorial process.

## The Concept of Symmorphosis and the Lung

When all the data were assembled and first drafts of the manuscripts written, the whole group met in Berne for a week of intense discussions to develop a coherent picture of the study. At this time we realized that we had actually engaged in a study of the overall design of the respiratory system, of the "pathway for oxygen,"[54] and that this required some formalization. We first set up an analytical model of the respiratory system that would relate $O_2$ flow rate to a set of structural and functional parameters, and this from the lung to the mitochondrial $O_2$ sink (Fig. 10). As a second step, we formulated a hypothesis on structure-function correlation that we could subject to testing: the hypothesis of *symmorphosis,* which we defined as "a state of structural design commensurate to functional needs resulting from regulated morphogenesis, whereby the formation of structural elements is regulated to satisfy but not exceed the requirements of the functional

system." We thought that symmorphosis—or economical design—should apply at all levels of the respiratory system so that it also meant that the lung's structural parameters must be matched to those of the circulation of blood and of the muscle's capillaries and mitochondria. The overall functional needs, in our case, should be the highest level of $O_2$ consumption that the organism can achieve, that is, $\dot{V}_{O_2}$max achieved by the muscle cells during running. We thus had collected the essential information for testing the hypothesis of symmorphosis.

What did this study of African mammals tell us about the relation between $O_2$ needs and the lung? Did it prove our prediction that $\dot{V}_{O_2}$max should vary linearly with body mass? Did it thus resolve the apparent paradox that $DL_{O_2}$ was matched to $\dot{V}_{O_2}$ when animals of the same size were compared but not in an allometric comparison across the size range? It did neither. Dick Taylor and his collaborators found that $\dot{V}_{O_2}$max was about proportional to resting $\dot{V}_{O_2}$, perhaps with a slightly steeper allometric exponent, 0.81 instead of 0.75.[43]

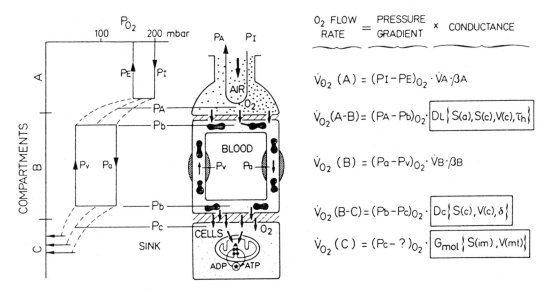

**Figure 10.** Model of respiratory system. (Reproduced with permission from reference 63.)

And our morphometric study of all these lungs revealed that morphometric $DL_{O_2}$ was linearly proportional to body mass, thus confirming my original result.[17] Thus $\dot{V}_{O_2}$ max and $DL_{O_2}$ have different allometric slopes when plotted against body mass (Fig. 11); as a consequence we had to conclude that the driving force for diffusive $O_2$ uptake, the alveolo-capillary $P_{O_2}$ difference, must become smaller as animal size increases. We hypothesized that this could be the result of the larger size of acini in larger lungs, which could reduce alveolar $P_{O_2}$ because of a longer diffusion path in the air phase or peripheral airways.[70] For comparison, it is worth noting that we did find a reasonable agreement between $\dot{V}_{O_2}$ max and mitochondrial volume as well as for muscle capillaries.[25,33] The hypothesis of symmorphosis was hence supported at these internal levels of the respiratory system, but apparently not in the lung.

## Looking at Athletic Species

The variation of metabolic rate observed between species in relation to their body size is related to their basal or standard metabolism.[32] Contrary to our expectations we found that animals of all sizes can apparently increase metabolic rate upon exercise by approximately the same relative amount, namely, by about tenfold, until they reach $\dot{V}_{O_2}$ max. This so-called aerobic scope, however, can vary considerably according to the prowess of an animal or a species. Thus, athletic species such as the dog or the horse have an aerobic scope of 30–50 fold above standard metabolism, on average 2.5 times that of more sedentary species of the same body size such as goats or cows, respectively. Because we had seen that our "little athletes," the Japanese waltzing mice, had a higher pulmonary diffusing capacity than their lazier counterparts, the Swiss

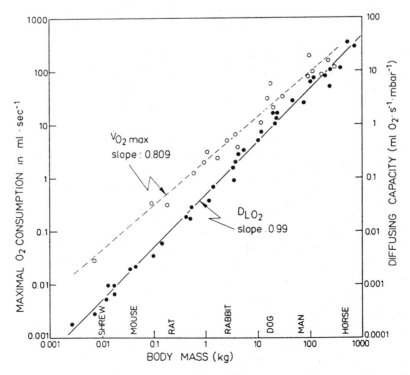

**Figure 11.** Allometric plots of pulmonary diffusing capacity $DL_{O_2}$ and maximal $O_2$ consumption show different slopes. (Reproduced with permission from reference 54.)

mice, we wondered whether this adaptive variation in $\dot{V}_{O_2}$max observed in larger species was associated with corresponding variations in the design of the respiratory system.

Together with Dick Taylor and his group we undertook a second series of studies in which we wished to test the hypothesis of symmorphosis by comparing dogs with goats, and ponies with calves, studies that again occupied us for about 5 years and involved as many investigators as those on allometry. The resulting eight papers were also published as a coherent sequence in *Respiration Physiology*.[44] Because we now had a consistent model of the respiratory system, the study could be more complete; in particular we now included measurements of physiological parameters that characterize $O_2$ transport by the circulation of blood,[30] a part of the study brilliantly performed by a young Ph.D. student at Harvard, Richard H. Karas, as part of his thesis work. These studies were later complemented by the comparison of standardbred race horses with steers, both weighing about 500 kg, a study done at the Veterinary School in Uppsala, a collaboration between a Swedish, an American, and a Swiss group, each chipping away in its own area of expertise.[9,28]

Table 2 provides a summary of the results of these studies; it compares the animals pairwise and calculates the ratio of parameters between the athletic and the sedentary species, e.g., dog/goat. We first observe that the ratio for body mass-specific $\dot{V}_{O_2}$max is 2.5 on average, as is the ratio for the total mitochondrial volume per unit body mass. From this we calculate that for $\dot{V}_{O_2}$max/V(mi), the ratio of athletic to sedentary species is about 1, i.e., it is invariant with adaptive variation or with different levels of $\dot{V}_{O_2}$max. In other words, the total volume of mitochondria in skeletal muscle is higher in athletic species in strict proportion to $\dot{V}_{O_2}$max. This led to the conclusion that the unit volume of mitochondria is capable of consuming the same amount of $O_2$ in athletic and sedentary species, which is to say that, in all species, muscle mitochondria are capable of the same maximal rate of oxidative phosphorylation, and this is also true in allometric variation. With respect to muscle capillaries, we must take into account that athletic species have a higher hematocrit (Table 2) and hence a higher $O_2$ capacity of the blood. The capillary volume is also higher, but it is the product of capillary volume and hematocrit, that is, the volume of capillary erythrocytes in the muscle that is proportional to the mitochondria of muscle cells and hence forms an invariant ratio to $\dot{V}_{O_2}$max. The differences in hematocrit also affect $O_2$ transport by the circulation, where we found the product of stroke volume (or ventricular volume) and hematocrit to be proportional to $\dot{V}_{O_2}$max, whereas maximal heart frequency is pairwise identical and depends only on body mass. But because maximal heart frequency varies with body mass it must be considered an additional functional factor.[69]

Studying the lungs we found that the athletic species had generally larger morphometric parameters so that, in the end, $DL_{O_2}$ was 1.7 times larger.[67] But this is clearly not proportional to the 2.5 times higher $\dot{V}_{O_2}$max (Table 2). In these studies we had obtained a reasonably complete set of physiological data so that we could have a closer look at what was happening in the lung during gas exchange (Fig. 12). By dividing alveolar capillary volume, obtained by morphometry, by cardiac output at $\dot{V}_{O_2}$max, obtained by the Fick principle, we could estimate the mean capillary transit time at $\dot{V}_{O_2}$max to be on the order of 0.3 s.[29] Alveolar $P_{O_2}$ could be calculated by the alveolar gas equation; mixed venous and arterial $P_{O_2}$ had been measured at $\dot{V}_{O_2}$max, and we had good estimates of the blood's $O_2$ reaction rate so that we could calculate the progression of capillary $O_2$ uptake by Bohr integration. This revealed, as shown

**Table 2**
Adaptive Variation of the Pathway for Oxygen. Ratios of Morphometric and
Physiologic Parameters of Muscle Mitochondria and Capillaries, and of Heart, Blood
and Lung in Relation to $\dot{V}_{O_2}$ max in Three Species Pairs

| | $\dot{V}_{O_2}max/M_b$ | Mitochondria | | Blood | Capillaries | | Heart | | | Lung | |
|---|---|---|---|---|---|---|---|---|---|---|---|
| | | $V(mt)/M_b$ | $[V(mt)]/[\dot{V}_{O_2}max]$ | $V_V(ec)$ | $V(c)/M_b$ | $[V(c)\cdot V_V(ec)]/[\dot{V}_{O_2}max]$ | $f_H$ | $VS/M_b$ | $[VS\cdot V_V(ec)]/[\dot{V}_{O_2}max/f_H]$ | $DL_{O_2}/M_b$ | $[DL_{O_2}]/[\dot{V}_{O_2}max]$ |
| | $ml\cdot s^{-1}\cdot kg^{-1}$ | $ml\cdot kg^{-1}$ | $ml\cdot ml^{-1}\cdot s$ | | $ml\cdot kg^{-1}$ | $ml\cdot ml^{-1}\cdot s$ | $min^{-1}$ | $ml\cdot kg^{-1}$ | $ml\cdot ml^{-1}$ | $ml\cdot s^{-1}\cdot mmHg^{-1}\cdot kg^{-1}$ | $mmHg$ |
| **25–30 kg** | | | | | | | | | | | |
| Dog | 2.29 | 40.6 | 17.7 | 0.50 | 8.2 | 1.79 | 274 | 3.17 | 3.16 | 0.118 | 0.052 |
| Goat | 0.95 | 13.8 | 14.5 | 0.30 | 4.5 | 1.42 | 268 | 2.07 | 2.92 | 0.080 | 0.084 |
| D/G | 2.4* | 2.9* | 1.2 | 1.68* | 1.8* | 1.26 | 1.02 | 1.53* | 1.08 | 1.48* | 0.61* |
| **150 kg** | | | | | | | | | | | |
| Pony | 1.48 | 19.5 | 13.2 | 0.42 | 5.1 | 1.45 | 215 | 2.50 | 2.54 | 0.079 | 0.053 |
| Calf | 0.61 | 9.2 | 15.1 | 0.31 | 3.2 | 1.63 | 213 | 1.78 | 3.21 | 0.050 | 0.082 |
| P/C | 2.4* | 2.13* | 0.9 | 1.35* | 1.6* | 0.89 | 1.02 | 1.40* | 0.79 | 1.57* | 0.65* |
| **450 kg** | | | | | | | | | | | |
| Horse | 2.23 | 30.0 | 13.5 | 0.55 | 8.3 | 2.05 | 202 | 3.11 | 2.58 | 0.108 | 0.048 |
| Steer | 0.85 | 11.6 | 13.7 | 0.40 | 5.3 | 2.49 | 216 | 1.52 | 2.58 | 0.054 | 0.064 |
| H/S | 2.6* | 2.6* | 1.0 | 1.4* | 1.6* | 0.82 | 0.94 | 2.1* | 1.00 | 2.0* | 0.76* |
| **Ath/Sed** | 2.5* | 2.5* | 1.03 | 1.5* | 1.7* | 0.99 | 1.0 | 1.7* | 0.96 | 1.7* | 0.67* |

*Note.* Data from references 9,28,43. Last line presents overall ratios for athletic/sedentary species. Asterisk denotes ratios significantly different from 1.[69]

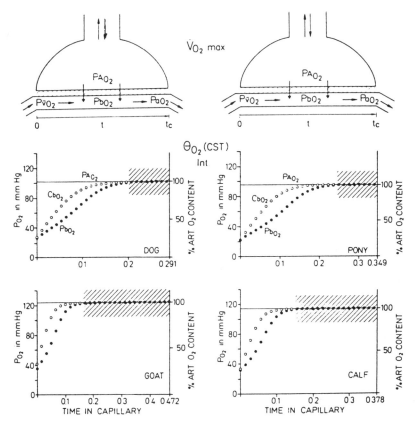

**Figure 12.** Increase in $O_2$ concentration, $C_{O_2}$ and $P_{O_2}$ of the blood during the time it transits the capillary bed. Athletic species (dogs and ponies) are compared with more sedentary goats and calves. The shaded areas indicate the "redundant" parts of the capillary path, which is shorter in athletic species. (Reproduced with permission from reference 29.)

in Figure 12, that equilibrium between capillary blood and alveolar air was completed, on average, before the blood left the capillary bed even at $\dot{V}_{O_2}$max. Thus we must conclude that the pulmonary gas exchanger maintains some redundancy or reserve diffusing capacity, but this redundancy appears to be smaller in the athletic than in the sedentary species.[29] This finding was confirmed when comparing horses and steers.[9] To check whether this conclusion is justified we subjected goats to a hypoxia test on the treadmill and found that they can run and maintain their $\dot{V}_{O_2}$max down to inspired $O_2$ fractions of 15%.[29] In contrast, we never succeeded in having dogs run near $\dot{V}_{O_2}$max when inspired $O_2$ was only slightly reduced; their small redundancy in $D_{L_{O_2}}$ may not give them enough reserve capacity. With respect to the human lung, where we had found a redundancy of about 50% (Table 1), it has been shown that the human lung can support high levels of $\dot{V}_{O_2}$ even at high altitude but that it can become the limiting factor for $\dot{V}_{O_2}$max in highly trained athletes who apparently also exploit some of this redundancy when they train for higher performance.[14,46]

Thus it appears that the pulmonary diffusing capacity is crudely matched to maximal metabolic rate but that it may not need to follow the $O_2$ demands of the body because it maintains a certain degree of redundancy, which can be a comfortable 50% in sedentary species, a value we had also found for the human lung (Table 1). Considering that the lung forms the interface to the environment where $P_{O_2}$ can vary, a "safety factor" of 2 is, in fact, reasonable and could conform well to what an engineer would build into such a vital organ, particularly because it appears that the lung is incapable of easily repairing any damage to its gas exchanger without a residual loss in functional capacity. And our environment, indeed, offers many opportunities for ill effects on this delicate structure.

## Conclusions

I have spent over three decades probing into the lung with all sorts of microscopes as well as with physiological and mathematical methods. I conclude that the beauty of this delicate and intricate structure is matched by the secrets it has not yet revealed. It still remains an exciting object of investigation. I have had the good fortune of a fantastic apprenticeship with great masters in the fields of morphology, respiration physiology, and cell biology, masters who have taught me to look beyond structure, as exciting as structure is for someone deeply committed to design and aesthetics. I have also had the opportunity of being put in charge of a sizable teaching and research department at the young age of 37 through which I could involve, in time, a large number of young and enthusiastic investigators. And, finally, I was more than lucky to find, at all times, partners for my research endeavors who brought in skills and expertise I did not have. Even the Atlantic Ocean and differences in the size and potential of the participating institutions and countries are no barrier to most fruitful collaboration—otherwise a partnership between the small University of Berne and the great Harvard University could not have

worked. All that counts is an open mind and a generous attitude toward one's partner. If you and your partner do not become friends it does not work.

The greatest lesson I have learned is that exciting research needs partnership because it is, in the long run, not productive to remain enclosed in one's narrow field. In my case, it would not have been productive to limit study to morphology or even morphometry; this tells only half the story, or less. Such studies must be closely combined with functional investigations true to the task I was given in 1959: "to do anything on the structure of the lung that is of interest for physiology." But I would like to now widen this task and ask morphologists and physiologists together to do anything on the structure and function of living creatures that is of interest for the understanding of life.

## Postscript

The preceding sounds like a happy success story, but for the sake of honesty and completeness I should perhaps mention that it was twice overshadowed by troubling experiences of scientific unfairness—to be more explicit: of persons who plagiarized but were never held responsible for their actions.

Before I moved from Columbia University to Rockefeller Institute in 1961 I introduced another fellow to the methods of lung morphometry that I had developed so that he could use them in the study of pathological specimens. I also gave him a copy of the draft of the methods section of "Morphometry of the Human Lung." By coincidence I found out in 1962 that he had written, based on this privileged information, a paper on these methods, which he submitted for publication one year after he left the laboratory. Although I tried to delay the publication of this paper until my own was published, it appeared in 1962 whereas mine carries the date of 1963. At the time I was shattered, for the date of publication sets the priority. I had been scooped.

A few years later I was working on $O_2$ toxicity in the lung, under contract with the U.S. Air Force Medical Research Division. Together with Peter Caldwell, then serving as captain in the air force, we exposed rats to pure $O_2$ breathing at Wright-Patterson Air Force Base. The analysis of tissues was conducted in my laboratory in Switzerland.[31] I was required to submit detailed quarterly reports to my contracting agency, giving results of our study to an air force captain who would review them and would serve as "monitor" of my contract. One day I received a paper for review that had been submitted to a prestigious journal by this captain, and to my dismay I found that it reported not only the general findings but also the main morphometric results of our study. We later found out that this officer had ordered a sergeant-technician, whom we had trained, to repeat our experiment on a few rats; given a contract to someone else to produce a few electron micrographs that matched our data; and written the paper based on our original confidential report. When I informed the journal's editor about the circumstances, the paper was rejected, but I was not allowed to inform air force authorities of this flagrant case of scientific fraud, because the paper I had received for review was "privileged information." The paper was then published, unaltered, in another journal. Some 15 years later, around 1980, this very person was involved in a major case of scientific fraud in the United States. The scenario closely resembled my own experience: a journal editor inadvertently referred the fraudulent manuscript for review to the original author of the abused data. In this instance, the story became public, and the brilliant if not soaring career of the man came to an abrupt end. What strikes me in this case is the pattern of repetition, and I wonder how much of this happens and remains unprosecuted, as it has in my own two cases. At the time of these incidents I was a young man with no established career, and these experiences hurt me deeply. In retrospect it appears, however, that persistence in honest work has greater rewards than fraudulent appropriation of another person's ideas.

**Acknowledgements:** My research has been continuously supported by generous grants from the Swiss National Science Foundation, as well as by many grants from other foundations. The Swiss Academy of Medical Sciences, the Swiss National Science Foundation, and the Fogarty International Center at the U.S. National Institutes of Health awarded me fellowships that gave me the opportunity for excellent postdoctoral training. I have been privileged to have had many enthusiastic collaborators. I cannot list them all, but their contributions are reflected by authorship in the reference list. And last, but not least, I have a wonderful wife who shared hardship and pleasure, excitement and frustration along this path.

# References

1. Bachofen, H., A. Ammann, D. Wangensteen, and E. R. Weibel. Perfusion fixation of lungs for structure-function analysis: credits and limitations. *J. Appl. Physiol.* 53: 528–533, 1982.
2. Bachofen, H., P. Gehr, and E. R. Weibel. Alterations of mechanical properties and morphology in excised rabbit lungs rinsed with a detergent. *J. Appl. Physiol.* 47: 1002–1010, 1979.
3. Bachofen, H., S. Schürch, M. Urbinelli, and E. R. Weibel. Relations among alveolar surface tension, surface area, volume, and recoil pressure. *J. Appl. Physiol.* 62: 1878–1887, 1987.
4. Bachofen, H., D. Wangensteen, and E. R. Weibel. Surfaces and volumes of alveolar tissue under zone II and zone III conditions. *J. Appl. Physiol.* 53: 879–885, 1982.
5. Bachofen, M., and E. R. Weibel. Alterations of the gas exchange apparatus in adult respiratory insufficiency associated with septicemia. *Am. Rev. Respir. Dis.* 116: 589–615, 1977.
6. Bolender, R. P., D. Paumgartner, D. Muellener, G. Losa, and E. R. Weibel. Integrated stereological and biochemical studies on hepatocytic membranes. I. Membrane re-

coveries in subcellular fractions. *J. Cell Biol.* 77: 565–583, 1978.

7. Burri, P. H., and E. R. Weibel. Morphometric estimation of pulmonary diffusion capacity. II. Effect of $P_{O_2}$ on the growing lung: adaptation of the growing rat lung to hypoxia and hyperoxia. *Respir. Physiol.* 11: 247–264, 1971.
8. Burri, P. H., J. Dbaly, and E. R. Weibel. The postnatal growth of the rat lung. I. Morphometry. *Anat. Rec.* 178: 711–730, 1974.
9. Constantinopol, M., J. H. Jones, E. R. Weibel, C. R. Taylor, A. Lindholm, and R. H. Karas. Oxygen transport during exercise in large mammals. II. Oxygen uptake by the pulmonary gas exchanger. *J. Appl. Physiol.* 67: 871–878, 1989.
10. Cournand, A. F. *From Roots . . . to Late Budding.* New York: Gardner, 1986.
11. Cruz-Orive, L. M., and E. R. Weibel. Recent stereological methods for cell biology: a brief survey. *Am. J. Physiol.* 258: L148–L156, 1990.
12. DeHoff, R. T. the quantitative estimation of mean surface curvature. *Trans. Metall. Soc. AIME* 239: 617, 1967.
13. Dejours, P. *Principles of Comparative Respiratory Physiology.* 2nd ed. Amsterdam: Elsevier, 1981, p. 93–108.
14. Dempsey, J. A. Is the lung built for exercise? *Med. Sci. Sports Exerc.* 18: 143–155, 1981.
15. Geelhaar, A., and E. R. Weibel. Morphometric estimation of pulmonary diffusion capacity. III. The effect of increased oxygen consumption in Japanese waltzing mice. *Respir. Physiol.* 11: 354–366, 1971.
16. Gehr, P., M. Bachofen, and E. R. Weibel. The normal human lung: ultrastructure and morphometric estimation of diffusion capacity. *Respir. Physiol.* 32: 121–140, 1978.
17. Gehr, P., D. K. Mwangi, A. Ammann, G. M. O. Maloiy, C. R. Taylor, and E. R. Weibel. Design of the mammalian respiratory system. V. Scaling morphometric pulmonary diffusing capacity to body mass: wild and domestic mammals. *Respir. Physiol.* 44: 61–86, 1981.
18. Gil, J., H. Bachofen, P. Gehr, and E. R. Weibel. Alveolar volume-surface area relation in air- and saline-filled lungs fixed by vascular perfusion. *J. Appl. Physiol.* 47: 990–1001, 1979.
19. Gil, J., and E. R. Weibel. Improvements in demonstration of lining layer of lung alveoli by electron microscopy. *Respir. Physiol.* 8: 13–36, 1969/70.

20. Gil, J., and E. R. Weibel. Morphological study of pressure-volume hysteresis in rat lungs fixed by vascular perfusion. *Respir. Physiol.* 15: 190–213, 1972.
21. Gomez, D. M. *Hémodynamique et Angiocinétique.* Paris: Hermann, 1941.
22. Gomez, D. M. A physico-mathematical study of lung function in normal subjects and in patients with obstructive pulmonary diseases. *Med. Thorac.* 22: 275–294, 1965.
23. Haefeli-Bleuer, B., and E. R. Weibel. Morphometry of the human pulmonary acinus. *Anat. Rec.* 220: 401–414, 1988.
24. Hoppeler, H., P. Lüthi, H. Claassen, E. R. Weibel, and H. Howald. The ultrastructure of the normal human skeletal muscle: a morphometric analysis on untrained men, women, and well-trained orienteers. *Pflügers Arch.* 344: 217–232, 1973.
25. Hoppeler, H., O. Mathieu, E. R. Weibel, R. Krauer, S. L. Lindstedt, and C. R. Taylor. Design of the mammalian respiratory system. VIII. Capillaries in skeletal muscles. *Respir. Physiol.* 44: 129–150, 1981.
26. Horsfield, K., G. Dart, D. E. Olson, G. F. Filley, and G. Cumming. Models of the human bronchial tree. *J. Appl. Physiol.* 31: 207–217, 1971.
27. Hugonnaud, C., P. Gehr, E. R. Weibel, and P. H. Burri. Adaptation of the growing lung to increased oxygen consumption. II. Morphometric analysis. *Respir. Physiol.* 29: 1–10, 1977.
28. Jones, J. H., K. E. Longworth, A. Lindholm, K. E. Conley, R. H. Karas, S. R. Kayar, and C. R. Taylor. Oxygen transport during exercise in large mammals. I. Adaptive variation in oxygen demand. *J. Appl. Physiol.* 67: 862–870, 1989.
29. Karas, R. H., C. R. Taylor, J. H. Jones, S. L. Lindstedt, R. B. Reeves, and E. R. Weibel. Adaptive variation in the mammalian respiratory system in relation to energetic demand. VII. Flow of oxygen across the pulmonary gas exchanger. *Respir. Physiol.* 69: 101–115, 1987.
30. Karas, R. H., C. R. Taylor, K. Rösler, and H. Hoppeler. Adaptive variation in the mammalian respiratory system in relation to energetic demand. V. Limits to oxygen transport by the circulation. *Respir. Physiol.* 65: 65–79, 1987.
31. Kistler, G. S., P. R. B. Caldwell, and E. R. Weibel. Development of fine structural damage to alveolar and capillary lining cells in oxygen-poisoned rat lungs. *J. Cell Biol.* 32: 605–628, 1967.

32. Kleiber, M. *The Fire of Life: An Introduction to Animal Energetics.* New York: Wiley, 1961, p. 454.

33. Mathieu, O., R. Krauer, H. Hoppeler, P. Gehr, S. L. Lindstedt. R. McN. Alexander, C. R. Taylor, and E. R. Weibel. Design of the mammalian respiratory system. VII. Scaling mitochondrial volume in skeletal muscle to body mass. *Respir. Physiol.* 44: 113–128, 1981.

34. Mead, J. Mechanical properties of lungs. *Physiol. Rev.* 41: 281–330, 1961.

35. Roughton, F. J. W., and R. E. Forster. Relative importance of diffusion and chemical reaction rates in determining rate of exchange of gases in the human lung, with special reference to true diffusing capacity of pulmonary membrane and volume of blood in the lung capillaries. *J. Appl. Physiol.* 11: 290–302, 1975.

36. Saltykov, S. A. *Stereometric Metallography.* 1st ed. Moscow: State Publishing House for Metals Sciences, 1945.

37. Schürch, S., H. Bachofen, and E. R. Weibel. Alveolar surface tensions in excised rabbit lungs: effect of temperature. *Respir. Physiol.* 62: 31–45, 1985.

38. Schwerzmann, K., L. M. Cruz-Orive, R. Eggmann, A. Saenger, and E. R. Weibel. Molecular architecture of the inner membrane of mitochondria from rat liver: a combined biochemical and stereological study. *J. Cell Biol.* 102: 97–103, 1986.

39. Schwerzmann, K., H. Hoppeler, S. R. Kayar, and E. R. Weibel. Oxidative capacity of muscle and mitochondria: correlation of physiological, biochemical, and morphometric characteristics. *Proc. Nat. Acad. Sci. USA* 86: 1583–1587, 1989.

40. Stäubli, W., R. Hess, and E. R. Weibel. Correlated morphometric and biochemical studies on the liver cell. II. Effects of phenobarbital on rat liver hepatocytes. *J. Cell Biol.* 42: 92–112, 1969.

41. Sterio, D. C. The unbiased estimation of number and sizes of arbitrary particles using the disector. *J. Microsc.* 134: 127–136, 1984.

42. Taylor, C. R. Energy cost of animal locomotion. In: *Comparative Physiology,* edited by L. Bolis, K. Schmidt-Nielsen and S. H. P. Maddrell. Amsterdam: North-Holland, 1973, p. 23–42.

43. Taylor, C. R., R. H. Karas, E. R. Weibel, and H. Hoppeler. Adaptive variation in the mammalian respiratory system in relation to energetic demand. *Respir. Physiol.* 69: 1–127, 1987.

44. Taylor, C. R., G. M. O. Maloiy, E. R. Weibel, V. A. Langman, J. M. Z. Kamau, H. J. Seeherman, and N. C. Heglund. Design of the mammalian respiratory system. III. Scaling maximum aerobic capacity to body mass: wild and domestic mammals. *Respir. Physiol.* 44: 25–37, 1981.

45. Tenney, S. M., and J. E. Remmers. Comparative quantitative morphology of the mammalian lung: diffusing area. *Nature* 197: 54–66, 1963.

46. Wagner, P. D., J. R. Sutton, J. T. Reeves, A. Cymerman, B. M. Groves, and M. K. Malconian. Operation Everest II: pulmonary gas exchange throughout a simulated ascent of Mt. Everest. *J. Appl. Physiol.* 63: 2348–2359, 1987.

47. Weibel, E. R. The early stages in the development of collateral circulation to the lung in rats. *Circ. Res.* 8: 353–376, 1960.

48. Weibel, E. R. *Morphometry of the Human Lung.* Berlin and New York: Springer and Academic, 1963.

49. Weibel, E. R. Principles and methods for the morphometric study of the lung and other organs. *Lab. Invest.* 12: 131–155, 1963.

50. Weibel, E. R. Morphometrics of the lung. In: *The Handbook of Physiology.* Washington, DC: American Physiological Society, Respiration Section, 1964, Vol. 1, Chap. 7, p. 285–307.

51. Weibel, E. R. Morphometric estimation of pulmonary diffusion capacity. I. Model and method. *Respir. Physiol.* 11: 54–75, 1970/71.

52. Weibel, E. R. Morphometric estimation of pulmonary diffusion capacity. V. Comparative morphometry of alveolar lungs. *Respir. Physiol.* 14: 26–43, 1972.

53. Weibel, E. R. *Stereological Methods.* Vol I: *Practical Methods for Biological Morphometry.* Vol 2: *Theoretical Foundations.* London: Academic, 1979/80.

54. Weibel, E. R. *The Pathway for Oxygen.* Cambridge, MA: Harvard University Press, 1984.

55. Weibel, E. R., H. Claassen, P. Gehr, S. Sehovic, and P. H. Burri. The respiratory system of the smallest mammal. In: *Comparative Physiology: Primitive Mammals,* edited by K. Schmidt-Nielsen, L. Bolis, and C. R. Taylor. Cambridge: Cambridge University Press, 1980, p. 181–191.

56. Weibel, E. R., and H. Elias. *Quantitative Methods in Morphology.* Heidelberg: Springer, 1967.

57. Weibel, E. R., and J. Gil. Electron microscopic demonstration of an extracellular duplex lining layer of alveoli. *Respir. Physiol.* 4: 42–57, 1968.
58. Weibel, E. R., and J. Gil. Structure-function relationships at the alveolar level. In: *Bioengineering Aspects of the Lung,* edited by J. B. West. New York: Marcel Dekker, 1977, p. 1–81.
59. Weibel, E. R., and D. M. Gomez. A principle for counting tissue structures on random sections. *J. Appl. Physiol.* 17: 343–348, 1962.
60. Weibel, E. R., and D. M. Gomez. Architecture of the human lung. *Science* 137: 577–585, 1962.
61. Weibel, E. R., and B. W. Knight. A morphometric study on the thickness of the pulmonary air-blood barrier. *J. Cell Biol.* 21: 367–384, 1964.
62. Weibel, E. R., and G. E. Palade. New cytoplasmic components in arterial endothelia. *J. Cell Biol.* 23: 101–112, 1964.
63. Weibel, E. R., and C. R. Taylor. Design of the mammalian respiratory system. *Respir. Physiol.* 44: 1–164, 1981.
64. Weibel, E. R., and A. Vidone. Fixation of the lung by formalin steam in a controlled state of air inflation. *Am. Rev. Respir. Dis.* 84: 856–861, 1961.
65. Weibel, E. R., G. S. Kistler, and W. F. Scherle. Practical stereological methods for morphometric cytology. *J. Cell Biol.* 30: 23–38, 1966.
66. Weibel, E. R., G. S. Kistler, and G. Töndury. A stereological electron microscope study of "tubular myelin figures" in alveolar fluids of rat lungs. *Z. Zellforsch.* 69: 418–427, 1966.
67. Weibel, E. R., L. B. Marques, M. Constantinopol, F. Doffey, P. Gehr, and C. R. Taylor. Adaptive variation in the mammalian respiratory system in relation to energetic demand. VI: The pulmonary gas exchanger. *Respir. Physiol.* 69: 81–100, 1987.
68. Weibel, E. R., W. Stäubli, H. R. Gnägi, and F. A. Hess. Correlated morphometric and biochemical studies on the liver cell. I. Morphometric model, stereologic methods and normal morphometric data for rat liver. *J. Cell. Biol.* 42: 68–91, 1969.
69. Weibel, E. R., C. R. Taylor, and H. Hoppeler. The concept of symmorphosis: a testable hypothesis of structure-function relationship. *Proc. Nat. Acad. Sci. USA* 88: 10357–10361, 1991.
70. Weibel, E. R., C. R. Taylor, P. Gehr, H. Hoppeler, O. Mathieu, and G. M. O. Maloiy. Design of the mammalian respiratory system. IX. Functional and structural limits for oxygen flow. *Respir. Physiol.* 44: 151–164, 1981.
71. West, B. J., V. Bhargava, and A. L. Goldberger. Beyond the principle of similitude: renormalization in the bronchial tree. *J. Appl. Physiol.* 60: 1089–1097, 1986.
72. Wicksell, S. D. The corpuscle problem: a mathematical study of a biometric problem. *Biometrika* 17: 84–99, 1925.
73. Wilson, T. A., and H. Bachofen. A model for mechanical structure of the alveolar duct. *J. Appl. Physiol.* 52: 1064–1070, 1982.

# 3

# Pulmonary Vascular Disease:
## A Joint Adventure

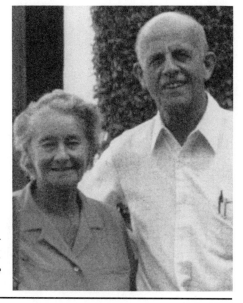

## C. A. Wagenvoort, M.D.

*Emeritus Professor of Pathology, University of Amsterdam. At present, Erasmus University, Rotterdam, The Netherlands*

It is difficult to say whether it was by fate, accident, or purpose that I became involved in studying the pulmonary circulation. It was probably by all three. I always wanted to be a biologist—well, not always. At the age of 3 years I decided to be a tulip vendor, at 6 nurseryman, at 10 a farmer, but from 12 on I wanted to be a biologist. However, when I was preparing to enter the university, it was pointed out to me, not without reason, that my employment prospects as a biologist would range from being unemployed to working as a school teacher. The latter possibility particularly filled me with horror, so I decided to embrace the medical study as a second choice.

That study was interrupted during the war and the German occupation of Hol-land. I had to hide from the Germans to avoid forced labor in our neighbor's country. For two years I was a farm laborer in the countryside; two of us had 18 cows to milk twice a day (Fig. 1). Only after the liberation could I pursue my studies.

In 1946 I became a student assistant at the histologic laboratory of Utrecht University. My research assignment involved counting ova in the ovaries of mice under various circumstances. But I also had to assist in the practical microscopic course. While screening a cross section of a lamprey (*Petromyzon fluviatilis*) for good examples of cartilage and chondroid tissue, I stumbled upon some very strange structures in the aorta of this fish (Fig. 2).

That afternoon had remarkable consequences. I received permission to drop the

From: Wagner WW, Jr, Weir EK (eds): *The Pulmonary Circulation and Gas Exchange.* ©1994, Futura Publishing Co Inc, Armonk, NY.

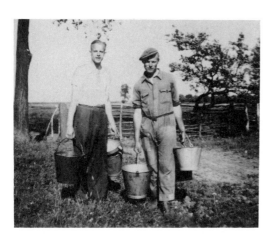

**Figure 1.** During World War II, I worked as a farm laborer milking cows.

eggs and to take up the arteries. I studied serial sections, made models (Fig. 3), and used them in the rheologic laboratory of the Technical Academy in Delft. In the meantime I graduated and got a job in the histology department.

The early fifties were exciting years for me, if only because three things happened within a short period: I married, finished my thesis, and decided to switch from histology to pathology.

A marriage may not seem essential to one's scientific career, but in my case it was. Noek, my wife, gave up her nursing job and, from the first day, became completely involved in my research, helping me in a thousand ways. When I say "from the first day," this may be taken literally. On the evening of the day we married, we left for Naples where I was going to work at the Zoological Station with a government grant.

My thesis, which I defended 10 days before my marriage, included a study of

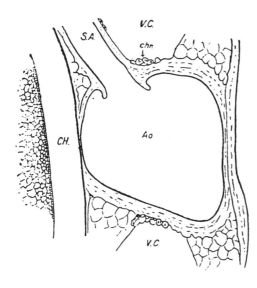

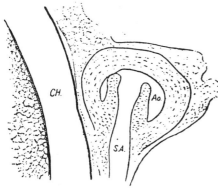

**Figure 2.** Cross section of lamprey aorta.

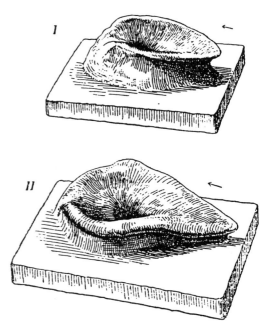

**Figure 3.** Model of structures found in lamprey aorta.

the structures found in the aorta of the lamprey. It appeared that these structures were also very numerous at branching points in other systemic arteries, although smaller and less spectacular (Fig. 4). Here they consisted of circularly arranged smooth muscle fibers around the orifice of a branch that protruded into the lumen of the parent artery. Except for the branchial arteries, we found them throughout the arterial tree, not only in the lamprey but also in other fishes and even in frogs. To a lesser extent they occur in mammals but only in systemic (Fig. 5) and not in pulmonary arteries.

Later it became clear that these ringlike structures can be found in pulmonary arteries of newborn infants and, in the presence of pulmonary hypertension, also in older children (Fig. 6) and adults. In other words they appeared whenever there was an increased pulmonary arterial muscularity. But that was later, after I switched to pathology.

The reason I made the move to pathology was that I thought that in histology the emphasis was turning more and more to biochemistry and biophysics and that I was losing contact with medicine. I never

regretted that decision. I received my training at the pathology department in Utrecht, and in 1956 we went to London with a grant for a year to study at the Postgraduate Medical School.

Any corpuscle entering the systemic circulation risks getting stuck in the pulmonary vasculature. This is what happened to me. In Professor Henry Dible's Department of Pathology I worked in particular with Vic Harrison (Fig. 7). In view of my interest in vessels, Harrison suggested that I have a close look at certain arterial alterations occurring in congenital heart disease with pulmonary hypertension. There were at that time contrasting opinions about these glomuslike, glomeruluslike, or plexiform lesions. Some believed that they were congenital malformations, others that they were acquired and the result of the high pressure in the pulmonary circulation, still others that they represented pulmonary arteriovenous anastomoses.

Vessels containing these peculiar alterations were traced over hundreds of serial sections, and reconstruction drawings were made (Fig. 8). I have always been fascinated by the plexiform lesions

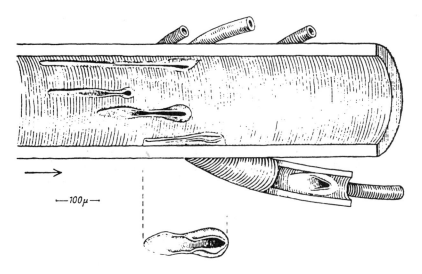

**Figure 4.** The structures were numerous at branching points in other septemis arteries.

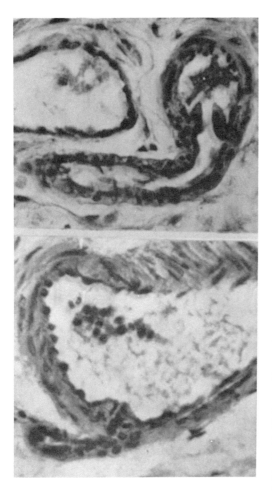

**Figure 5.** Photomicrographs of circularly arranged smooth muscle fibers around the orifice of a branch that protruded into the lumen of the parent artery.

and still believe that observations from that study give a clue to their pathogenesis. Their location immediately after an arterial ramification, the same spot where fibrinoid necrosis is found in these cases, and the destruction of the media in the area occupied by the plexus suggest a causal relationship between arterial necrosis and the resulting fibrin clot and the plexiform lesion.[5]

On my return to Holland in 1957, I moved from Utrecht to Leiden University, where there was a very active department of pathology. What did not change was my interest in pulmonary vascular pathology. I started to do morphometry of pulmonary arteries and developed a method for distinguishing medial hypertrophy from vasoconstriction.[6]

Professor Gerard Brom, the thoracic surgeon in Leiden, was very interested in hypertensive pulmonary vascular disease, and over the years I received more and more lung biopsies, taken routinely during cardiac surgery for congenital heart disease, later also for acquired heart disease. This material formed the basis for a great deal of research in close cooperation with Jan Nauta and Hans Weeda and led to several publications.[11–13]

Then the faculty invited Jesse Edwards (Fig. 9) to Leiden. I was familiar with his work, in particular with his Lewis O'Connor Memorial Lecture,[4] and I very much wanted to talk to him. I devised a strategy, but it was not as easy to implement as I had thought. During the reception following his lecture, a solid mass of faculty members surrounded him, impenetrable for a beginning pathologist. Fortunately, the inevitable moment came at which he absented himself, and I managed to meet up with him in the corridor and guide him to my room, where I had laid out a small exposition of my work on the pulmonary vasculature. His reaction was positive, and I asked him if I could come to Rochester to work with him.

One year later, in 1959, Noek and I went to the Mayo Clinic. It was the beginning of a marvelous year. Although we both worked very hard, it felt to us like one long holiday. Noek started to work as a nurse in St. Mary's Hospital and in the evenings and weekends helped me with my work. As a research assistant I was employed in the morbid anatomy department and spent every moment I could

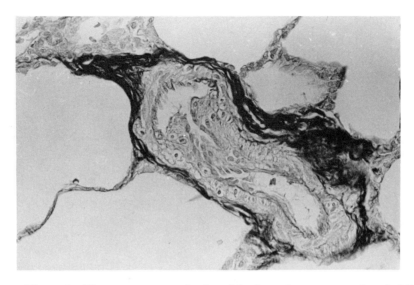

**Figure 6.** These ringlike structures can be found in the pulmonary arteries of children with pulmonary hypertension.

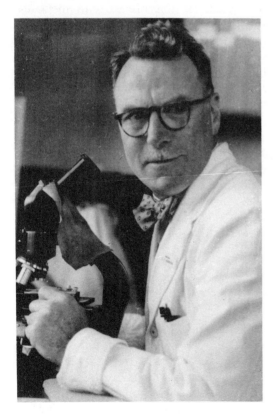

**Figure 7.** Vic Harrison.

spare from the routine work on the morphology of the lung vessels.

Our experience with morphometry was very useful. However, it was such time-consuming work that I could not do what I hoped and thus I asked Noek to help me. It soon was evident that she enjoyed this work and did it very meticulously. She always refused to learn anything about the condition of the patient until she had produced the final data, so as to avoid bias. Because all records have always been kept, the number of vessels morphometrically assessed over the whole period can be estimated as over 500,000. Some of my friends used to say "She is doing the work; he is just talking about it." I do not think this is a fair assessment, but it certainly illustrates the magnitude of the work.

In our first publications from the Mayo Clinic, her work was acknowledged as "with the technical assistance of . . . ." Her input in subsequent studies certainly was not limited to technical assistance, so from then on she became a full coauthor. I

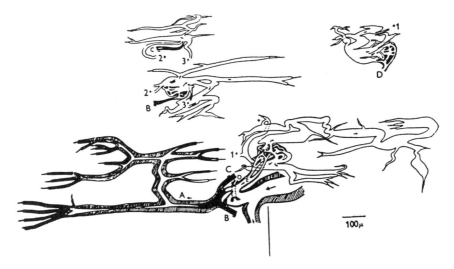

**Figure 8.** Reconstruction of plexiform lesion from serial sections.

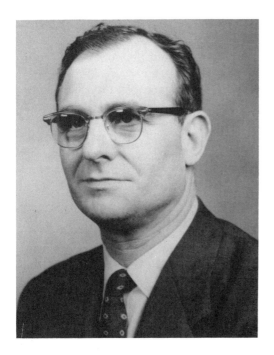

**Figure 9.** Jesse Edwards.

insisted on this point; Noek herself had no ambitions in this direction but enjoyed sharing the adventure.

To have Jesse Edwards as a teacher was a privilege and to work with him a pleasure. He was always relaxed and helpful, whatever the pressure of his own work. My study of the pulmonary circulation brought me in contact with many others engaged in the same field, including Howard Burchell, Jim DuShane, Henry Neufeld, and John Shepherd, all of whom contributed to my education.

In 1960 I returned to Leiden, but with an assignment: write a book with Edwards and Heath on the pathology of the lung vessels.[10] This project took up much of my time and was almost finished when, in 1962, I was appointed professor of pathology at the University of Amsterdam. So that I could finish the book I requested and was given a delay in my appointment until January 1, 1963.

The Department of Pathology of the University Hospital in Amsterdam was built in 1930. Although not practical in all respects, with its large rooms and wide corridors, it was a beautiful building (Fig. 10). The department was understaffed and underequipped. There were, however, compensations. Several cupboards were full of microscopes, all dated from before 1930 and many were early nineteenth-century specimens, some outfitted with candlelight illumination. I really got excited with I found an eighteenth-century sun microscope (Fig. 11) in prime condition. It was to be used in a dark room and had a mirror projecting through a hole in the shutter, catching the sunlight and projecting an image of whatever is put on the object holder on the opposite wall. There were also some nineteenth-century microtomes, in which the object was moved by means of a screw (Fig. 12).

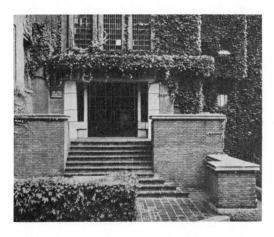

**Figure 10.** Department of Pathology of the University Hospital in Amsterdam.

The department also had an enormous library but one almost devoid of books less than 20 years old. I did have a treasure of antique medical books and atlases from Van Leeuwenhoek and Bonet to Cruveilhier and Virchow. While taking good care of the antiquities, I was handicapped by the lack of people and modern equipment and books. Nonetheless this meant that I had a free hand to shape the department according to my own views, particularly because in the early sixties money was not a major problem.

Over the years some diversity developed in our department with regard to scientific topics, but cardiovascular pathology took priority and pulmonary vascular pathology remained my personal interest. At this time we paid much attention to the normal lung vessels, arteries, veins, and anastomoses, in all age groups.

Noek had experience tracing vessels in serial sections and applied this to the study of anastomoses. Always working at home, she worked her way through 44 series with over 20,000 histologic sections. Venovenous anastomoses appeared to be numerous, but anastomoses between

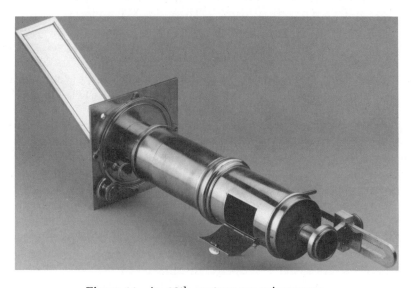

**Figure 11.** An 18th-century sun microscope.

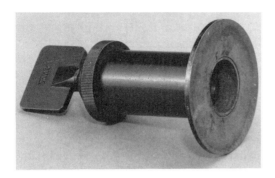

**Figure 12.** A 19th-century microtome.

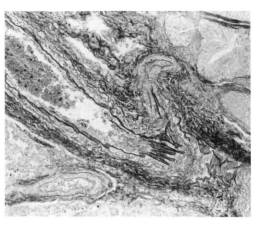

**Figure 13.** Photomicrograph of pulmonary artery supplying bronchial wall.

pulmonary arteries were not found in normal lungs, and those between bronchial and pulmonary arteries were very scarce.

One day Noek told me that she regularly found branches of pulmonary arteries supplying the interstitium of the lung and the bronchial walls (Fig. 13) and branches of bronchial arteries ending up in alveolar capillaries. I found this difficult to believe, so I checked the vessels she had marked. I had to admit that she was right; we published the findings of these pulmobronchial and bronchopulmonary arteries together.[14]

Another subject that fascinated us was primary pulmonary hypertension. The reports on its morphology dealt with a few cases at best and were often confusing or contradictory. In some cases, the lung vessels were described as being completely normal. It was evident that more material was needed for an adequate evaluation.

We started collecting all publications on primary pulmonary hypertension that we could find. This was a lot of work because in the sixties the literature was not as computerized as it is now. We found approximately 600 cases in over 200 papers. Between 1967 and 1969 we sent hundreds of circular letters to colleagues all over the world requesting slides or paraffin blocks from their cases, particularly from the ones that had been published. The response was very satis-

factory. We received material from 162 cases out of 51 departments in 14 countries. In 156 cases the material was adequate and subjected to morphometry.

In 110 out of these 156 patients, the morphology of the lung vessels was identical to that observed in congenital heart disease with a shunt. In 31 patients there were only thrombotic lesions, while in the remaining 15 cases there was a variety of patterns of vascular changes, including veno-occlusive disease and lesions of pulmonary venous hypertension (Table 1). Thus, in our material there were more than three times as many cases of what was later called plexogenic arteriopathy than cases with exclusively thrombotic changes. Although in our publication on this topic[15] we warned against the inevitable selection in the material, this ratio has sometimes been cited as a realistic proportion. However, in the 1960s the term "primary pulmonary hypertension" referred to the primary form of plexogenic arteriopathy. Those were the cases we requested, and so was it generally understood.

Later the term "primary pulmonary hypertension" received a completely different meaning. In October 1973, at a meeting in Geneva of a World Health Organization committee on primary pulmo-

**Table 1**
Cases Submitted Under Diagnosis Primary
Pulmonary Hypertension[a]

| Diagnosis | No. of cases |
|---|---|
| Chronic thromboembolism | 31 |
| Chronic pulmonary venous hypertension | 5 |
| Pulmonary venoocclusive disease | 5 |
| Sarcoidosis | 1 |
| Chronic bronchitis and emphysema | 3 |
| Pulmonary schistosomiasis | 1 |
| Vasoconstrictive primary pulmonary hypertension[a] | 110 |
| Total | 156 |

[a]Later called "plexogenic arteriopathy."
*Note.* (Reprinted with permission from reference 15.)

nary hypertension, two recommendations were made with regard to terminology. First, it was decided that the morphologic entity characterized by concentric-laminar intimal fibrosis, fibrinoid necrosis, and plexiform lesions should have its own name. For that reason, the two pathologists on the committee, Donald Heath and I, were asked to come up with a suggestion. While having lunch together, we invented the term "plexogenic arteriopathy"—*plexogenic* to indicate that this condition potentially would lead to one of its final and certainly most characteristic alterations: the plexiform lesion. Our proposal was accepted that afternoon. The other recommendation was to no longer use the term "primary pulmonary hypertension" for the morphologic entity of plexogenic arteriopathy but for all cases in which there were no clinical indications for the cause of the elevation of pressure.

In retrospect I think that this was an unfortunate decision. If the clinicians are unable to explain the elevated pressure, it should be called "unexplained pulmonary hypertension."[2] By using the term "primary pulmonary hypertension," clini-

cians suggest that they have made a diagnosis rather than having failed to do so. Maybe that is the reason the term used in this sense has become so popular.

The report of the committee meeting[3] pointed out that clinically unexplained pulmonary hypertension usually appears to be based on one of three morphologic conditions: plexogenic arteriopathy, thromboembolic arteriopathy, and pulmonary veno-occlusive disease. Although this may be so usually, whatever the form or whatever the underlying morphology, the cause of an elevated pulmonary arterial pressure may sometimes elude the clinician's diagnostic possibilities. This can happen not only with very rare diseases, such as capillary hemangiomatosis or pulmonary arterial medial defects, but also occasionally with more common conditions that present in an unusual fashion, such as tumor embolism. Occasionally unexplained pulmonary hypertension appears at autopsy to be caused by tumor embolism, usually from a gastric or mammary carcinoma that had remained asymptomatic. In a case like that the term "primary," as used in the World Health Organization's definition, seems out of place.

A direct consequence of our involvement in primary pulmonary hypertension was the analysis of various histologic patterns and thereby a classification of morphologic entities in pulmonary vascular disease.[7] For a thorough and systematic study of a case with abnormal lung vessels, with or without pulmonary hypertension, classification is of great help. It certainly helped us get an overview of what to expect in the way of vascular lesions in the lungs and under what circumstances these might occur. Noek joined me in publishing a book on pulmonary vascular pathology. This book, which appeared in 1977,[8] has always been particularly dear to me.

With increasing frequency we received open lung biopsy specimens, taken not during correction of cardiac disease but as a separate procedure. In part, this was done in patients with unexplained pulmonary hypertension to establish a diagnosis. However, we also received many biopsy specimens from patients with known congenital cardiac defects to decide whether pulmonary vascular disease was reversible and correction of the defect permissible. Our experience with hundreds of peroperative biopsies in such cases and comparing there specimens in the same patient with those taken during a banding procedure of the pulmonary artery, and subsequently during corrective surgery, appeared very important in this respect.[9,16]

Other activities included the production of experimental pulmonary hypertension by hypoxia or by application of fulvine, and in particular the morphology of vasoconstriction. These electron-microscopic studies were done in cooperation with Kurt Dingemans.[1]

Since my retirement in 1985 from the University of Amsterdam, I have been fortunate to have the opportunity to work in the Department of Pathology of the Erasmus University in Rotterdam. Although this is a part-time job and I do only pulmonary and pulmonary vascular pathology, it keeps me busy in a pleasant way with diagnostic and experimental work.

Traveling is often a consequence of involvement in scientific work. Some like it and others do not. I liked it, but I had a great advantage: I never went alone. Noek and I traveled to all continents. Together

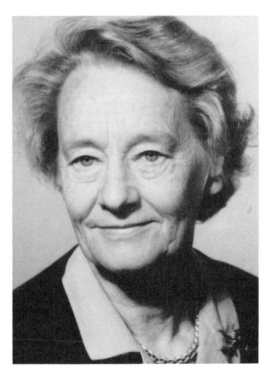

**Figure 14.** Noek Wagenvoort.

we have had many adventures, both unpleasant and delightful. We shared a great hobby—birdwatching—and, wherever we were, we used any opportunity after the congress or symposium for that purpose. Another important dividend of traveling was that we made good friends all over the world. We were always grateful for that.

Noek died very suddenly a couple of months ago. A joint venture has come to an end. I am grateful for the opportunity to pay a tribute to her and to the work she did over almost 40 years (Fig. 14).

## References

1. Dingemans, K. P., and C. A. Wagenvoort. Ultrastructural study of contraction of pulmonary vascular smooth muscle cells. *Lab. Investig.* 35: 205–212, 1976.
2. Fishman, A. P. Editorial. Unexplained pulmonary hypertension. *Circulation* 65: 651–652, 1982.
3. Hatano, S., and T. Strasser (Editors). Primary Pulmonary Hypertension. Report of Committee, World Health Organization, Geneva, 1975.
4. Edwards, J. E. Functional pathology of the pulmonary vascular tree in congenital cardiac disease. *Circulation* 15: 164–196, 1957.
5. Wagenvoort, C. A. The morphology of cer-

tain vascular lesions in pulmonary hypertension. *J. Pathol. Bacteriol.* 78: 503–511, 1959.

6. Wagenvoort, C. A. Vasoconstriction and medial hypertrophy in pulmonary hypertension. *Circulation* 22: 535–546, 1960.

7. Wagenvoort, C. A. Classifying pulmonary vascular disease. *Chest* 64: 503–504, 1973.

8. Wagenvoort, C. A. N. Wagenvoort, *Pathology of Pulmonary Hypertension.* New York: J. Wiley & Sons, 1977.

9. Wagenvoort, C. A. Open lung biopsies in congenital heart disease for evaluation of pulmonary vascular disease: predictive value with regard to corrective operability. *Histopathology* 9: 417–436, 1985.

10. Wagenvoort, C. A., D. Heath, and J. E. Edwards. The Pathology of the Pulmonary Circulation. Springfield, IL: Ch. C. Thomas, 1964.

11. Wagenvoort, C. A., J. Nauta, P. J. van der Schaar, H. W. H. Weeda, and N. Wagenvoort. Effect of flow and pressure on pulmonary vessels. A semiquantitative study based on lung biopsies. *Circulation* 35: 1028–1037, 1967.

12. Wagenvoort, C. A., J. Nauta, P. J. van der Schaar, H. W. H. Weeda, and N. Wagenvoort. Vascular changes in pulmonic stenosis and tetralogy of Fallot studied in lung biopsies. *Circulation* 36: 924–932, 1967.

13. Wagenvoort, C. A., J. Nauta, P. J. van der Schaar, H. W. H. Weeda, and N. Wagenvoort. The pulmonary vasculature in complete transposition of the great vessels, judged from lung biopsies. *Circulation* 38: 746–754, 1968.

14. Wagenvoort, C. A., and N. Wagenvoort. Arterial anastomoses, bronchopulmonary arteries and pulmobronchial arteries in perinatal lungs. *Lab. Investig.* 16: 13–24, 1967.

15. Wagenvoort, C. A., and N. Wagenvoort. Primary pulmonary hypertension: a pathologic study of the lung vessels in 156 clinically diagnosed cases. *Circulation* 42: 1163–1184, 1970.

16. Wagenvoort, C. A., N. Wagenvoort, and Y. Draulans-Noë. Reversibility of plexogenic pulmonary arteriopathy following banding of the pulmonary artery. *J. Thorac. Cardiovasc. Surg.* 87: 876–886, 1984.

# 4

# Pulmonary Edema
# Then and Now

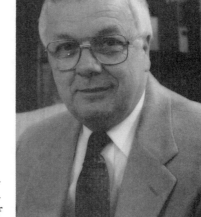

## Norman C. Staub, M.D.

*Professor of Physiology, Cardiovascular Research Institute and Department of Physiology, University of California, San Francisco, California*

When I began investigating lung liquid and solute exchange in 1962, I needed to study only two papers. One was the monumental review by Visscher, Haddy, and Stephens[57]; the other was the study by Guyton and Lindsey[19] on the intravascular forces in Starling's hypothesis as applied to pulmonary edema.

In 1967 two other extensive papers appeared: one by Levine and colleagues[27] and ours on the sequence of events in edema liquid accumulation.[52] These and nearly all other experimental studies had a common motif—namely, to study lung liquid and solute exchange one had to induce overwhelming edema.

The requirement for massive liquid infusions or severe, irreversible chemical injury bothered me because it made study-ing the early, potentially reversible events leading to edema nearly impossible. This stimulated my subsequent work in Australia to develop the unanesthetized sheep chronic lung lymph fistula model.[48,49] Drinker[12] and later Uhley and his associates[56] had managed to cannulate the right lymph duct in anesthetized dogs and sample lung lymph, but they could only do so for a few hours.

An interesting historical sidelight about how discoveries are really made in contrast to how they are reported is that the experiments that led to our first edema paper, published in 1967, were not designed to study the pattern of edema liquid accumulation.[52] Rather, their purpose was to measure pulmonary capillary blood volume by the carbon monoxide diffusing

From: Wagner WW, Jr, Weir EK (eds): *The Pulmonary Circulation and Gas Exchange.* ©1994, Futura Publishing Co Inc, Armonk, NY.

capacity method to test the hypothesis that edema filled the alveoli in a quantal (all-or-none) manner, a hypothesis first proposed by my mentor, Dr. Robert Forster, in a seminar at the Department of Physiology and Pharmacology in the Graduate School of Medicine, University of Pennsylvania (personal communication, 1958) (Fig. 1). Nineteen fifty-eight marks the beginning of my interest in several aspects of intrathoracic liquid and protein exchange which my colleagues and I continue to investigate.

The sequence of events in the accumulation of edema, which is why our 1967 paper is so often cited, was added in retrospect. It was entirely an accidental finding, as are most discoveries in biomedical research, Congress and NIH policymakers notwithstanding.

By 1968 we knew that pulmonary edema could be produced in lab animals by a variety of techniques. Clinically, a new syndrome had appeared[4] called the adult respiratory distress syndrome, characterized by rapid onset of respiratory failure in patients who had not previously shown significant lung abnormalities. The ubiquitous finding was that the pulmonary edema was not due to elevated lung microvascular pressure or to low plasma protein osmotic pressure. Terminally, the alveolar architecture was usually badly deranged. The alveoli and interstitium were filled with proteinaceous liquid and inflammatory cells. Early fibrosis was frequently present.

An example of how quickly a field can develop after a technological breakthrough is the case of the creation of the chronic lung lymph fistula in sheep.[46,51] Figure 2 shows one of the first published experiments in sheep.[45] In 1974 we published our first complete paper on the

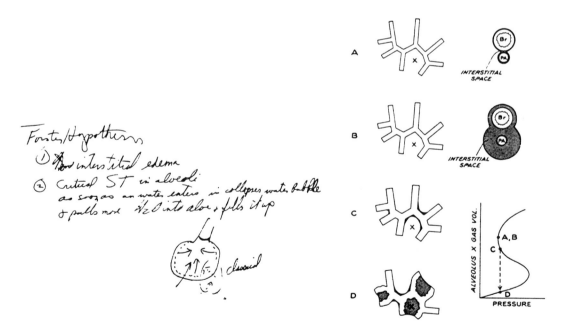

**Figure 1.** Left: Theory of all-or-none filling of alveoli by edema liquid from unedited notes I took during a seminar by R. E. Forster, University of Pennsylvania, Graduate School of Medicine in the spring of 1958. Right: Final form of the all-or-none theory (see cartoons c & d and inset graph). This is the most frequently reproduced of all my figures. (Reproduced with permission from reference 52.)

## BLOOD AND PULMONARY LYMPH
## EFFECTS OF BLOOD INFUSION

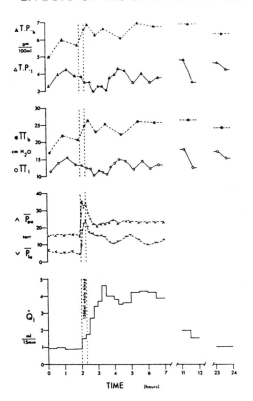

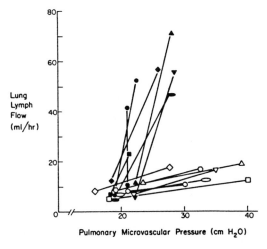

**Figure 3.** Effect of pseudomonas bacterial infusion on the lung's microvascular barrier in seven pairs of unanesthetized sheep. Effects of microvascular pressure are compared before (open symbols) and after (filled symbols) the bacteremia. In those days we had no idea why the lung of the sheep was so sensitive to bacteremia. (Reproduced with permission from reference 10.)

**Figure 2.** Time course of a reversible microvascular injury in an unanesthetized sheep. Note the large increase in lymph flow for a modest rise in pulmonary arterial mean pressure (Ppa) while the lymph protein osmotic press (πl) increased. The experiment was an accident due to an incompatible blood transfusion response. Other abbreviations: T. P. is total protein concentration in blood (b) and caudal mediastinal node efferent lymph (l), respectively; π is protein osmotic pressure; P is hydrostatic pressure; Q is flow. (Reproduced with permission from reference 45.)

pseudomonas model of increased lung microvascular permeability in the sheep (see Fig. 3).[10] A year later we published our classic study of increased pressure in chronic unanesthetized sheep (Fig. 4).[15] I was recently told (Charles Hales, personal communication) that in the early 1970s ours were the only papers dealing with edema in sheep but that by 1990 there

were over 180 papers using the sheep lung lymph fistula.

By 1991 much more is known about the pathophysiology of lung liquid and solute exchange. Lung edema can be induced minimally and reversibly or massively and irreversibly by vascular hydrostatic and osmotic pressure changes or by injury to the pulmonary microvascular endothelial barrier. Hypoxia, up to 48 hours in awake adult sheep (Fig. 5), did not affect filtration, even though pulmonary arterial pressure doubled.[9] Transient overpressurization of the microvessels is probably the common basis for neurogenic[44] and hypoxic edema,[34] although it is difficult to physically damage the lung's capillaries[25] (Fig. 6); indeed heroic measures are required to cause injury.[13,23]

Chemical injury to the microvessels occurs by several agencies. Whether these have a common basis is not clear. Even in 1991 I find it difficult to believe that hydrochloric acid aspiration[35] (Fig. 7) and

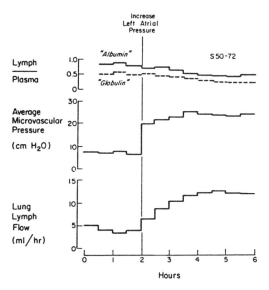

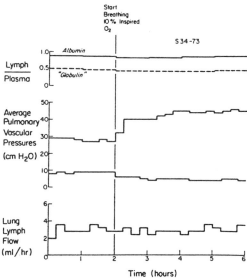

**Figure 4.** Effect of increased left atrial pressure in an unanesthetized sheep. The characteristic slow, modest rise in lymph flow and the fall in the lymph protein concentration are shown. These experiments showed conclusively that the awake sheep can be used to study the effects of lung liquid filtration in a reversible manner without injuring the animal. Most earlier investigations of lung edema had required massive interventions to obtain observable responses because measurement methods were primitive. Consequently, the subtle early changes were missed. (Reproduced with permission from reference 15.)

**Figure 5.** Acute alveolar hypoxia affects only the arterial resistance in the unanesthetized sheep, as shown by the stable lymph flow, which is a sensitive measure of microvascular pressure. This paper also proved that sheep have a strong, sustained hypoxic vasoconstrictor response for up to 48 hours. (Reproduced with permission from reference 9.)

intravenous air emboli[36] (Fig. 8) share a common mechanism, as some claim.

One thing we have learned is that adult respiratory distress syndrome is not primarily a lung disease. The lung manifestations are real enough, but they are secondary to events occurring elsewhere in the body that pour potent bioactive compounds, activated leucocytes, or microdebris into the venous circulation—first stop, the lung's microvascular sieve.

## Cell Biology

Although it is important to know where we came from, it is even more important to know where we are going. The remainder of this chapter describes some of the new directions I am taking in studying the cellular biology of pulmonary edema. As my understanding of lung liquid and solute exchange has increased, my investigations have been moving toward unraveling the interactions among cells. This does not mean I have abandoned whole animal physiology for cell or molecular biology. Nothing will displace physiology as the queen of biological sciences. Everything discovered in test tubes, on culture dishes, or in isolated tissues has to be confirmed and assigned its proper role in the whole animal. Even the most ardent biotechnologists agree on that. But as a problem-oriented physiologist, I will use whatever disciplines or techniques are necessary to solve the problem I am investigating.[49]

LUNG OVERPERFUSION AND HYPOXIA

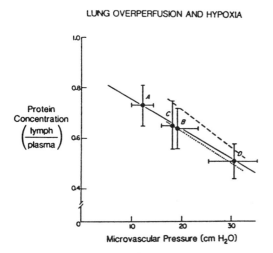

ACID ASPIRATION

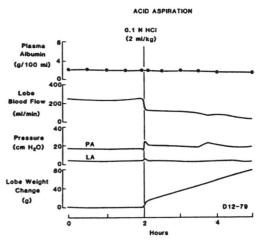

**Figure 6.** Attempts to find evidence in support of the overperfusion theory of high-altitude pulmonary edema failed. The lung endothelial barrier proved to be remarkably resistant to physical damage by increased blood flow [resection of 65% of lung mass (B)], acute alveolar hypoxia (C) and increased left atrial pressure (D). (A) is baseline. All of the labeled points fall along the same line as seen in unanesthetized sheep with increased pressure only. (Reproduced with permission from reference 25.)

**Figure 7.** Hydrochloric acid injury in an isolated perfused dog lung lobe. Note the increase in lung weight even though flow is reduced and the pulmonary arterial and left atrial pressures were kept fairly constant. The injury, as measured by weight gain, occurs instantly and is an acid burn to the alveolar capillary barrier. (Reproduced with permission from reference 35.)

## Endothelium

### Organ-Specific Endothelial Restrictions to Liquid and Solute Flow

The endothelial cells of the hepatic sinusoids have characteristic sieve plates with openings of about 0.1 μm, which permit convective transport of molecules and particles up to the size of small chylomicrons and their remnants. Endocrine organ capillaries have fenestrated endothelium, presumably to give lipophilic hormones easier access to circulating blood.

The lung's microvascular endothelium also has special, if less obvious, characteristics. It forms a continuous barrier with intercellular junctions that markedly restrict protein flow.[47] In contrast to many systemic beds, the postcapillary venular endothelium is insensitive to histamine-

induced gap formation. But immediately adjacent lies the bronchial circulation, and it, being a systemic vascular bed, is histamine sensitive.[38] In the adult the pulmonary microcirculation has essentially no power of regeneration, but the bronchial circulation does. How are these organ-specific differences controlled?

The fact that in some of its functional attributes the pulmonary microcirculation behaves in a manner contrary to or at least differently from the systemic microcirculation is a challenging problem.

### Phagocytosis by Endothelium

In the early 1920s, several workers investigating the intravascular clearance of bacteria and test particles showed that in some species the lung retained a large fraction of the infused material.[22] A remarkable quantitative study of manganese oxide particle distribution by Lund, Shaw, and Drinker[30] showed this dramatically for the cat (Fig. 9). We owe much to the

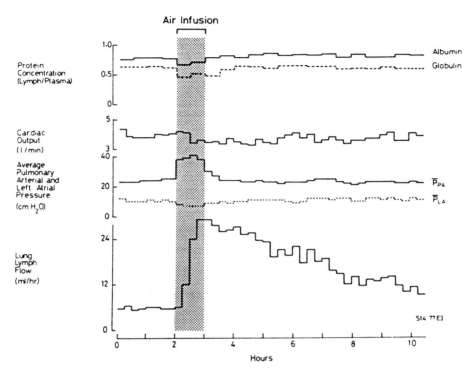

**Figure 8.** Prolonged reversible controlled lung microvascular injury by air emboli. Except during the 1-hour air infusion, the pulmonary vascular pressures were normal. The lung lymph flow rise was sometimes spectacular, as shown here, and persistent. We now believe that the time course of the recovery of the lymph flow to baseline corresponds to the healing of the endothelial barrier. (Reproduced with permission from reference 36.)

early physiologists, whose discoveries are often overlooked.

Some endothelium, such as in the liver sinusoids, is constitutively able to endocytize a variety of small particles, but in the pulmonary circulation we have found little evidence for such activity. In two independent electron microscopic searches by my collaborators, Dr. Kurt Albertine[2] has never and Dr. Anne Nicolaysen (personal communication, 1991) has only rarely seen endocytosis of tracer particles (such as Monastral blue, liposomes, microspheres) by pulmonary microvascular endothelium.

Because endocytic activity by endothelial cells occurs avidly in culture, it must be normally repressed in the intact

lung's microvessels. One likely possibility is that some component of the extracellular matrix inhibits endoethelial cell endocytosis. The endothelium of the liver sinusoids lacks a basement membrane, which may explain its endocytotic and phagocytic properties. I mention this theme of local environmental regulation because it may also have something to do with the signaling that controls the tightness of the intercellular junctions between endothelial cells.

Equally important for regulating endothelial barrier leakiness are physical factors. For example, there is considerable controversy about whether diffusive permeability measurements on endothelial monolayer cultures has any physiological

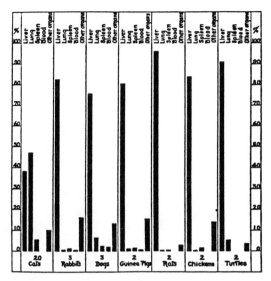

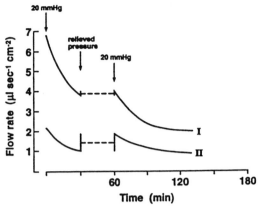

**Figure 9.** Quantification of manganese dioxide microparticle distribution among various mammals. The remarkable retention in the lung of cats (left panel) was attributed to "activated" endothelium. We now know that the effect is due to phagocytosis by the resident population of pulmonary intravascular macrophages. (Reproduced with permission from reference 30.)

**Figure 10.** Physical forces may significantly modulate hydraulic conductivity measured across cultured endothelium. Two-time courses (I & II) of the effect of 20 mmHg filtration pressure applied over 2 hours with a 30-min halt as shown. (Reproduced with permission from reference 5.)

significance.[1,43] Already in 1983 Baetscher and Brune had published evidence showing that modest hydrostatic pressure (20 mmHg) applied to monolayers increased their protein reflection coefficient in a reversible manner[5,5a] (Fig. 10). Likewise, other investigators find that flow (shear) over cultured endothelial cells modifies their phenotypic characteristics. Maybe endothelial cells need to be leaned on to function normally.

Although I do not know how the endothelial barrier is controlled, I do know this is a problem of the greatest importance in microvascular physiology. We should use whatever tools are required to solve it.

## Neutrophils

The total blood leucocyte pool is divided roughly 40:60 between the *circulating* and *sequestered* pools, which are readily exchangeable.[60] Intravital microscopy and rheological analysis have long indicated that most of the sequestered pool consists of leucocytes marginated in the postcapillary venules, where hydrodynamic forces push the leucocytes toward the wall as the main bulk of red cells burst forth from the confinement of the capillaries.[5,40] However, we have never found any significant leucocyte margination in pulmonary venules, even under conditions of low flow, which ought to promote it. Table 1 shows that in sheep most of the neutrophils are located in the capillaries, and some are located in the arterioles. When we reported these data in 1982, neither we nor others were able to explain the lack of venular margination in the lung (Fig. 11).[53]

Most of the sequestered pool in the lung is caused by delayed capillary transit due to the fact that the spherical leucocytes are about the same size as the widest diameter of the alveolar wall capillaries, which are actually elliptical, not circular, in cross section.

Because the lung capillaries are as large as or larger than systemic capillaries, the delayed lung transit must be due to the

**Table 1**
Relative Concentration of Neutrophils in Two Normal Sheep Lungs

| Predicted based on peripheral blood concentration | Small arteries & arterioles (100–1,000 μm diameter) | Alveolar wall (capillaries) | Small veins & venules (100–1,000 μm diameter) |
|---|---|---|---|
| 36 ± 2* | 183 ± 122 | 520 ± 155 | 49 ± 28 |

*Note.* Values refer to number per mm² of blood or alveolar wall in fixed 1-μm-thick sections. Reprinted with permission from reference 53.

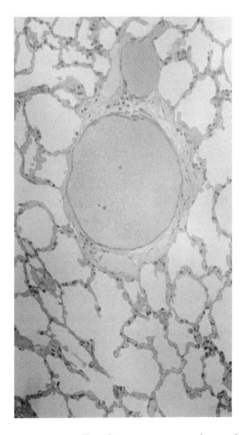

**Figure 11.** Small pulmonary vein and venule showing absence of leukocyte margination under normal conditions. Two large and two small lymphatics (pale gray filled outlines) can be seen in the perivenular adventitia. (Reproduced with permission from reference 53.)

low pulmonary arterial pressure. To confirm this, Hogg and his colleagues have shown that the lung transit time of labeled neutrophils is markedly blood-flow dependent at low flows.[31] Because of their

**Table 2**
Lung Neutrophil Transit Time and Sequestration

| Transit time, s | Sequestration, % of circulating pool |
|---|---|
| 15 | 25 |
| 30 | 50 |
| 60 | 100 |
| 120 | 200 |
| 180 | 300 |
| 360 | 600 |

*Note.* Assumes total circulation time is 60 s.

high overall viscosity, leucocytes must deform before they can pass through the capillaries. The upstream hydrostatic pressure is the driving force. Slow deformation delays their transit relative to erythrocytes and plasma. For example, because all of the cardiac output flows through the lung every minute, a delay in leucocyte transit of 1 min would account for 50% of the total leucocyte pool being retained in the lung. Table 2 lists the effect of various lung-capillary transit time delays on the fraction of neutrophils sequestered in the pulmonary capillaries.

Through a pleural window and using video microscopy, Lien and associates[28] found the *median* pulmonary capillary transit time of fluorescent-labeled neutrophils was about 25 s; a substantial fraction remained for more than 1 min. The median time (half the cells) is probably a better estimate of the normal transit delay than is the mean because the mean transit times are not normally distributed.[42]

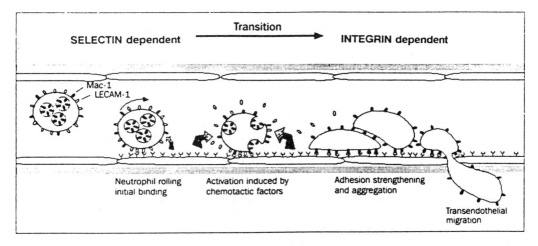

**Figure 12.** Model of neutrophil binding to endothelium. The initial sticking is transient and due to expression of a selectin on the endothelium or cell surface. (Modified from reference 24.)

There is even a possible explanation for the absence of venular margination in the lung. Fiebig and coworkers have evidence that neutrophil sticking and rolling in systemic postcapillary venules probably does not occur normally either. It is, unfortunately, the effect of low-level stimulation during the intravital microscopy preparation procedures.[16]

### What Makes Neutrophils Adhere to Endothelium?

Some new discoveries about cell surface adhesion molecules may explain neutrophil adhesion, although I know of no direct experiments on lung endothelium that have been published.

Among the three main classes of adherence molecules, *immunoglobulin superfamily, integrins,* and *selectins,* the *selectins* mediate the initial binding of leucocytes to endothelium. The known selectins (E for ELAM-1, L for MEL-14, and P for GMP-140) have carbohydrate (lectin) domains at their tips. P-selectin is stored in the α-granules of platelets and in Weibel-Palade bodies of endothelial cells. When systemic venular endothelium is perturbed, either E- or P-selectin is rapidly expressed in large quantities on the luminal surface, which enhances the adherence of neutrophils via counterreceptors on the leucocyte surface.[26] The selectin binding is transient, as these receptors are rapidly shed from the cell surface, a process necessary to permit migration through the intercellular junctions[24] (Fig. 12).

The significance of all this with respect to pulmonary edema may have to do with histamine. Endothelial gaps form transiently and reproducibly in many systemic venules following histamine H-1 receptor activation. Also, the P-selectin (GMP-140) is cycled to the endothelial cell surface after histamine stimulation. However, the pulmonary vascular endothelium is *not* histamine sensitive in terms of histamine-induced gap formation. Is it a coincidence that the lung's venules do not cause leucocytes to stick? Is there a relation between gap formation and histamine-triggered selectin expression?

### How Large is the Lung-Marginated Leucocyte Pool?

The lung appears to have been overemphasized as the main site of normal neutrophil sequestration. As I am partly responsible for that belief, I think I should help correct it. In 1982 we presented quantitative histologic data showing a large sequestered pool of neutrophils in the pulmonary capillaries of normal sheep. We estimated the excess lung pool was about three times the circulating pool. Because we used unactivated native cells, our conclusion seemed to be as certain as is possible in physiological research.[53]

Our work was confirmed, which always makes one feel good, and vastly extended by Hogg's group.[21] However, such a large pool requires a very long neutrophil residence time—3 min, according to Table 2, which is much longer than the median time found by Lien.[28]

This discrepancy caused us to try to confirm our original results. In anesthetized goats we perfused the leucocytes out of the pulmonary vascular bed with saline followed by Ca- and Mg-free media containing chelators. We recovered leucocytes in excess of the estimated residual blood volume, but the excess amounted to only 25%, not 300%, of the circulating pool (see Table 3). Twenty-five percent is equivalent to a 15-s median transit time delay for leucocytes in the lung's capillaries (Table 2); a finding similar to Lien's results.[54]

While we were gathering these data, Peters and coworkers, using total body scanning of labeled neutrophils in humans, obtained evidence that sequestration in the lung constitutes about 10–15% of the circulating pool.[37]

## Lung Endothelial Injury May Be Neutrophil-Dependent

The important role played by neutrophils in acute lung microvascular injury has been partially clarified over the last 15 years. Haslett has described priming of neutrophils by endotoxin and activation of neutrophil-killing functions by a variety of agencies.[20]

**Table 3**
Neutrophils Washed Out of Normal
Goat Pulmonary Circulation

|  | Recovery in excess of residual lung blood volume, millions | Recovery, % of circulating pool |
|---|---|---|
| Saline washout | 799 ± 326 | 18 |
| Chelator washout | 401 ± 137 | 9 |

*Note.* Data are mean ± *SD* for 6 anesthetized goats. Reprinted with permission from reference 50.

Even earlier, we demonstrated an important role for neutrophils in the acute lung injury caused by air emboli, as summarized in Figure 13.[17] The special significance of our data is that Binder and colleagues[7,8] had already excluded fibrinogen and platelets.

Yet several unsolved problems remain. For example, acute lung injury and, of course, adult respiratory distress syndrome can occur in leucopenic patients. The mere presence of neutrophils at an inflammatory site does not prove their involvement in the genesis of the lesion. Neutrophils go to sites of inflammation to protect, not harm us. Harmful actions of neutrophils are the exception, not the rule. We need to keep a proper perspective about these valuable scavengers.

Other leucocytes may also be activated inappropriately. Circulating monocytes are recruited to sites of inflammation in much the same manner as neutrophils. They differentiate into macrophages, which are much better, more efficient killers than neutrophils. In fact, there is good evidence that in acute lung infections the macrophages phagocytize and digest the inflammatory neutrophils, thus preventing their tissue disintegration and the consequent release of proteolytic enzymes.

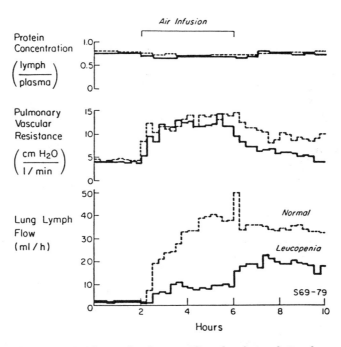

**Figure 13.** Evidence for the specific role of circulating leucocytes in the lung microvascular injury caused by microemboli. Time course of two experiments using acute air embolism induced acute lung injury in an unanesthetized sheep. Dashed lines, control study; solid lines, neutrophil depletion study. (Reproduced with permission from reference 17.)

## Macrophages

### The Unusual Sensitivity of Some Species to Endotoxin

Most readers may know that the sheep and the pig are the favorite experimental models of acute septic lung microvascular injury. For nearly two decades we and others ignored the fact that these species have unusually severe pulmonary hemodynamic responses to bacteria, endotoxin, and a variety of foreign particulates. The lethal intravenous dose of E. coli endotoxin in sheep and pig ranges between 10 and 50 µg/kg. The cause of death is pulmonary vascular hypertension with very low cardiac output or microvascular injury and edema.

On the other hand, the pulmonary circulation of most species is insensitive to bacteremia or endotoxin (Fig. 14). For example, the baboon is at least 1,000 times more resistant to the lethal effects of E. coli endotoxin than is the sheep. The endotoxin-insensitive animals die from general systemic shock, not pulmonary vascular disturbances. In spite of repeated claims that humans are exquisitely sensitive to endotoxin, human sensitivity is unknown because only infinitesimal doses (a few nanograms/kg) have been given.[55] I am not convinced that the human lung circulation is sensitive to endotoxin.

How can these differences in endotoxin sensitivity among species be explained? The first physiological clue came from a comparison of pigs and dogs by Crocker and colleagues,[11] who showed that pseudomonas bacteremia causes profound hemodynamic changes in pigs but

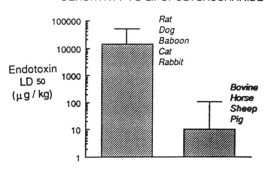

SENSITIVITY TO LIPOPOLYSACCHARIDE

**Figure 14.** The remarkable species-specific sensitivity to endotoxin. Those animals with reactive pulmonary intravascular macrophages form the sensitive group. They die quickly of pulmonary vascular shutdown, whereas the low-sensitivity animals have a delayed death due to systemic shock.

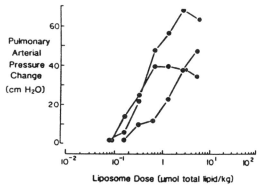

**Figure 15.** Dose-response curve for pulmonary arterial pressure as a function of test liposome particle dose in three unanesthetized sheep. The threshold dose is approximately 0.1 μmol total lipid per kg body weight. With the large doses the sheep showed signs of respiratory distress. (Reproduced with permission from reference 24.)

not in dogs because pigs have a large resident population of macrophages living in their pulmonary capillaries. My associate, Kenji Miyamoto, using liposomes as test particles in sheep, has confirmed Crocker's results[33] (Fig. 15).

Schneeberger was the first to show the presence of macrophages in the capillaries of the cat lung,[41] but Rybicka[39] was the first to recognize them in cattle as a distinct resident population. After Crocker's pioneering work, several investigators reported the existence of macrophages in various species of the order *artiodactyla* (pigs, sheep, bovine, goat).

We reported them independently in 1986,[3] although we did not show their full physiological significance until 1988.[33] In 1989, I concluded on functional grounds that horses, order *perissodactyla* must have pulmonary intravascular macrophages.[50] This year we found intravascular macrophages in the reindeer (Fig. 16) (*artiodactyla*) (Staub, unpublished).

By the way, remember the phagocytic endothelium of cats and lambs reported in the 1920s? It turns out that it was not endothelium at all but intravascular macrophages that could not be resolved by light microscopy in those days, mainly because the histologic sections were too thick.

## Are Intravascular Macrophages Responsible for the Extreme Sensitivity of Some Species to Foreign Particles or Endotoxin?

To prove cause and effect between a suspected agent and its putative action in the body, Koch's postulates (Table 4) must be fulfilled. Thus far, two of Koch's three postulates have been established. The intravascular macrophages are always present when foreign particles induce pulmonary hypertension, thromboxane secretion from the lung, and lung retention of foreign particles.

Data from several labs using putative macrophages washed out of the pulmonary circulation of pigs indicate that these cells do release thromboxane and other eicosinoids in response to appropriate stimuli.[6,18]

We are testing Koch's third postulate by studying the newborn lamb, which, like the newborn piglet, has few lung intravascular macrophages.[29,59] We have found that 1- to 3-day-old lambs have little

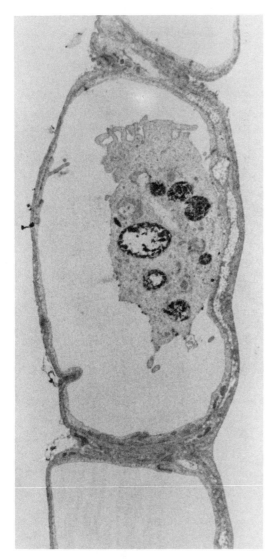

**Table 4**
Koch's Postulates

1. Cells are present whenever phenomenon occurs.
2. Isolated cells are responsive to specific stimuli.
3. Responses cease when cells are removed or inhibited, but responses return when cells are restored.

**Figure 16.** Electron micrograph of a resident pulmonary intravascular macrophage in a reindeer (Order: *artiodactyla*). The macrophage, containing several phagosomes with tracer particles of Monastral blue pigment, is permanently adherent to the microvascular endothelium (From A. Nicolaysen, previously unpublished, 1991.)

lation between the secretion of thromboxane within the pulmonary circulation and the rise in pulmonary arterial pressure or calculated resistance.[14,29]

In most species, including humans, liver macrophages (Kupffer cells) constitute the main mass of the reticuloendothelial system, which is the intravascular component of the mononuclear phagocytic system. Kupffer cells provide a good model because in form and function they are similar to pulmonary intravascular macrophages. They both phagocytize the same types of particles, including endotoxin, which is ordinarily thought of as specific for Kupffer cells.

Warner and Brain have shown in sheep that radioactively labeled endotoxin is taken up predominantly by liver macrophages when infused into the portal vein but by lung intravascular macrophages when infused intravenously.[58] In animals without lung intravascular macrophages, of course, Kupffer cell uptake accounts for nearly all of the infused endotoxin.

## What Do the Intravascular Macrophages Have To Do With Pulmonary Edema?

I believe that the microvascular leak seen in sheep and pigs after sepsis or endotoxin depends on some function of the intravascular macrophages. Meyrick and Brigham[32] located the main lung vascular lesions of endotoxemia in the capillaries and associated the lesions with a

or no response to test particles in doses that cause a large effect at 2 weeks of age, when intravascular macrophages abound.

The fascinating story of the lung intravascular macrophages is just beginning to unfold. For example, there is a close corre-

variety of leucocytes, including "activated" lymphocytes. Although they did not identify intravascular macrophages in their lung sections, at least two of their figures show mononuclear cells that look suspiciously like macrophages.

When we tested endotoxin in 1-day-old lambs, we did not detect any pulmonary hemodynamic changes, whereas an equal or lesser dose of endotoxin markedly affects 2-week-old lambs; this again parallels the rapid growth of the intravascular macrophage population.

## Summary

It was not possible to write a grant application to study endothelium, neutrophils, or intravascular macrophages in 1958, when I became interested in pulmonary edema. My objective in those days was to examine, the early pathophysiology of edema. I accidentally discovered how to make chronic lung lymph fistulas in sheep. In fact almost every important discovery emanating from my lab over 30 years has been fortuitous or serendipitous. However, as Pasteur said, chance favors the prepared mind. In 1991 we are more sensitized to cellular and molecular physiology because of great theoretical and technical advances in molecular and cellular biology, which have made it possible to analyze cellular and subcellular mechanisms.

I have briefly described three kinds of cells that are intimately related to understanding the mechanisms of pulmonary edema and acute lung microvascular injury. These cells are the microvascular endothelium (which behaves differently than systemic endothelium in some important ways), the circulating neutrophils (when inappropriately activated), and the still-mysterious pulmonary intravascular macrophages. Understanding the cellular biology of these cells will, when placed in context with physiological studies in whole animals, allow a fuller understanding of the pathophysiology of pulmonary edema than can be achieved by either the cell biologist or the whole animal physiologist alone.

## References

1. Albelda, S. M., P. M. Sampson, F. R. Haselton, J. M. McNiff, S. N. Mueller, S. K. Williams, A. P. Fishman and E. Levine. Permeability characteristics of cultured endothelial cell monolayers. *J. Appl. Physiol.* 64: 308–322, 1988.
2. Albertine, K. H., S. A. Decker, E. L. Schultz, and N. C. Staub. Clearance of monastral blue by intravascular macrophages in pulmonary microvessels of sheep, goat and pig. *Anat. Rec.* 281: 6a, 1987.
3. Albertine, K. H., and N. C. Staub. Vascular tracers alter hemodynamics and airway pressure in anesthetized sheep. *Microvasc. Res.* 32: 279–288, 1986.
4. Asbaugh, D. G., D. B. Bigelow, T. L. Petty, and B. E. Levine. Acute respiratory distress in adults. *Lancet* 2: 319–323, 1967.
5. Atherton, A., and G. V. R. Born. Quantitative investigations of the adhesiveness of circulating polymorphonuclear leucocytes to blood vessel walls. *J. Physiol. (London)* 222: 447–474, 1972.
5a. Baetscher, M., and K. Brune. An in vitro system for measuring endothelial permeability under hydrostatic pressure. *Exp. Cell Res.* 148: 541–547, 1983.
6. Bertram, T. A., L. H. Overby, A. R. Brody, and T. E. Eling. Comparison of arachidonic-acid metabolism by pulmonary intravascular and alveolar macrophages exposed to particulate and soluble stimuli. *Lab. Invest.* 61: 457–466, 1989.
7. Binder, A. S., W. Kageler, A. Perel, M. R. Flick, and N. C. Staub. Effect of platelet depletion on lung vascular permeability after microemboli in sheep. *J. Appl. Physiol.* 48: 414–420, 1980.
8. Binder, A. S., K. Nakahara, K. Ohkuda, W. Kageler, and N. C. Staub. Effect of heparin or fibrinogen depletion on lung fluid balance in sheep after emboli. *J. Appl. Physiol.* 47: 213–219, 1979.

9. Bland, R. D., R. H. Demling, S. L. Selinger, and N. C. Staub. Effects of alveolar hypoxia on lung fluid and protein transport in unanesthetized sheep. *Circ. Res.* 40: 269–274, 1977.

10. Brigham K. L., W. C. Woolverton, L. H. Blake, and N. C. Staub. Increased sheep lung vascular permeability caused by pseudomonas bacteremia. *J. Clin. Invest.* 54: 792–801, 1974.

11. Crocker, S. H., D. O. Eddy, R. N. Obenauf, B. L. Wismar, and B. D. Lowery. Bacteremia: host-specific lung clearance and pulmonary failure. *J. Trauma* 21: 215–219, 1981.

12. Drinker, C. K. *Pulmonary Edema and Inflammation.* Cambridge, MA: Harvard University Press, 1945.

13. Egan, E. A. Lung inflation, lung solute permeability and alveolar edema. *J. Appl. Physiol.* 53: 121–125, 1982.

14. Enzan, K., Y. Wang, E. Schultz, F. Stravos, M. D. Mitchell, and N. C. Staub. Pulmonary hemodynamic reaction to foreign blood in goats and rabbits. *J. Appl. Physiol.* 71: 2231–2237, 1991.

15. Erdmann, A. J., T. R. Vaughan, K. L. Brigham, W. C. Woolverton, and N. C. Staub. Effect of increased vascular pressure on lung fluid balance in unanesthetized sheep. *Circ. Res.* 37: 271–284, 1975.

16. Fiebig, E., K. Ley, and K.-E. Arfors. Rapid leukocyte accumulation by "spontaneous" rolling and adhesion in the exteriorized rabbit mesentery. *Int. J. Microcirc. Clin. Exp.* 10: 127–144, 1991.

17. Flick, M. R., A. Perel, and N. C. Staub. Leukocytes are required for increased lung microvascular permeability after microembolization in sheep. *Circ. Res.* 48: 344–351, 1981.

18. Fowler, A. A., P. D. Carey, C. J. Walsh, C. N. Sessler, V. R. Mumaw, D. E. Bechard, S. K. Leeper-Woodford, B. J. Fisher, C. R. Blocher, T. K. Byrne, and H. J. Sugarman. *In situ* pulmonary vascular perfusion for improved recovery of pulmonary intravascular macrophages. *Microvasc. Res.* 41: 328–344, 1991.

19. Guyton, A. C., and A. M. Lindsey. Effect of elevated left atrial pressure and decreased plasma protein concentration on the development of pulmonary edema. *Circ. Res.* 7: 649–657, 1959.

20. Haslett, C., L. A. Guthrie, M. M. Kopamiak, R. B. Johnston, Jr., and P. M. Henson. Modulation of multiple neutrophil functions by preparative methods and trace concentrations of bacterial lipopolysaccharide. *Amer. J. Pathol.* 119: 101–110, 1985.

21. Hogg, J. C. Neutrophil kinetics and lung injury. *Physiol. Rev.* 67: 1249–1295, 1987.

22. Hopkins, J. G., and J. T. Parker. The effect of injections of hemolytic streptococci on susceptible and insusceptible animals. *J. Exp. Med.* 27: 1–26, 1918.

23. Hultgren, H. N. High altitude pulmonary edema. In *Lung Water and Solute Exchange,* edited by N. C. Staub. New York: Marcel Dekker, 1978, p. 437–469.

24. Kishimoto, T. K. A dynamic model for neutrophil localization to inflammatory sites. *J. NIH Res.* 3: 75–77, 1991.

25. Landolt, C. C., M. A. Matthay, K. H. Albertine, P. J. Roos, J. P. Wiener-Kronish, and N. C. Staub. Overperfusion, hypoxia and increased pressure cause only hydrostatic pulmonary edema in anesthetized sheep. *Circ. Res.* 52: 335–341, 1983.

26. Lawrence, M. B., and T. A. Springer. Leukocytes role on a selectin at physiologic flow rates: distinction from and prerequisite for adhesion through integrins. *Cell* 65: 859–873, 1991.

27. Levine, O. R., R. B. Mellins, R. M. Senior, and A. P. Fishman. The application of Startling's law of capillary exchange to the lung. *J. Clin. Invest.* 46: 934–944, 1967.

28. Lien, D. C., W. W. Wagner, Jr., R. L. Capen, C. Haslett, W. L. Hanson, S. E. Hoffmeister, P. M. Henson, and G. S. Worthen. Physiological neutrophil sequestration in the lung: visual evidence for localization in the capillaries. *J. Appl. Physiol.* 62: 1236–1243, 1987.

29. Longworth, K. E., J. Y. Westcott, D. Lei, A. Westgate, and N. C. Staub. Development of pulmonary intravascular macrophages in lambs: hemodynamics and uptake of particles. *J. Appl. Physiol.* 73: 2608–2615, 1992.

30. Lund, C. C., L. A. Shaw, and C. K. Drinker. Quantitative distribution of particulate material (manganese oxide) administered intravenously to dog, rabbit, guinea pig, rat, chicken and turtle. *J. Exp. Med.* 33: 231–238, 1921.

31. Martin, B. A., J. L. Wright, H. Thommasen, and J. C. Hogg. Effect of pulmonary blood flow on the exchange between the circulating and marginating pool of polymorphonuclear leukocytes in dog lungs. *J. Clin. Invest.* 69: 1277–1285, 1982.

32. Meyrick, B., and K. L. Brigham. Repeated

Escherichia coli endotoxin-induced pulmonary inflammation causes chronic pulmonary hypertension in sheep—structural and functional changes. *Lab. Invest.* 55: 164–176, 1986.

33. Miyamoto, K., E. Schultz, T. Heath, M. D. Mitchell, K. H. Albertine, and N. C. Staub. Pulmonary intravascular macrophages and hemodynamic effects of liposomes in sheep. *J. Appl. Physiol.* 64: 1143–1152, 1988.

34. Moss, G., C. Staunton, and A. A. Stein. Cerebral etiology of the "shock lung syndrome". *J. Trauma* 12: 885–890, 1972.

35. Nanjo, S., J. Bhattacharya, and N. C. Staub. Concentrated albumin does not affect lung edema formation after acid instillation in the dog. *Am. Rev. Respir. Dis.* 128: 884–889, 1983.

36. Ohkuda, K., K. Nakahara, A. Binder, and N. C. Staub. Venous air emboli in sheep: reversible increase in lung microvascular permeability. *J. Appl. Physiol.* 51: 887–894, 1981.

37. Peters, A. M., S. H. Saverymuttu, R. N. Bell, and J. P. Lavender. Quantification of the distribution of the marginating granulocyte pool in man. *Scand. J. Haematol.* 34: 111–120, 1985.

38. Pietra, G. G., J. P. Szidon, M. M. Leventhal, and A. P. Fishman. Histamine and interstitial pulmonary edema in the dog. *Circ. Res.* 29: 323–337, 1971.

39. Rybicka, K., B. D. T. Daly, J. J. Migliore, and J. C. Norman. Intravascular macrophages in normal calf lung: an electron microscopic study. *Am. J. Anat.* 139: 353–368, 1974.

40. Schmid-Schoenbein, G. W., S. Usami, R. Skalak, and S. Chien. Interaction of leukocytes and erythrocytes in capillary and post-capillary vessels. *Microvasc. Res.* 19: 45–70, 1980.

41. Schneeberger-Keeley, E. E., and E. J. Burger. Intravascular macrophages in cat lungs after open chest ventilation. *Lab. Invest.* 22: 361–369, 1970.

42. Shellito, J., C. Esparza, and C. Armstrong. Maintenance of the normal rat alveolar macrophage cell population. *Am. Rev. Respir. Dis.* 135: 78–82, 1987.

43. Siflinger-Birnboim, A., P. Del Vecchio, J. A. Cooper, P. A. Blumenstock, J. M. Shepard, and A. B. Malik. Molecular sieving characteristics of the cultured endothelial monolayer. *J. Cell Physiol.* 132: 111–117, 1987.

44. Simon R. P. Pulmonary lymphatic flow alterations during intracranial hypertension in sheep. *Ann. Neurol.* 15: 188–194, 1984.

45. Staub, N. C. The pathophysiology of pulmonary edema. *Human Path.* 1: 419–432, 1970.

46. Staub, N. C. Steady-state transvascular water filtration in unanesthetized sheep. *Circ. Res.* (Suppl. 1) 28/29: 135–139, 1971.

47. Staub, N. C. Pulmonary edema. *Physiol. Rev.* 54: 678–811, 1974.

48. Staub, N. C. The lymphatics of the sheep lung. In: *Festschrift for F. C. Courtice,* edited by D. Garlick. NSW, Australia: University of New South Wales, Kesington, 1981, p. 184–194.

49. Staub, N. C. Tell it like it was: part II. *Am. Rev. Resp. Dis.* 136: 1018–1024, 1988.

50. Staub, N. C. Pulmonary vascular reactivity: a status report. In: *The Pulmonary Intravascular Macrophage,* edited by N. C. Staub. Mt. Kisco, NY: Futura, 1989. p. 123–139.

51. Staub, N. C., R. D. Bland, K. L. Brigham, R. H. Demling, and A. J. Erdmann III. Preparation of chronic lung lymph fistulas in sheep. *J. Surg. Res.* 19: 315–320, 1975.

52. Staub, N. C., H. Nagano, and M. L. Pearce. Pulmonary edema in dogs, especially the sequence of fluid accumulation in the lungs. *J. Appl. Physiol.* 22: 227–240, 1967.

53. Staub, N. C., E. L. Schultz, and K. H. Albertine. Leucocytes and pulmonary microvascular injury. In: *Mechanisms of Microvascular Injury,* edited by A. B. Malik and N. C. Staub. *Ann. NY Acad. Sci.* 384: 332–343, 1982.

54. Staub, N. C., E. L. Schultz, K. Longworth, and Y. Wang. Quantification of leucocytes washed from the pulmonary circulation of goats. *Am. Rev. Respir. Dis.* 139: A297, 1989.

55. Suffredini, A. F., P. E. Fromm, M. M. Parker, M. Brenner, J. A. Kovacs, R. A. Wesley, and J. E. Parrillo. The cardiovascular response of normal humans to the administration of endotoxin. *N. Engl. J. Med.* 321: 280–287, 1989.

56. Uhley, H., S. E. Leeds, J. J. Sampson, and M. Friedman. Some observations on the role of lymphatics in experimental acute pulmonary edema. *Circ. Res.* 9: 688–693, 1961.

57. Visscher, M. B., F. J. Haddy, and G. Stephens. The physiology and pharmacology of lung edema. *Pharmacol. Rev.* 8: 389–434, 1956.

58. Warner, A. E., M. M. De Camp, R. M.

Molina, and J. D. Brain. Pulmonary removal of endotoxin results in acute lung
injury in sheep. *Lab. Invest.* 59: 219–230,
1988.

59. Winkler, G. C. Pulmonary intravascular
macrophages in domestic animal species:
review of structural and functional properties. *Am. J. Anat.* 181: 217–234, 1988.

60. Wintrobe, M. M., G. R. Lee, D. R. Boggs, T.
C. Bithell, J. Foerster, J. W. Athens, and J.
N. Lukens. *Clinical Hematology.* 8th ed.
Philadelphia: Lea & Febiger, 1981.

# 5

# Structural Remodeling of the Pulmonary Vasculature by Environmental Change and Disease

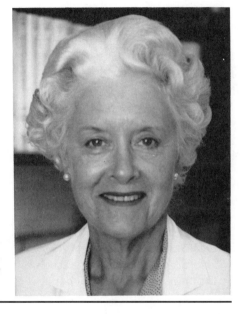

**Lynne M. Reid, M.D.**

*S. Burt Wolbach Professor of Pathology, Department of Pathology, Children's Hospital, Harvard Medical School, Boston, Massachusetts*

I was born in Melbourne, Australia, of Scottish extraction, from farming and commercial folk. This meant that education was important, although I had no professional people among my immediate relatives. "You must be able to earn your own living," was the only requirement from my parents.

I paid my first visit to America as a teenager. It was during the Second World War—a fascinating if somewhat scarey journey—after Dunkirk but before Pearl Harbor. I had been at school in London for several years, and we were on our way back to Australia. I attended the World's Fair and went across Canada by train.

In 1942, I started medical school at Melbourne University. The Australian army had already lost so many doctors that during our first year being a "medical student" became a reserved occupation, and the course of study was compressed to process us as doctors more quickly. After the compressed medical course, our resident years were extended as the troops returned. During my second year I became resident and registrar to the new Department of Thoracic Surgery. This was headed by John Hayward, who had just returned

From: Wagner WW, Jr, Weir EK (eds): *The Pulmonary Circulation and Gas Exchange.* ©1994, Futura Publishing Co Inc, Armonk, NY.

from the war in the Pacific. In those days to see inside the chest was just as exciting and, to the public, just as glamorous as transplantation is today.

One of my duties—a taste of things to come—was to inflate and fix the surgical specimens with formalin. This often occurred late at night, because we operated on Friday afternoon and in those days a lobectomy or pneumonectomy often took eight hours. In was on Tuesday morning that the team gathered for the pathologist, E. S. J. King, to cut the specimen, and woe betide me if any segment, any part of that lung was not perfectly fixed or inflated. "Tut tut, hardly up to Brompton's standards," would be Hayward's comment. He had trained there before the war. This hospital embodied the history of thoracic medicine and represented its new challenges.

At that time the pattern for postgraduate medical education in Australia was for new physicians to take advanced exams first in Australia and then again in England. Several of the older generation, Hume Turnbull, a senior physician at the Royal Melbourne Hospital; Sir Alan Newton, an early president of the Royal Australasian College of Surgeons, now active in reforming medical teaching; and Ivan Maxwell, also a senior physician and one of my special teachers, were encouraging us to try research instead.

Bronchiectasis and lung cancer were the most common diseases treated surgically. One day I asked Hayward what happened in bronchiectasis to the bronchi that did not opacify in the bronchogram—the method we used in those days to diagnose bronchiectasis. "Nobody knows," he said. "Perhaps you had better find out and tell us." This led to my first research grant with the National Health and Medical Research Council of Australia. I would learn later from Professor King that it was the first given to pathology. One of the important questions to be answered at that time was whether bronchiectasis was congenital or acquired.

To tackle this question, it was necessary to first establish the normal anatomy of the lung. How many airways does it have? How do they really branch? It was not enough to fit pattern to botanical models, as had previously been done by bearded professors and discussed in various dusty tomes available to me in the basement of the university library. Cotyledons, dichotomy, trichotomy, equal and unequal—all melted into abstract models. First I dissected the leathery and uninflated lungs that I harvested from the cadavers in the anatomy school. It was about this time that the lung segmental anatomy was established by Boyden and Brock to fill practical surgical needs.

This epitomizes the start of the new specialty of thoracic medicine and surgery. It was necessary to discover the relevant practical lung anatomy and function. New journals appeared—*Thorax* in England, the *Journal of Thoracic and Cardiovascular Surgery* in the United States. A multidisciplinary approach was now being harnessed to understand and treat diseases of that paired organ, the lung. Did you put a paper on lung pathology in a general pathology journal or in a lung journal? This was a practical question that perhaps some recognize for cellular pathology today.

In 1950 I went back to England for further postgraduate work, unsure of whether I would be able to continue in research or would go back to clinical medicine. Even if I continued in lung research I wanted more clinical background, and so it was on to Brompton Hospital planning a medical residency. At this time Neville Oswald, with the support of F. H. Young (both were physicians at Brompton and at St. Bartholomew's), was putting together a team to tackle a pulmonary problem that surfaced after the war once antibiotics had controlled acute infectious lung diseases. They were interested in me because of my research experience. I had two papers, one in press and one submitted, so I was enrolled as pathologist to the group. What is chronic bronchitis? What is emphysema? Are they different, or are they the same and these words are just the different English and American names? These were the questions to be answered.

This led to my link to Sir Roy Cameron, professor of pathology at London University and head of the Department of Pathology at University College Hospital, Fellow of the Royal Society, and later first president of the Royal College of Pathologists. University College was probably the only hospital in the United Kingdom that had experimental research as a major activity in its pathology department—and it was an outstanding one. For example, Professor Howard Florey's department at Oxford had no hospital link. From Cameron I learned many things, among them the way he educated, helped, and supervised his research trainees and that it was possible to move from the pathology of human disease to experiment and to animal models.

George Simon, a great radiologist and wonderful person, was an important and challenging colleague. He specialized in lung radiology at the Brompton and at St. Batholomew's Hospital (Barts) in London. "You can always tell a Barts man, but you can't tell him much" is the quip for the graduates of that oldest of hospitals, founded by Rahere. He was part of the multidisciplinary approach and demanded reliable and precise pathological information. "What causes that Shaaadow?" he fired at me in his characteristic voice. He had been deaf since medical student days. Many a time I found in the middle of my desk a scruffy slice of lung in a plastic lunch bag, brought from some other hospital, to help him interpret some interesting "shaaadow." He raised critical questions from examining the chest radiograph that we could explore in the surgical specimen.

To give more precision to the analysis of arteries, we followed a method, already in the literature, of concentrating on a selected anatomic level in the pattern of branching to compare the normal with diseased lung.[87] This revealed a greater complexity in structure of the peripheral vascular bed than expected and new facts about the branching pattern. The next round of questions included: How did these structures develop? How did these branches grow?

Cardiac surgery had by now budded from thoracic surgery, so the effect of congenital heart lesions on vascular structure was important, as was the question of whether surgical correction of the cardiac lesion would be followed by structural and functional correction of the lung's vessels.

The airway and arterial anatomy kept us in touch with Edward Allen Boyden, a true New Englander and the doyen of lung anatomists. For many years he was a summer visitor for several precious weeks when he alighted at Brompton on his flight from Seattle to Athens to spend his summer holiday in Greece.

In the 1960s I made a special return flight to America. It was the same year the Beatles made their first. They went to Carnegie Hall, and I went to Aspen to meet Roger Mitchell and his colleagues and to attend the first official Aspen Conference. I also recall alighting in New York during several journeys to visit Dorothy Andersen at Presbyterian Babies Hospital to share her experience in cystic fibrosis, which meant retrieving formalin-fixed lung specimens from the dungeons of the hospital.

These were years when young colleagues from England and abroad joined me and we formed a department. Mucus, or *Schleimstoff,* as the Germans more picturesquely call it, was still a major interest. What causes hypersecretion? What prevents it? These were questions we explored in animal experimental studies, in organ culture, and by biochemical analysis in our laboratory and in collaboration with colleagues such as R. A. Gibbons and Scott Blair. "How can you let these pretty girls work on something as unpleasant as sputum?" a French colleague once chided me.

We had added a new model for study relevant to lung and heart disease—hypoxia. Our physiological colleagues could tell us that hypoxia made arteries twitch, but what did it do to structure? For the first time we showed in detail the structural remodeling it induced.

As we focus on the pulmonary vascular bed, we will see that as for the airways it was necessary to establish the appropriate normal anatomy before proceeding to identify abnormality of disease. The challenge came from the cardiac surgeons who needed help with interpretation of biopsy material from patients with congenital heart lesions. From understanding the effects of growth as well as other changes in the pulmonary vascular bed, outcome could be more reliably predicted and evolution of disease better understood and interpreted.

## Quantitative Analysis of Pulmonary Circulation— Preacinar Arterial Branching

To analyze quantitatively structural features of the pulmonary circulation, the first concern is choice of technique. It is intuitive that the external diameter and wall thickness of an artery reflect its state of constriction. To obtain a consistent and defined artifact so that normal pulmonary arteries at different ages and at various levels within the lung can be characterized and then compared with disease, it is first necessary to distend the arteries before fixation (Fig. 1).

The increased understanding of the systemic circulation achieved in the last century was based on vessels distended before fixation. Bright[11] and his succes-

sors studied systemic hypertension in distended vessels. For some reason, in the early years of this century this habit, certainly for the pulmonary bed, was lost. In the decade after World War II Short[114], a radiologist, used a radio-opaque barium gelatine mixture for preparing angiograms of the excised lung, developing a method that gives good filling of the precapillary side of the pulmonary circulation, provides an excellent angiogram and permits light microscopic examination and quantitation (Fig. 1) Histologically, veins are identified as unfilled. If the injection is into the veins, then filling stops at post capillary venules and the arteries are identified as unfilled.

I visited J. Schilling at Hammersmith Hospital: he was interested in the coronary microcirculation. The old pharmacy—in my memory it seems it was in a dungeon—had many great vats that should have been used for wine or beer fermentation but in which barium was being washed to leave a consistent charge, because this influenced the viscosity of the mixture. I think Dr. Schilling's purpose was to fill the capillary bed, and such technical aspects were critical. We adopted the method of Short using the mixture of barium sulphate—gelatin relatively liquid when warm but of a viscosity that did not penetrate capillaries. As the medium cools it sets into a firm gel that can be sectioned in a paraffin block—a big advantage over corosion casts, although at certain times these are useful.

In their study of biopsy material O'Neil, Thomas, and Hartroft[87] focused on arteries running with bronchioli to achieve some consistency. Max Elliott, a newly fledged pulmonary physician from Sydney, wanted to prepare a Ph.D. thesis.[28] Our plan for Dr. Elliott's study—as it turned out an ambitious one—was to establish in several normal adult lungs the structure, diameter, and wall thickness of arteries along the course of an axial pathway, that is, an arterial channel running from a seg-

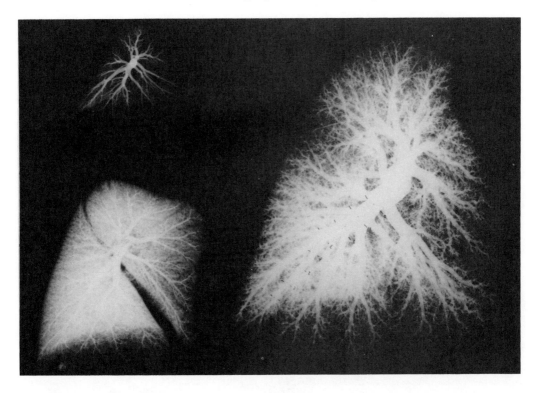

**Figure 1.** Arteriogram of the human lung at thee ages. Top left: Newborn. Bottom left: 18 months. Right: Adult. All preacinar arteries are present at birth. The increase in peripheral filling and in background haze represents an increase in density of intraacinar arteries (From reference 99.)

mental hilum to the distal pleural surface of the segment. If we "landmarked" the artery by its accompanying airway, this would allow comparison at similar levels of branching and provide a precise basis of comparison between lungs of various ages and between the normal and diseased lung. We expected some range of size and structure in large or small, young or old, male or female, but we were not prepared for the complexity and interesting new facts his study revealed (Fig. 2).

In addition to the expected pulmonary artery branch that accompanies each bronchial branch, Elliott found two to three times as many additional ones that ran a short course independent of the branching airways (Fig. 3).[29,95,100,106] The former we called "conventional," the latter "supernumerary." In the distended bed the lumen area of the preacinar supernumeraries is about one third of the total area of all preacinar side branches, conventional added to supernumerary. So these supernumerary arteries represent a significant volume.[23]

The supernumerary branches arise from all preacinar arteries as well as from arteries that run with the identified intraacinar prealveolar airways, the respiratory bronchioli and alveolar ducts. At a given level the supernumeraries tend to be smaller than the adjacent conventional arteries, but over the whole length of an artery some supernumeraries are larger than some conventional.[15,28,29,50,51] At the preacinar level all arteries, whether conventional or supernumerary, have a muscular structure. In the adult it is possible to predict structure from external diameter, that is, if diameter measurement is made in an injected specimen.

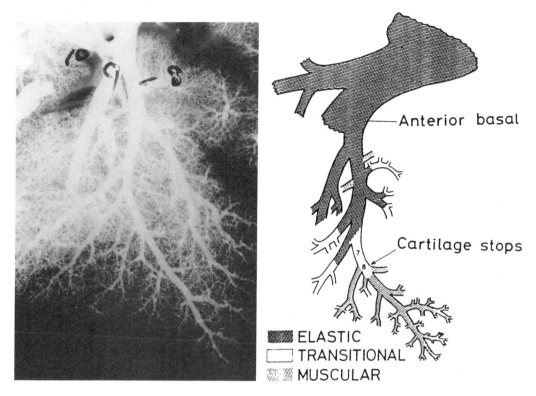

**Figure 2.** Left: Postmortem arteriogram of anterior basal segmental artery in a slice of adult lung 1-cm thick from a normal male of 39 (prepared by injection of barium sulfate-gelatin mixture). The number of arteries arising from the axial artery shown here is about three times as many as the number of branches that arise from the accompanying airway. Right: Diagrammatic representation of the structure of the anterior basal segmental artery shown in the left-hand figure. At generation 8 cartilage stops in accompanying airway. The region distal to the arrow represents the cluster of acini making up a lobule. (From reference 29.)

It is intriguing to speculate on the special function of these arteries. First, how do they contribute to recruitment? Over a given stretch of artery the diameter of adjacent branches varies, implying a different critical opening or closing pressure. Do these relatively minor differences in successive branches contribute to the "instability" at a given level so that increased local flow and pressure progressively recruit more branches. We know from a single pass angiogram that many more arteries are present than show as large branches in the clinical angiogram. Whether this means that even large arteries rotate function through successive heart beats or whether, at low basal flow, some pathways receive so little blood that the lumen is below resolution has not really been addressed.

Another important function of these arteries is that they represent a short cut to regions of lung whose main supply arrives after a longer and roundabout course. If there is a block in more distal channels, these short ones provide a collateral flow—through the back door. If one imagines a block anywhere along an axial artery, the downstream lung does not receive its "central" supply. Insofar as the distal lung abuts against the more proximal stretch of pulmonary artery, it re-

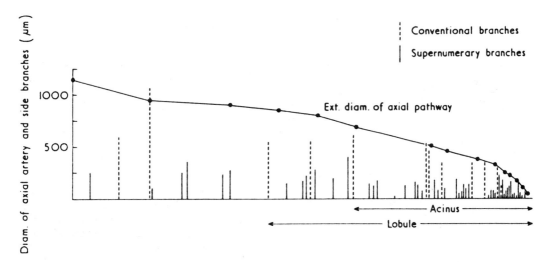

**Figure 3.** Reconstruction of the arterial branching pattern within a lobule and its immediate prelobular region from a lung of a 5-year-old child. The external diameter of the axial pathway and of the conventional and supernumerary arteries is shown. The length of the pathway traced is 1.26 cm. (From reference 58).

ceives short side branches from the proximal artery that enter one side of that respiratory unit. Such collateral flow opens further connections to the vascular bed distal to the block.

Such a block could be from a thrombus or the intimal injury of pulmonary vascular obstructive disease that develops under conditions of high flow. The opening of channels larger than capillaries between pulmonary artery and pulmonary artery produces "arcades," seen in a number of conditions—congenital heart lesions, interstitial fibrosis of the idiopathic variety[74] and emphysema associated with antiprotease deficiency to mention a few. We do not know how long these arcades take to develop.

A similar arrangement of conventional and supernumerary is seen in the veins.[23] Venous tributaries are even more numerous than pulmonary artery branches. From each point of branching of the bronchial tree two veins pass in opposite directions. Always drainage is to the periphery of a unit, be it acinus, lobule, or segment. Effectively then a venogram or arteriogram shows a similar tapering pattern of large vessels, like the main branches of a tree, as well as a "whiskered" look of shorter vessels between the main branchings that are distributed for supply or drainage to the sheath of respiratory lung enclosing each major vessel.

## Intraacinar—Pulmonary Circulation—Pre- and Postcapillary

The pulmonary microcirculation has a characteristic structure that I like to think is as characteristic as the glomerulus. It is an epithelial–vascular unit. Here we concentrate on its microvessels. Along any arterial pathway, whether short and close to the hilum or long and running to the furthest pleural surface, we pass from a muscular structure to one in which the muscular coat is incomplete in a cross section appearing "partially muscular" (Figs. 4 and 5). This continues into an artery that, by light microscopy, has no muscle, is "non-muscular."[99,102,105] These structural features appear in arteries bigger than capillaries. The part of the wall

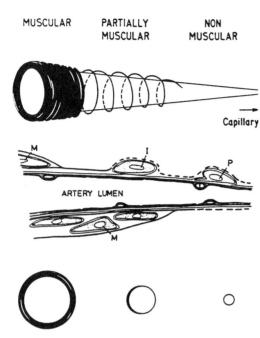

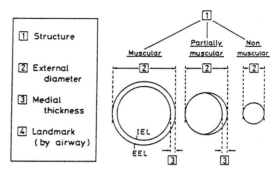

**Figure 5.** Morphometric analysis of pulmonary artery profiles: (1) vessel structure is noted—muscular, partially muscular, nonmuscular; (2) the external diameter is measured—the distance between the two edges of the external lamina; (3) the medial thickness is measured—the distance between the internal (IEL) and the external (EEL) elastic lamina, and the accompanying airway is recorded as a landmark—bronchus or terminal bronchiolus (preacinar), respiratory bronchiolus, alveolar duct, or alveolar wall (intraacinar). (From reference 67.)

**Figure 4.** Diagrammatic representation of the end of any arterial pathway within the lung. Top and bottom drawing shows appearance by light microscopy, in longitudinal and transverse section, respectively. Middle drawing includes additional features shown by electron microscopy: in the muscle-free region of the wall, a pericyte (P) is found in the nonmuscular artery and an intermediate cell (l) in the partially muscular artery. These are precursor smooth muscle cells. E = endothelial cell; M = muscle. Dr. Anderson (see iv) once started a talk with the top and bottom of this slide and the remark "by which you will know that I am one of Professor Reid's muscle men." I should explain that in England this means a "chucker-outer" or "bouncer." (From reference 101.)

that is nonmuscular has the structure of a capillary and is doubtless part of the gas exchanging surface. Electron microscopy, particularly when coupled with dissection reconstruction, reveals additional features.[20,80] The nonmuscular stretches of wall also include muscle cell: often the cell processes of this subintimal layer are even thinner than the endothelium or Type I epithelial cell. This is a critical region because it undergoes significant and widespread remodeling in disease, particularly in hypertension, both primary

or idiopathic and secondary varieties, where the cause can be identified.

A similar structure is seen on the venous side. Like a mirror image, the capillary opens into a nonmuscular vein that passes to a partially and then to a fully muscular vein. The unit that is important to consider here is the mesh between the end of the muscular pulmonary artery and the start of the first pulmonary muscular vein. This model therefore includes a unit that can be identified by its ports of ingress and egress. Probably the unit really starts with the smallest muscular artery, which has the thickest wall for its diameter and thus is a resistance artery. From their cross communication in disease, we know that these units are not isolated. Just as collateral ventilation occurs between a unit and its neighbors, so the capillary bed between adjacent vascular units is an open mesh, at least potentially.

The change or transition from one arterial structure to another does not always occur in arteries of the same size. In any one size range there is a mixed population of arteries—muscular, partially muscular, and nonmuscular—so to analyze in a given lung the structural features of the microvasculature, the proportion of each structural type of a given size must be assessed.[28,101,102,105] The behavior of this part of the lung in response to disease or change in ambient conditions indicates that, in spite of similarity in structure between microartery and microvein, their receptors are different.

## New Features: Internal and External Elastic Laminae in Pulmonary Arteries— Contracture in Disease

The quantitative techniques I have described, including vascular injection, are time consuming, but their advantage for research is not in doubt. Artery "size" is usually measured as the diameter be-

tween the external elastic laminae. It was a reasonable hope that the injection procedure could be sidestepped if an artery could be characterized by the length of an elastic lamina(e). For this reason Fernie and Lamb, for example, have tried to characterize artery size by external lamina length.[31,32] But this expectation is not fulfilled by findings.

By serendipity, Paul Davies found that the lengths of internal and external laminae seem discordant. Surprisingly, in some arteries, the larger ones, the internal lamina is longer than the external (Fig. 6): in small arteries it is the reverse (Fig. 7). The length relationship between the laminae varies with artery size: even more seriously this relationship is changed by hypoxia. In the normal lung this method might be justified if landmarking is included: as a basis for comparing normal with diseased it fails.

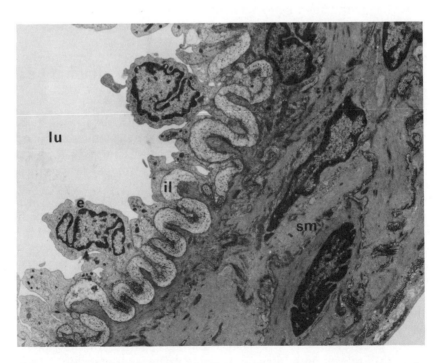

**Figure 6.** Electron micrography of a distended preacinar, muscular artery of a normal rat showing persistence of crenations in the internal elastic lamina (il), the external lamina being smooth; e = endothelium; lu = lumen; sm = medial smooth muscle cell (X8,400). (From reference 22).

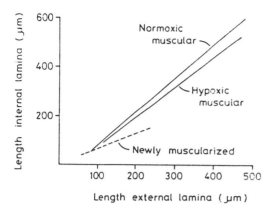

**Figure 7.** Regression lines of internal to external lamina length for cross sections of muscular arteries from normal rats and of muscular and newly muscularized arteries from rats exposed for 14 days to hypobaric hypoxia. (From reference 19.)

Davies was investigating in vitro reactivity by the partially and nonmuscular small arteries, by placing tissue into physiological medium with added constrictor drugs.[18,19] The arteries he studied are much smaller than can be analyzed by threading on a wire and applying strain. Certainly small vessels without smooth muscle respond to a constrictor by lumen area reduction and by thickening or crinkling their walls. It is also of interest that the response by the remodeled hypoxic bed, expressed in relation to wall mass, is no greater than in the normal.

That the internal lamina is usually longer than the external suggests the external lamina is the one smoothed first and is the restraint to distension. At maximum distension the inner lamina is never smoothed out, so that the endothelium lines a series of corrugations that must provide a special microenvironment for these cells. The physiological implications of this and the way local changes in intraluminal pressure and flow are transduced to wall effects pose intriguing questions.

In the smaller vessels the internal lamina is the shorter one and presumably determines distensibility. Hypoxic remodeling changes this relationship (Fig. 7). Meyrick had shown that contracture of the large arteries is associated with increase in collagen and hyperplasia of adventitial fibroblasts.[56,81] The laminae have not been specifically studied. In some small muscular arteries, where normally the internal lamina is longer than the external, under conditions of hypoxia it becomes the shorter one. This is part of the overall infringement on the luminal space by wall hypertrophy and restructuring. Some injuries cause a vessel dilation and increase in microvascular volume as in cirrhosis of liver (4), whereas in the pulmonary hypertensions the typical injury is vascular lumen narrowing and restriction of microvascular volume. Recently, Ohar and colleagues have demonstrated contracture of the elastic laminae in small vessels in a model of pulmonary hypertension after platelet activating factor administration.[86] The laminar length is an unsatisfactory way to characterize an artery.

## Primary Pulmonary Artery Hypertension

The technique of injection and the new facts it revealed about normal pulmonary vessels permitted quantitative exploration of a variety of serious diseases. The first I mention is primary pulmonary artery hypertension and whether it is a separate disease. When I started our studies this was fiercely debated.

Nothing so frustrates a physician as the inability to diagnose and to treat, preferably to cure, a patient. With this I sympathize, but it sometimes leads to illogical and unfeeling behavior on the part of the clinician. To say "primary" is to admit ignorance, a difficult thing for a great physician. The leading cardiologists of the day considered primary pulmonary artery hypertension a microthromboembolic disease missed by the pathologist. In London cardiologists at the Heart Hospital and the Hammersmith Hospitals subscribed to this view. Paul Wood was certainly in the vanguard. As a clinician/pathologist I had seen cases where it seemed clear that pulmonary hypertension was idiopathic (or "essential"), that is, without an identified cause. I had seen "primary" cases in which, during their clinical course, right heart failure had led to peripheral thrombus and then embolus, but this complication hardly justifies the idea of spectrum. Certainly to invoke "missed" thromboembolic disease seems unnecessary, but many pathologists were playing into the hands of the cardiologist.

Series of primary pulmonary artery hypertension and thromboembolic hypertension were being reported with, in general, the conclusion that they represent a "spectrum of change." I shudder intellectually when I hear the word "spectrum" or "continuum." Logic and reasoning go out the window. "Spectrum" usually means that the right questions have yet to be asked to identify the distinguishing characteristics of either end of that spectrum. A separate question arises as to why there should be overlap in the middle.

I well recall Paul Wood hoping to enlist my support in a request to the surgeons to place a collecting filter in the inferior vena cava of an adolescent girl to collect clots that he believed were being "thrown off" by her pelvic veins. The patient, now diagnosed as having pulmonary hypertension, was short of breath going up stairs during her first menstrual period. The history also included two or three such incidents a month apart, the last preceeding her first period by about a month. Such was the conviction of the cardiologists (perhaps faith is the word) that Paul Wood was prepared to see this as an example of thromboembolism.

Over several years I had collected for vascular injection and quantitative study three "early" cases of primary and three of thromboembolic pulmonary hypten-sion, in each of which there seemed no doubt as to the diagnosis because there were no confounding symptoms or signs. All had a short history, so as far as possible we were looking at the earliest cases of the disease that could be collected. Of course this does not tell us about the duration of the disease; the best we can do is to select short duration of symptoms.

This small group of carefully selected patients was important.[1,2] It established the separateness of the pathological findings in the two conditions. As Plopper has emphasized, we do not "prove" a hypothesis; rather, we "fail to disprove" it. For this the critical case has great value: numbers are not everything. Gerald Anderson, now a distinguished consultant physician in the United Kingdom, made a quantitative assessment of the lungs of these six cases and presented them as thesis for his M.D. at London University. The time came for oral examination of the thesis. It was to be held at Hammersmith Hospital with three external examiners (not from our hospital). "There are only four people in the world I don't want to examine my thesis, and I have three of them," Anderson announced to me when he received his notification from London University. After his exam he was to call at my home near the Brompton to tell me the outcome and, we hoped, to quaff a glass of champagne. I had expected him about 5 o'clock. At 6 o'clock I thought perhaps he had gone straight home, I hoped wishing to celebrate, not needing to be comforted by his delightful physician wife and family. At 7 he rang the doorbell. The exam that had been expected to last about an hour had gone for nearly three, but he was successful, now an accredited M.D. It had taken all that time for the physicians to overcome their discomfort at the results and conclusions of this research.

Primary pulmonary artery hypertension has continued to suffer from unfortunate attitudes. As a result of the work of the committee of the World Health Organization called to consider pulmonary hypertension, it was decided to call primary pulmonary artery hypertension plexogenic or plexiform.[39] I feel like Cassandra when I deplore the unfortunate results of this, but it put the "cause" back decades. Even elementary logic confirms that this lesion is not an appropriate way to characterize the disease. Certainly it does get at the cause of primary pulmonary artery hypertension even if it has some bearing on its pathophysiology. The plexiform lesion is found in secondary hypertensions as well as in the so-called primary hypertension (synonyms: essential, idiopathic), and it is not found in all cases of primary hypertension. Members of that committee have recently stated that the way the terms have been used misrepresents the position of the pathologists on that committee. Be that as it may, perhaps we can begin to investigate the disease without conditioning by these preconceived ideas.

A more cheerful part of this story is that Dr. Anderson found special features in those three cases of primary pulmonaryarterial hypertension.[15] At least one subgroup is characterized by an obliterative lesion of the small arteries (those less than 40μ: the nonmuscular and some of the partially muscular arteries disappear (Figs. 8, 9, and 10). When seen in an early stage, affected vessels are detected as "ghost" arteries, but these ultimately leave no trace; only quantitative assessment reveals their loss. At least sometimes the obliterative lesions appear quickly. Untrastructural studies in a further case[75] also showed these obliterative changes.

Collaboration with George Simon made an important contribution to the study. Anderson and I analyzed with Simon the radiographic features of the six cases but we also studied a much larger series of pulmonary artery hypertension patients.[2] This included presumptive cases of primary and of thromboembolic as well as those that were clinically less

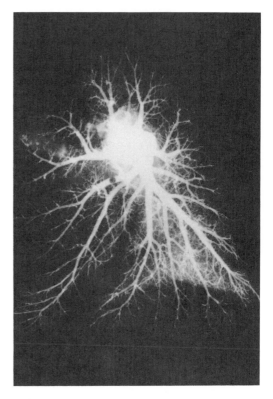

**Figure 8.** Angiograms of the left lung of a patient with idiopathic pulmonary arterial hypertension. Fine peripheral pruning is apparent throughout the lung. Case 1 in Figure 10. (From reference 1.)

clear. In this way we included some late cases in which the picture and the pathology were doubtless mixed. The pathophysiology of dilatation of central arteries in some cases is still not clear.

George Simon was a brilliant and popular teacher. He also struck delicious terror into the hearts of his audience as he orchestrated a film-reading session. It was difficult to choose between closeness to the film as better for learning and the comfort of the relative anonymity of the back row. Even there, however, one was likely to be passed that long grey aero knitting needle, particularly if the patient had tuberculosis and the student clearly saw a cavity. "Show me the caaaarvity," he would say. That clear, perfect ring you outlined would be progres-

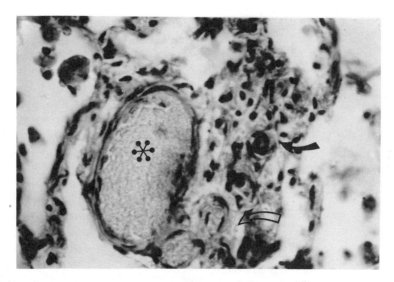

**Figure 9.** Photomicrograph of lung section from patient with idiopathic pulmonary arterial hypertension who died within 6 months of the first symptom. Filling of small muscular artery (*) and its side branch *(open arrow)* with another branch *(closed arrow)* being replaced by concentric arrangement of fibrils and nuclei (4-µm section; Verhoff's elastic van Gieson, original magnification x 500). (From reference 1.)

sively dismissed as "rib," "clavicle," "blood vessel."

One day Tracy Harold, registrar to Oswald's firm, an experienced chest physician (he had been the youngest major in the British Army at the time of his recent demobilization), and a highly intelligent and analytical investigator, asked me to join him and several other members of our "firm" (I was now attached to Oswald's group) to visit Simon at his home. I learned that he had recently had his annual chest radiograph, a check up for long standing apical scarring. This time it was found to have spread. In those days bed rest and soon antibiotics would be treatment. Out of this visit it emerged that Simon would write a book and we at the hospital would help in any way we could. So started a series of valuable and stimulating collaborations, and the precious friendship with George and Joanna Simon and their family. Ultimately, George's book was written and the first of several

editions of it appeared in 1956.[115] It is outstanding for the rigor of the pathological correlations he demanded.

## Hypoxia

When I started in the study of lung disease, there was little research beyond physiological studies and epidemiological/physiological studies. Thoracic Society meetings were dominated by papers and discussions of lung function and of the techniques used. I recall once thinking, "Heavens, this is like an argument as to whether Sahli, Talquist, or Haldane technique is better for measuring haemoglobin—and almost as boring. Why don't we use lung function techniques to find out something about disease?" Looking globally there were bright spots of pulmonary experimental studies, for example, on pulmonary and bronchial circulatory interactions by Averill Liebow. Other ex-

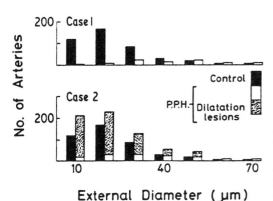

**Figure 10.** Reduction in the number of nonmuscular arteries less than 40 μm in diameter in primary pulmonary hypertension (PPH). Case 1: the patient with the shortest clinical history had no dilatation lesions. Case 2: a patient with a longer clinical history did have dilatation lesions. (From reference 1.)

perimental studies were surgeon conducted and directed to problems of practical significance in the surgical field.

When Ted Badger was president of the American Thoracic Society, I was a visiting professor in Boston. In response to his question as to where I thought the society should be putting its money, I recall saying something like, "Not into proving that chronic bronchitis is the same in New York as London, Pittsburgh as Sheffield, Dallas as Pittsburgh. I think experimental pathology, using animal models of disease, could help us." For I had been privileged to be accepted by Sir Roy Cameron as an extramural student in pathology to the University College Hospital and had watched and learned from him the way to use and work in experimental pathology and to use this to train physicians or pathologists. Quickly Ted Badger came back to me with the fact that well over 90% of their funding was going into just such lung function studies as I had mentioned.

Some years later I heard, on what to

me was a red letter day, a talk by Julius Comroe in which he questioned the value of respiratory function tests in the clinical setting. As we might expect from Comroe, he also put his criticism in perspective. Normal human lung function is so dependent on the voluntary cooperation of the subject that animal studies are of little use, and the hospital setting is in fact the only place where a captive population is available. Perhaps my disillusionment with the function studies had started when my pulmonary physiological colleagues would not allow me to deduce from the fascinating reduction in diffusing capacity, as in primary pulmonary artery hypertension or a probably hypoplastic vascular bed, that there was something defective in the microcirculation. In this physiological climate it was the vasoconstrictive response to hypoxia[107] rapidly reversed on return to air, that occupied students of hypoxia, whether at altitude or for the patient.

Thus in search of structure, that yang to the yin of function, we investigated an animal model of chronic hypoxia—half atmospheric pressure gave us a hypobaric model. Our chamber did not have the glories that I have now seen from Natick to Shanghai, but was a converted small autoclave about a yard high and a couple of feet across. Practical advice for this conversion was given by Coats, a hematologist (the sister of Coats, the physiologist) who had used such an autoclave to develop a model of polycythemia.

The structural changes that Hislop found were surprising and represented a response and remodeling of that precapillary arterial segment that we had identified in the normal adult human lung.[56] After a few days in hypoxia, structural change in the rat precapillary segment is apparent by light microscopy. The structural effects of hypoxia we could then correlate with the functional changes of pulmonary hypertension and right ventricular hypertrophy. These correlations became a major research interest and contribution of the department, first in London and then in Boston. But a model of disease is only as good as how you use it, as the questions you ask. One of the questions we asked was whether recovery occurred. At least partial recovery occurred as assessed by light microscopy: later we would know that "baggage" was still carried by the lung even after some months back in air.

The paper was sent to a cardiological journal, selected as first choice because these studies had been supported by the Heart Foundation. To our surprise and consternation, the reviewers gave us the message, "This paper must not be published since it contradicts the conclusions of the World Health Organization on Pulmonary Hypertension." Their conclusion had been that there is no recovery from hypertension. I can remember from my philosophical vantage of 45 years of age reassuring Hislop.

"This is life, and strangely it does not detract from the results—rather the reverse! The more genuinely new, the more discomforting the fact, the harder for the scientific establishment to accept it."

From the susceptibilities of someone in their twenties came the reply, "Oh I am glad you're here! I would have jumped into the Thames."

I contacted the editor, prepared to answer the editorial questions but demurring over rejection. It was clear he would be discomforted if I pressed the point; the policy evidently was "to let the reviewers have last word." This was an occasion on which I wished for a colleague with at least a little "fire in the belly." I called the *Journal of Experimental Pathology,* the main peer-reviewed publication in this field, explained to the editor what had happened, and offered to send a copy of the review in question. I received the encouraging reply, "Just send us the paper. We don't want the review." It was soon published.[56]

From subsequent studies at light and ultrastructural level,[56,76,78,100] combined with functional investigation explored by additional pharmacological perturbation[71,72,73,79,88,91] the interesting facts emerge. One of the advantages of coming to Harvard was that we developed and applied appropriate catheterization of the rat heart[87] thanks to the skills of Mark Aronwitz, and the collaboration of Walter Gamble and Marlene Rabinovitch, and the participation of Barbara Meyrick, Ruth Ellen Fried, Paul Davies, David Langleben, and Rosemary Jones.

The hypoxic model revealed rapid changes in the precursor muscle cells at the periphery (Figs. 11a,b, and 12). Hypertrophy, then hyperplasia, remodels the microcirculation, lengthening the resistance segment, thickening the wall, and narrowing the lumen—a structural restriction of volume in addition to any constrictor response.[78,79] The simulated ascent of Everest indicates that similar changes occur in man.[38]

This effect falls predominantly on the arteries, and arteries at all levels are affected, the large arteries as early as the peripheral.[81] Centrally the striking change is an increase in labeling index of the advential fibroblast (i.e., cell division increases, a measure of hyperplasia) (Figs. 12A & B). This change occurs when pressure rise is slight. In a given vessel the timing of the hyperplastic response is different for each layer and for a given layer different at different levels of branching (Figs. 13 and 14). This diversity of receptor and receptor activity of a given cell type reflects the structural diversity along a vessel and the changes in cytokine/mediator soup stimulated by acute and continuing change in partial pressure of oxygen in airway gas and oxygen tension in tissue. The separate significance of these is still not quite defined.

It is as safe as most generalizations in medicine to say that in all species some individuals, "nonresponders," do not react to acute hypoxia by vasoconstriction.

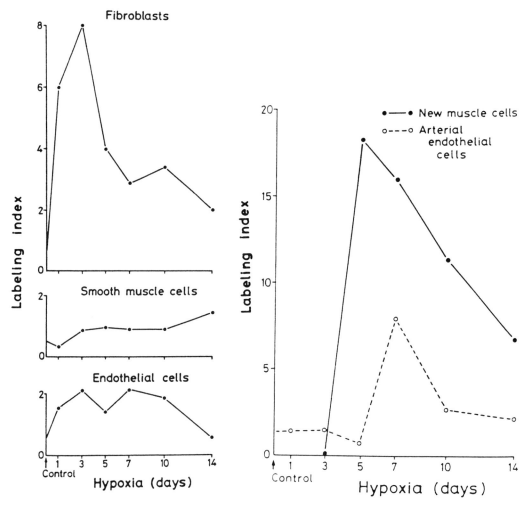

**Figure 11.** Labeling index of vascular cells after exposure to hypoxia. **A** Adventitial fibroblasts, medial smooth muscle cells, and endothelial cells of the hilar muscular artery. **B** Intraacinar new muscle cells (solid circles) and arterial endothelial cells (open circles) of intraacinar arteries. (From reference 79.)

We have never found an animal that does not show structural remodeling. Even in a series of animals with structural remodeling from chronic hypoxia, nonresponders to the acute challenge are identified.[60] Vasoconstriction is not necessary to structural change. The gradually increasing pulmonary arterial pressure that persists when animals are returned to room air correlates with increase in severity of structural change. Polycythemia when present also makes a significant contribution to elevated blood pressure.[34]

In the media, it is hypertrophy of the smooth muscle cell rather than hyperplasia that predominates. Elastin increases so that the laminae are thicker, and the interstitial matrix thickens, separating the smooth muscle cells more widely. In large arteries endothelial cells increase in number and size. In the nonmuscular part of small arteries the precursor smooth muscle cells change with little effect seen on the endothelium.[79]

Recovery means that pressure will reach the normal level within months, and

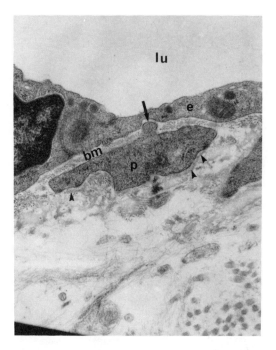

**Figure 12.** Electron micrograph of an artery running within the alveolar wall external diameter, 13 μm. A process *(arrow)* of the pericyte (p) passes through the single basement membrane separating it from the endothelial cell (X40,500). (From reference 22.)

there will be reversal of the peripheral remodeling detected by light microscopy.[35] Return to air is seen as further injury, however. Barbara Meyrick would show that endothelial cells, while still attached to the basement membrane at their periphery, are separated centrally from the basement membrane by a bulla of fluid.[81] Return to air is seen thus as relative hyperoxia, with edema the marker of this injury.

Cor pulmonale was helpfully defined by the World Health Organization as right ventricular hypertrophy in contrast to the usual definition of right heart failure. This has the virtue of separating cardiac failure from hypertrophy, the latter being an adaptation by the right ventricle to high pulmonary vascular resistance, emphasizing the need to distinguish right ventricular hypertrophy from failure.

Cystic fibrosis[16,37,97,111] and chronic bronchitis[112,113] are diseases of chronic hypoxia that cause vascular remodeling, but of course at the autopsy the lungs are a palimpsest of so many accidents that it is difficult to analyze them with the precision of an experiment. In the lung it was taught that emphysema and fibrosis cause right ventricular hypertrophy because of loss of vascular bed, but by no means does this always occur.[101,111,112] Arcades open up between pulmonary arteries and provide "run-off." In fibrosis it may be that the level of hypoxic constriction is critical. In emphysema it seems that resistance arteries are lost so that there is a different reaction by the vascular bed from that of a normal lung.

The role of constriction in structural remodeling is difficult to analyze. We have tried giving a dilator but found that the effect of isoproterenol itself is to cause restructuring.[36] One "growth" pathway then is provoked by its receptors.

In cystic fibrosis, right ventricular hypertrophy occurs very late. In a group of children and young adults we studied it was within the last year or so of life that right ventricular hypertrophy could be identified.[110] It is curious and unexplained that polycythemia seems virtually not to occur in cystic fibrosis patients.

## Hyperoxia

When we moved to Boston, I was encouraged by Harvard and Children's to maintain an interest in adult disease. We continued with organ culture and biochemical studies to study bronchial mucus, to follow the nature and control of mucus secretion in the normal and in the hypersecretory airway, as of chronic bronchitis and cystic fibrosis. We added an interest in "shock lung" or adult respiratory distress syndrome, as it was soon to be called as part of a fruitful collaboration with Warren Zapol and his special center of research based at the Department of

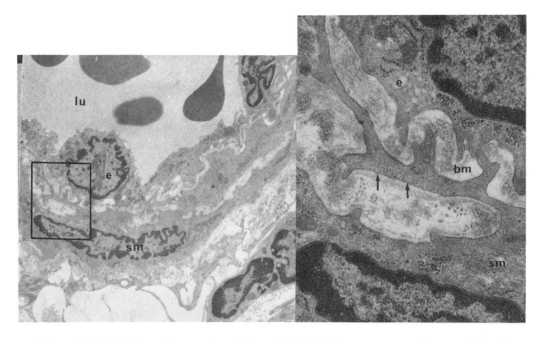

**Figure 13.** **A** Electron micrography of the wall of a distal rat artery, newly muscularized after 14 days hypoxia, fixed undistended: e = endothelial cell; sm = new muscle cells. Area in rectangle is shown at higher magnification in **B**; lu = lumen (X10,200). **B** High power electron micrograph of the area enclosed by a rectangle in **A**. A thin, branched extension of the new muscle cell (sm) projects toward the endothelium (e). Like the main part of the cell, the extension bears many caveolae (*arrows*), mainly along the abluminal membrane. bm = basement membrane (X40,500). (From reference 22.)

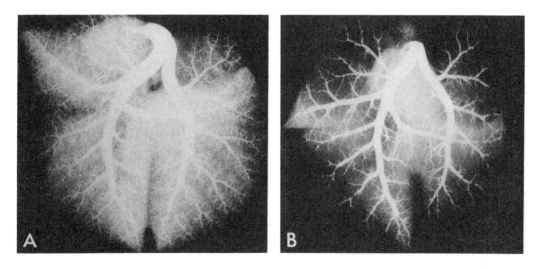

**Figure 14.** Exposure to hyperoxia causes pulmonary hypertension by widespread obliteration of small arteries. Rat pulmonary arteriogram (original magnification X2.5): **A** Normal. **B** Showing narrowing of main axial pathways and loss of filling of small branches after 87% $O_2$ for 28 days. (From reference 63.)

Anesthesia at Massachusetts General Hospital.[67,118] The devastating response of the lung to severe peripheral trauma poses intriguing questions about normal lung function, the products of severe tissue damage, and the susceptibility of the lung to injury by such products. Clearly the lung's vascular bed is central in this problem, both as the route by which cytokines arrive and as the first site of the severe injury that leads to lung congestion, edema, and hemorrhage and starts the often fatal amplification of inflammation produced by the early injury.

Oxygen administration, while life saving, is likely a player in ongoing injury, and so we set ourselves to identify its contribution, as well as to explore other models of injury. Rosemary Jones became the authority on the vascular injury of high oxygen[61,62,63] as well as of sepsis and endotoxemia.[66,67] She was able to develop models of each of these, both as acute as well as the more difficult and challenging one of continuing injury. Orlando Kirton worked with her on the sepsis and endotoxemia models: his surgical skill, coupled with his hard work led to significant biological results relating to these particular models as well as to the nature of injury in general.

But back to hyperoxia. In the alveolar region Crapo has described the necrotizing injury.[14] Jones's first concern was analysis of the vascular structures we have described above (Fig. 15). Major differences between hyperoxia and hypoxia emerged. Hyperoxia affects the vessels upstream and downstream from the capillary bed, causing significant injury to the veins[13,59]: it produces an obliterative lesion—an injury different from the metabolic or hypertrophic response during hypoxia. The residual patent bed is remodeled, perhaps in response to high pressure and flow through the persisting patent channels, perhaps to cytokines released by cells of the injured tissue and activated inflammatory cells. The patent

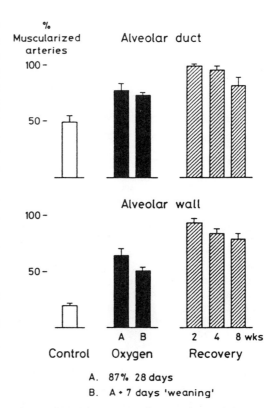

**Figure 15.** Percentage of muscularized (muscular and partially muscular) alveolar duct and alveolar wall arteries (mean ± SEM) in control rats and in five groups of rats exposed to 87% $O_2$ for 28 days (hyperoxia). **A** Hyperoxia alone. **B** Hyperoxia plus weaning to air over 7 days by daily 10% reduction in oxygen concentration. Recovery equals **B** plus 2, 4, or 8 weeks of breathing air. (From reference 63.)

vessels in the rat alveolar wall are restructured to form muscular arteries.[61,62]

Dr. Jones studied recovery from hyperoxic pulmonary hypertension.[63] Animals only survived return to air if weaned to it gradually—a drop of $FIO_2$ from 0.8 to 0.2 over 7 or more days. The extraordinary result was that during this time right ventricular hypertrophy, as well as muscularization of small arteries, continued to increase (Fig. 16): hemodynamic studies revealed the pulmonary arterial pressure continued to rise during this period and identified the rapid constrictive response of too fast a return to air. Animals, accli-

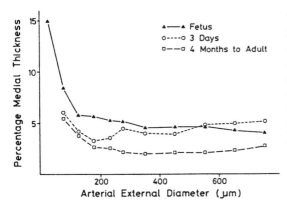

**Figure 16.** Arterial wall thickness (WT) as percentage of external diameter (ED) calculated by (2 x WT/ED) x 100. Arteries of all sizes are thicker in the fetus than in the adult. Soon after birth, the increase in compliance of small arteries is apparent by a decrease in wall thickness and an increase in external diameter (judged at similar level in branching pattern). (Modified from reference 58.)

matized to high oxygen, identified return to air as relative hypoxia and a vasoconstrictor response occurred. The abnormal now represents homeostasis: shift this, even a little, and it represents new injury.

The obliterative lesions put this injury with the group of primary pulmonary artery hypertension (1), some cases of venous hypertension,[17,22] and experimental models such as that caused by monocrotaline injury.[53,72,77] These are different from either hypoxia or the early stages of high flow, where change can be considered hypertrophic and metabolic rather than obliterative and necrotic.

Recently Jones has written a new chapter in our understanding of structural remodeling. In high oxygen injury two main types of restructuring are seen.[69,72] In the first the precursor smooth muscle cells in the nonmuscular stretches of artery wall (i.e., part of the partially muscular and nonmuscular walls) remodels to produce a muscular artery with internal and external elastic laminae. The second type is at present identified only for hyperoxia. Here some nonmuscular stretches of

vessel remodel from migration and alignment of an interstitial fibroblast, which changes its phenotype to a contractile cell and produces an internal and external elastic lamina, changing the structure of the microvessel to that of a muscular artery. Evolution of this response has been followed in a series of elegant electron microscopic reconstructions.[68]

## Persistent Pulmonary Hypertension of the Newborn

Although the Brompton was primarily an adult hospital, pediatric patients, medical and surgical, called for analysis of lung disease affecting growth. The McLeod syndrome, congenital heart lesions, lobar emphysema of the newborn and childhood, cystic fibrosis, and scoliosis all challenged us to understand lung growth in a way that would help us diagnose and interpret disease, follow its treatment, and understand compensatory growth. For persistent pulmonary hypertension of the newborn, our move to Harvard provided us with critical material.

In London I had received consult material on several infants who had died a few weeks after birth from unexplained pulmonary hypertension.[40] Our expectation was that perinatal adaptation[54,58] had failed, but microscopic sections revealed an abnormal structure to the alveolar wall arteries.[40,83,84] In the newborn, these are normally nonmuscular whereas in the cases of hypertension they are well muscularized. Because within a few weeks hypoxia can produce structural changes, apparent by light microscopy, we were cautious in interpreting the structural findings. Perhaps these changes had been acquired after birth and were not present at birth. At Children's Hospital, Boston, we examined the lungs of the six fatal cases of persistent pulmonary hypertension of the newborn that died over a 12-

month period. John Murphy, a cardiological fellow, was responsible for the arterial injections and quantification of vascular arterial structure, and Gordon Vawter was responsible for the general pathological interpretation. I would never have made the move from the adult to the pediatric setting if Gordon Vawter had not been there with special responsibility for the diagnostic services. He was a superb diagnostic pediatric pathologist, a thoughtful and inspiring clinical investigator, and a loyal and warm colleague.

Because these patients had died within 3 days of birth, our hypothesis was that the lung, including the vasular bed, would be normal but that the perinatal adaptation of thinning of the resistance arteries had failed. This thinning reflects an increase in compliance exquisitely localized to the resistance segment: in the small resistance muscular arteries, normally situated near the beginning of the acinus in the newborn, external diameter increases and wall thickness drops.[49,50,52,58] To our surprise structural changes in excessive muscularization of arteries within the acinus were found. This change had been present not only at birth, but also a significant time before birth.[84,85] The intraalveolar wall arteries were smaller than normal, had thick muscular walls, and often had two elastic laminae and a thick collagen adventitia. In some patients upstream preacinar arteries were smaller than normal and also had increased collagenous adventitia. In at least one case numerous thrombi were present. This, then, was a new disease, a new syndrome. No wonder dilators did not help these infants.

We now looked at fatal cases of meconium aspiration.[85] Here surely the hypothesis would hold—normal structure but the accident of aspiration, associated with hypoxia and hypoxemia, preventing normal perinatal adaptation. In 10 of the 11 consecutive deaths from this syndrome we found the same excessive arterial muscularization. "Precocious musculariza-

tion" is convenient shorthand to describe this finding.[84,85] Hypoxemia in utero does not cause these changes[83], nor does administration of indomethacin.[24]

This finding is consistent with the clinical study carried out at Children's Hospital of Philadelphia[33]: that report does not include pathological examination. The clinicians were frustrated that they could not predict which babies with meconium passage or aspiration would have clinical problems. Some with seemingly severe meconium aspiration had a benign course, whereas others in whom it was expected to cause little problem were dead within a few days and with relatively clear radiographs. They found that only those babies who had persistent pulmonary hypertension caused clinical concern, that the deaths were in this group, and that about half of these infants died.

So it seemed that meconium passage and aspiration, rather than the cause, is a marker of persistent pulmonary hypertension of the newborn. The term "meconium aspiration syndrome" is used increasingly. The results of these studies have significant medical and legal implications. A cesarean section an hour or two earlier will not prevent the structural changes characteristic of this persistent pulmonary hypertension of the newborn: more aggressive tracheal suction by the neonatologist will not prevent the structural basis of the persistent pulmonary hypertension. The obstetrician and neonatologist have some protection.

The move to Harvard came at a time when I was dean of the Cardio Thoracic Institute in London. The Wolfson Foundation had recently given money toward a new four story animal facility and designated    one floor for our department. We were at the stage when the vascular work was burgeoning, and we needed to expand, so all seemed set favorably. But I knew that London University was running at about 30% inflation a year, largely due to the catch-up in salaries, particularly of technicians. Twice as much money had to be raised to do the same amount of work as three years earlier, and this when the Medical Research Council Grants, mostly now for only three years, came with the proviso that no year-end adjustment for inflation need be requested. A three-year grant was virtually becoming 18 months. The department was at least 16; myself, a secretary, and two technicians were the only ones on "hard money." Recently my department had been first on our institute's list for the next established academic appointment of a lecturer. This would have been for an assistant to me, but that was the year a Conservative government canceled any university expansion and our department was frozen without a second academic appointment.

The invitation to Harvard included the invitation to bring any of my colleagues. Of course that assumed that we could raise research funds because no funds are provided from Harvard or Children's for research. But I would have enough seed money to justify that leap of faith to cross the Atlantic. Twenty and a half souls crossed—me, nine of my colleagues, and their families: the half was "in utero."

It was a heady time joining Children's and Harvard. Mary Ellen Avery was head of pediatrics and Alex Nadas, head of pediatric cardiology. These were two colleagues with special interest and relevance for our coming and our work. I was greeted in one welcoming speech: "We now feel good. We have had a lady for the first breath and now we have one for the last gasp." On another occasion Dr. Avery admitted, "It was so good to be the first woman M.D. to be full professor at a Harvard Hospital, but what if they had not appointed a second?"

## Lung Growth

Hypoplastic lungs at birth as in Potter's syndrome,[55] hyperlucent lungs after birth as in McLeod's syndrome[74,92,93,95] the effect on lung growth of the abnormal hemodynamics of congenital heart disease,[41,42,43,44,48,89,90] the mechanical embarassment to lung by a congenital diaphragmatic hernia, and compensatory growth after correction of these conditions each pose questions concerning normal and abnormal lung growth.[16,58,89,106,108,109,110]

Quantification was needed to analyze airway and alveolar as well as vascular growth. As part of my first study of bronchiectasis I analyzed the branching pattern of the airways and established the number of airway generations along axial pathways in the various segments.[45,46] Dr. Urs Bucher from Berne had made further studies using quantification methods to establish the pattern of growth.[12] Stereological methods were being successfully applied to counting alveoli and measuring features of the gas exchange surface. Cournand had told me of Gomez, the Cuban exile, who had been his friend of student days in Paris and who had worked with Homer Smith in quantifying renal structure. Cournand had also told me of his dream to one day interest Gomez in the lung. This dream was realized, and Weibel[116] and Dunnill[26,27] were brought in to work with Gomez.[116] These investigators established the total alveolar number. Boyden with his reconstructions explored the intraacinar arrangement of the alveoli.[5,6,8,9,10] Emery and Mithal[30] developed a quick way to check alveolar development—by counting the alveoli transected by a radian passing from a respiratory bronchiolus to the distal acinar edge.

And now we had techniques that enabled us to quantify growth of the vascular bed.[14,43,45,46,47] With quantitative data, in a time frame we formulated the Laws of Lung Development that summarize airway, alveolar, and vessel growth. Each dances to a different drummer.

**Law I: Airways.** The airways—bronchi and bronchioli—are present by the 16th week of intrauterine life. They develop before birth during the pseudoglandular stage[96,98] (Fig. 17).

**Law II: Alveoli.** At birth the "alveolar" spaces are more primitive than in the adult and are described as "primitive saccules" by Boyden.[5] Of these saccules, about $20 \times 10^6$ are present at birth.[15,25,27] After birth the alveoli appear and multiply so that by the age of about 8 years, their number is about $300 \times 10^6$ and are within the adult range.

**Law III: Vascular.** The "vascular law" reflects the first two. The preacinar branches of the pulmonary artery, that is, those that accompany bronchi or bronchioli, appear at the same time as the accompanying airways. These include conventional and supernumerary. The intraacinar vessels appear as alveoli grow[14] (Figs. 18 and 19). The number of venous tributaries resembles the number of pulmonary artery branches. These veins also appear early as successive airway branches appear.[23]

The airways are a prenatal story, the alveoli mainly a postnatal one: the vascular tree partakes of both. The similarity between the central arterial branching pattern of siblings is an intriguing feature identified by Dr. Hislop.[57]

Lung development includes growth in mass and volume as well as maturation of function: it is marked by sudden and dramatic shifts in template, to which development conforms. These changes in template represent changes in signal and control. It is not necessary for the whole of one stage of development to be complete before the switch is thrown and the program shifts. The normal number of airways is not necessarily achieved before the lung switches to alveolar development. Dissociation between airway and alveolar multiplication is seen in many conditions—diaphragmatic hernia, renal agenesis[55,98] and the lung in rhesus isoimmunization, to name but a few. Scoliosis, cystic fibrosis, and McLeod syndrome are examples of disturbed postnatal growth.

Congenital heart disease is a vascular story.[41,42,43,44,48,89,90] Abnormal hemody-

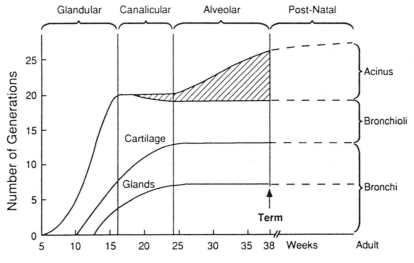

**Figure 17.** Diagrammatic representation of the development of the bronchial tree. Lobar bronchi appear at the 6th week of gestation. By 16 weeks all nonrespiratory airways are present. Most respiratory ones appear between 16 weeks and birth, some in infancy. Cartilage and glands appear later. (From reference 11.)

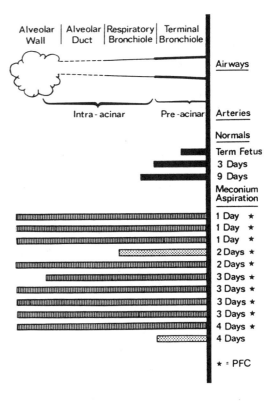

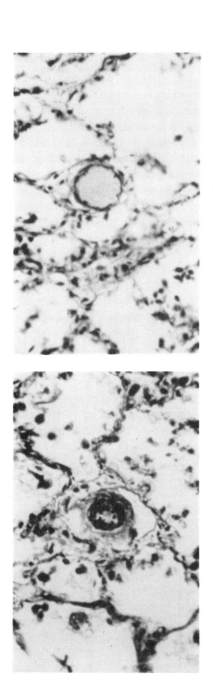

**Figure 18.** A normal intraacinar pulmonary artery (**top**) and one from a newborn infant with persistent pulmonary hypertension (**bottom**) showing a well-developed medial muscle layer and dense collagen sheath including a lymphatic vessel. (From reference 84.)

**Figure 19.** Diagram of muscle extension along pulmonary arterial branches (*shaded bars*). In the normal newborn infant, virtually no intraacinar artery is muscular. In 9 of 10 infants with meconium aspiration and persistent pulmonary hypertension (PPH), muscle extended into more peripheral arteries; the infant with meconium aspiration without PPH (case 11) had normal intraacinar arteries. PFC = persistent fetal circulation (From reference 85.)

namic function before birth modulates vascular growth (Fig. 20). And yet the airspaces typically grow normally and appear normal: some lesions are associated with abnormal hemodynamic growth only after birth, so that while alveoli multiply normally the vessels do not. Quantitative assessment makes it possible to detect such disturbance in lung growth, an additional feature to the ones described by Heath and Edwards[47] for pulmonary vascular obstructive disease. This permits assessment of any effect on growth by congenital heart lesions and assessment of adaptation and growth that occurs after

### Peripheral Pulmonary Arterial Development

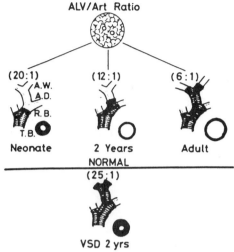

**Figure 20.** Biopsy analysis of structural changes in ventricular septal defect. The number of alevoli (ALV) and the number of arteries (Art) per unit area are given as a ratio. **A** A. W. = alveolar wall; A. D. = alveolar duct; R. B. = respiratory bronchiolus; T. B. = terminal bronchiolus. The progressive extension to the periphery is illustrated at three ages. The size and wall thickness of the artery with terminal bronchiolus is shown in cross section. **B** Findings in a case of ventricular septal defect (VSD) in a patient aged 2 years. The number of arteries is decreased, the arterial muscle is abnormally far to the periphery, and the artery is smaller, with an abnormally thick wall. (From reference 99.)

their repair. A new dimension could be detected in the biopsy that paid back our debt to O'Neal and Hartroft.[87]

Professor Allen Boyden is linked closely to study of lung growth. My first meeting with him was after he had just given a guest lecture at the Institute of Diseases of the Chest, Brompton Hospital. I was too new and too low in the pecking order to have been asked to the sherry after the lecture served in the Institute Library. The small ladies cloak room—one toilet, one wash basin, one mirror,—was crammed with the few women present at the lecture. There was a commanding knock on the door. Nervously the girl nearest to it opened the door. There stood in all his glory Norman Barrett (of Barrett's esophagus) with his commanding surgical presence and Etonian background!

"Is Lynne Reid there? Professor Boyden has asked to meet her. He thinks she's a man!"

So secretly rather chuffed but appropriately demure I was conducted to the library and presented.

Allen Boyden, the doyen of lung anatomists, described in more detail than any other anatomist the distribution and variation of the broncho-pulmonary segments, units critical to the conduct of thoracic surgery. Also he had used the Born wax plate method to reconstruct the acinus at various ages and in various species. After the illness and death of his wife, he used to spend his summer holidays in Greece and the Eastern Mediterranean visiting and studying classical sites and artifacts. One year he went to Turkey, to Halicarnassus, to see the Greek medical school older than Cos. He developed the agreeable habit of visiting our department for several weeks or a month on his way to Greece. He became harbinger of summer and reason for a series of delightful dinners when we would go to his favorite French restaurant, Chez Solange near Leicester Square, eat scampi provençale and drink a bottle of Lanson champagne, all of this punctuated by sketches on the back of a bill, or even a linen table napkin. These were mainly sketches of the acinus as its development unfolded progressively or of interesting cases of developmental anomalies, such as tracheo-oesophageal fistulae. We were often a source of considerable curiosity to our fellow diners, which was a cause of embarassment to that shy and somewhat staid New Englander.

Professor Boyden had another love beside the lung—the gall bladder. In opposition to another of my mentors and heroes Sir Gordon Gordon-Taylor, Boyden believed, and then demonstrated, that the gall bladder has a sphincter. He often regaled and enthraled me with stories of how he developed the fatty Boyden egg meal to relax that sphincter. At 6 o'clock in the morning he was allowed into the department of radiology of his hospital with his cats, colleagues, and the egg meal, on condition that all was clear by 8 o'clock when patients arrived.

His beautiful work with acini had been done on a number of animal species.[8,9]

"Allen, please give us a reconstruction of the human lung?"

"Oh no, Lynne, I can never get a perfect series of sections on human material."

He was calling for thousands of truly serial sections, and even if a few in the thousands were missing, for him this was failure—"not perfect." If I was persuasive it was because I could tell him how much more useful it would be to the understanding of lung growth in health and disease in the human patient if he could overcome his aversion to anything less than perfection and give us even a 90% perfect view of the human acinus. He happily gave us several important reconstructions of the human lung before, still in harness, he died at the age of 95.[5,6,10]

The systemic arteries in so-called sequestrated segments and the systemic arteries seen in some cases of congenital heart disease were a puzzle. In our attempt to interpret some systemic vessels associated with congenital heart lesions, I had searched the literature. After I questioned him one day on these reports, he shook his head in the special solemn, sad way he had and said, "Oh, yes, but that and the literature is wrong."

"Please then, go and tell us definitively, what does happen for the bronchial arteries?"

He contacted administrators at the Carnegie Foundation, who waived their rules and allowed him to take special series of slides home with him for his reconstruction work. From these slides came his paper describing the early "primitive" systemic arteries to the lung arising from the aorta in the neck, close to the celiac axis.[7] These normally disappear at about 6 weeks of fetal life, and the definitive bronchial arteries do not grow in from the aorta until about the 10th to the 12th week. If the primitive arteries persist, they migrate with the celiac axis to below the diaphragm. The elastic artery that commonly supplies the sequestrated segment arising typically from the aorta below the diaphragm represents persistence of this primitive system.

## Pathways of Cellular Control

To understand remodeling of nonmuscular and partially muscular arteries we need to understand the control of cell phenotype. Intercellular communication is critical, and this is modulated by interstitial matrix.

When I talked of pulmonary hypertension, I became tired of hearing from some of my colleagues that pulmonary hypertension was really just the atheroma/atherosclerosis of the lung. I admit that signals are likely to be conserved but emphasize that the differences are so great that this is an irrelevant way to describe pulmonary hypertension. Atheroma is essentially a disease of large and systemic arteries, pulmonary hypertension a disease of the lung's microcirculation. Care must be taken in transferring information from the systemic to the pulmonary circulation. Certainly most of the studies that have been done with cellular control use systemic vessels and cells.

If we wanted to study the lung in organ culture, I believed strongly that we must use lung cells. And so we started cell culture of lung cells. At that time Judah Folkman was studying endothelium but threw away the pericytes: we said we found pericytes even more interesting than the things he kept. We could use available techniques to recover pericytes[21] and also, with ingenuity, grow endothelial cells, smooth muscle cells, and fibroblasts from the lung, in some instances from both the hilum and periphery.[21,64,101,103,104]

A working hypothesis is that in the nonmuscular precapillary arteries, the normal endothelial cell inhibits the pericyte: in hypoxia and other types of excessive muscularization the pericyte breaks free and in some way develops further to change its phenotype.[104]

Paul Davies grew these cells and showed that the endothelial cell substrate has an autocrine/paracrine stimulatory effect on endothelial cell culture, no effect on smooth muscle, and an inhibitory effect on the pericyte.[21] This was a success (Fig. 21). Here we were poised to explore the inhibitory control in the lung, clearly important to understanding normal function and its modification in disease. We were due for a three-year review of this project in the Specialized Center of Research on pulmonary hypertension. At the beginning of the grant the three-year review had been understandable because it was explicitly requested to confirm that we could do technically what we had hoped and claimed. Because we had done what we said we would do, I was prepared to waive a site visit and have the decision made by a conference call. I should not have done so. It was a great disappointment that we were turned down. In an apologetic call from a member of the committee and also in the "pink sheets' was included the remark that there was no need for anyone else to grow endothelial cells. I would have thought that it was the questions asked that were critical. Many of the issues that we would have addressed have still not been dealt with.

But it is good to be active during this explosion of cytokines and mediators. We will likely learn more of the critical systems of control in the next few years.[82–84] And yet there must be concern at the

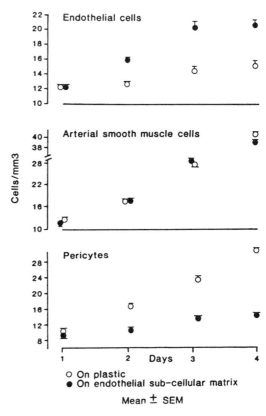

**Figure 21.** The effect on pulmonary vascular cell growth in vitro of substrate derived from rat lung microvascular endothelial cells. The endothelial cells were grown to postconfluence and treated with 0.5% aqueous Triton–X. • = cells plated on substrate; ○ = cells placed on plastic. Each point is the mean ± SEM. The pericyte multiplication is inhibited, that of muscle cell unaffected, and of endothelial cells enhanced. (From reference 21.)

uncritical approach of some investigators to results of in vitro studies. The ultimate appeal must be to tissue, to the in vivo preparations either of the normal subject or patient or in the experimental animal model. We need something on the order of Koch's postulates for infectious disease to keep us on the rails in assessing the significance of cellular events.[103–105]

## Cirrhosis of the Liver

Not all disease is restriction or constriction. Some injuries cause dilatation, flaccidity of the vessel wall: dilatation is also injury.

Even as a medical student the topic of spider nevi had intrigued me as presented in the elegant studies and monograph of William Bean.[3] In the 1950s in London hypoxemia in patients with cirrhosis of the liver was much discussed. I was not impressed with the theory of vascular shunting giving venous admixture. After pulmonary artery injections, the intraacinar microcirculation of the lungs of patients dying from cirrhosis of the liver was analyzed. In some of these patients the pleura was covered with hundreds of spider nevi.[4,69] None were seen in control specimens, yet in most cases there was virtually no cross filling to the veins (Fig. 22). The small arteries of the lung were affected by diffuse dilatation. These were evidently like the spider nevi in the skin as described by Bean: dilatation is on the arterial side of the capillary bed. Our injection techniques revealed this picture, although we knew from the clinical use of radiolabeled media that there is a degree of capillary dilatation that allows more and larger particulate matter to pass the capillary bed than in the normal. The finding of spider nevi was especially gratifying as it extended Bean's findings; he had considered that there were no spider nevi in deep organs.

The colleague involved in this study was P. Bertholet from Paris. He had come to work on liver disease with Professor Sheila Sherlock. I believe it was planned that he would use radioactive markers to investigate vascular shunting as the cause of hypoxemia in liver cirrhosis. Sadly, or I might say happily, for him and us, it was found that an accident had caused such radioactive contamination to the laboratory where he was to work that the studies were not now possible. An urgent call came from Professor Sherlock. Could I include Bertholet in our study? So a serious but crestfallen young French academic traveled across London and arrived at our laboratory. I could reassure him that Professor

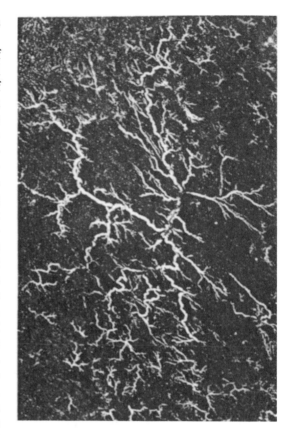

**Figure 22.** Pleural surface showing the numerous, mostly discrete spider naevi injected with Micropaque barium suspension present over the surface of the lung. (From reference 69.)

Sherlock would also have her name on the paper.[4] It seemed that in the eyes of his professor in Paris the sine qua non for his visit to be successful was coauthorship of a paper with Professor Sherlock.

His next disappointment was when he presented his results to me, saying he could see no rhyme or reason to them. But analyzing beyond standard statistics of the mean, it became clear that there was one case of biliary cirrhosis mistakenly included that alarmingly distorted the data and that the characteristic change was indeed a diffuse dilatation.

Later, against my better judgement, we would agree to look at fatal cases of fulminant hepatic necrosis.[117] Fortunately, I was mistaken. These patients are also hypoxemic, but I presumed that the other problems of overdose with paracetamol caused the hypoxemia. To our surprise we found that in these patients within a few days of the injury, diffuse arterial dilatation had developed. What cytokine is responsible for this? Even now I do not think it has been established. But the change is not only rapid in onset but rapidly reversible. Several of the hypoxemic patients whose lungs we did *not* receive survived, and as they recovered the hypoxemia disappeared. Here was a vicarious experiment. And now liver transplant is giving us additional information on this story.

These years have seen what Kuhn would call a shift in paradigm that represents nothing short of a scientific revolution.[70] The most recent one is the shift to the study of cytokines and mediators. Kornberg, in opening his autobiography, *The Odyssey of an Enzyme Biochemist,* considers that this century of science is characterized by a series of successive hunts, each about two decades long.[74] First he recognizes the microbe hunters, then vitamin hunters, enzyme hunters, and gene hunters. Finally he considers neurobiology so successful a subject that the end of this century may well become the time of the "head hunters." I would rather make this a little broader and say that it looks very much as if the last decades go to the "cytokine meddlers and mediator peddlers." Structure and function are a yang and yin, particularly as we try to understand the normal pulmonary vascular bed, its response to growth and environment, and its disturbance by disease. Each of the more biochemical and

molecular hunts must ultimately be incorporated into cellular structure.

This had been quite an odyssey and I feel privileged to have made it. I suppose the Golden Fleece has been understanding the pathogenesis of disease in order to improve diagnosis and treatment. The actual journey has been from patient to laboratory and experimental model and back again to the bedside. I have enjoyed it—mostly—and I can wish you no better.

It is my colleagues who have made the journey possible and who have been its reward. I thank them all for their hard work, shared insights, and commitment to our joint venture and for the jokes and friendships we have shared along the way and still share.

When I was younger, I sometimes thought that if ever asked to tell it "how it was," I *would* mention the bad and gloomy patches—the unprofessional and mean behavior I have seen and experienced, the self-doubts that assailed me. You could read between the lines of this account and realize that there were sloughs of despond, times of uncertainty. But the overall impression is of sunny uplands. Now I am older, and I choose to give it this way—sunny uplands where events and people come together in rewarding, useful, and successful activity. It is the good fortune, the good luck I celebrate—these are the gifts of grace. And I have had so many of this kind—the loving care of parents, the nurture of school teachers, the inspiration and encouragement from my chiefs and seniors, and the warm support and comradeship of colleagues of all ages. It is these that give the golden glow.

---

## References

1. Anderson, G., G. Simon, and L. Reid. Primary and thrombo-embolic pulmonary hypertension. A quantitative pathological study. *J. Pathol.* 110: 273–293, 1973.
2. Anderson, G., L. Reid, and G. Simon. The radiographic appearances in primary and in thromboembolic pulmonary hypertension. *Clin. Radiol.* 24: 113–120, 1973.
3. Bean, W. B. Vascular Spiders and Related Lesions of the Skin. Oxford: Blackwell Scientific Publications, 1959.
4. Berthelot, P., J. G. Walker, S. Sherlock, and

L. Reid. Arterial changes in the lungs in cirrhosis of the liver—lung spider nevi. *N. Engl. J. Med.* 274: 291–298, 1966.

5. Boyden, E. A. Development and growth of the airways. In: *Development of the Lung,* edited by W. A. Hodson. In: *Lung Biology in Health and Disease,* edited by C. Lenfant. New York: Marcel Dekker, 1977, vol. 6, p. 3–35.

6. Boyden, E. A. The mode of origin of pulmonary acini and respiratory bronchioles in the fetal lung. *Am J. Anat.* 141: 317–328, 1974.

7. Boyden, E. A. The developing bronchial arteries in a fetus of the 12th week. *Am J. Anat.* 129: 357–368, 1970.

8. Boyden, E. A. The development of the lung in the pigtail monkey (Macaca nemestrina L). *Anat. Rec.* 186: 15–37, 1976.

9. Boyden, E.A., and D. H. Tompsett. The postnatal growth of the lung in the dog. *Acta Anat.* 47: 185–215, 1961.

10. Boyden, E. A., and Tompsett, D. H. The changing patterns in the developing lungs of infants. *Acta Anat.* 61: 164–192, 1965.

11. Bright, R. *Guy's Hosp. Rep.* 1:338, 1836.

12. Bucher, U. G., and L. Reid. Development of the intrasegmental bronchial tree. The pattern of branching and development of cartilage at various stages of intra-uterine life. *Thorax* 16: 207–218, 1961.

13. Coflesky, J. T., R. Jones, L. Reid, and J. N. Evans. Mechanical properties and structure of isolated pulmonary arteries remodelled by hyperoxia. *Am. Rev. Respir. Dis.* 136: 388–394, 1987.

14. Crapo, J. D., M. Peters-Golden, J. Marsh-Salin, and J. S. Shelburne. Pathologic changes in the lungs of oxygen-adapted rats: a morphometric analysis. *Lab. Invest.* 39: 640–653, 1978.

15. Davies, G., and L. Reid. Growth of the alveoli and pulmonary arteries in childhood. *Thorax* 25: 669–681, 1970.

16. Davies, G. Lung damage, hypoplasia and right ventricular hypertrophy in cystic fibrosis. In: *Proceedings of the Fifth International Cystic Fibrosis Conference, Churchill College, Cambridge, 1969,* edited by D. Lawson. London: Cystic Fibrosis Research Trust, 1969, p. 350–360.

17. Davies, P., and L. Reid. Pulmonary veno-occlusive disease in siblings: case reports and morphometric study. *Hum. Pathol.* 13: 911–915, 1982.

18. Davies, P., F. Maddalo, and L. Reid. The response of microvessels in rat lung ex-plants to incubation with norepinephrine. *Exp. Lung Res.* 7: 93–100, 1984.

19. Davies, P., F. Maddalo, and L. Reid. Effect of chronic hypoxia on structure and reactivity of rat lung microvessels. *J. Appl. Physiol.* 58: 795–801, 1985.

20. Davies, P., G. Burke, and L. Reid. The structure of the wall of the rat intraacinar pulmonary artery: an electron microscopic study of microdissected preparations. *Microvasc. Res.* 32: 50–63, 1986.

21. Davies, P., B. T. Smith, F. B. Maddalo, D. Langleben, D. Tobias, K. Fujiwara, and L. Reid. Characteristics of lung pericytes in culture including their growth inhibition by endothelial substrate. *Microvasc. Res.* 33: 300–314, 1987.

22. Davies, P., R. Jones, B, Schloo, and L. Reid. Endothelium of the pulmonary vasculature in health and disease. In: *Pulmonary Endothelium in Health and Disease,* edited by U. S. Ryan. In: *Lung Biology in Health and Disease,* edited by C. Lenfant. New York: Marcel Dekker, 1987, vol. 32, p. 375–445.

23. deMello, D. and L. M. Reid. Arteries and veins. In: *The Lung. Scientific Foundations,* edited by R. G. Crystal and J. B. West. New York: Raven, 1991, vol. 1, p. 767–777.

24. deMello, D. E., J. D. Murphy, M. J. Aronovitz, P. Davies, and L. Reid. Effects of indomethacin *in utero* on the pulmonary vasculature of the newborn guinea pig. *Pediatr. Res.* 22: 693–697, 1987.

25. deMello, D. E., P. Davies, and L. M. Reid. Lung growth and development. In: *Current Pulmonology,* edited by D. Simmons. Chicago: Year Book Medical Publishers, 1989, vol. 10, p. 159–208.

26. Dunnill, M. A. Quantitative methods in the study of pulmonary pathology. *Thorax* 17: 320–328, 1962.

27. Dunnill, M. S. Postnatal growth of the lung. *Thorax* 17: 329–333, 1962.

28. Elliott, F. M. The pulmonary artery system in normal and diseased lungs—structure in relation to pattern of branching (Dissertation). London University, 1964.

29. Elliott, F. M., and L. Reid. Some new facts about the pulmonary artery and its branching pattern. *Clin. Radiol.* 16: 193–198, 1965.

30. Emery, J. L., and A. Mithal. The number of alveoli in the terminal respiratory unit of man during late intrauterine life and childhood. *Arch. Dis. Child* 35: 544–547, 1960.

31. Fernie, J. M., and D. Lamb. A new method for measuring intimal component of pulmonary arteries. *J. Clin. Pathol.* 38: 1374–1379, 1985.

32. Ferni, J. M., and D. Lamb. A new method for quantitating the medial component of pulmonary arteries: the measurements. *Arch. Pathol. Lab. Med.* 109: 156–162, 1985.

33. Fox, W. W., M. H. Gewitz, R. Dinwiddie, W. H. Drummond, and G. J. Peckham. Pulmonary hypertension in the perinatal aspiration syndromes. *Pediatrics* 59: 205–211, 1977.

34. Fried, R., B. Meyrick, M. Rabinovitch, and L. Reid. Polycythemia and the acute hypoxic response in awake rats following chronic hypoxia. *J. Appl. Physiol.* 55: 1167–1172, 1983.

35. Fried, R., and L. Reid. Early recovery from hypoxic pulmonary hypertension: a structural and functional study. *J. Appl. Physiol.* 57: 1247–1253, 1984.

36. Fried, R., and L. Reid. The effect of isoproterenol on the development and recovery of hypoxic pulmonary hypertension: a structural and hemodynamic study. *Am. J. Pathol.* 121: 102–111. 1985.

37. Geggel, R., A. Dozor, D. Fyler, and L. Reid. The effect of vasodilators at rest and during exercise in young adults with cystic fibrosis and chronic cor pulmonale. *Am. Rev. Respir. Dis.* 131: 531–536, 1985.

38. Groves, B. N., J. T. Reeves, J. R. Sutton, P. D. Wagner, A. Cymerman, M. K. Malconian, P. B. Rock, P. M. Young, and C. S. Houston. Operation Everest II: elevated high-altitude pulmonary resistance unresponsive to oxygen. *J. Appl. Physiol* 63: 521–530, 1987.

39. Hatano, S., T. Strasser (Editors). *Primary Pulmonary Hypertension: Report on a WHO Meeting.* Geneva; World Health Organization, 1975.

40. Haworth, S. G., and L. Reid. Persistent fetal circulation: newly recognized structural features. *J. Pediatr.* 88: 614–620, 1976.

41. Haworth, S. G., and L. Reid. Structural study of pulmonary circulation and of heart in total anomalous pulmonary venous return in early infancy. *Br. Heart J.* 39: 80–92, 1977.

42. Haworth, S. G., and L. Reid. Quantitative structural study of pulmonary circulation in the newborn with aortic atresia, stenosis or coarctation. *Thorax* 32: 121–128, 1977.

43. Haworth, S. G., and L. M. Reid. Quantitative structural study of pulmonary circulation in the newborn with pulmonary atresia. *Thorax* 32: 129–133, 1977.

44. Haworth, S. G., U. Sauer, K. Buhlmeyer, and L. Reid. Development of the pulmonary circulation in ventricular septal defect: a quantitative structural study. *Am. J. Cardiol.* 40: 781–788, 1977.

45. Hayward, J., and L. Reid. Observations on the anatomy of the intrasegmental bronchial tree. *Thorax* 7: 89–97, 1952.

46. Hayward, J., and L. Reid. The cartilage of the intrapulmonary bronchi in normal lungs, in bronchiectasis, and in massive collapse. *Thorax* 7: 98–110, 1952.

47. Heath, D., and J. E. Edwards. The pathology of hypertensive pulmonary vascular disease: a description of six grades of structural changes in the pulmonary arteries with special reference to congenital cardiac septal defects. *Circulation* 18: 533–547, 1958.

48. Hislop, A., S. G. Haworth, E. A. Shinebourne, and L. Reid. Quantitative structural analysis of pulmonary vessels in isolated ventricular septal defect in infancy. *Br. Heart J.* 37: 1014–1021, 1975.

49. Hislop, A. The non-muscular phase of the pulmonary circulation in the child. In: *Proceedings of the Fifth International Cystic Fibrosis Conference, Churchill College, Cambridge, 1969,* edited by D. Lawson. London: Cystic Fibrosis Research Trust, 1969, p. 340–349.

50. Hislop, A., and L. Reid. Pulmonary arterial development during childhood: branching pattern and structure. *Thorax* 28: 129–135, 1973.

51. Hislop, A., and L. Reid. Fetal and childhood development of the intrapulmonary veins in man—branching pattern and structure. *Thorax* 28: 313–319, 1973.

52. Hislop, A., and L. Reid. Development of the acinus in the human lung. *Thorax* 29: 90–94, 1974.

53. Hislop, A., and L. Reid. Arterial changes in Crotalaria spectabilis-induced pulmonary hypertension in rats. *Br. J. Exp. Path.* 55: 153–163, 1974.

54. Hislop, A., and L. Reid. Formation of the pulmonary vasculature. In: *Development of the Lung,* edited by W. A. Hodson. In: *Lung Biology in Health and Disease,* edited by C. Lenfant. New York: Marcel Dekker, 1977, vol. 6, p. 37–86.

55. Hislop, A., E. Hey, and L. Reid. The lungs in congenital bilateral renal agenesis and

dysplasia. *Arch. Dis. Child* 54: 32–38, 1979.

56. Hislop, A., and L. Reid. New findings in pulmonary arteries of rats with hypoxia-induced pulmonary hypertension. *Br. J. Exp. Pathol.* 57: 542–554, 1976.

57. Hislop, A., and L. Reid. The similarity of the pulmonary artery branching system in siblings. *Forensic Sci.* 2: 37–52, 1973.

58. Hislop, A., and L. Reid. Growth and development of the respiratory system: Anatomical development. In: *Scientific Foundation of Paediatrics.* 2nd ed. edited by J. A. Davis and J. Dobbing, London: Heinemann Medical Publications, 1981, p. 390–431.

59. Hu, L-M., and R. Jones. Injury and remodeling of distal pulmonary veins by high oxygen––a morphometric study. *Am. J. Pathol.* 134: 253–262, 1989.

60. Hu, L-M., R. Geggel, P. Davies, and L. Reid. The effect of heparin on the haemodynamic and structural response in the rat to acute and chronic hypoxia. *Brit. J. Exp. Pathol.* 70: 113–124, 1989.

61. Jones, R., W. M. Zapol, and L. Reid. Pulmonary arterial wall injury and remodelling by hyperoxia. *Chest* 83: 40S–42S, 1983.

62. Jones, R., W. M. Zapol, and L. Reid. Pulmonary artery remodeling and pulmonary hypertension after exposure to hyperoxia for 7 days: a morphometric and hemodynamic study. *Am. J. Pathol.* 117: 273–285, 1984.

63. Jones, R., W. M. Zapol, and L. Reid. Oxygen toxicity and restructuring of pulmonary arteries—a morphometric study: the response to 4 weeks' exposure to hyperoxia and return to breathing air. *Am. J. Pathol.* 121: 212–223, 1985.

64. Jones, R., Y. Yang, S. deMarinis, and A. Carvalho. Release of tissue plasminogen activator inhibitor and eiscosanoids by cultured endothelial cells and pericytes from rat pulmonary microvessels and pulmonary artery smooth muscle cells. *Am. Rev. Respir. Dis.* 135: 100A, 1987.

65. Jones, R. Ultrastructural analysis of contractile cell development in hyperoxic pulmonary hypertension: fibroblasts and intermediate cells selectively reorganize non-muscular segments. *Am. J. Pathol.* 141: 491–1505, 1992.

66. Jones, R., O. Kirton, W. M. Zapol, and L. Reid. Rat pulmonary artery wall injury by chronic intermittent infusions of Escherichia coli endotoxin: obliterative vasculitis and vascular occlusion. *Lab. Invest.* 54: 282–294, 1986.

67. Jones, R., W. M. Zapol, J. F. Tomashefski, Jr., O. C. Kirton, K. Kobayashi, and L. M. Reid. Pulmonary vascular pathology: human and experimental studies. In: *Acute Respiratory Failure,* edited by W. M. Zapol and K. J. Falke. In: *Lung Biology in Health and Disease,* edited by C. Lenfant. New York: Marcel Dekker, 1985, vol. 24, p. 23–160.

68. Jones, R. Ultrastructural analysis of contractile cell development in lung microvessels in hypertensive pulmonary hypertension: fibroblast and intermediate cell selectively reorganize non-muscular segments. *Am. J. Pathol.* 141: 6, 1992.

69. Karlish, A. J., R. Marshall, L. Reid, and S. Sherlock. Cyanosis with hepatic cirrhosis: a case with pulmonary arteriovenous shunting. *Thorax* 22: 555–561, 1967.

70. Kuhn, T. S. The Structure of Scientific Revolutions. 2nd ed. Chicago: University of Chicago Press, 1970.

71. Langleben, D., R. Jones, M. Aronovitz, N. Hill, L-C. Ou, and L. Reid. Pulmonary artery structural changes in two colonies of rats with different sensitivity to chronic hypoxia. *Am. J. Pathol.* 128: 61–66, 1987.

72. Langleben, D., J. L. Szarek, J. T. Coflesky, R. Jones, L. M. Reid, and J. N. Evans. Altered artery mechanics and structure in monocrotaline pulmonary hypertension. *J. Appl. Physiol.* 65: 2326–2331, 1988.

73. Langleben, D., R. B. Fox, R. C. Jones, and L. M. Reid. Effects of dimethlythiourea on chronic hypoxia-induced pulmonary arterial remodelling and ventricular hypertrophy in rats. *Clin. Invest. Med.* 12(4): 235–240, 1989.

74. Livingstone, J.L., J. G. Lewis, L. Reid, and K. E. Jefferson. Diffuse interstitial pulmonary fibrosis: a clinical, radiological and pathological study based on 45 patients. *O. J. Med.* 33: 71–103, 1964.

75. Meyrick, B., S. W., Clarke, C. Symons, D. J. Woodgate, and L. Reid. Primary pulmonary hypertension: a case report including electron microscopic study. *Br. J. Dis. Chest* 68: 11–20, 1974.

76. Meyrick, B., J. Miller, and L. Reid. Pulmonary oedema induced by ANTU, or by high or low oxygen concentrations in rat—an electron microscopic study. *Br. J. Exp. Pathol.* 53: 347–358, 1972.

77. Meyrick, B., and L. Reid. Development of pulmonary arterial changes in rats fed with Crotalaria spectabilis. *Am. J. Pathol.* 94: 37–50, 1979.

78. Meyrick, B., and L. Reid. The effect of continued hypoxia on rat pulmonary arte-

rial circulation: an ultrastructural study. *Lab. Invest.* 38: 188–200, 1978.

79. Meyrick, B., and L. Reid. Hypoxia and incorporation of ³H-thymidine by cells of the rat pulmonary arteries and alveolar wall. *Am J. Pathol.* 96: 51–70, 1979.

80. Meyrick, B., and L. Reid. Ultrastructural features of the distended pulmonary arteries of the normal rat. *Anat. Rec.* 193: 71–97, 1979.

81. Meyrick, B., and L. Reid. Hypoxia-induced structural changes in the media and adventitia of rat hilar pulmonary artery, and their regression. *Am. J. Pathol.* 100: 151–178, 1980.

82. Meyrick, B., and L Reid. Normal postnatal development of the media of the rat hilar pulmonary artery and its remodeling by chronic hypoxia. *Lab. Invest.* 46: 505–514, 1982.

83. Murphy, J., M. Aronovitz, and L. Reid. Effects of chronic in utero hypoxia on the pulmonary vasculature of the newborn guinea pig. *Pediatr. Res.* 2: 292–295.

84. Murphy, J.D., M. Rabinovitch, J. D. Goldstein, and L. Reid. The structural basis of persistent pulmonary hypertension of the newborn infant. *J. Pediatr.* 98: 962–967, 1981.

85. Murphy, J. D., G. Vawter, and L. Reid. Pulmonary vascular disease in fatal meconium aspiration. *J. Pediatr.* 104: 758–762, 1984.

86. Ohar, J. A., K. S. Waller, D. E. deMello, and R. O. Webster. Platelet activating factor (PAF) induces progressive pulmonary hypertensive changes. *FASEB J.* 2a: 1579, 1988.

87. O'Neal, R. M., W. A. Thomas, and P. M. Hartroft. Media of small muscular pulmonary arteries in mitral stenosis. *Arch. Path.* 60: 267, 1955.

88. Rabinovitch, M., W. Gamble, A. S. Nadas, O. S. Miettinen, and L. Reid. Rat pulmonary circulation after chronic hypoxia: Hemodynamic and structural features. *Am. J. Physiol.* 236: H818–H827, 1979.

89. Rabinovitch, M., S. Haworth, A. Castaneda, A. Nadas, and L. Reid. Lung biopsy in congenital heart disease: a morphometric approach to pulmonary vascular disease. *Circulation* 58: 1107–1122, 1978.

90. Rabinovitch, M., S. Haworth, Z. Vance, G. Vawter, A. Castaneda, A. Nadas, and L. Reid. Early pulmonary vascular changes in congenital heart disease studied in biopsy tissue. *Hum. Pathol.* (Suppl.) 11: 499–509, 1980.

91. Rabinovitch, M., M. Konstam, W. Gamble, N. Papanicolaou, M. Aronovitz, S. Treves, and L. Reid. Changes in pulmonary blood flow affect vascular response to chronic hypoxia in rats. *Circ. Res.* 52: 432–441, 1983.

92. Reid, L., and G. Simon. Unilateral lung transradiancy. *Thorax* 17: 230–239, 1962.

93. Reid, L., and G. Simon. The role of alveolar hypoplasia in some types of emphysema. *Br. J. Dis. Chest* 58: 158–168, 1964.

94. Reid, L. The angiogram and pulmonary artery structure and branching (in the normal lung and with reference to disease). *Proc. Roy. Soc. Med.* 58: 681–684, 1965.

95. Reid, L., G. Simon, P. A. Zorab, and R. Seidelin. The development of unilateral hypertransradiancy of the lung. *Br. J. Dis. Chest* 61: 190–192, 1967.

96. Reid, L. The laws of lung development. In: *Proceedings of the Fifth International Cystic Fibrosis Conference, Churchill College, Cambridge, 1969,* edited by D. Lawson. London: Cystic Fibrosis Research Trust, 1969, p. 333–339.

97. Reid, L., and D. Ryland. The pulmonary circulation in cystic fibrosis. In: *Fundamental Problems of Cystic Fibrosis and Related Diseases,* edited by J. A. Mangos and R. G. Talamo. Miami: Symposia Specialists Medical Books, 1973, p. 195–208.

98. Reid, L. M. The lung: Its growth and remodeling in health and disease. B. D. Edward. Neuhauser Lecture. *AJR* 129: 777–788, 1977.

99. Reid, L. The pulmonary circulation: remodeling in growth and disease. The 1978 J. Burns Amberson Lecture. *Am. Rev. Respir. Dis.* 119: 531–546, 1979.

100. Reid, L., and B. Meyrick. Hypoxia and pulmonary vascular endothelium. In: *Metabolic Activities of the Lung.* Ciba Foundation Symposium, new series 78. Amsterdam: Excerpta Medica, 1980, 37–61.

101. Reid, L. *Structure and Function in Pulmonary Hypertension: New Perceptions.* Seventh Simon Rodbard Memorial Lecture. *Chest* 89: 279–288, 1986.

102. Reid, L., R. Fried, R. Geggel, and D. Langleben. Anatomy of pulmonary hypertensive states. In: *Abnormal Pulmonary Circulation.* In: *Contemporary Issues in Pulmonary Disease,* edited by N. S. Cherniak and N. H. Edelman. New York: Churchill Livingstone, 1986, vol. 4, p. 221–263.

103. Reid, L. M. Overview. The Third Grover Conference on the Pulmonary Circulation: The control of cellular proliferation in the pulmonary circulation. *Am. Rev. Respir. Dis.* 140: 1490–1493, 1989.

104. Reid, L. M., and P. Davies. Control of cell proliferation in pulmonary hypertension. In: *Pulmonary Vascular Physiology and Pathophysiology,* edited by E. K. Weir and J. T. Reeves. In: *Lung Biology in Health and Disease,* edited by C. Lenfant. New York: Marcel Dekker, 1989, vol. 38, p. 541–611.

105. Reid, L. Vascular remodeling. In: *The Pulmonary Circulation Normal and Abnormal: Mechanisms, Management, and the National Registry,* edited by A. P. Fishman. Philadelphia: University of Pennsylvania Press. 1990, p. 259–282.

106. Reid, L. Pathological changes in the lungs in scoliosis. In: *Scoliosis,* edited by P. A. Zorab. Springfield, IL: Charles C. Thomas, 1969, p. 67–86.

107. Rendas, A., M. Branthwaite, S. Lennox, and L. Reid. Response of the pulmonary circulation to acute hypoxia in the growing pig. *J. Appl. Physiol.* 52: 811–814, 1982.

108. Rendas, A., M. Branthwaite, and L. Reid. Growth of the pulmonary circulation in the normal pig—structural analysis and cardiopulmonary function. *J. Appl. Physiol.* 45: 806–817, 1978.

109. Rendas, A., S. Lennox, and L. Reid. Aorta-pulmonary shunts in growing pigs: Functional and structural assessment of the changes in the pulmonary circulation. *J. Thorac. Cardiovasc. Surg.* 77: 109–118, 1979.

110. Rendas, A., and L. Reid. Pulmonary vasculature of piglets after correction of aorta-pulmonary shunts. *J. Thorac. Cardiovasc. Surg.* 85: 911–916, 1983.

111. Ryland, D., and L. Reid. The pulmonary circulation in cystic fibrosis *Thorax* 30: 285–292, 1975.

112. Semmens, M., and L. Reid. Pulmonary arterial muscularity and right ventricular hypertrophy in chronic bronchitis and emphysema. *Br. J. Dis. Chest* 68: 253–263, 1974.

113. Shelton, D. M., E. Keal, and L. Reid. The pulmonary circulation in chronic bronchitis and emphysema. Nineteenth Aspen Lung Conference. *Chest* 71: 303S–306S, 1977.

114. Short, D. S. Post-mortem pulmonary arteriography with special reference to the study of pulmonary hypertension. *J. Fac. Radiol.* 8: 118–131. 1956.

115. Simon, G. *Principles of Chest X-ray Diagnosis.* 1st ed. London: Butterworths, 1956.

116. Weibel, E. R. *Morphometry of the Human Lung.* Berlin: Springer, 1963.

117. Williams, A., P. Trewby, R. Williams, and L. Reid. Structural alterations to the pulmonary circulation of fulminant hepatic failure. *Thorax* 34: 447–453, 1979.

118. Zapol, W. M., and K. J. Falke (Editors). *Acute Respiratory Failure.* In: *Lung Biology in Health and Disease,* edited by C. Lenfant. New York, Marcel Dekker, 1985.

# 6

# A Personal View of Neonatal Pulmonary Hypertension

**John T. Reeves, M.D.**

*Professor of Medicine and Pediatrics, Department of Medicine, University of Colorado Health Sciences Center, Denver, Colorado*

. . in the embryo . . . the two ventricles . . . as in a double nut . . . are nearly equal in all respects . . . And this is so, because in the fetus . . . blood . . . flows by the foramen ovale and ductus arteriosus directly from the vena cava into the aorta, whence it is distributed to the whole body. Both ventricles have therefore the same office to perform, whence their equality of constitution. It is only when the lungs are used, and it is requisite that the passages indicated should be blocked up, that the difference . . . of strength . . . between the two ventricles begins to be apparent. In the altered circumstances, the right has only to drive the blood through the lungs, whilst the left has to propel it through the whole body.
—William Harvey, 1628[21]

Life takes unexpected turns. When I came to Denver in June 1957 to learn clinical cardiology from Gil Blount, my plan had been to spend one year at the University of Colorado and then return to my home in Hazard, Kentucky, to take up the practice of medicine. However, one reason I began a fellowship was to see what research might be like. I had always liked science, and my B.S. degree in biology from MIT had reflected a heavily scientific curriculum. In view of that back-

From: Wagner WW, Jr, Weir EK (eds): *The Pulmonary Circulation and Gas Exchange.* ©1994, Futura Publishing Co Inc, Armonk, NY.

ground, Gil assigned me to the cardiac catheterization laboratory rather than to the clinical cardiology service. The assignment meant that I would work under the direction of Bob Grover, the newly appointed head of the laboratory. Out of the opportunity to work with Bob grew an enduring friendship, and the excitement of the laboratory changed the direction of my life. I would no longer pursue my plan of returning to the Appalachian region of Kentucky to practice internal medicine and cardiology.

Gil's practice included infants and children. One of the first catheterizations in which I participated was in J. J., a 14-month-old child with ventricular septal defect and pulmonary hypertension. Bob had been finding that tolazoline (an imidazoline with sympatholytic, parasympathomimetic, and histaminelike actions) lowered pulmonary arterial pressure and caused pulmonary vasodilation in young children and some infants such as J. J.[19] (Fig. 1). It was known that pulmonary arterial pressure could be lowered by a pharmacologic agent,[15,18] but studies like

those in J. J. seemed important because they were showing for the first time that vasoconstriction contributed to pulmonary hypertension in congenital heart disease.

Our excitement was tempered by findings from sea level that tolazoline was ineffective in pulmonary hypertensive children with ventricular septal defects.[32] One possibility was that the lower barometric pressure ($P_B$, 630 mmHg) at Denver's altitude (1,600 m) was causing pulmonary vasoconstriction not present at sea level and that the tolazoline was reversing this constrictive component. The inspired oxygen tension in Denver is 122 mmHg compared to 150 mmHg at sea level. In infants with increased lung blood flows, the lower oxygen levels could cause the small pulmonary arteries to constrict.

A decade earlier, U. S. von Euler (Fig. 2) had shown that hypoxia caused pulmonary vasoconstriction in adult cats (Fig. 3). The discussion section in his paper addressed the question of the "purpose" of a pulmonary vasoconstriction by low oxygen. Those who are afraid it is not appro-

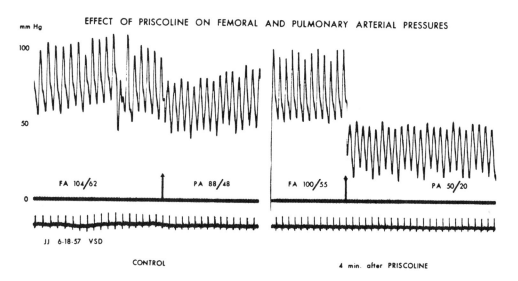

**Figure 1.** Femoral and pulmonary arterial pressures before (CONTROL) and 4 min after tolazoline (PRISCOLINE), from J. J., a 14-month-old infant with ventricular septal defect and pulmonary hypertension. At the arrow, pressure was switched from femoral to pulmonary artery. (Reproduced with permission from reference 19.)

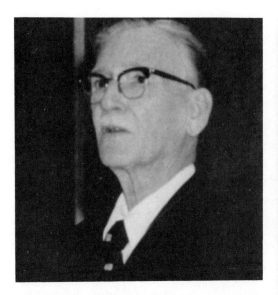

**Figure 2.** U. S. von Euler approximately 6 months before his death. Although this celebrated scientist had discovered and named the slow-reacting substance of anaphylaxis (later identified as leukotriene), discovered and named prostaglandin, and received the Nobel prize for his work on the sympathetics, this lecture given in Denver, at the invitation of Wiltz Wagner, was the only one he ever gave on hypoxic pulmonary hypertension.

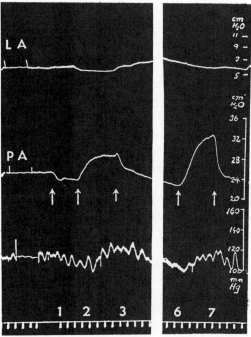

**Figure 3.** A portion of the original pressure tracing of hypoxic pulmonary vasoconstriction. From above downward are left atrial (LA), pulmonary arterial (PA), and systemic arterial pressure. Pressure scales are shown at the right. Time marks are at 30-s intervals. Arrows indicate a switch: 1. from air to oxygen; 2. from oxygen to 6.5% carbon dioxide in oxygen; 3. back to oxygen; 6. from oxygen to 10.5% oxygen in nitrogen; 7. back to oxygen. Interventions no. 4 and no. 5 are not shown. (Reproduced with permission from reference 17.)

priate to discuss purpose in scientific papers might take heart from his original article[17]:

> *It is required . . . that the blood becomes distributed to the different parts of the lung in such a way, that the alveolar air will give off oxygen and take up carbon dioxide fairly evenly throughout the lungs. . . . If the blood flow becomes inadequate in relation to the ventilation in some parts of the lungs, the corresponding alveolar air will become richer in oxygen and poorer in carbon dioxide than the rest of the lungs. But this will lead to a dilatation of the blood vessels in that part of the lung with a redistribution of the blood as a consequence. It is interesting to note that oxygen want and carbon dioxide ac-*

> *cumulation have exactly the reverse local effects on the vessels of the systemic and pulmonary circulations respectively; in both cases, however, they seem to be adapted for their special purposes.*

As appealing as von Euler's suggestion might be, local matching of ventilation to perfusion within the air-breathing lung does not explain the function of hypoxia in the fetal lung. There a somewhat different function must be served, because intrapulmonary ventilation-perfusion relationships are irrelevant to gas exchange when the lung is filled with fluid. Rather, it seems that pulmonary vasoconstriction in the fetal lung is a part of a bodywide strategy to maintain flow to the placenta, the fetal organ of oxygenation. As is now clear, hypoxic pulmonary vasoconstriction is well developed in the fetal lung.[6,7,10] The greater pulmonary vasoconstrictor responses in young animals compared to older animals[8,22] suggested "that the relatively weak hypoxic pulmonary pressor response seen in the adult mammal may be a remnant of a mechanism which existed in utero."[29] If so, it is important to consider the control of the fetal lung circulation.

Two classical series of studies relating to the lung circulation of fetal sheep had been done at the Nuffield Institute of Medical Research in Oxford, England. The institute was housed in a building designed as an astronomical observatory by Wyatt and Keene, two famous eighteenth-century architects who based their design on the Temple of the Winds at Athens (Fig. 4). With the introduction of gas lighting in an adjacent street, the telescopes were moved to South Africa. Supported by a generous grant from Lord Nuffield in the twentieth century, the building came to house the Nuffield Institute and be used for medical research. There, with collaboration between Oxford and Cambridge scientists, the foundation was laid for our modern understanding of the fetal circulation.

Since the late 1920s, Barcroft at Cambridge had sought to establish the true course of fetal blood flow, attempting thereby to bring order to the unbelievable welter of preexisting theories. Relative to the lung circulation, it was necessary to confirm that the two ventricles in utero really were "a double nut," "with the same office to perform," and were therefore pumping blood in parallel. Historical

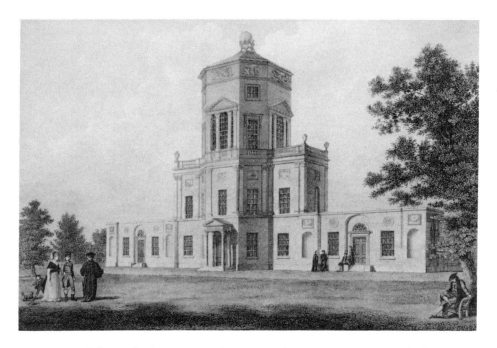

**Figure 4.** A lithograph from 1794 of Wyatt and Keene's astronomical observatory designed after the Temple of the Winds in Athens. Subsequently the building housed the Nuffield Institute for Medical Research. It included Barclay's radiographic laboratory in the 1930s and Dawes's laboratory from 1948 to 1970. (Courtesy of G. S. Dawes.)

review has indicated the inadequacies of earlier approaches[3,10] Barcroft enlisted the help of Barclay and Franklin from Oxford. Dawes (personal communication) recalled the circumstances:

*Barclay was a radiologist who was retired but was interested in the technology of X-ray cinematography for a variety of purposes. He joined up with Dr. K. J. Franklin, a fellow of Oriel College and tutor in Physiology who had moved with Professor Gunn (my predecessor) from the Department of Pharmacology to apply this new technology in the study of the venous circulation. The story that I was told was that Barcroft had an engagement in Oxford and happened to travel down from London in the same compartment of the train as K. J. Franklin after Franklin had just given an illustrated communication of the application of X-ray cinematography to the study of the venous system of experimental animals and it was, of course, Barcroft's idea to apply this technique to the fetal lamb.*

Possibly, the first cardiac cinematography ever performed was done to examine the fetal circulation in the lamb.[3,4] The result was that superior caval blood was seen to flow primarily into the right ventricle, the pulmonary artery, and through the ductus to the descending aorta (Fig. 5). The inferior caval blood was seen to flow primarily into the left atrium, left ventricle, and out the ascending aorta (Figs. 6A and 6B). Because the two ventricles both pumped blood directly into the aorta, they

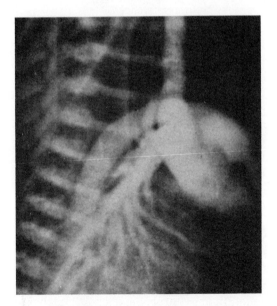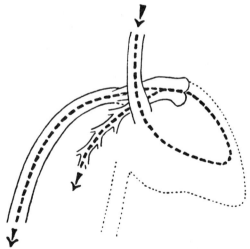

**Figure 5.** One frame from a series of rapid-sequence radiographs following injection of radiopaque contrast into the superior vena cava of a mature fetal lamb with an intact umbilical circulation. On the left is a reproduction of the actual radiograph. On the right is the author's interpretation of the path of the contrast from the superior vena cava, through the right heart, resulting in nearly simultaneously filling of the pulmonary arteries and the descending aorta. The path from the pulmonary artery to the descending aorta, not shown in this radiograph, was demonstrated in other studies. Note absence of opacification of the ascending aorta and the arteries supplying the head. (Reproduced with permission from reference 3.)

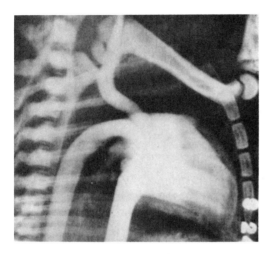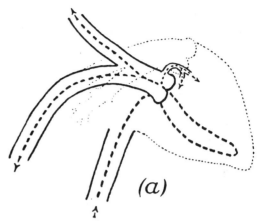

**Figure 6.** One frame from a series of rapid-sequence radiographs following injection of radiopaque contrast into the inferior vena cava of a mature fetal lamb with an intact umbilical circulation. On the left is a reproduction of the actual radiograph. From above downward are the densely opacified brachiocephalic artery to the head, the ascending and descending aorta, and the inferior vena cava. Barely seen is faint opacification of the pulmonary artery. On the right is the author's interpretation of the path of the contrast from the inferior vena cava, through the left heart, resulting in filling of the ascending aorta and the brachio-cephalic artery. Note position of the main pulmonary artery is shown by the broken lines. (Reproduced with permission from reference 3.)

could be considered to be in parallel and to develop similar pressures, consistent with Harvey's views.

However, these superb radiographs of functional anatomy did not reveal the pressures in the ventricles, the magnitude of pulmonary blood flow, or the changes in pressures and flows at birth. Direct measurements of pressure and flow were required, and Oxford's Temple of the Winds was again the setting for ground-breaking medical research. In 1948, Geoffrey Dawes (Fig. 7) became director of the Nuffield Institute. He developed into a high art the study of the living, exterior-ized fetus. His measurements in lambs showed that fetal pulmonary arterial pressure was as high, or higher, than that in the fetal aorta (Fig. 8), confirming the similar-ity of the pressures in the two great arter-ies. Pulmonary arterial pressure fell on ventilating the lung with air, but the aortic pressure did not, indicating relative pul-monary hypertension in the fetus. Occlu-sion of the ductus caused pulmonary arte-

rial pressure to fall further, while aortic pressure rose (Fig. 8), demonstrating that blood now flowed from aorta to pulmo-nary artery. These concepts have been repeatedly confirmed in laboratories around the world using sophisticated in vivo recording techniques. Thus, within the space of a few years, measurements in Dawes's laboratory had cleared the fog of uncertainty that for centuries had clouded the fetal circulation.

A further series of experiments, done with impeccable measurements of pres-sure and flow, showed the several factors that contributed to the high fetal resis-tance and its decrease at birth.[13] Gaseous inflation of the lung, the decrease in alveo-lar carbon dioxide and the increase in alveolar oxygen all occur with the first breath, and all were found to play a role in decreasing resistance to blood flow (Fig. 9). In addition, in the fetus, high sympa-thetic tone contributed to the high pulmo-nary vascular resistance. Hypoxia in-creased pulmonary arterial pressure in the

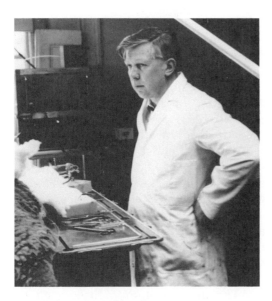

**Figure 7.** Photograph of Professor G. S. Dawes taken in 1968 during an experiment on the fetal lamb in his Nuffield Institute laboratory in the Oxford Temple of the Winds.

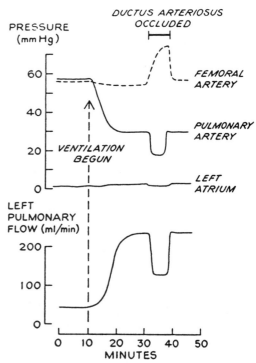

**Figure 8.** Schematic pulmonary arterial, femoral arterial, and left atrial pressures, top, and left pulmonary arterial flow, bottom, in the exteriorized mature fetus with an intact placental circulation. Before the onset of ventilation, mean pulmonary arterial pressure is slightly higher than that in the femoral artery, and left pulmonary arterial flow is low. Following the onset of ventilation, pulmonary arterial pressure falls, but not that in the femoral artery or left atrium. Pulmonary flow rises. Occlusion of the ductus arteriosus is accompanied by a sharp rise in femoral arterial pressure and falls in pulmonary arterial and left atrial pressure and in pulmonary arterial flow. (Reproduced with permission from reference 10.)

isolated, perfused fetal lung, indicating the pressor response was inherent within the lung itself. While mechanical (a collapsed and fluid-filled lung) and neural (high sympathetic tone) factors contributed to the high vascular resistance in the fetal lung, chemical factors (high carbon dioxide, low oxygen) were clearly important. Multiple mechanisms often operate to preserve a vital function, as, for example, in maintenance of systemic arterial pressure in the adult. In the fetus, the normally low fetal oxygen tension, assisted by other factors, maintains high pulmonary arterial pressure and resistance in the collapsed, water-filled lung.

The high lung vascular resistance, in turn, may be important for the maintenance of fetal oxygenation. If the low fetal oxygen levels maintain constriction in certain vascular beds such as the lung, blood flow is directed toward the relatively passive placental bed, which is not constricted by hypoxia. The distribution of blood flow is not only important for normal development of the fetus, but may

also become essential in times of hypoxic stress, because cardiac output in the fetus is relatively fixed[14] and placental flow is determined by arterial pressure.[5] To raise pressure, redistribution of flow away from less essential organs must occur. Thus, hypoxia markedly constricts the femoral arterial bed, and the effect is abolished by denervation of the aortic chemoreceptors (Fig. 10). Apparently during the latter part of gestation the maintenance of high resis-

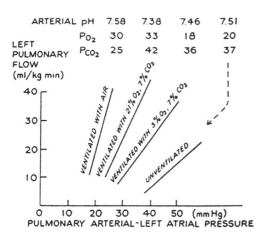

**Figure 9.** Pulmonary arterial pressure-flow curves redrawn from tracings obtained in a mature fetal lamb with intact placental circulation. Systemic arterial blood gases in this fetus are indicated above for the various interventions. With pulmonary ventilation using a gas designed not to change the fetal oxygen and carbon dioxide tensions, the lung vascular bed vasodilates, i.e., the curve shifts to the left. Upon ventilation with a mixture higher in oxygen but with no decrease in fetal alveolar oxygen there is further dilation. When the fetus was ventilated with air (high oxygen and no carbon dioxide), there is still more pulmonary vasodilation. (Reproduced with permission from reference 10.)

tance in the femoral arterial bed depends on hypoxia-mediated activity from the aortic[11] and, to a lesser extent, carotid chemoreceptors.[12] Hypoxia acts directly to constrict flow to the lung and acts via the nervous system to constrict flow to the lower body. In both instances the net result is increased arterial pressure, which should increase flow to the placenta and facilitate oxygen transport to the fetus. Therefore, in the fetus,

> *"as in the adult, blood flow is redistributed to maintain the circulation through the heart, brain and organs of gas exchange at the expense of blood supply to those tissues which are, in the short term, more expendable."*[10]

In 1967 and 1968, I had the opportunity to work on some of these studies, with Dawes, in the Nuffield Institute, then housed in the Temple of the Winds.

It is possible that the hypoxic vasoconstriction of the lung arteries evolved primarily as a mechanism for fetal survival. If so, a powerful mechanism in the fetus might persist after birth and be stronger in the newborn period than in the adult. Our findings in the young calf suggested that such might be the case (Fig. 11). Perhaps the hypoxia of Colorado's altitude constricted the lung arteries in our young patients with ventricular septal defect. Such constriction could be relieved by a vasodilating drug.

The unique features of the lung circu-

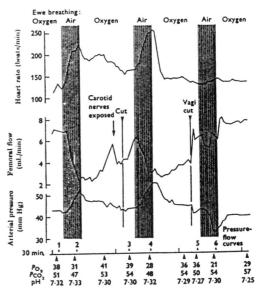

**Figure 10.** Heart rate, femoral flow, and systemic arterial pressure in a mature fetal lamb with an intact placental circulation. The shaded areas indicate the times the ewe is breathing air, as indicated along the top of the figure. The fetal arterial blood-gas tensions and pH are indicated along the abscissa. Time marks are at 30-min intervals. In the fetal lamb, carotid body denervation follows cutting of the carotid nerves, and aortic body denervation follows cutting of the vagi. (Reproduced with permission from reference 11.)

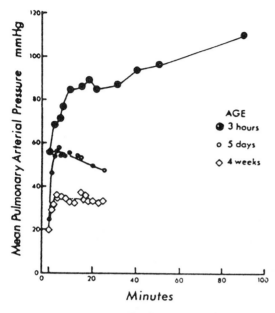

**Figure 11.** Mean pulmonary arterial pressure during hypoxia is greater in a calf 3 hours after birth than at 4 weeks of age. Intermediate pressures were observed at 5 days of age. (Reproduced with permission from reference 29.)

lation around the time of birth are underscored by the occasionally turbulent transition from fetal life to air breathing. At birth, the lungs must expand with air, the lung arteries must relax for pulmonary arterial pressure to fall, the blood must flow to well-oxygenated alveoli, and all of this must occur within minutes. In approximately 1 of 1,500 live human births, the transition is faulty and neonatal pulmonary hypertension results. The cause is unknown, but precipitating factors often considered are high pulmonary vascular resistance in utero (premature ductal constriction), asphyxia or meconium aspiration during birth, or noxious stimuli in the newborn period (hypoxia, infection). For those newborns not responding to tracheal intubation and hyperventilation with high oxygen mixtures, treatment involves expensive, risky heart-lung bypass for several days. Even so, mortality approaches 20%.

In the early 1980s Kurt Stenmark, a pediatric pulmonary critical care specialist, asked us if we could develop an animal model of severe pulmonary hypertension in the newborn period. He wished to replicate certain features of the human disease, including pulmonary arterial pressure at or above systemic arterial levels, right to left intracardiac shunting, and severe hypoxemia. Also, the small pulmonary arteries should show remarkably thickened walls, particularly with adventitial proliferation, because such vessels are found in infants dying with neonatal pulmonary hypertension (Fig. 12A). The newborn's capacity to develop pulmonary hypertension, combined with the potential for rapid tissue growth, could produce life-threatening lung vessel thickening. We wondered whether severe hypoxia in the newborn calf could induce similar findings. The newborn calf was a convenient size for study, and previous work at Colorado State University in Fort Collins had indicated that the bovine species seemed susceptible to hypoxic pulmonary hypertension,[35] particularly when compared to other species.[31]

We had experience extending back many years with brisket disease of cattle, which is caused by pulmonary hypertension at high altitude. In the 1950s, Pierson and Jensen[25] with Alexander[1,2] and Will,[35] had reactivated the study of brisket disease at Colorado State University. In 1958 Grover and I joined forces with these scientists at Colorado State University in collaborative research that continues to this day. The first fruit of the collaboration was to show that cattle brought from Kansas to 10,000 feet in South Park, Colorado, developed severe pulmonary hypertension over a period of several months[35] compared to low-altitude cattle.[28] Two years later Bob Grover and I, with the help from his wife Estelle, constructed a corral (Fig. 13) and set it up at 12,700 feet on the summit flats of Mt. Evans, Colorado, for the study of cattle[20] and sheep.[27] Don Will joined us for that experiment, and my

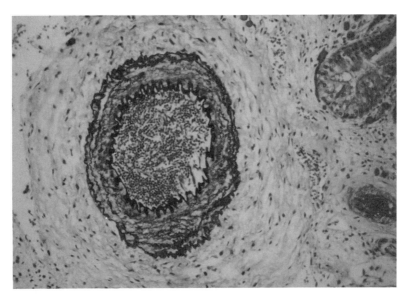

**Figure 12a.** Photomicrograph of a pulmonary arteriole from an infant dying at 5 days of age from neonatal pulmonary hypertension.

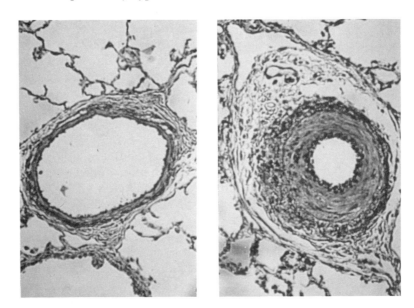

**Figure 12b, c.** Left: Photomicrograph of a pulmonary arteriole from a normal 2-week-old calf raised at 1,500 m. Right: Photomicrograph of a pulmonary arteriole from a 2-week-old calf that had been at 4,300 m altitude from birth.

wife, Carol, did the cooking for the research crew. Our infant daughter, Catherine, first learned to stand on Mt. Evans during our time there. Hard physical labor, intellectual activity, and collegial collaboration—all while having one's family around—must be one of the most satisfying combinations human beings can experience. And so it was for me in that summer of 1960 on Mt. Evans.

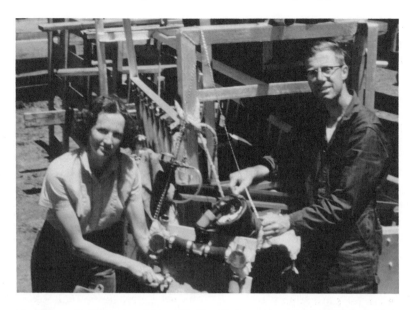

**Figure 13.** Robert F. Grover and his wife Estelle in 1960 at the corral that was set up at 12,700 feet on Mount Evans to study the effect of altitude on cattle and sheep.

A result of that research was that the magnitude of the pulmonary hypertension and the rate at which it developed was greater than what we had observed two years earlier at 10,000 ft in steers of the same age. Thus, the greater the stimulus, the greater the response. Later my study of newborn calves placed in an altitude chamber at 11,000 ft showed even more rapid development of pulmonary hypertension,[30] indicating the important contribution of young postnatal age to the response.

To create an animal model that replicated some of the features of human neonatal pulmonary hypertension, it seemed appropriate to extend our previous experience. Therefore, to accelerate further the development of pulmonary hypertension, we placed newborn calves at even higher altitudes, of 14,000 to 14,500 ft.[33] When we combined the results from all of these studies, it was clear that the rate and severity of the pulmonary hypertension increased with the severity of the hypoxia and with the youth of the cattle (Fig. 14). In particular, putting the day-old calf for 2

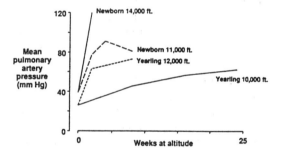

**Figure 14.** Mean pulmonary arterial pressures over time in cattle exposed to actual or simulated altitude. Pulmonary hypertension in yearling steers develops at a slower rate and with a lesser magnitude at 10,000 ft[35] than at 12,700 ft.[20] Newborn male calves more rapidly develop more severe pulmonary hypertension at 11,000 ft[30] than do yearling steers. The most severe and most rapid pulmonary hypertension was seen in newborns at 14,000 ft.[24,33]

weeks at 4,300 to 4,500 m, as reported by Kurt Stenmark[33,34] and Chris Orton,[24] resulted in suprasystemic pulmonary hypertension, right to left shunting through the foramen ovale and the ductus arteriosus, poor responses to vasodilators, and extreme thickness of the walls of small pulmonary arteries (Figs. 12B and C). Such findings resembled those in infants dying of neonatal pulmonary hypertension, suggesting that the newborn calf might be a good model for some aspects of the disease in humans.

Through this model, new insights have been gained into vascular wall biology, particularly by Kurt Stenmark, Norbert Voelkel, and our collaborators, which include the investigative team headed by Bob Mecham at Washington University in St. Louis.[16,23,26] Primary questions relate to the relative roles of hypoxia and elevated pressure in producing the vascular abnormalities in the calves and to the cells initiating the changes. The answers are sought in vivo, in vitro, and in isolated cellular systems. In vivo studies utilizing coarctation of pulmonary arterial branches in calves at high altitude suggest that the lower arterial pressure distal to the coarctation is associated with less vascular wall thickening. Also, pulmonary veins, which are hypoxic but have normal intraluminal pressures, remain normal. Culture of whole vessel rings under stretched and nonstretched conditions indicates greater mitotic activity in the stretched vessels. Although such studies do not rule out a role for hypoxia, they do emphasize that pressure per se plays a crucial role in the vascular changes accompanying neonatal pulmonary hypertension.

Although we do not know which cells initiate the wall thickening, we have been surprised at the activation of the adventitia in the hypertensive calves. Such activation occurs early and is of large magnitude. Using bromo-deoxy-uridine, Chris Orton has found greatly increased numbers of adventitial fibroblasts undergoing cell division in the hypertensive calves relative to the numbers of smooth muscle cells. In situ hybridization for RNA of matrix proteins, such as collagen I and fibronectin, also indicate much greater secretion from adventitial cells than from

the media in the fetus and in the hypertensive calves. Although there is intense activity in the adventitia, the media is not quiescent in hypertension. For example, in hypertension the normal regression of elastin gene expression is not confined to the inner third of the media but, rather, reverts to the fetal pattern that shows expression across the full thickness of the intralobar arterial wall. By combining physiological techniques with the cellular and molecular biological tools available today, insights not dreamed of a few decades ago may be gained into pulmonary circulatory control under normal and abnormal conditions.

The discoveries appear to proceed at an ever-increasing rate. Looking back over the long reach of history, if I can see more distant horizons, it is because "Dwarfs on the shoulders of giants see further than the giants themselves." The early Greek and Roman philosophers did the best they could with the tool they had at hand, namely, morbid anatomy. The great advance by Harvey combined a receptive mind with observations in the living ani-

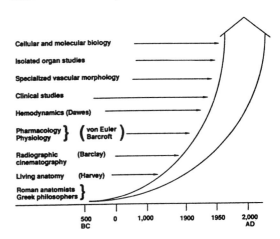

**Figure 15.** The evolution of understanding in neonatal pulmonary hypertension proceeds at an ever-increasing pace with the utilization of new techniques from different scientific disciplines.

mal. The modern era was ushered in by physiologists—von Euler, Barcroft, Barclay, and Dawes. Today we have available sophisticated tools of pathology, morphometric histology, cellular and molecular biology and a host of talented investigators who communicate constantly with each other. Each period in history has kept the best of the preceding period while adding advances of its own (Fig. 15). The understanding in the neonatal pulmonary circulation will grow at an ever-increasing rate as long as scientists continue collaborating within and across institutions, within and across disciplines, and within and across the centuries.

**Acknowledgments:** For the quote, I am indebted to S. Marsh Tenney, who wrote, *"The widely quoted, . . . 'on the shoulders of giants . . .' is most often attributed to Robert Burton, but it seems to have originated with Stella Didachus (16th C.)."* Pygmaeos gigantum humeris impositos plusquam ipsos gigantes videre. *(Dwarfs on the shoulders of giants see farther than the giants themselves.)*
*I think that this catchy observation has been repeated in various modified forms by many writers . . . —Marsh*

# References

1. Alexander, A. F., and R. Jensen. Gross cardiac changes in cattle with high mountain (Brisket) disease and in experimental cattle maintained at high altitudes. *Am. J. Vet. Res.* 20: 680, 1959.

2. Alexander, A. F., D. H. Will, R. F. Grover, and J. T. Reeves. Pulmonary hypertension and right ventricular hypertrophy in cattle at high altitude. *Am. J. Vet. Res.* 21: 199, 1960.

3. Barclay, A. E., J. Barcroft, D. H. Barron, and K. J. Franklin. A radiographic demonstration of the circulation through the heart in the adult and in the foetus, and the identification of the ductus arteriosus. *Br. J. Radiol.* 12: 505–517, 1939.

4. Barclay, A. E., K. J. Franklin, and M. M. L. Pritchard. *The Foetal Circulation.* Springfield, IL: Charles C. Thomas, 1945.

5. Born, G. V. R., G. S. Dawes, and J. C. Mott. Oxygen lack and autonomic nervous control of the foetal circulation of the lamb. *J. Physiol. (London)* 134: 149–166, 1956.

6. Cassin, S., G. S. Dawes, J. C. Mott, B. B. Ross, and L. B. Strang. The vascular resistance in the foetal and newly ventilated lung of the lamb. *J. Physiol. (London)* 171: 61–79, 1964.

7. Colebatch, H. J. H., G. S. Dawes, J. W. Goodwin, and R. A. Nadeau. The nervous control of the circulation in the foetal and newly expanded lungs of the lamb. *J. Physiol. (London)* 178: 544–562, 1965.

8. Dawes, G. S. Physiological effects of anoxia in the foetal and newborn lamb. *Lect. Sci. Basis Med.* 5: 53, 1955–56.

9. Dawes, G. S. Physiological changes in the circulation after birth. In: *Circulation of the Blood,* Men and Ideas, edited by A. P. Fishman and D. W. Richards. New York: Oxford University Press, 1964.

10. Dawes, G. S. *Foetal and Neonatal Physiology.* Chicago: Year Book Medical Publishers, 1968.

11. Dawes, G. S., S. L. B. Duncan, B. V. Lewis, C. L. Merlet, J. B. Owen-Thomas, and J. T. Reeves. Hypoxaemia and aortic chemoreceptor function in foetal lambs. *J. Physiol.* 210: 105–116, 1969.

12. Dawes, G. S., S. L. B. Duncan, B. V. Lewis, C. L. Merlet, J. B. Owen-Thomas, and J. T. Reeves. Cyanide stimulation of the systemic arterial chemoreceptors in foetal lambs. *J. Physiol. (London)* 210: 117–128, 1969.

13. Dawes, G. S., J. C. Mott, J. G. Widdicombe, and D. G. Wyatt. Changes in the lungs of the newborn lamb. *J. Physiol. (London)* 121: 141–162, 1953.

14. Downing, S. E., N. S. Talner, and T. H. Gardner. Ventricular function in the newborn lamb. *Am. J. Physiol.* 208: 931–937, 1965.

15. Dresdale, D. T., R. J. Michtom, and M. Schultz. Recent studies in primary pulmonary hypertension, including pharmacodynamic observations on pulmonary vascular resistance. *Bull. NY. Acad. Med.* 30: 195, 1954.

16. Durmowicz, A. G., D. B. Badesch, W. C. Parks, and K. R. Stenmark. Hypoxia induced inhibition of tropoelastin synthesis by neonatal calf pulmonary artery smooth muscle cells. *Am. J. Respir. Cell. Mol. Biol.* 5: 464–469, 1991.

17. Euler, U. S. von and G. Liljestrand. Observations on the pulmonary arterial blood pressure in the cat. *Acta Physiol. Scand.* 12: 301–320, 1947.

18. Gardiner, J. M. The effect of "Priscol" in

pulmonary hypertension. *Aust. Ann. Med.* 3: 59, 1954.

19. Grover, R. F., J. T. Reeves, and S. G. Blount, Jr. Tolazoline hydrochloride (Priscoline): An effective pulmonary vasodilator. *Am. Heart J.* 61: 5–15, 1961.

20. Grover, R. F., J. T. Reeves, D. H. Will, and S. G. Blount, Jr. Pulmonary vasoconstriction in steers at high altitude. *J. Appl. Physiol.* 18: 567–574, 1963.

21. Harvey, W. *On the Motion of the Heart and Blood in Animals.* [Willis's translation, revised and edited by A. Bowie.] London: George Bell and Sons, 1889, p. 82.

22. James, L. S., and R. D. Rowe. The pattern of response of pulmonary and systemic arterial pressures in newborn and older infants to short periods of hypoxia. *J. Pediatr.* 51: 5, 1957.

23. Mecham, R. P., L. A. Whitehouse, D. S. Wrenn, W. C. Parks, G. L. Griffin, R. W. Senior, E. C. Crouch, K. R. Stenmark, and N. F. Voelkel. Smooth muscle-mediated connective tissue remodeling in pulmonary hypertension. *Science* 237: 423–426, 1987.

24. Orton, E. C., J. T. Reeves, and K. R. Stenmark. Pulmonary vasodilation with structurally altered pulmonary vessels and pulmonary hypertension. *J. Appl. Physiol.* 65: 2459–2467, 1988.

25. Pierson, R. E., and R. Jensen. Brisket Disease. In: *Diseases of Cattle.* Evanston, IL: American Veterinary, 1956.

26. Prosser, I. W., K. R. Stenmark, M. Suthar, E. C. Crouch, R. P. Mecham, and W. C. Parks. Regional heterogeneity of elastin and collagen gene expression in intralobar arteries in response to hypoxic pulmonary hypertension as demonstrated by in situ hybridization. *Am. J. Pathol.* 135: 1073–1088, 1989.

27. Reeves, J. T., E. B. Grover, and R. F. Grover. Pulmonary circulation and oxygen transport in lambs at high altitude. *J. Appl. Physiol.* 18: 560–566, 1963.

28. Reeves, J. T., R. F. Grover, D. H. Will, and A. F. Alexander. Hemodynamics in normal cattle. *Circ. Res.* 10: 166–171, 1962.

29. Reeves, J. T., and J. E. Leathers. Circulatory changes following birth of the calf and the effects of hypoxia. *Circ. Res.* 15: 343–354, 1964.

30. Reeves, J. T., and J. E. Leathers. Postnatal development of pulmonary and bronchial arterial circulations in the calf and the effects of chronic hypoxia. *Anat. Rec.* 157: 641–656, 1967.

31. Reeves, J. T., W. W. Wagner, I. F. McMurtry, and R. F. Grover. Physiological effects of high altitude on the pulmonary circulation. *Int Rev Physiol: Environ Physiol III* 20: 289–310, 1979.

32. Rudolph, A. M., M. H. Paul, L. S. Sommer, and A. S. Nadas. Effects of tolazoline hydrocholoride (Priscoline) on circulatory dynamics of patients with pulmonary hypertension. *Am. Heart J.* 55: 424, 1958.

33. Stenmark, K. R., J. Fasules, D. M. Hyde, N. F. Voelkel, J. Henson, A. Tucker, H. Wilson, and J. T. Reeves. Severe pulmonary hypertension and arterial adventitial changes in newborn calves at 4300 m. *J. Appl. Physiol.* 62: 821–830, 1987.

34. Stenmark, K. R., E. C. Orton, J. T. Reeves, N. F. Voelkel, E. C. Crouch, W. C. Parks, and R. P. Mecham. Vascular remodeling in neonatal pulmonary hypertension. *Chest* 93: 127–133, 1988.

35. Will, D. H., A. F. Alexander, J. T. Reeves, and R. F. Grover. High altitude-induced pulmonary hypertension in normal cattle. *Circ. Res.* 10: 172–177, 1962.

# 7

# Search for Diffusion Limitation in Pulmonary Gas Exchange

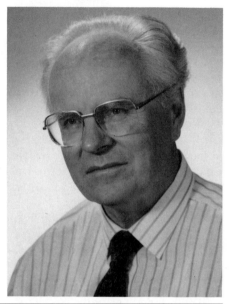

**Johannes Piiper, M.D.**

*Director, Department of Physiology, Max Planck Institute for Experimental Medicine, Göttingen, Germany*

I dedicate this chapter to the memory of those who introduced me to physiology and guided and promoted me through the years: Wolfgang Schoedel, long-time head of the Department of Physiology and my predecessor; Kurt Kramer, head of the Department of Physiology at Göttingen University (later at the University of Munich) and my academic promoter, whose enthusiasm for physiology inspired me; and Hermann Rahn, of Buffalo, New York, who was unsurpassed as a questor of things physiological.

## From Estonia to Germany, Through War and Peace

My father was born in a poor family in Tallinn, capital city of the Government of Estonia in the Russian Empire. With the support of well-off relatives, he was able to complete secondary school in Tallinn and study biological sciences at the University of St. Petersburg. He became professor of zoology at the University of Tartu when it reopened as an Estonian university in 1919, after Estonia had won its independence from czarist Russia after fighting both the Germans and the Red Army in the years following World War I.

I was born in 1924 and grew up in a free country during a peaceful time of economic growth and cultural development. All this came to an end with the establishment of Soviet military bases in Estonia in the fall of 1939 and the annexation of Estonia by the Soviet Union in the summer of 1940. After the onset of the

From: Wagner WW, Jr, Weir EK (eds): *The Pulmonary Circulation and Gas Exchange.* ©1994, Futura Publishing Co Inc, Armonk, NY.

German-Soviet war in June 1941, many Estonians were arrested and deported to northern Russia, and young Estonians were drafted into the Red Army. Being one year too young, I escaped the draft.

The German forces advanced quickly, but when they reached Tartu, they were halted for several weeks by the river that flowed through the city. During that time a large part of the city was destroyed by the fires resulting from artillery shelling and arson by Red partisans. In 1942 I graduated from secondary school in Tartu, after which I had to join the Luftwaffe, first as an auxiliary serviceman, but soon thereafter as a regular soldier stationed in Estonian territory.

As the German army retreated from the Baltic countries in September 1944, my unit was shipped across the Baltic to East Prussia. I was wounded on the outskirts of Königsberg, escaped from the encircled city on horse cart, and was taken on board a hospital ship to the port of Sassnitz on Rügen Island. There the less seriously wounded were immediately disembarked and taken on a hospital train. The severely wounded stayed on board the ship, which left the port and headed to the roadstead for safety, but it was hit by bombs dropped by Allied aircraft the following night and sank with all the severely wounded. My remarkable luck was that, though graded as severely wounded, I had been helped by lightly wounded German soldiers to the train, thereby escaping the shipwreck. During the following four days the hospital train traveled across the whole of war-torn Germany, from north to south. Finally we stopped near Garmisch-Partenkirchen in Bavaria and were put into an auxiliary hospital.

Soon after American forces occupied Bavaria, my wound had healed sufficiently, and I was taken to an American prisoner-of-war camp in Garmisch-Partenkirchen. Being Estonian, I could not be released due to lack of regulations, whereas Germans were continually discharged. But a fellow professor of my father had come as refugee to Göttingen and searched for me by advertising in a refugee newspaper, which was smuggled into the camp. Finally, by the end of 1946, I was discharged along with a number of Estonians, Latvians, and Lithuanians. The reason I went to Göttingen, where a large camp for Baltic refugees was located, was that I wanted to enter the university's medical school. This had been my parents' wish, and I never hesitated to comply with it, although I was attracted more by biology than medicine.

I had lost all my documents including school certificates, and it was utterly impossible to obtain substitutes from Estonia. All I could do was procure written declarations from two of my former teachers who had come as refugees to Germany. But the main reason I was accepted was the extraordinary considerateness of Göttingen University's counselor for foreign students, Dr. Wienert, who, after having heard my story, arranged my admission pending my passing an oral admission examination. Because of my long absence from school and my poor mastery of scientific German, this was the most difficult exam I have ever taken. My examiner in mathematics and physics was Professor Hans Loeschcke, the well-known respiratory physiologist. I remember one of the problems he gave me was determining the height of Egyptian pyramids using a yardstick but without climbing the structures (Luckily I had always been good in geometry.)

With much luck I had survived the war and was admitted to medical school, but I was alone. My parents and my sister remained in Estonia. I received some support from Estonian refugees, and I lodged clandestinely in a Displaced Persons' camp supported by refugee organizations. I could not obtain official permission to stay there, because of my military past. Later I was admitted to a student home supported by a Lutheran church organization. After finishing two and a half years of my preclinical studies, I applied for immigration to the United States but was denied because of my military involvement on the wrong side. About one year later I was requested to come to an emigration camp for a new interview, but then I was the one who declined, intending to finish medical school in Germany.

After passing the state medical examination I looked for a place to work and to prepare my medical doctor thesis. After some unsuccessful applications, I was introduced by Professor Loeschcke to Professor Schoedel, the director of the physiology laboratory of the research institute (later named the Max Planck Institute), where I was accepted in January 1953. An important asset was that I could get a fellowship, worth about 100 German marks a month, which at that time and in my circumstances was a good income. I never felt as rich since then. Today I am still working in that institute, and since 1973 I have served as director of the Department of Physiology.

## Steady-State Gas Exchange: Diffusion Limitation versus Ventilation/Perfusion Inequality and Shunt

In September 1958 I came to the United States to work for one year with Hermann Rahn in the Department of Physiology at the University of Buffalo, later called the State University of New York at Buffalo. The timing was awkward because my wife was expecting our first child, and I could not afford to take her to the United States. In Buffalo, I was introduced to the American way of life and to the analysis of pulmonary gas exchange by Pierre Haab, who had come to Rahn from the laboratory of Alfred Fleisch at Lausanne a year earlier. (An interesting coincidence is that Fleisch had invented the pneumotachograph as professor of physiology at

the Estonian University of Tartu). I was fortunate to find in Pierre Haab not only an indispensable coworker in Buffalo, but also a scientific companion and a friend for life.

I learned that the alveolar-arterial $P_{O_2}$ difference ($AaD_{O_2}$) was conventionally attributed to three mechanisms: ventilation-perfusion ($\dot{V}_A/\dot{Q}$) inequality, shunt, and diffusion limitation, which were not easily differentiated (Fig. 1). Hermann Rahn's idea was to demonstrate the effect of ventilation-perfusion inequality by an experiment that had a simple and straightforward design but could not be easily performed. According to Farhi and Rahn[10] the $AaD_{O_2}$ due to $\dot{V}_A/\dot{Q}$ inequality should be much reduced when $N_2$ is eliminated from inspired gas. This could be achieved by breathing 100% $O_2$ in a hypobaric chamber at a total pressure reduced to such a level that alveolar and arterial $P_{O_2}$ stayed normoxic, i.e., at a total pressure of about 197 Torr, equivalent to 10 km of altitude. The result of the exciting experiments we carried out, with all three of us (the experimental dog, Pierre Haab, and myself) confined in the hypobaric chamber for many hours, was unexpected and disappointing: the $AaD_{O_2}$ in anesthetized, artificially ventilated dogs remained unchanged after elimination of $N_2$ from inspired gas.[17] We considered several possible "loopholes" such as incomplete elimination of $N_2$, accelerated development of atelectatic shunt in the absence of $N_2$, and $\dot{V}_A/\dot{Q}$ inequality of a mainly alveolar dead space-like character (the $AaD_{O_2}$ due to alveolar dead space would be little affected by elimination of $N_2$). We also considered the possibility that the $AaD_{O_2}$ in dogs in our experimental conditions was not due to $\dot{V}_A/\dot{Q}$ inequality but to another kind of maldistribution, unequal distribution of diffusing capacity to blood flow ($D/\dot{Q}$ inequality) (Fig. 2).[44]

I had developed the concept of $D/\dot{Q}$ ratio to explain the experimentally determined absorption rates of inert gases of

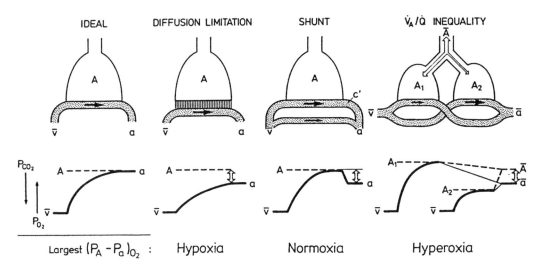

**Figure 1.** Models showing the mechanisms of the alveolar-arterial $P_{O_2}$ difference ($AaD_{O_2}$) by diffusion limitation, shunt, and $\dot{V}_A/\dot{Q}$ inequality. *Lower panel:* $P_{O_2}$ profiles in alveolar gas and pulmonary capillary blood. $AaD_{O_2}$ is indicated by open arrows.

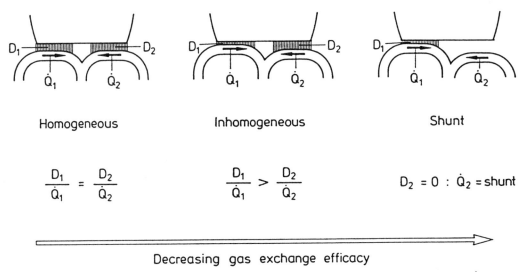

**Figure 2.** Models for unequal distribution of diffusing capacity (D) to blood flow ($\dot{Q}$). D is distributed to the two compartments in such a manner that total, $D = D_1 + D_2$, remains constant. The decreasing gas exchange efficiency is caused by the inability of increased $D/\dot{Q}$ in one unit to compensate for the reduced $D/\dot{Q}$ in the other unit.

varied solubility and diffusivity from subcutaneous gas pockets in rats that Canfield and Rahn observed prior to my arrival in Buffalo.[50] When allowing for variance of the $D/\dot{Q}$ ratio in lungs, the dependence of $AaD_{O_2}$ on alveolar $P_{O_2}$ found in our experiment could indeed be explained. In normoxia the $AaD_{O_2}$ was mainly attributable to a lung compartment with low $D/\dot{Q}$. In hyperoxia there would be no diffusion limitation in this compartment (no $AaD_{O_2}$), and in deep hypoxia the blood flow of this compartment would be functionally close to a complete shunt.[53]

As the $CO_2$ electrode became available (after 1960), we and others showed that there existed an arterial-to-end-expired $P_{CO_2}$ difference in anesthetized dogs that explained part of the total $AaD_{O_2}$ not attributable to shunt or (evenly distributed) diffusion. The larger part of $AaD_{O_2}$ measured in normoxia could not, however, be explained by this factor (e.g., reference 2). Yet by the elegant multiple inert gas elimination technique (MIGET),[66,67] $AaD_{O_2}$ in man and dog has been shown to be mainly explainable by $\dot{V}A/\dot{Q}$ variance. From my perspective today, our results with elimination of $N_2$ may have been mistaken, but they did stimulate us to look for other solutions and thus led to the concept of $D/\dot{Q}$ and its variance. On the other hand, it would be strange if the sizable variance of pulmonary capillary transit time, as measured by videofluorescence microscopy in subpleural, pulmonary vessels by Wiltz Wagner,[4,69,70] had no effect on $O_2$ exchange. Moreover, the pulsatile pulmonary capillary blood flow as demonstrated by Grant de Jong Lee and associates[29] is expected to have effects analogous to those of local blood flow variance.

The combination of $D/\dot{Q}$ inequality with that of $\dot{V}A/\dot{Q}$ inequality in a "$\dot{V}/\dot{Q}=D/\dot{Q}$ field"[45] remained theory for a long time. Only recently have Yamaguchi and coworkers attempted to apply this concept. Combining experimental results of MIGET with $CO_2$, $O_2$, and CO exchange data obtained from pulmonary patients, Yamaguchi and coworkers[74] have been able to estimate quantitatively both $\dot{V}A/\dot{Q}$ and $D/\dot{Q}$ inequality.

Back in Europe from Buffalo, Pierre Haab and I returned to the conventional analysis of alveolar gas exchange in anesthetized dogs. To increase the relative diffusion limitation effects on $AaD_{O_2}$, we measured gas exchange variables in deep hypoxia (Fig. 1). This time we used the recently available blood $P_{CO_2}$, electrodes and mass spectrometry for continuous gas analysis.[16] The results showed only a very small $AaD_{O_2}$ to be attributable to diffusion limitation (Fig. 3). But this was a maximal effect based on the assumption that alveolar dead space was the only effective mode of $\dot{V}A/\dot{Q}$ heterogeneity. When other modes of $\dot{V}A/\dot{Q}$ inequality were assumed, the diffusion limitation component of $AaD_{O_2}$ approached zero.

Also, measurements of $O_2$ exchange in isolated, blood-perfused dog lung lobes in hypoxia led to results that were not easily explained by diffusion limitation.[46] Following an idea of Masaji Mochizuki (with whom I had interminable discussions as he worked with Heinz Bartels in the physiology department of the University of Göttingen 1953 and 1954), we performed measurements with varied hematocrit. The $AaD_{O_2}$ was found to be independent of hematocrit, in agreement with Mochizuki and coworkers[40] and correspondingly the calculated $D_{O_2}$ came out proportional to hematocrit. This could be explained by a model with all resistance to $O_2$ uptake in red blood cells (and no resistance in the blood-gas barrier or plasma). But the same effect would be produced by a shunt beside a major compartment exhibiting no diffusion limitation. The shunt model could also explain the independence of $AaD_{O_2}$ of blood flow, which led to a directly proportional relationship between $D_{O_2}$ and blood flow.[46]

It followed from all the theoretical models and experimental results that an $AaD_{O_2}$ due to diffusion limitation was not easily evaluated. Even its existence could not be convincingly demonstrated, apparently due to disturbing influences of functional inhomogeneities like ventilation-perfusion and other inequalities.

## Rebreathing: Attempt to Isolate Diffusion Limitation

The stimulus came from Paolo Cerretelli, from the laboratory of Rodolfo Margaria in Milan (now in Geneva), with

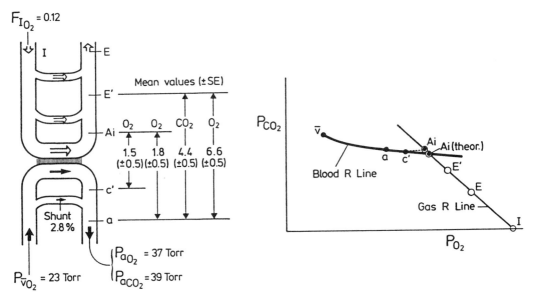

**Figure 3.** Analysis of alveolar gas exchange in hypoxia. *Left:* model of lung with series dead space, alveolar dead space, and effective alveolar ventilation, capillary, and shunt blood flow. Mean values (± SE) of $P_{O_2}$ and $P_{CO_2}$ differences, obtained in 11 anesthetized, paralyzed, artificially ventilated dogs are indicated. After Haab et al.[16]. *Right:* $P_{CO_2} - P_{O_2}$ diagram with blood and gas R lines underlying the analysis of alveolar gas exchange according to the model at left.

whom I had collaborated since 1962 on studies of $O_2$ supply to stimulated isolated muscles and exercising animals. With Hermann Rahn and Leon Farhi, he had attempted to determine mixed venous $P_{O_2}$ in man by rebreathing, using mass spectrometry.[6] Be selecting a gas mixture of appropriate composition and volume, he and his coworkers attempted to obtain mixed venous $P_{O_2}$ and $P_{CO_2}$ from rebreathing plateau values of $CO_2$ and $O_2$. But in most cases this ideal condition of true plateau could not be achieved. Instead, the mixed venous $P_{O_2}$ had to be extrapolated or interpolated from a plot of rate of change of $P_{O_2}$ against $P_{O_2}$: the true value was assumed where the rate of change of $P_{O_2}$ became zero[7].

I became involved when Cerretelli asked me to analyze the factors that might determine the kinetics of the approach of lung gas $P_{O_2}$ toward the equilibrium value, i.e., mixed venous $P_{O_2}$. According to the theory, in an ideal system these kinetics were determined by the ratio of the overall $O_2$ conductance, determined by pulmonary diffusing capacity for $O_2$ ($D_{O_2}$), pulmonary capillary blood flow, and the slope of the blood $O_2$ dissociation curve, to the $O_2$ capacitance, given by the total gas volume of lungs and rebreathing bag.[51] Because an infinitely high ventilation cannot be achieved, in practice the effective ventilation and the partitioning of the total gas to lungs and rebreathing bag also had to be taken into account (Fig. 4). The feasibility of the method was tested in experiments on anesthetized dogs[1] and on man at rest and during exercise.[64]

The method could be improved by introducing a stable isotope of $O_2$, $^{18}O_2$, in low concentration (0.07% in the rebreathing mixture) as test gas.[37] This had two important advantages. First, mixed venous partial pressure of the isotope could be neglected. Second, the effective blood dissociation curve of the isotopic $O_2$ against its partial pressure could be re-

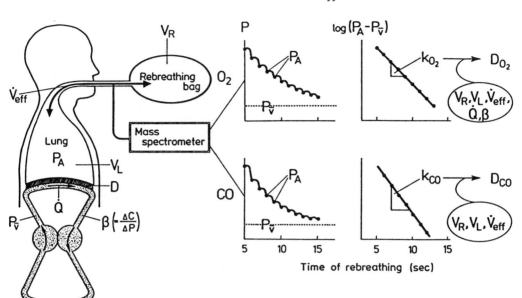

**Figure 4.** Determination of diffusing capacities (D) for $O_2$ and CO by rebreathing: model and recordings of partial pressures in rebreathing gas by mass spectrometry. $V_R$, (average) volume of rebreathing bag; $V_L$, (average) lung volume; $\dot{V}_{eff}$, effective alveolar ventilation; $\dot{Q}$, pulmonary blood flow; $\beta$, slope of effective blood dissociation curve. For $D_{CO}$, $\dot{Q}$ and $\beta$ are not required because CO uptake may be regarded as not limited by blood flow. Time available for measurement is limited by onset of recirculation (about 12th s).

garded as a straight line through the mixed venous point of the abundant isotope ($O^{16}_2$). From simultaneous determination of CO diffusing capacity, a stable isotope of CO, $^{13}CO$, was used, again to be able to neglect CO in mixed venous blood and, more important, to be able to separate CO from $N_2$ when using continuous respiratory mass spectrometry with relatively low mass resolution.

The advantage of rebreathing is the homogenization of lung gas by rebreathing, thus reducing or even practically eliminating the effects of unequal distribution of ventilation to blood flow. Simultaneous determination of $D_{O_2}$ and $D_{CO_2}$ in normal man showed that the resting values were higher than usually reported (using other methods), their increase in exercise was moderate, a plateau value was reached, and the ratio $D_{O_2}/D_{CO}$ was about 1:2, i.e., close to the ratio of Krogh diffusion constants for tissue[37] (Fig. 5). The last finding was taken to indicate

that simple diffusion was the main factor involved.

Recently a group in Oxford[3] and a group in Bordeaux[14] have reported measurements of pulmonary diffusing capacity in patients using a new test gas, nitric

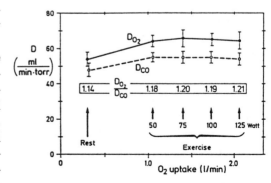

**Figure 5.** Simultaneous determinations of the diffusing capacities for $O_2$ and CO ($D_{O_2}$, $D_{CO}$) by rebreathing in man at rest and during bicycle ergometer exercise. Mean values ± SE obtained in 6 normal males, 20–33 years of age. After Meyer *et al.*[37]

oxide (NO).[36] The advantage of NO is that it reacts much faster with hemoglobin than does CO. But NO is a highly reactive and toxic gas, and it must be used in very low concentrations. It could be measured in gas samples using highly sensitive chemiluminescence detectors developed for monitoring atmospheric pollution. Using mass spectrometry, we had to go to considerably higher concentrations than used in man by the other groups (600 ppm vs. 10 to 40 ppm), and therefore we preferred to work on dogs. Because of the reactivity and instability of NO, particular measures had to be taken for its continuous recording by the mass spectrometer during rebreathing.

Simultaneous rebreathing of NO and CO yielded average $D_{NO}$ in anesthetized dogs about four times higher than $D_{CO}$[39] (Fig. 6). According to literature data, the Krogh diffusion constant ratio NO/CO is close to 2. The higher figure for the $D_{NO}/D_{CO}$ ratio probably is due to the slow reaction of CO with hemoglobin. Even in hypoxia, where substantial free Hb is also present in arterialized blood, the $D_{NO}/D_{CO}$ ratio averaged 3.2. The inference that CO uptake is strongly reaction limited evidently is disagreement with our conclusions from simultaneous measurements of $D_{CO}$ and $D_{O_2}$ in humans (see above). Because the ratio $D_{O_2}/D_{CO}$ was found close to the Krogh diffusion constant ratio $O_2/CO$, it was concluded that both $O_2$ and CO were limited by simple diffusion. The high $D_{NO}/D_{CO}$ ratio would mean that true $D_{CO}$ was higher than measured and the estimated $D_{O_2}$ was an underestimation, possibly due to remaining inhomogeneity effects (D/Q̇ inhomogeneity?).

Of particular interest was a small but significant increase of $D_{NO}$ in hypoxia and decrease in hyperoxia.[39] Because the reaction of Hb with NO is known to be very fast, we would like to attribute these changes to real changes in D (increase in size or number of perfused pulmonary capillaries).

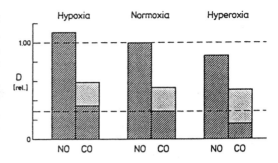

**Figure 6.** Simultaneous determinations of the diffusing capacities (D) for NO and CO by rebreathing in 8 anesthetized, artificially ventilated dogs. Mean values relative to $D_{NO}$ in normoxia. The differences between normoxia and hypoxia and between normoxia and hyperoxia are statistically significant for both $D_{NO}$ and $D_{CO}$. After Meyer *et al.*[39]

The problem of $CO_2$ equilibration kinetics of blood in pulmonary capillaries has been experimentally investigated by Hyde and coworkers[24] in humans. They applied a breath-holding method in which the kinetics of $^{13}CO_2$ equilibration was compared with that of acetylene. But the equilibration limitation effect on $^{13}CO_2$ uptake was too small to be measurable. The effective diffusing capacity, $D_{CO_2}$, was estimated to be higher than 200 ml/(min·Torr). Using the same $CO_2$ isotope and acetylene but applying rebreathing and continuous recording of $^{13}CO_2$ and acetylene during rebreathing by mass spectrometry, we could estimate the $CO_2$ diffusing capacity at 180 ml/(min·Torr) at rest and at 300 ml/(min·Torr) during moderate exercise.[54]

Our main interest was comparing $D_{CO_2}$ with $D_{O_2}$, both measured by rebreathing in similar experimental conditions. The mean ratios $D_{CO_2}/D_{O_2}$ were 3.3 at rest and 4.7 during exercise, thus averaging 4. But the Krogh diffusion constant ratio $K_{CO_2}/K_{O_2}$ is about 20–25. Thus the capillary-alveolar equilibration of $CO_2$ was found to be much slower than expected on the basis of $CO_2$ diffusion. It is well known that the blood-gas $CO_2$ transfer in lungs is a complex process consisting of many component processes. The bicarbonate-chloride exchange between red blood cells and plasma, the dehydration of carbonic acid to $CO_2$ in plasma, and the same reaction in the red cells (in spite of the presence of carbonic anhydrase) are known or suspected to be relatively slow. Thus the diffusion of $CO_2$ may lead to a rapid equilibration of $CO_2$ in blood with alveolar gas, but the subsequent slow reequilibration between $CO_2$, $HCO_3^-$, and $H^+$ in red cells and plasma would lead to an elevation of $P_{CO_2}$ in arterialized blood after it has left the lungs (to be eventually completed as the blood is in a $CO_2$ electrode) (Fig. 7).

## Diffusion/Perfusion Model: Extent and Site of Diffusion Limitation

In the analysis of gas exchange, a basic question is to what extent gas transfer is limited by perfusion and by diffusion. The simplest model, applicable to many situations (such as absorption from tissue gas pockets, gas transfer through skin, gas transfer in lungs), is a gas phase maintained at constant composition having gas exchange with flowing blood, of a certain effective solubility for the gas considered, across a barrier constituting a resistance to diffusion.[55] The calculated partial pressure profiles are shown in Figure 8. They are determined by the ratio of diffusing capacity (D) and the product of blood flow ($\dot{Q}$) and the effective solubility ($\beta$), which is the slope of blood dissociation curves in terms of concentration (content) versus partial pressure ($\beta = dC/dP$). The ratio, $D/(\dot{Q}\beta)$, may be termed the equilibration index. For the relative equilibration deficit of arterial blood $(P_A-P_a)/(P_A-P\bar{v})$, the following equation holds:

$$\frac{P_A - P_a}{P_A - P\bar{v}} = e^{-\frac{D}{\dot{Q}\beta}} \qquad (1)$$

Clearly for $D/\dot{Q} \to \infty$, $P_A - P_a \to 0$, meaning absence of diffusion limitation. With decreasing $D/\dot{Q}$, $P_A - P_a$ increases, denoting increasing diffusion limitation. The relationship of Equation (1) can be applied to any gas including $O_2$.

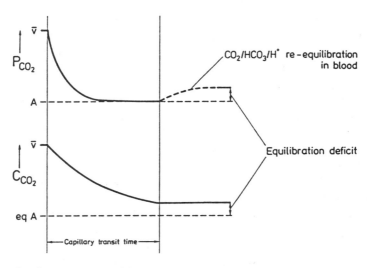

**Figure 7.** Blood-gas $CO_2$ equilibration in lungs. Qualitative model to explain the experimental finding that the $CO_2/O_2$ ratio of diffusing capacities was much smaller than the corresponding Krogh diffusion constant ratio for tissue. The equilibration of $CO_2$ proper is rapid and practically complete during the pulmonary capillary transit time, but the equilibrium for total $CO_2$ content is not reached.

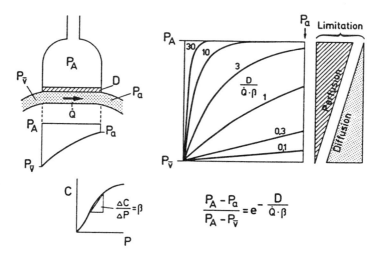

**Figure 8.** Diffusion-perfusion limitation in alveolar-capillary gas transfer. Model, partial pressure profiles for various values of $D/(\dot{Q} \cdot \beta)$, and a dissociation curve (concentration, C, as function of partial pressure, P) showing definition of the capacitance coefficient $\beta = \Delta C/\Delta P$. After Piiper and Scheid.[55]

Whereas in the normoxic and slightly hypoxic regions the assumption of a constant $\beta$ is problematic because of the evident curvature of the $O_2$ dissociation curve, and a procedure like Bohr integration should be applied, in deep hypoxia the $O_2$ dissociation is sufficiently linear. The effects of the curvature of blood $O_2$ dissociation curves have been recently investigated.[27,28] With the value of $D_{O_2}$ determined in our laboratory in deep hypoxia and $\dot{Q}$ and $\beta$ calculated after the values estimated by Cerretelli[5] in man in the base camp of Mt. Everest (altitude 5,350 m), a strong diffusion limitation results for rest (12%) and an even stronger one for maximum $O_2$ uptake exercise (64%). The $AaD_{O_2}$ estimated therefrom (2 Torr at rest, 27 Torr at maximum $O_2$ uptake exercise) is in rough agreement with measurements performed by Wagner and coworkers in normobaric or hypobaric simulated altitude.[19,63,65,68]

There is also growing evidence for diffusion limitation of pulmonary $O_2$ uptake in very strenuous exercise in human athletes in normoxia.[9] In these cases the $D/\dot{Q}$ inhomogeneity may play a role, as the transit times in some pulmonary capillaries may be reduced so much as to turn their flow to functional shunt flow.

Let us make a short excursion to lower vertebrates (indeed, the comparative physiology of gas exchange in vertebrates has been in the center of my research interest for a long time). In amphibians, cutaneous gas exchange is important, particularly for $CO_2$ elimination, but also for $O_2$ uptake. Because skin must have a certain thickness to provide mechanical protection, diffusion limitation in cutaneous gas exchange is expected to be much more prominent than in lungs. Remarkably, in various groups of salamanders lungs have been reduced so that all exchange occurs through skin (and oral and pharyngeal mucosa).

Randall Gatz and Eugene Crawford, zoologists from Lexington, Kentucky, took lungless salamanders captured in the Alleghenies to Göttingen to study their cutaneous gas exchange. We could measure $P_{O_2}$ and $P_{CO_2}$ in blood sampled from the single ventricle and roughly estimate the blood flow and diffusing capacity of the skin using soluble inert gases. Calculations with the values thus obtained revealed a strong degree of diffusion limitation for both $O_2$ uptake and $CO_2$ output.[52] Remarkably, animals are highly tolerant of hypoxia[13] and can substantially increase their cutaneous $O_2$ uptake during exercise. Evidently the diffusing capacity can be adaptively increased.[11]

Estimation of the pulmonary equilibration deficit of $CO_2$ in human lungs by introducing values of D, $\dot{Q}$, and $\beta$ into Equation (1) yielded 2% for rest but 18% for maximum $O_2$ uptake exercise.[54] The corresponding arterial-to-alveolar $P_{CO_2}$ differences were 0.2 Torr and 7 Torr, respectively. Thus, against what is usually believed, blood-gas $CO_2$ equilibration in lungs may play an important role in limiting the efficiency of $CO_2$ elimination.

## Site of Resistance to Gas Transfer: Red Blood Cells versus "Membrane"

The role of $O_2$ transfer resistance of the red blood cells in alveolar $O_2$ uptake (and $O_2$ delivery in tissues) has been discussed for many years. It was fortunate for us that in 1981 Robert Holland from Sydney, Australia, came to us for a sabbatical and initiated a number of studies on $O_2$ kinetics of red cells using an improved stopped-flow technique. Our attention was directed toward determining the extracellular resistance to $O_2$ transfer in stopped-flow experiments and to obtaining, by subtraction of the extracellular resistance, a better estimate of the true $O_2$ transfer resistance of red blood cells or its reciprocal, the specific $O_2$ transfer conductance, $\Theta$.[25] As expected the $\Theta_{O_2}$ values corrected for perierythrocyte $O_2$ transfer resistances were considerably larger than previously published values.[75]

Using the well-known Roughton-Forster relationship, which is based on the additivity of intraerythrocyte (RBC) and extraerythrocyte ("membrane") transfer resistances,

$$\frac{1}{D_L} = \frac{1}{D_M} + \frac{1}{V_C \cdot \theta} \qquad (2)$$

where $D_L$ is pulmonary D; $D_M$, "membrane" D; and $V_C$, pulmonary capillary blood volume. We calculated for the ratio $D_L/D_M$, equivalent to the fraction of extraerythrocyte $O_2$ uptake resistance in total $O_2$ uptake resistance, 0.88 (assuming $D_{O_2} = 54$ ml/(min · Torr) and $V_C = 100$ ml). With a previously determined value of $\Theta$, 1.5,[20] the figure would be 0.67. Thus a major part of the $O_2$ uptake resistance in lungs appears to be located outside the red cells, in the plasma and tissue barrier. This conclusion is not in good agreement with morphometric data, which show that diffusion distances within red cells are larger than those across the air-blood tissue barrier.[71] But in red cells $O_2$ transport appears to be facilitated by hemoglobin (diffusion of $O_2$-hemoglobin). Moreover, intracapillary hematocrit is generally lower than large vessel hematocrit. Because $\Theta$ is defined for normal hematocrit (0.45), a lower hematocrit (lower $\Theta$) would lead to an increased $D_M$ for a given (measured) $D_L$. Another factor that is difficult to assess is the convective mixing of red cell interior and plasma during blood flow through pulmonary microvessels in vivo.

In other studies using the stopped-flow apparatus we attempted to further analyze the factors determining the $O_2$ transport within the red blood cells. Using a particular model for evaluation of measurements, we concluded that the diffusion coefficients of $O_2$ and hemoglobin were the most important variables, but $O_2$ reaction kinetics of hemoglobin also had a limiting effect.[23] In contrast, measurements of $O_2$ uptake kinetics at varied temperature left very little space for a limiting role of the chemical reaction.[73] Both studies may be considered as evidence for a minor role of the kinetics of the chemical reaction of hemoglobin with $O_2$ in limiting $O_2$ uptake.

Many years ago, I had tried to measure the red cell–plasma equilibration of $CO_2$-bicarbonate in vitro using the rapid mixing–continuous flow technique combined with filtration for plasma sampling. At that time I looked for a possible explanation of the relatively large arterial-alveolar $P_{CO_2}$ differences found in anesthetized dogs. But the results showed the kinetics of bicarbonate to be very rapid, leading to 90% equilibration in 0.11 s on the average.[47] Because the usually assumed transit time of pulmonary capillaries, 0.3 to 1 s, is longer, a discrepancy appears to exist: the in vitro results suggest no measurable equilibration limitation in contrast to the in vivo $^{13}CO_2$ equilibration results. But both in vivo and in vitro techniques are difficult and fraught with potential errors. A reevaluation using improved methods would be welcome.

## Blood-Gas Equilibrium of $CO_2$: "Anomalous" versus Conventional

In the Symposium on $CO_2$: Chemical, Biochemical and Physiological Aspects, which took place in Philadelphia in August 1968 (as a satellite to the International Congress of Physiological Sciences in Washington, D.C.) a remarkable finding was presented by Gail Gurtner (at that time in Buffalo). He showed experimental data obtained in anesthetized dogs in rebreathing equilibrium, exhibiting large negative $P_{CO_2}$ differences between alveolar gas and mixed venous blood, averaging about 10 Torr but reaching up to 28 Torr.[15] Moreover, he presented an elegant physiochemical theory, which came to be known as the charged membrane hypothesis, to

explain the experimental data. This remarkable paper gave rise to a lively debate in which two discussants, Gabriel Laszlo (London) and Jack Hackney (Downey, California) reported that they had not been able to reproduce the negative blood-gas $P_{CO_2}$ differences in alveolar gas-blood $CO_2$ equilibrium.

In the wake of the Gurtner paper, a number of studies have been performed, most of them confirming negative mixed venous-to-alveolar or arterial-to-alveolar $P_{CO_2}$ differences in rebreathing equilibrium in varied experimental conditions (reviewed in references 49 and 57). The excitement about this finding was understandable. There was every reason to believe that this phenomenon of a negative blood-gas $P_{CO_2}$ difference would not be confined to rebreathing equilibrium but would be operative also in steady-state gas exchange (Fig. 9). But this would invalidate the classical approach to the analysis of alveolar gas exchange in which the equality of $P_{CO_2}$ between alveolar gas and end-capillary blood in equilibrium was a central, seemingly obvious, assumption.

Indeed, soon Donald Jennings (Kingston, Ontario) claimed that negative blood-gas $P_{CO_2}$ differences occurred in anesthetized dogs during steady-state gas exchange in hypercapnia.[25] Having spotted this paper, my coworkers and I immediately set out to repeat the experiments, essentially duplicating the experimental conditions. But we could not reproduce the results: there were no negative arterial-to-alveolar $P_{CO_2}$ differences.[56] Soon after the completion of these experiments, I had the opportunity to present the results at the 1978 fall meeting of the American Physiological Society in St. Louis.[48] Donald Jennings was present, and our discordant experimental results were discussed. After the session, we continued the discussion with some beer. The outcome was a visit by Peter Scheid and myself to Jennings's laboratory at Kingston, followed by joint experiments in Göttingen.

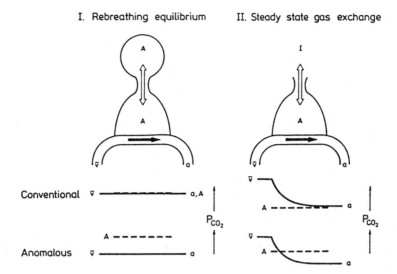

I. Rebreathing equilibrium    II. Steady state gas exchange

**Figure 9.** Models for blood-gas equilibrium of $CO_2$. In *rebreathing equilibrium,* conventionally an equality of mixed venous, arterial, and alveolar $P_{CO_2}$ is assumed; in the "anomalous" case, mixed venous and arterial $P_{CO_2}$ are lower than alveolar $P_{CO_2}$. In *steady-state gas exchange,* conventionally close to complete equilibration, with arterial close to alveolar $P_{CO_2}$, is assumed; in the "anomalous" case, an equilibrium with $P_{CO_2}$ in blood lower than $P_{CO_2}$ in gas is supposed to be approached, leading to arterial $P_{CO_2}$ being lower than alveolar $P_{CO_2}$.

The experiments were performed on awake dogs prepared with a chronic tracheostomy and exteriorized carotid loop (exactly as done in Kingston) but using our mass spectrometer for alveolar-expired $P_{CO_2}$ and our blood electrodes for $P_{CO_2}$. The result was that in hypercapnia no single measurement in any dog had a negative value of the arterial-to-end-expired $P_{CO_2}$ difference: with 5% inspired $CO_2$ the mean value was +0.9 Torr (significantly different from zero), with 10% $CO_2$, +0.1 Torr (not significantly different from zero). The results were published in a joint communication (26), although Jennings was not quite convinced. We planned a later continuation of the research in Kingston, but it did not occur.

Thereafter another North American physiologist who had found indirect evidence for negative blood-gas $P_{CO_2}$ differences in dogs in steady-state gas exchange came to us, initially with the intention of restudying the phenomenon, but then he drifted to other experiments. Other ac-

tions and reactions in this campaign followed. Steinbrook and coworkers[62] reported large negative blood-gas $P_{CO_2}$ differences, averaging −12 Torr in 178 measurements during long-lasting rebreathing in awake goats. We repeated the experiments on awake dogs in similar conditions but found no significant blood-gas $P_{CO_2}$ difference (average −0.4 Torr in 266 measurements).[60] Because previously larger anomalous blood-gas $P_{CO_2}$ differences had been reported to occur in exercise, we repeated measurements in dogs rebreathing while running on a treadmill. The result was the same: no negative blood-gas $P_{CO_2}$ differences were observed.[30]

During these years I frequently asked colleagues their opinions on the controversial matter of negative blood-gas $P_{CO_2}$ differences, or they approached me about it. The opinions fell into two opposite camps. Many encouraged us to continue our efforts, with improved methodology, to reproduce this interesting phenomenon, which we evidently had failed to find. Others wondered why we wasted time and effort trying to reproduce something that was nonexistent because it evidently contradicted physicochemical laws. In the last few years some reports of small negative $P_{CO_2}$ differences have appeared, but studies explicitly aimed at checking the phenomenon, with negative results, have also been published.[8,12]

In a detailed analysis of potential sources of error it seemed that more factors led to falsely negative than to falsely positive blood-gas $P_{CO_2}$ differences, the simplest and possibly most important one being loss of $CO_2$ from blood during sampling or transfer into the electrode.[57] But it was practically impossible to explain the large differences amounting to tens of Torr $P_{CO_2}$. It seems wise to consider this interesting issue to be open, and I encourage all students of $CO_2$/acid-base balance to look out for evidence pro or con.

It is important to point out that the equilibration kinetics of labeled $CO_2$, discussed in a preceding section, concerns a fundamentally different aspect: the kinetics of approach to an equilibrium that, in principle, is independent of the position of the equilibrium. Thus the kinetic data and their interpretation are compatible with any constellation of blood-gas $P_{CO_2}$ differences in the equilibrium state.

## Diffusion Resistance in Gas Phase: Conflicting Evidence

There has been considerable controversy, revived recently about what part of the overall diffusion resistance to movement of $O_2$ and $CO_2$ between inspired gas and pulmonary capillary blood may be located in the alveolar gas. The consequence of such a transfer resistance would be a partial pressure gradient in the terminal airways, often referred to as stratification. This gradient could be detected during a prolonged expiration as a rising

(falling) alveolar plateau of $CO_2$ ($O_2$) or of inert foreign gases previously inspired.

These problems were investigated half a century ago by, among others, my teacher and predecessor, Wolf Schoedel, then at the Department of Physiology, University of Göttingen, headed by Hermann Rein.[41,59] It was realized that not only stratification proper, but also continuing gas transfer between blood and alveolar gas and sequential emptying of lung areas with varied gas concentrations might be involved in producing sloping alveolar plateaus (Fig. 10). With the advent of rapid gas concentration recording techniques like infrared absorption and mass spectrometry, the shape of expirograms of various gases could be recorded more accurately.

The simultaneous measurement of several gas species of different diffusivities is of particular interest for the detection of diffusion limitations. Because of its great contrast in diffusivity, the pair He/$SF_6$ has been frequently used, the ratio of their diffusivities amounting to 6.0 from Graham's Law (diffusivity inversely proportional to the square root of molecular weight). After measurements in our laboratory, the ratio of diffusion coefficients of He and $SF_6$ in a gas mixture of 14% $O_2$, 6% $CO_2$, and 80% $N_2$ was 7.2.[72] For a simple diffusion resistance model, one expects the gradient per transfer rate to be inversely proportional to diffusivity. Because the transfer rate is proportional to the end-expired-to-inspired (or mixed-expired-to-inspired) partial pressure difference, the relative slope of the alveolar plateau (i.e., standardized to the above-mentioned partial pressure differences) should be inversely proportional to diffusivity, i.e., the $SF_6$/He ratio of standardized alveolar slopes should be about 7.

Scherer's group in Philadelphia has studied the expirograms of $CO_2$ and intravenously infused He and $SF_6$ in man. The reported $SF_6$/He ratios of the standardized slopes were 3:13[58] and later, with im-

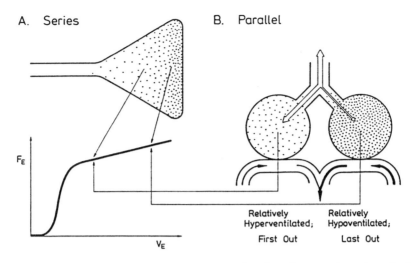

**Figure 10.** Alternative mechanisms of sloping alveolar plateaus. Density of stippling indicates gas concentration. A. *Series* inhomogeneity or stratification. Upon expiration, the sloping alveolar plateau directly reflects the stratification is alveolar space. B. *Parallel* inhomogeneity, e.g., produced for $CO_2$ by unequal distribution of ventilation to blood flow. If relatively hyperventilated lung areas expire earlier and relatively hypoventilated areas expire later, a sloping alveolar plateau is generated.

proved technique, 1.85.[42] As pointed out by the same group, due to the trumpetlike shape of the lung airways (when considered as total airways cross section as function of length), the expected ratio is considerably smaller than the diffusivity ratio and may reach the values that were experimentally found. The authors concluded that diffusion resistance in the airways is the main factor in producing the alveolar slope.

In our laboratory we found in anesthetized dogs well-established alveolar slopes, but $SF_6$/He slope ratios were much closer to unity, and in many conditions the ratios were even below unity.[34] This finding indicated that the slopes were due to other factors besides incomplete diffusional equilibration in gas phase. Because the effects of continuing gas exchange were compensated for by a special technique, only sequential expiration of lung areas of differing gas composition, due to $\dot{V}_A/\dot{Q}$ or $\dot{V}_A/V_A$ inequalities, was a possible explanation. The simplest model to explain the experimental data consisted of two peripheral compartments connected to a central common compartment. The gas exchange between the central and each of the peripheral compartments was implemented by both diffusion and ventilation, characterized by a diffusive and a ventilatory conductance.[22] In subsequent experiments on dogs, the sloping alveolar plateaus of $CO_2$, $O_2$, and intravenously infused acetylene and Freon-22 were determined.[35] In another series, the alveolar slopes of He and $SF_6$ administered through inspired gas and through venous blood were comparatively studied[38] (Fig. 11). In all cases only a minor dependence of the test gas alveolar slopes on diffusivity was found.

The picture emerging from these experiments performed in Göttingen is that the alveolar slope is mainly due to continuous gas exchange (particularly for well-soluble gases, but also for little-soluble gases like He and $SF_6$ when intravenously infused), secondarily to sequential expiration from lung areas with differing test gas composition (due to ventilation-perfusion or ventilation-volume inequalities). Finally, but to a lesser extent, the slope is

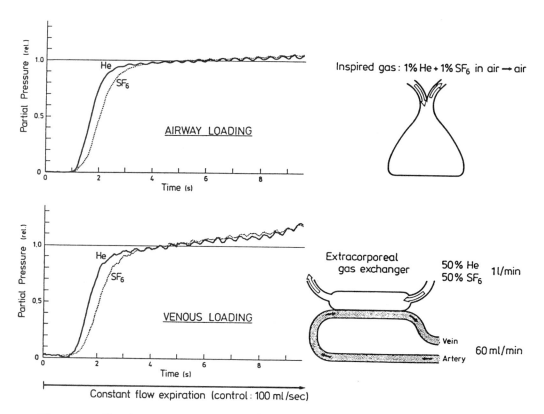

**Figure 11.** Simultaneous expirograms of He and $SF_6$ obtained in anesthetized, artificially ventilated dogs during constant flow expiration. *Airway loading:* first breath after wash-in equilibration with 1% He and 1% $SF_6$ in air. *Venous loading:* continuous administration of He and $SF_6$ by equilibration of blood using an extracorporeal gas exchanger. The following findings are evident: larger dead space for $SF_6$ than for He; slightly higher alveolar slopes for $SF_6$ than for He; higher alveolar slopes for venous loading compared to airway loading. After Meyer *et al.*[38]

due to diffusion resistance in gas phase (as indicated by dependence on the diffusion coefficient).

The differing results from Philadelphia and Göttingen have led to discussions, reciprocal laboratory visits, and a joint symposium at a meeting of the Federation of American Societies for Experimental Biology (FASEB, Washington, D.C., April 1990). What we could agree on was that the source of the discrepancies might be sought in the species (humans in Philadelphia vs. dog in Göttingen) and in the experimental conditions (spontaneous breathing in Philadelphia vs. artificial ventilation with prolonged, linear expira-

tion in Göttingen). An interesting aspect of this story should be mentioned: both the Philadelphia group and the Göttingen group had difficulty getting their papers accepted for publication by a leading journal of respiratory physiology, apparently because the concepts, models, and interpretations of both groups were in disagreement with the views of influential referees. Indeed, other attractive lung models producing sloping alveolar plateaus are models with asymmetrically branching "trumpets" of different lengths leading to locally varying diffusion resistances.[31,43] We have not tried to apply such models because of their complexity and a lack of information about the anatomy, preferring simpler models composed of a few compartments as functional analogs.

According to model calculations, the relative alveolar slopes due to incomplete diffusive mixing are expected to increase with increased breathing frequency and reduced total volume and have been found to do so during rapid shallow breathing in humans.[42] An extreme form of rapid shallow breathing is panting in the dog, with breathing frequencies of about 5/s and tidal volumes close to anatomical dead space. Using a special technique, expirograms during panting could be obtained.[33] They showed a very steeply rising $P_{CO_2}$ (falling $P_{O_2}$) during expiration, immediately followed by a rapid fall of $P_{CO_2}$ (rise of $P_{O_2}$) during inspiration (Fig. 12). This could be described in two ways: absence of an alveolar plateau or an extremely steeply sloping alveolar plateau,

not differentiable from phase II of the normal expirogram. Moreover, the arterial $P_{CO_2}$ was much higher than the peak expired $P_{CO_2}$.

This looked very much like a well-developed stratification. But the expirograms of two intravenously infused gases of equal solubility but different diffusivity, acetylene and Freon 22, were close to identical.[61] (Fig. 12). Moreover, the multiple breath washout kinetics of helium and $SF_6$ were very similar.[18] This points to a relatively small role for diffusion limitation, and the prevalent role of convection, probably a "stratified ventilation" in a serial system. But unequal parallel ventilation with relatively hypoventilated areas expiring last could not be excluded. Similar results and conclusions were reached from experiments with high-frequency ventilation in anesthetized dogs, with respiratory frequencies varied from 10 to 40/s.[32]

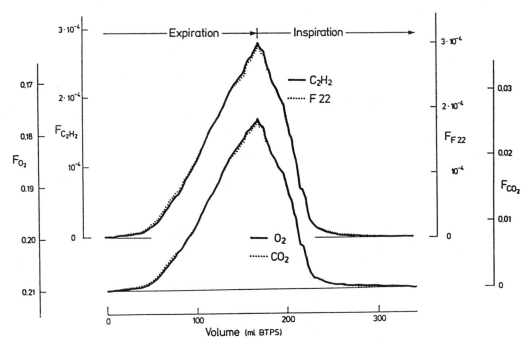

**Figure 12.** Gas concentration profiles of intravenously infused acetylene ($C_2H_2$), Freon 22 (F22), and of $O_2$ and $CO_2$ during a single respiratory cycle in dogs during panting ($\approx$ 5 breaths/s), plotted against respired volume (abscissa). Note reversed scale for $O_2$ as compared to other gases. After Šipinková *et al.*[61]

It is rather difficult to separate airway diffusion gradients proper (stratification) from unequal distribution effects due to inhomogeneity of ventilation and diffusion among parallel and serial airway elements.

## Epilogue

This is a fleeting report of the main features of my meandering, erratic journey through diffusion problems in lungs. No aspect has been completely clarified, but my coworkers and I had in many cases the pleasure of experimentally verifying what we expected and, what is at first less gratifying but more fruitful in the long run, finding unexpected results. Of fundamental importance were personal contacts with scientists from other laboratories. Most of our contributions have arisen from such contacts, which gave rise to reciprocal visits and joint projects.

**Acknowledgment:** The work reported here could not have been performed without the collaboration of many coworkers whose names appear as coauthors of the publications in the reference list. I am particularly grateful to Dr. Peter Scheid (now in the Department of Physiology, University Bochum) and Dr. Michael Meyer, who participated, in many cases as principal investigators in most of the recent studies on which this report is based.

## References

1. Adaro, F., P. Scheid, J. Teichmann, and J. Piiper. A rebreathing method for estimating pulmonary $D_{O_2}$: theory and measurements in dog lungs. *Respir. Physiol.* 18: 43–63, 1973.
2. Aoyagi, K., J. Piiper, and F. May. Alveolärer Gasaustausch und Kreislauf am narkotisierten Hund bei Spontanatmung und bei künstlicher Beatmung. *Pflügers Arch.* 286: 311–316, 1965.
3. Borland, C. D. R., and T. W. Higenbottam. A simultaneous single breath measurement of pulmonary diffusing capacity with nitric oxide and carbon monoxide. *Eur. Respir. J.* 2: 56–63, 1989.
4. Capen, R. L., W. L. Hanson, L. P. Latham, C. A. Dawson, and W. W. Wagner, Jr. Distribution of pulmonary capillary transit times in recruited networks. *J. Appl. Physiol.* 69: 473–478, 1990.
5. Cerretelli, P. Limiting factors to oxygen transport on Mount Everest. *J. Appl. Physiol.* 40: 658–667, 1976.
6. Cerretelli, P., J. C. Cruz, L. E. Farhi, and H. Rahn. Determination of mixed venous $O_2$ and $CO_2$ tensions and cardiac output by a rebreathing method. *Respir. Physiol.* 1: 258–264, 1966.
7. Cerretelli, P., P. E. Di Prampero, and D. W. Rennie. Measurement of mixed venous oxygen tension by a modified rebreathing procedure. *J. Appl. Physiol.* 28: 707–711, 1970.
8. Clark, J. S., A. G. Cutillo, M. J. Criddle, D. V. Collins, F. L. Farr, A. H. Bigler, and A. D. Renzetti, Jr. Gas-blood $P_{CO_2}$ and $P_{O_2}$ equilibration in a steady-state rebreathing dog preparation. *J. Appl. Physiol.* 56: 1229–1236, 1984.
9. Dempsey, J. A., P. G. Hanson, and K. S. Henderson. Exercise-induced arterial hypoxaemia in healthy human subjects at sea level. *J. Physiol.* 355: 161–175, 1984.
10. Farhi, L. E., and J. Rahn. A theoretical analysis of the alveolar-arterial $O_2$ difference with special reference to the distribution effect. *J. Appl. Physiol.* 7: 691–703, 1955.
11. Feder, M. E., R. J. Full, and J. Piiper. Elimination kinetics of acetylene and Freon 22 in resting and active lungless salamanders. *Respir. Physiol.* 72: 229–240, 1988.
12. Fordyce, W. E., and R. K. Kanter. Arterial-end tidal $P_{CO_2}$ equilibration in the cat during acute hypercapnia. *Respir. Physiol.* 73: 257–272, 1988.
13. Gatz, R. N., and J. Piiper. Anaerobic energy metabolism during severe hypoxia in the lungless salamander *Desmognathus fuscus (Plethodontidae)*. *Respir. Physiol.* 38: 377–384, 1979.
14. Guénard, H., N. Varène, and P. Vaida. Determination of lung capillary blood volume and membrane diffusing capacity in man by the measurements of NO and CO transfer. *Respir. Physiol.* 70: 113–120, 1987.
15. Gurtner, G. H., S. H. Song, and L. E. Farhi. Alveolar to mixed venous $P_{CO_2}$ difference under conditions of no gas exchange. *Respir. Physiol.* 7: 173–187, 1969.
16. Haab, P., G. Duc, R. Stucki, and J. Piiper. Les échanges gazeux en hypoxie et la capacité de diffusion pour l'oxygène chez le

chien narcotisé. *Acta Helv. Physiol.* 22: 203–227, 1964.

17. Haab, P., J. Piiper, and H. Rahn. Attempt to demonstrate the distribution component of the alveolar-arterial oxygen pressure difference. *J. Appl. Physiol.* 15: 235–240, 1960.

18. Hahn, G., I. Šipinková, C. Buess, M. Meyer, and J. Piiper. Multiple breath washout of He and $SF_6$ in panting dogs. *Respir. Physiol.* 82: 39–46, 1990.

19. Hammond, M. D., G. E. Gale, K. S. Kapitan, A. Ries, P. D. Wagner. Pulmonary gas exchange in humans during normobaric hypoxic exercise. *J. Appl. Physiol.* 61: 1749–1757, 1986.

20. Holland, R. A. B., W. van Hezewijk, and J. Zubzanda. Velocity of oxygen uptake by partly saturated adult and fetal human red cells. *Respir. Physiol.* 29: 303–314, 1977.

21. Holland, R. A. B., H. Shibata, P. Scheid, and J. Piiper. Kinetics of $O_2$ uptake and release by red cells in stopped-flow apparatus: effects of unstirred layer. *Respir. Physiol.* 59: 71–91, 1985.

22. Hook, C., M. Meyer, and J. Piiper. Model simulation of single-breath washout of insoluble gases from dog lungs. *J. Appl. Physiol.* 58: 802–811, 1985.

23. Hook, C., K. Yamaguchi, P. Scheid, and J. Piiper. Oxygen transfer of red blood cells: experimental data and model analysis. *Respir. Physiol.* 72: 65–82, 1988.

24. Hyde, R. W., R. J. M. Puy, W. F. Raub, and R. E. Forster. Rate of disappearance of labeled carbon dioxide from the lungs of humans during breath holding: a method for studying the dynamics of pulmonary $CO_2$ exchange. *J. Clin. Invest.* 47: 1535–1552, 1968.

25. Jennings, D. B., and C. C. Chen. Negative arterial-mixed expired $P_{CO_2}$ gradient during acute and chronic hypercapnia. *J. Appl. Physiol.* 38: 382–388, 1975.

26. Jennings, D. B., M. Meyer, T. Stokke, J. Piiper, and P. Scheid. Blood-gas $CO_2$ equilibration in lungs of unanesthetized dogs during hypercapnia. *J. Appl. Physiol.* 52: 1177–1180, 1982.

27. Kobayashi, H., B. Pelster, J. Piiper, and P. Scheid. Diffusion and perfusion limitation in alveolar $O_2$ exchange: shape of the blood $O_2$ equilibrium curve. *Respir. Physiol.* 83: 23–34, 1991.

28. Kobayashi, H., J. Piiper, and P. Scheid. Effect of the curvature of the $O_2$ equilibrium curve on alveolar $O_2$ uptake: theory. *Respir. Physiol.* 83: 255–260, 1991.

29. Lee, G. de J., and A. B. DuBois. Pulmonary capillary blood flow in man. *J. Clin. Invest.* 34: 1380–1390, 1955.

30. Loeppky, J. A., P. Scotto, H. Rieke, M. Meyer, and J. Piiper. Arterial-alveolar $CO_2$ equilibration in exercising dogs during prolonged rebreathing. *J. Appl. Physiol.* 58: 1654–1658, 1985.

31. Luijendijk, S. C. M., A. Zwart, W. R. de Vries, and E. M. Salet. The sloping alveolar plateaus at synchronous ventilation. *Pflügers Arch.* 384: 267–277, 1980.

32. Meyer, M. Gas mixing in dog lungs during high frequency ventilation studied by partial washout–single exhalation technique. *Respir. Physiol.* 82: 11–28, 1990.

33. Meyer, M., G. Hahn, C. Buess, U. Mesch, and J. Piiper. Pulmonary gas exchange in panting dogs. *J. Appl. Physiol.* 66: 1258–1263, 1989.

34. Meyer, M., C. Hook, H. Rieke, and J. Piiper. Gas mixing in dog lungs studied by single-breath washout of He and $SF_6$. *J. Appl. Physiol.* 55: 1795–1802, 1983.

35. Meyer, M., M. Mohr, H. Schulz, and J. Piiper. Sloping alveolar plateaus of $CO_2$, $O_2$, and intravenously infused $C_2H_2$ and $CHC1F_2$ in the dog. *Respir. Physiol.* 81: 137–151, 1990.

36. Meyer, M., and J. Piiper. Nitric oxide (NO), a new test gas for study of alveolar-capillary diffusion. *Eur. Respir. J.* 2: 494–496, 1989.

37. Meyer, M., P. Scheid, G. Riepl, H.-J. Wagner, and J. Piiper. Pulmonary diffusing capacities for $O_2$ and CO measured by a rebreathing technique. *J. Appl. Physiol. (Respirat. Environ. Exer. Physiol.)* 51: 1643–1650, 1981.

38. Meyer, M., K.-D. Schuster, H. Schulz, M. Mohr, and J. Piiper. Alveolar slope and dead space of He and $SF_6$ in dogs: Comparison of airway and venous loading. *J. Appl. Physiol.* 69: 937–944, 1990.

39. Meyer, M., K.-D. Schuster, H. Schulz, M. Mohr, and J. Piiper. Pulmonary diffusing capacities for nitric oxide and carbon monoxide determined by rebreathing in dogs. *J. Appl. Physiol.* 68: 2344–2357, 1990.

40. Mochizuki, M., T. Anso, H. Goto, A. Hamamoto, and Y. Makiguchi. The dependence of the diffusing capacity on the $HbO_2$ saturation of the capillary blood and on anemia. *Japan J. Physiol.* 8: 225–233, 1958.

41. Mundt, E., W. Schoedel, and H. Schwartz. Über die Gleichmässigkeit der Lungenbelüftung. *Pflügers Arch.* 244: 99–119, 1940.

42. Neufeld, G. R., S. Gobran, J. E. Baumgardner, S. J. Aukburg, M. Schreiner, and P. W. Scherer. Diffusivity, respiratory rate and tidal volume influence inert gas expirograms. *Respir. Physiol.* 84: 31–47, 1991.

43. Paiva, M., and L. A. Engel. The anatomical basis for the sloping alveolar plateau. *Respir. Physiol.* 44: 325–337, 1981.

44. Piiper, J. Unequal distribution of pulmonary diffusing capacity and the alveolar-arterial $P_{O_2}$ differences: theory. *J. Appl. Physiol.* 16: 493–498, 1961.

45. Piiper, J. Variations of ventilation and diffusing capacity to perfusion determining the alveolar-arterial $O_2$ difference: theory. *J. Appl. Physiol.* 16: 507–510, 1961.

46. Piiper, J. $O_2$-Austausch der isolierten Hundelunge im hypoxischen Bereich bei Veränderungen der Erythrocytenkonzentration und der Durchblutung. *Pflügers Arch.* 275: 193–214, 1962.

47. Piiper, J. Geschwindigkeit des $CO_2$-Austausches zwischen Erythrocyten und Plasma. *Pflügers Arch.* 278: 500–512, 1964.

48. Piiper, J. Blood-gas equilibration of $CO_2$ in pulmonary gas exchange of mammals and birds. *The Physiologist* 22: 54–59, 1979.

49. Piiper, J. Blood-gas equilibrium of carbon dioxide in lungs: a continuing controversy. *J. Appl. Physiol.* 60: 1–8, 1986.

50. Piiper, J., R. E. Canfield, and H. Rahn. Absorption of various inert gases from subcutaneous gas pockets in rats. *J. Appl. Physiol.* 17: 268–274, 1962.

51. Piiper, J., P. Cerretelli, D. W. Rennie, and P. E. di Prampero. Estimation of the pulmonary diffusing capacity for $O_2$ by a rebreathing procedure. *Respir. Physiol.* 12: 157–162, 1971.

52. Piiper, J., R. W. Gatz, and E. C. Crawford. Gas transport characteristics in an exclusively skin-breathing salamander, *Desmognathus fuscus (Plethodontidae).* In: *Respiration of Amphibious Vertebrates,* edited by G. M. Hughes. London: Academic, 1976, pp. 339–356.

53. Piiper, J., P. Haab, and H. Rahn. Unequal distribution of pulmonary diffusing capacity in the anesthetized dog. *J. Appl. Physiol.* 16: 499–506, 1961.

54. Piiper, J., M. Meyer, C. Marconi, and P. Scheid. Alveolar-capillary equilibration kinetics of $^{13}CO_2$ in human lungs studied by rebreathing. *Respir. Physiol.* 42: 29–41, 1980.

55. Piiper, J., and P. Scheid. Model for capillary-alveolar equilibration with special reference to $O_2$ uptake in hypoxia. *Respir. Physiol.* 46: 193–208, 1981.

56. Scheid, P., M. Meyer, and J. Piiper. Arterial-expired $P_{CO_2}$ differences in the dog during acute hypercapnia. *J. Appl. Physiol.* 47: 1074–1078, 1979.

57. Scheid, P., and J. Piiper. Blood-gas equilibrium of carbon dioxide in lungs: a critical review. *Respir. Physiol.* 39: 1–31, 1980.

58. Scherer, P. W., S. Gobran, S. J. Aukburg, J. E. Baumgardner, R. Bartkowski, and G. R. Neufeld. Numerical and experimental study of steady-state $CO_2$ and inert gas washout. *J. Appl. Physiol.* 64: 1022–1029, 1988.

59. Schoedel, W. Alveolarluft. *Ergebnisse der Physiologie* 39: 449–488, 1937.

60. Scotto, P., H. Rieke, H. J. Schmitt, M. Meyer, and J. Piiper. Blood-gas equilibration of $CO_2$ and $O_2$ in lungs of awake dogs during prolonged rebreathing. *J. Appl. Physiol.* 57: 1354–1359, 1984.

61. Šipinková, I., G. Hahn, A. Hillebrecht, M. Meyer, and J. Piiper. Expirograms of $O_2$, $CO_2$, and intravenously infused $C_2H_2$ and Freon-22 during panting in dogs. *J. Appl. Physiol.* 68: 2344–2357, 1990.

62. Steinbrook, R. A., V. Fencl, R. A. Gabel, D. E. Leith, and S. E. Weinberger. Reversal of arterial-to-expired $CO_2$ partial pressure differences during rebreathing in goats. *J. Appl. Physiol.* 55: 736–741, 1983.

63. Torre-Bueno, J. R., P. D. Wagner, H. A. Saltzman, G. E. Gale, and R. E. Moon. Diffusion limitation in normal humans during exercise at sea level and simulated altitude. *J. Appl. Physiol.* 58: 989–995, 1985.

64. Veicsteinas, A., H. Magnussen, M. Meyer, and P. Cerretelli. Pulmonary $O_2$ diffusing capacity at exercise by a modified rebreathing method. *Eur. J. Appl. Physiol.* 35: 79–88, 1976.

65. Wagner, P. D., G. E. Gale, R. E. Moon, J. R. Torre-Bueno, B. W. Stolp, and H. A. Saltzman. Pulmonary gas exchange in humans exercising at sea level and simulated altitude. *J. Appl. Physiol.* 61: 260–270, 1986.

66. Wagner, P. D., R. B. Laravuso, R. R. Uhl, and J. B. West. Continuous distributions of ventilation-perfusion ratios in normal subjects breathing air and 100% $O_2$. *J. Clin. Invest.* 54: 54–68, 1974.

67. Wagner, P. D., H. A. Saltzman, and J. B. West. Measurement of continuous distributions of ventilation-perfusion ratios: theory. *J. Appl. Physiol.* 36: 588–599, 1974.

68. Wagner, P. D., J. R. Sutton, J. T. Reeves, A. Cymerman, B. M. Groves, and M. K. Malconian. Operation Everest II: pulmonary gas exchange during a simulated ascent of Mt. Everest. *J. Appl. Physiol.* 63: 2348–2359, 1987.

69. Wagner, W. W., Jr., L. P. Latham, M. N. Gillespie, J. P. Guenther, and R. L. Capen. Direct measurement of pulmonary capillary transit times. *Science* 218: 379–381, 1982.

70. Wang, P. M., Q.-H. Yang, and S. J. Lai-Fook. Effect of positive airway pressure on capillary transit time in rabbit lung. *J. Appl. Physiol.* 69: 2262–2268, 1990.

71. Weibel, E. R. *Morphometry of the Human Lung.* New York: Springer, 1963.

72. Worth, H., and J. Piiper. Diffusion of helium, carbon monoxide and sulfur hexafluoride in gas mixtures similar to alveolar gas. *Respir. Physiol.* 32: 155–166, 1978.

73. Yamaguchi, K., J. Glahn, P. Scheid, and J. Piiper. Oxygen transfer conductance of human red blood cells at varied pH and temperature. *Respir. Physiol.* 67: 209–223, 1987.

74. Yamaguchi, K., A. Kawai, M. Mori, K. Asano, T. Takasugi, A. Umeda, and T. Yokoyama. Continuous distributions of ventilation and gas conductance to perfusion in the lungs. In: *Oxygen Transport to Tissue XII,* edited by J. Piiper, T. K. Goldstick, and M. Meyer. New York: Plenum, 1990, p. 625–636.

75. Yamaguchi, K., D. Nguyen-Phu, P. Scheid, and J. Piiper. Kinetics of $O_2$ uptake and release by human erythrocytes studied by a stopped-flow technique. *J. Appl. Physiol.* 58: 1215–1224, 1985.

# 8

# Pulmonary Mechanics and the Pulmonary Blood Vessels

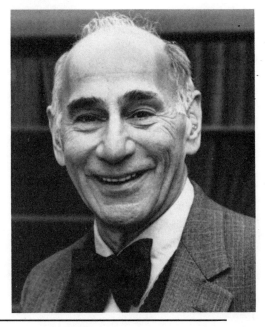

**Solbert Permutt, M.D.**

*Professor, Department of Medicine, Johns Hopkins Asthma and Allergy Center, Francis Scott Key Medical Center, Baltimore, Maryland*

When I was five years old, my mother took me to a movie called *Arrowsmith,* based on the great novel by Sinclair Lewis about a physician who became a medical scientist. From the time I saw that movie, I dreamed of becoming a medical scientist like Arrowsmith. The scenes in which Arrowsmith was conducting a clinical trial of a possible new therapy for bubonic plague were extremely frightening to me. From the book, which I read in my early teens, I know that the trial was being carried out on a native population of an island in the Caribbean. There were striking scenes of misery and death everywhere, and I was very sad when his wife who was a nurse died of the plague. My mother told me that I had great trouble

sleeping during the next week and continually awoke with horrible nightmares. The most vivid recollection I have of the movie is of the ending. Martin Arrowsmith is obviously leaving his hospital and laboratory for good, but then, remembering that he has forgotten something, he runs back into his laboratory and picks up a strange object that my mother told me was a microscope. I had assumed that when he was leaving the laboratory and hospital, he was giving up his dangerous work, and I was glad, but it was apparent to me, even at the age of five, that his going back for the microscope meant that he was going to continue his work. My feelings must have been a mixture of grave concern for him and even greater admiration for

From: Wagner WW, Jr, Weir EK (eds): *The Pulmonary Circulation and Gas Exchange.* ©1994, Futura Publishing Co Inc, Armonk, NY.

his bravery and dedication. When my mother explained to me what a microscope was, it took on special significance for me, because an instrument that made it possible to see invisible objects was something very powerful indeed, and I knew that when I grew up I wanted to be able to work with just such powerful instruments. Although the work might be dangerous, it would also be adventurous, and I was willing to take the risks in the same way that a policeman or fireman does.

At about the same age, I remember coloring pictures of biblical scenes in our Sunday School class. We got a gold star if we colored a picture well, a blue star if not so well, and no star if it was colored poorly. I do not think I got many gold stars because, as I later discovered, I was colorblind. Nevertheless, one day while coloring a picture of Adam and Eve in the Garden of Eden, my friend Melvin Cohen remarked that this was not the way that Adam looked but that he really looked like an ape. I did not believe him, but when we looked in his sister's high school history textbook, we saw a strange picture of what I presume was a Neanderthal man, and the caption under the picture was "the first man." I had absolutely no doubt that the history book was accurate, and I concluded that what I was being taught in Sunday School was false. I did not think my Sunday School teachers were intentionally lying to me, but still I knew that what they were teaching me was not true. Why I was so much more ready to accept historical over biblical information I do not know, but from then on I had more confidence in scientific models than in explanations that invoked burning bushes, parted seas, and going to heaven in a fiery chariot. I read everything I could get my hands on about science, especially medical science and evolution.

Parallel to my interests in science, I began to develop an interest in mathematics. I was no more competent in arithmetic or mathematics than any of my classmates,

but I was more intensely interested and puzzled by a number of strange mysteries. Marvin Udelson, a friend of mine who was a few years ahead of me in school, kept showing me strange things that he was learning that bewildered me. He must have enjoyed my failure to understand what he clearly grasped. Did I know that there could be numbers that were less than nothing? All you had to do was put a minus sign in front of a regular number. How could there be something less than nothing? Did I know that you could divide a smaller number by a larger number? How could you divide a smaller number by a larger number? Did I know that if you didn't know what the answer was, you could substitute an $x$ for the answer and then by some magical process come out with the answer? I began to look at mathematical books in the library that were filled with the most beautiful and mysterious symbols. I then learned that these symbols were the language of science. I knew that if I could learn to use such symbols along with instruments like microscopes, I could make important discoveries and probably have lots of fun at the same time. That is what I wanted to do when I grew up. In essence, it is what I have tried to do with my life, but I encountered some major detours along the way.

After a year of premedicine at the University of Alabama, I was drafted into the army in 1943 at 18 years of age. The army sent me to school in uniform for both premedicine and one year of medical school before the war was over in 1945. In 1949, after receiving my M.D. degree, I took a year's medical internship at the University of Chicago. I loved the exhilarating intensity of housestaff training, but clinical medicine was not what I had pictured for myself. I wanted to be working at "the cutting edge of science." So instead of continuing with my housestaff training, I went to work in the Department of Anatomy at the University of Chicago on the properties of the intercellular matrix, then called the ground substance, in the laboratory of Isadore Gersh. Even by today's standards, I was working at least near the cutting edge.

The next two years were pure misery. It was not that I had no moments of great joy in the work—on the contrary, I could sometimes feel pure ecstasy, but that was part of the problem. I could not control the rapid oscillations between feeling that my work was on the verge of being outstanding and that all of my endeavors were completely worthless, that I was second rate, and that medical science was for someone else, not me. I probably could not have chosen a field for which I was more unsuited. Most of my time was spent describing microscopic sections. Besides my color blindness, something more fundamental was in my way than having chosen the wrong field. I was not mature enough to know how to cope with the problems of working in science as a professional and doing what had to be done without inspiration. For me it was ecstasy or nothing. I began spending more and more of my time in the university commons playing chess and bridge and less time in the laboratory.

I also became heavily involved in what were then considered left-wing political activities right at the time the whole country was responding with mass hysteria to the dangers of communism, "the great Red scare." My rather mild political activities, such as supporting friendship with the Soviet Union and China and outlawing the atom bomb, put me into direct conflict with Joe McCarthy and his ilk.

During this awful period of my life, when the future looked so dismal, I met Loretta, my wife for more than 40 years. I was amazed then, and am still amazed today, that she had no concerns about a future with me. We got married in January of 1952.

In July of that year I gave up all notions of ever doing medical science and went back to my house staff training at the University of Chicago, but, by January of 1953, because of the doctor's draft, because we were involved in a shooting war with Korea, because I had my medical education at government expense during the Second World War, and because I refused to inform on my friends and associates in the political movements in which I had been involved, I was drafted into the army as a private. After finishing 12 weeks of basic training for enlisted men at Camp Pickett in Virginia as a medical corpsman, I was sent to Fitzsimmons Army Hospital in Denver at the rank of private.

Fitzsimmons Army Hospital was one of the outstanding institutions in the entire world in the field of tuberculosis, and I was lucky to have been sent there, even as an enlisted man. After a while, when the authorities saw that I was not interested in subverting the army, they assigned me as an assistant to William Harris, a remarkable physician, trained by Amberson, who later became the chief of the unit that Amberson had founded at Bellevue. My life was changed forever. He was an inspiring teacher. After a few months of exposure to him, I never wanted to do anything except pulmonary medicine, and I would have been perfectly happy to spend the rest of my career in the field of tuberculosis. Bill wanted to set up a nontuberculous chest service at Fitzsimmons, and he apparently persuaded the establishment at Fitzsimmons that I was capable of running the large tuberculosis ward of which he had been in charge. This I was allowed to do as a private with the help of a nurse who was a major. Bill went on to create the first nontuberculous chest unit at the hospital. During this same period of time, I also received outstanding support from William Stead, now the director of the tuberculosis programs of the Arkansas Department of Health, who taught me how to use pulmonary function tests in the clinical evaluation of patients with respiratory impairment.

I now was very happy. I rejected the notion of becoming a medical scientist like Martin Arrowsmith; being a good pulmonary clinician was more than enough to satisfy my now considerably modified ambitions. I still had a few obstacles to overcome, however. The principal one was that McCarthy accused the army of employing communists. This was the basis of the Army-McCarthy Hearings at that time. The army responded in a most courageous and forthright manner—after drafting me, they gave me an undesirable discharge.* This was in April 1954, and I now had a serious problem. If I was going to be a pulmonary physician, I needed more house staff training and more clinical training in pulmonary medicine. It should not be surprising that there were essentially no jobs whatsoever available to me when I informed the selection committees of my dubious relations with the United States Army, which I believed I had to do because I knew my story would come out later anyway. I had outstanding letters of support from Bill Harris, Bill Stead, and even the general in charge of Fitzsimmons Army Hospital, but no house staff positions or fellowships were offered. Late in June of 1954, Robert Bloch, a former professor of medicine at the University of Chicago whom I had known and who was then head of the Pulmonary Division of Montefiore Hospital in New York, telegraphed me that he would like me to be his chief resident, but he could not offer me the position unless I was willing to come to New York at my expense and be interviewed by the board of trustees of the hospital. I went to New York, the board of trustees approved of me, and I finished my formal house staff training there.

My 2 years at Montefiore Hospital were very happy ones. The first year I supervised the interns and residents who rotated through the Pulmonary Division as part of their required house staff training in medicine. The following year I became the chief resident of the Department of Medicine. I was asked to consider a part-time or full-time clinical position in the Pulmonary Division following my training, and it was my firm intention to remain in New York in clinical pulmonary disease.

While at Montefiore Hospital I became interested in several scientific questions that grew out of my clinical activities. What controlled the size of a tuberculous cavity? Did pneumothorax decrease the size of the cavity because the pressure within the cavity decreased relative to the pressure at the pleural surface of the lobe, or did the cavity decrease in size because the surrounding lung tissue was under less elastic tension? I was fascinated with the controversies I read about in the medical literature. Some favored pressure, others tension, but it seemed to me that elastic tension was more important. A hole in a rubber membrane gets smaller when it is not stretched even though there is no change in pressure. I could not have realized at the time that the relationship between the size of the cavity as a function of distending pressure versus elastic tension of the surrounding tissue would become a major focus of my later scientific work: mechanical interdependence of the elements of the lungs.

As I read more about how the partial pressures of oxygen and carbon dioxide in the arterial blood were dependent on the state of pulmonary function, it seemed to me that the gas pressures of the venous blood would reflect the state of systemic function. I started spending some time in the cardiac catheterization laboratory and even carried out a few unfocused projects on oxygen saturation in venous blood.

My intense interest in scientific ques-

---

*In keeping with the increasing recognition of the perniciousness of McCarthyism, the *Undesirable Discharge* I received on April 29, 1954, was changed to a *General (under honorable conditions) Discharge* on November 12, 1957, and to an *Honorable Discharge* on April 14, 1958. By the end of 1958, I had received back pay as a medical officer with the rank of captain.

tions and my enthusiastic communication of these ideas in numerous conversations with my colleagues at Montefiore led a number of my advisors to conclude that I showed considerable promise for creative scientific work in medicine. They suggested that I would do well to consider training with one of the groups that was applying modern concepts of respiratory physiology and pulmonary function testing to the newly developing field of pulmonary medicine.

I would have liked to believe that my advisors were correct, but I felt that my knowledge and enthusiasm for science that I had since a young child were overrated as predictors of success. I thought I had already had the opportunity to become a medical scientist, and I had failed. I did not want to fail again. My advisors, persuaded me, however, that one or two years of research training in respiratory physiology would make me a better clinician and teacher if I chose to return to Montefiore. Loretta also encouraged me to try one more time to see if I might have a future as a medical scientist.

In early 1956, I visited several groups that were at the forefront of modern respiratory physiology and pulmonary medicine. I decided to apply for a fellowship with Richard L. Riley's group at Johns Hopkins because Riley had developed the only method of measuring blood $O_2$ and $CO_2$ tensions then in use and also had been involved with the development of cardiac catheterization through his work with Cournand and Richards. I thought work in his laboratory would provide me an opportunity to test my ideas about the significance of venous gas tensions. Riley offered me a fellowship starting in July 1956 with support from the National Foundation for Infantile Paralysis.

What a magnificent place was Riley's laboratory! There were not yet clinical subspecialty divisions of the Department of Medicine at Hopkins. Riley's laboratory was part of the Physiological Division of the Department of Medicine, which contained the pulmonary function laboratories and the heart station of the Johns Hopkins Hospital. Only two members of the faculty were at Riley's laboratory: Riley himself and Richard Shepard. Riley's laboratory was filled with fellows from all over the world; the interaction between the fellows with each other and with Riley and Shepard was unforgettably exciting and productive. A few large projects in clinical investigation were being pushed forward by Shepard and Riley with the participation of the fellows. The fellows also were responsible for consulting and performing pulmonary function studies on patients from the Johns Hopkins Hospital. Most of their activities, however, arose spontaneously through their contacts with each other.

After I had been in the laboratory for a few months, Harry Martin, a fellow in his second year of training, asked me if I would be interested in working with him on measuring the static pressure-volume relations of adult subjects to see if the lungs lost elastic recoil with age. I accepted the invitation. I had first met Harry Martin at Fitzsimmons Army Hospital, and I had great affection for him because he had never let the difference between his rank of captain and my rank of private interfere with warm and friendly relations between us and our families.

We assumed the pressure in a balloon in the esophagus would approximate the pressure on the pleural surface of the lungs, and the difference between airway and pleural pressure when there was no air flow would be a measure of the elastic recoil pressure of the lungs. We measured the pressure-volume relations throughout the entire vital capacity range and measured residual volume by helium dilution. We thought the shape of the curves and the magnitude of hysteresis represented a fundamental property of the lungs.[20] In a sense, this is true, but it was not as simple as we thought.

J. B. L. (Jack) Howell, another fellow in the department, and I were assigned the task of giving demonstrations of pulmonary function tests to Hopkins medical students in the spring of 1957. Howell was an expert in pulmonary mechanics. In addition to his medical degree, he had received a Ph.D. in physiology from studies on the mechanical properties of the lungs of human subjects while working in the laboratory of Sampson Wright at the Middlesex Hospital in London. We both thought it would be a great idea to show the medical students how to measure the elastic properties of the lungs, as Martin and I had just done and Howell had done for his Ph.D. degree. We thought it would be much simpler and much more reproducible to carry out these measurements in open chest anesthetized dogs, and we would not have to do a hard sell to the medical students to get them to swallow balloons. But we never made the demonstration to the students because we could never get a single reproducible curve. We got markedly different recoil pressures at the same lung volume depending on the inflation history to achieve the volume (Fig. 1).

A lung was degassed in vacuo, inflated to 30 cm $H_2O$, then deflated to 0 cm $H_2O$. An inflation-deflation procedure was then carried out as shown in Figure 1. The pressure was changed by 2 cm water steps, and the volume was measured at 1 min following the change. In 11 of 13 dogs, we produced marked degrees of trapping. It was clear that the trapping was due to airway closure occurring at progressively higher airway pressures, as indicated by the deflation inflections moving progressively to the right and the progressively higher opening pressures on inflation.

John Clements, who was then working at the Army Chemical Center, fre-

quently visited Riley's department, just at the time he was forming his ideas on the significance of surfactant. We assumed the overinflated state that was produced by the slow inflation-deflation cycles was a function of altered surface tension, because the whole cycle could be repeated if the lung was degassed in vacuo and a new surface formed. Further, the saline pressure-volume curve (which John Clements showed us how to carry out) was normal.

I presented these findings at the fall meetings of the Physiological Society in Iowa in 1957.[18] It was my first presentation of a paper at a scientific society. Speaking for both Jack Howell and myself here is what I said:

*The fact that repeated inflation-deflation cycles lead to a condition where bronchi are occluded with positive pressure across the lung is somewhat surprising. Certainly, it would appear unlikely that the properties of the bronchial wall have been altered in such a manner to cause them to close at higher pressures across the lung. One possibility is that the critical closing pressure across the bronchi remains the same, but the interstitial pressure surrounding the bronchi has increased above the ambient pressure of the lung.\**

What Howell and I were getting at was a model of the lung that was essentially a system of small bubbles within an elastic tissue matrix. We thought that the slow and repeated inflation-deflations led to an accumulation of so much of John Clements's surfactant that the bubbles had virtually no recoil pressure on deflation. Nevertheless, the recoil of the stretched tissue elements produced a high interstitial pressure that squeezed on the bronchi

---

\*In retrospect, the relationship between critical closure and surrounding pressure, which has dominated my thinking for 35 years, was implicitly considered in my first presentation of a paper at a scientific society.

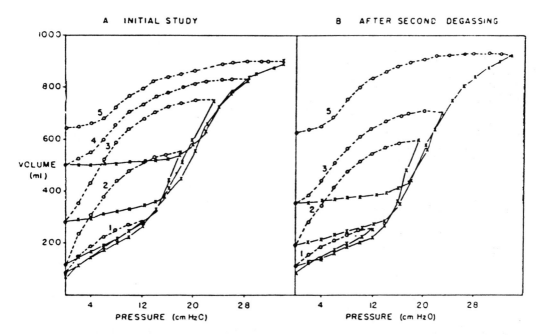

**Figure 1.** The lung from a dog was degassed in vacuo and placed in a plethysmograph with the trachea connected to an external spirometer. The lobe was inflated by lowering the pressure within the plethysmograph. It was first inflated to a transpulmonary pressure of 30 cm $H_2O$, then deflated to zero transpulmonary pressure. Then a series of five inflation-deflation cycles were carried out. These relations are shown on the left. Pressure is equal to atmospheric minus plethysmographic pressure (transpulmonary pressure), and the volume of the lobe is determined from the spirometer. The entire process was repeated for the curves shown on the right, except that the fourth inflation-deflation cycle was omitted. (From presentation at fall meeting of the American Physiological Society in 1957.)

and caused them to close at high lung volumes. If the positive interstitial pressure were squeezing on the airways, it must also be squeezing on blood vessels, and if we could attach a manometer to the blood vessels under conditions where their volume was held constant, we could use the blood vessels like an esophageal balloon—but a balloon within the interstitium of the lung rather than within the pleural cavity. Donald Proctor, who had worked with Harry Martin on the pressure-volume relations of excised bronchi,[10] joined us for these experiments.

The method we used is shown in Figure 2. We inflated the lobes by lowering the pressure within the box: negative-pressure inflation. At the time we carried out this work, there was still widespread belief that positive and negative pressure inflation had different effects on pulmonary blood vessels. We showed that the effects were identical as long as the vascular and airway pressures had the same relation to each other as is shown in the figure.

The vein and artery of a lobe of a dog's lobe were connected to a common tube, which in turn was connected to one end of a water-filled manometer. Between the vessels and manometer was a small air-filled syringe, which created an air space between the vessel and manometer. The vascular pressure at a transpulmonary pressure of zero was set by controlling the level of the liquid meniscus in the vertical tube relative to the top of the lobe. As the lobe was inflated, the meniscus was kept

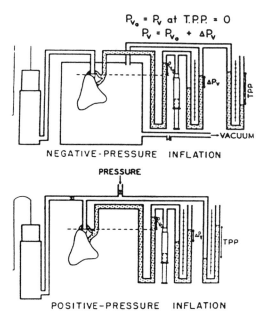

$P_{V_0} = P_V$ at T.P.P. $= 0$
$P_V = P_{V_0} + \Delta P_V$

NEGATIVE-PRESSURE INFLATION

POSITIVE-PRESSURE INFLATION

**Figure 2.** Diagram of apparatus to measure changes in vascular pressure when vascular volume is held constant. Vascular volume is assumed to be constant when meniscus in manometer nearest lobe is kept at a fixed level. Level of meniscus can be controlled by pushing or withdrawing plunger of syringe. Change in pressure necessary to keep vascular volume constant is shown by $\Delta P_V$. Total vascular pressure ($P_V$) is the algebraic sum of $PV_0$ and $\Delta P_V$. $PV_0$ is the vascular pressure measured relative to the top of the lobe at a transpulmonary pressure of zero. (From reference 19.)

at the same level by pulling or pushing the barrel of the syringe and recording the pressure on the manometer necessary to keep the level fixed. We believed that most people would think that the pressure in the manometer would not change because they would assume that the interstitial pressure would remain constant and equal to pleural pressure. We were hoping to see a rise in the pressure around the vessels due to an increase in the interstitial pressure, and because of our nearly complete ignorance of the pulmonary circulation, we believed that this would be a big discovery. And that is exactly what happened—in the first experiment.

I remember vividly how we called in other fellows to share with us these momentous findings. The same results happened on several more occasions, but then one day, when we grabbed hold of some unsuspecting (and probably bored) colleague to show him *truth,* exactly the opposite happened: with lung inflation, the pressure fell. This was a jarring emotional experience consisting of a mixture of some surprise, some disappointment, and utter confusion.

After a while we learned how to make the pressure go either way or hardly change at all by setting the initial level of the meniscus a little above, a little below, or right at the top of the lobe (Fig. 3). With the initial level just a few centimeters above the top of the lobe, we had to apply more than 20 cm $H_2O$ positive pressure from the syringe, and with the initial level a few centimeters below the top of the lobe, we had to apply more than 20 cm $H_2O$ negative pressure. These results established that lung inflation could either squeeze or pull on the pulmonary vessels. Although we could control the direction of the change, we did not know why a small change in the initial pressure could have such a profound difference on the response.

Now other people became interested in what was going on. Dick Shepard referred to this as the "flower pot" experiment because that is what he was reminded of when he looked at the symmetrical arrangement of the curves of Figure 3. Jack Howell and I would take the graphs of the experimental data to Dick Riley's house to discuss them with him. He was staying at home taking chemotherapy for a mild flare-up of his tuberculosis. It was Riley who figured out what was going on. He said that the shape of a lobe during inflation changed from something like a thin slice of pie to a thick slice with the point of the slice analogous to the hilum. He believed that during inflation the wid-

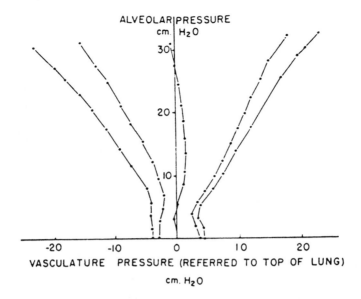

**Figure 3.** Vascular pressure relative to the pressure at the pleural surface of a dog's lobe required to maintain a constant vascular volume, plotted against alveolar pressure relative to pleural pressure. The hydrostatic level is the top of the lobe. (From reference 23.)

ening of the lobe would exert a traction on the larger blood vessels, while the smaller peripheral vessels would be compressed by the increasing pressure in the alveolar spaces. He said that we should be able to model this with a Krogh spirometer by having struts pull on an elastic tube traversing the spirometer from its axis and terminating inside of a balloon within the body of the spirometer itself. We would see that the conducting tube was widened by the attached struts while at the same time that portion of the tube within the balloon would be compressed. We made a transparent Krogh spirometer, but we never had to put the struts in place, for when a balloon was inflated inside the spirometer, we could see the fluid level rise (Figure 4)!

This seemed then and even now both beautiful and amazing, but the explanation is simple. The space around the balloon was essentially constant, and the enlargement of the spirometer produced by

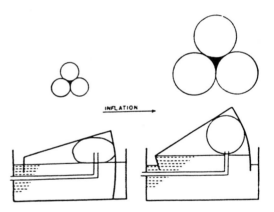

**Figure 4.** As the pressure in the balloon within the Krogh spirometer was inflated with positive pressure, the fluid level within the spirometer rose, indicating that the pressure on the outer surface of the balloon had become negative relative to atmospheric pressure at the same time that the pressure within the balloon became positive relative to atmospheric pressure. Similarly, the pressure within the space confined by three cylindrical balloons became increasingly negative relative to atmospheric pressure as the pressure within the balloons became increasingly positive. (From reference 23.)

the positive pressure in the balloon produced a negative pressure of the surrounding air. In an analogous way, we reasoned that the constancy of the interstitial volume of the lung tissue required a negative pressure as the alveoli enlarged with positive pressure. We also showed that if we put three cylindrical balloons inside a third balloon, simultaneous inflation of the three balloons caused the pressure between the balloons to become negative.

We now reversed our initial concept of interstitial pressure: rather than being positive, we inferred that it is usually negative and becomes increasingly so with lung inflation. Only years later did Ed Faridy and I figure out what caused the closure of the airways in the overinflated state.[2]

This is how we explained the flower pot experiment: inflation always pulled on the larger vessels and squeezed on the smaller ones. At low initial pressure, there was not much liquid in the small vessels, so inflation was dominated by what happened to the larger ones. At high initial pressure, more liquid was pushed out of the small vessels than could be accommodated by the expanding larger ones. At intermediate pressures, the opposing effects on simultaneously compressed and expanded vessels was balanced. We became confident in the soundness of this concept when we examined the effect of lung inflation on vascular volume at constant vascular pressure (Fig. 5).[19] The top panel shows the effect of a change in vascular volume on the abscissa against lung volume on the ordinate. The lower panel shows the change in vascular volume against transpulmonary pressure. Each panel shows three curves for three different vascular pressures. The vascular pressure was held constant by connecting the vein and artery to a horizontal burette held at a fixed level relative to the top of the lobe. On the left, the burette was 4 cm above the top of the lobe; on the right, 4 cm below the top of the lobe; and for the

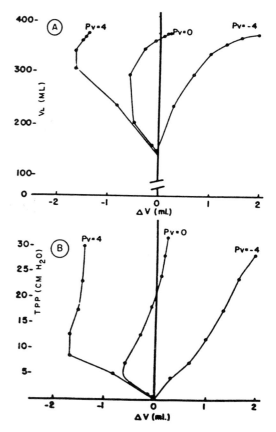

**Figure 5.** A: relationship between air volume of lobe ($V_L$) and changes in vascular volume ($\Delta V$) at three different vascular pressures ($P_v$) in a typical experiment. B: same experiment as in 5A, showing relationship between transpulmonary pressure (TPP) and changes in vascular volume ($\Delta V$) at three different vascular pressures ($P_v$). (From reference 19.)

middle curve, the burette was at the top of the lobe.

Consider first the left-hand curves. As the lung was inflated, more liquid was squeezed from the small vessels than could be accommodated by the larger ones, and liquid moved from the vessels to the burettes. With a sufficiently high level of inflation, there was no more liquid to be squeezed out, so only the expansion of the larger vessels was apparent, and liquid moved from the burettes into the pulmonary vessels. For the middle curve, qualitatively the pattern was the same, but there was less liquid in the compressed vessels so the expansion of the larger vessels became apparent at a lower state of inflation. On the right, with still less liquid in the compressed vessels, the expansion of the larger vessels was apparent throughout the range of inflation.

These curves were fairly convincing, but there was only a limited range of inflation to demonstrate the expansion when the vascular pressure was high. We wanted to study the larger vessels independently and show that they expanded throughout inflation regardless of the vascular pressure. To do this we needed a way to block the smaller vessels from the larger. It was again through sheer ignorance that we were led to a method that worked. For reasons not at all apparent to me now, we thought that it would be better to do experiments with the blood vessels containing dextran solution rather than blood. We later showed that the experiments worked perfectly well with blood in the vessels, so I do not know why we felt compelled to remove it and replace it with something else. Nevertheless, the experiments were always preceded by a prolonged washout of the blood with the dextran solution, and often the lungs became somewhat edematous. Jack said that he remembered reading that an excised kidney perfused with kerosene instead of blood did not become edematous.* We purchased some kerosene from a small nearby store, but we found that we could not get it to pass through the pulmonary vessels even with very high pressures, presumably because of interfacial surface tension. After many unsuccessful attempts to establish a block with plastic microspheres or lycopodium spores between the small and the large blood vessels, it occurred to us that the kerosene, still sitting around the lab, might provide just the type of block we needed for the same reason that we could not perfuse the lung with it. We emptied the small pulmonary vessels by high inflation pressure and then replaced the dextran with kerosene, which filled only the larger vessels while the small vessels remained unfilled. Kerosene always moved into the pulmonary vessels with inflation regardless of whether the burettes were above or below the top of the lobe.[4]

We now had a method of dividing the pulmonary vessels into two compartments, and we could show that the two compartments responded in an exactly opposite fashion to lung inflation. The pressure-volume relations of the vascular bed when the blood vessels were filled with kerosene were those of the large vessels, which were expanded by lung inflation. The pressure-volume characteristics of the small blood vessels, which were compressed with lung inflation, could be studied by subtracting the kerosene pressure-volume curve from the dextran pressure-volume curve (Fig. 6). We called the two compartments the *expanded* and *compressed* compartments. Jere Mead wrote a review article for the *Handbook of Physiology* on lung inflation and hemodynamics in 1964[11] and designated the vessels that composed our two compartments *alveolar* and *extra-alveolar* vessels, much more suitable words than what we chose, and these words have stuck.

We later found that Charles Clifford Macklin had used a latex solution in much the same way that we had used kerosene. He had understood the significance of our major findings in 1946,[9] but his work had been given almost no consideration in the literature on pulmonary circulation. Macklin not only anticipated the compartmentalization of the pulmonary blood vessels, but he also contributed to our

---

*I think I know where Jack might have gotten the idea. Eleven pages after the abstract of reference 18 in *The Physiologist* of 1957 is the following abstract: *Effect of perfusion pressure on the "circulating volume" of the isolated canine kidney perfused with a kerosene–mineral oil mixture* by Irving Green et al.!

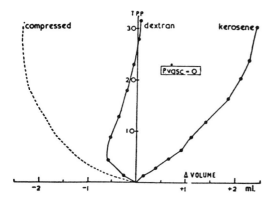

**Figure 6.** Relationship between transpulmonary pressure and change in vascular volume at a vascular pressure of 0 cm $H_2O$ (hydrostatic reference at top of lobe). Center and right-hand curves represent volume changes in dextran-containing and kerosene-containing vascular bed, respectively. Curve representing volume change of compressed portion of vascular bed (broken line) is constructed from difference between these two curves. (From reference 4.)

knowledge of pulmonary surface-active material. This work too had been unappreciated. In 1976, Staub, Clements, Proctor, and I held a symposium of the work of Charles Clifford Macklin that unfortunately had not been appreciated during his life.[24] He had died in 1959.

Up to this point, we had studied the pulmonary vessels only under static conditions. We then became interested in how lung inflation affected flow through the pulmonary vessels. If the small pulmonary vessels did not resist collapse and were functionally surrounded by the gas pressure in the alveoli, we predicted that inflating a lobe at constant vascular pressure would cause a decrease in the flow because of the greater effect of compression of small vessels than expansion of the larger ones and complete cessation of flow when the alveolar pressure equaled the pulmonary arterial pressure measured relative to the most dependent portion of the lobe. Such an experiment is shown in Figure 7.[23]

The lobe was perfused from an arterial reservoir 12 cm above the most dependent portion of the lobe to a venous reservoir at a lower level. We predicted that the flow would cease when the alveolar pressure was raised to 12 cm $H_2O$. This is where the arrow is placed. It was apparent that there was virtual cessation of the flow at that point, but a small amount of flow still remained until the alveolar pressure was raised to a considerably higher level. We suggested that this remaining flow might be occurring through vessels at the junctions of the alveolar septa (corner vessels)[22] because they would be protected against the full transmission of alveolar pressure due to the highly curved surfaces. But this small amount of flow did not keep us from feeling rather certain that most of the vessels of the compressed compartment, or alveolar vessels, as they were later called, were surrounded by pressure equal to alveolar pressure.[4]

In 1958, I went to the National Jewish Hospital in Denver as the director of both the pulmonary function and cardiac catheterization laboratories. Jack Howell went back to England, where he later became

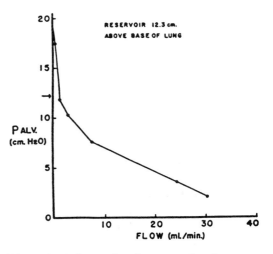

**Figure 7.** Relationship between alveolar pressure relative to pleural pressure (Palv) and pulmonary vascular flow and the lobe of a dog perfused from a reservoir 12.3 cm above the most dependent part. The horizontal arrow is at Palv = 12.3 cm $H_2O$. (From reference 23.)

chairman of medicine and then dean of the medical school at Southamptom. He has been a recent president of the British Medical Society. I now began working with Baruch Bromberger-Barnea and Harry Bane in a fine animal research facility (Fig. 8). We wanted to know how lung inflation affected the pulmonary circulation during life. We hoped to show that the highly artificial experiments on excised lobes with the blood replaced by dextran or kerosene had some relevance.

We measured pulmonary blood flow by the Fick principle using steady-state

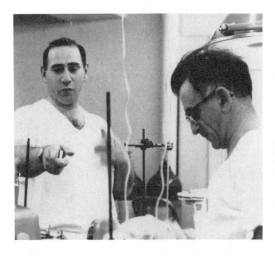

**Figure 8a.** Solbert Permutt (left) and Baruch Bromberger-Barnea working at the National Jewish Hospital in Denver in 1958.

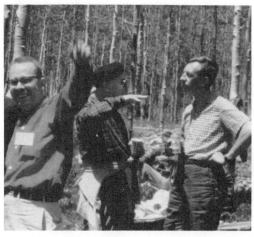

**Figure 8b.** Harry Bane, André Cournand, and John West. Aspen conference, 1962.

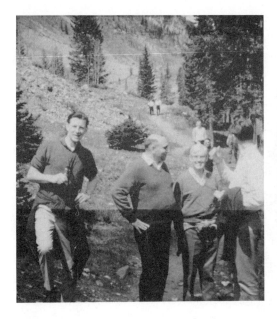

**Figure 8c.** J. B. L. Howell, Sol Permutt, and Dick Riley. Aspen conference, 1962.

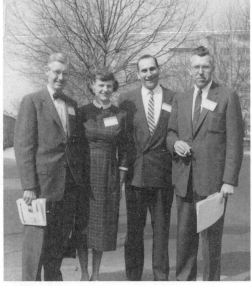

**Figure 8d.** Dick Riley, his wife Polly, Sol Permutt, and Richard Shephard. Federation meeting, Philadelphia, 1958.

oxygen consumption and the difference in arterial oxygen content between the systemic and pulmonary arteries, and we attempted to systematically study how lung inflation affected pulmonary vascular resistance in anesthetized dogs. We made measurements with the dogs breathing either spontaneously or with intermittent positive pressure ventilation at various levels of end-expiratory pressure. We devised methods of increasing transpulmonary pressure at constant pleural pressure or increasing pleural pressure at constant transpulmonary pressure. We could change cardiac output by adding or withdrawing blood. We made 90 measurements of pulmonary vascular resistance in 14 dogs at various levels of transpulmonary pressure, pleural pressure, and cardiac output. I presented these findings at the fall meetings of the American Physiological Society in 1960[13]:

*Where lung size was increased, pulmonary vascular resistance showed* *an inverse relationship to left atrial minus alveolar pressure. . . . To us this suggests that the site of the increase in vascular resistance associated with increasing transpulmonary pressure is located in small vessels whose intraluminal pressure is approximated by left atrial pressure and whose extraluminal pressure is approximated by alveolar pressure.*

We considered the pulmonary circulation to have two resistances in series (Fig. 9). $R_1$ is the resistance of the arterial extra-alveolar vessels. $R_2$ is the resistance of the alveolar vessels. We assumed that the intraluminal pressure of the alveolar vessels was equal to left atrial pressure, and the pressure on the outer surface of the alveolar vessels was equal to the alveolar pressure. We believed that these two pressures algebraically summed to create some sort of graded constriction of the alveolar vessels to account for the negative correlation between pulmonary vascular

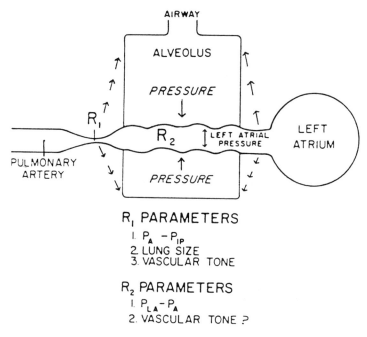

**Figure 9.** This is from the original slide shown at the fall meetings of the American Physiological Society in 1960 (reference 13). I think the model is still useful today.

resistance and left atrial minus alveolar pressure.

One afternoon between the fall meeting in 1960 and the spring meeting in 1961 of the American Physiological Society, it suddenly dawned on me that this was not how the system acted. I became convinced that our results were not explained by graded constrictions but, rather, by the effect of alveolar pressure on the back pressure to flow. When the left atrial pressure was greater than the alveolar pressure, it was the back pressure to flow through the pulmonary vessels, but when the alveolar pressure was greater than the left atrial pressure, the alveolar pressure was the back pressure to flow. It suddenly seemed inescapable that when alveolar pressure was higher than left atrial pressure, the pressure at the downstream end of the alveolar vessels could be neither higher nor lower than the alveolar pressure and therefore must be equal to the alveolar pressure.

I suddenly realized that afternoon that in effect a "waterfall" exists between the collapsible alveolar vessels and the left atrium, and raising or lowering the left atrial pressure when it was lower than alveolar pressure has no more influence on flow through the system than raising or lowering a bathtub affects the water coming out of a shower. That same afternoon, Baruch Bromberger, Harry Bane, and I started replotting the data we had presented at the fall meetings. If the waterfall idea were correct, there would be a single pressure-flow curve for each of the 14 dogs if the appropriate back pressure were used. That is essentially what we found, and we presented our ideas of the vascular

waterfall at the spring meeting of the American Physiological Society in 1961.[14]

We next tried to see if we could demonstrate an absence of the effect of a change in left atrial pressure when it was below alveolar pressure. We cannulated the pulmonary vein to the left lower lobe in open chest, anesthetized dogs and recorded on an x–y oscilloscope instantaneous changes in flow from the pulmonary vein as the pressure in the vein was slowly changed. The flow through the rest of the lungs was left undisturbed. Pulmonary arterial pressure was held constant at any desired level by either varying venous return or connecting a reservoir to the main pulmonary artery.

An example of the effect of varying pulmonary venous pressure on the flow through a pulmonary lobe at constant pulmonary arterial pressure is shown in Figure 10.[15] The lower curve was obtained first as venous pressure was slowly raised. Flow ceased when pulmonary venous pressure equaled pulmonary arterial pressure. The upper curve was then obtained as pulmonary venous pressure was slowly lowered. The dashed vertical curve is at the level of the alveolar pressure, which was held constant.

We were satisfied that the predictions of the waterfall model were supported, but we noted these exceptions: (1) hysteresis was present, (2) the point of maximum flow occurred at a higher level than alveolar pressure, and (3) as venous pressure was lowered below the level of alveolar pressure there was a significant decrease in flow.*

The most impressive support for the waterfall model came from the effect of a

---

*Several years ago, Fung and Yen attempted to account for the hysteresis and the decrease in flow as venous pressure was lowered beyond the level of the maximum flow. They used a distributive model that had the added feature of recruitment and derecruitment of alveolar vessels. (Fung, Y. C., Yen, R. T. New theory of pulmonary blood flow in zone 2 condition. *J. Appl. Physiol.* 60: 138–150, 1986). The reason the maximal flow occurred at a level higher than alveolar pressure suggested to us that tone in alveolar vessels could be additive to the effect of alveolar pressure. This certainly appears to be so in hypoxic pulmonary vasoconstriction in the pig (see reference 19).

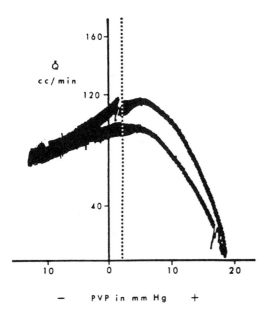

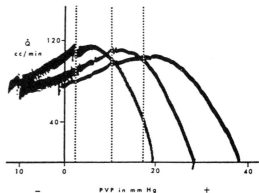

**Figure 11.** The relationship between flow ($\dot{Q}$) and pulmonary venous pressure (PVP) at three different pulmonary arterial pressures and alveolar pressures in the left lower lobe of an open chest dog. (From reference 15.)

**Figure 10.** The relationship between flow ($\dot{Q}$) and pulmonary venous pressure (PVP) at constant pulmonary arterial pressure in the left lower lobe of an open chest dog. The broken vertical line represents the level where alveolar pressure in the lobe was held constant. The lower curve was obtained first, as venous pressure was raised; the upper curve was then obtained, as venous pressure was lowered. (From reference 15.)

change in alveolar pressure on the relationship between pulmonary venous pressure and flow. If the waterfall model is correct, a change in alveolar pressure should only change the position of the curve, not its shape. We were impressed (and I still am) that the effect of increasing alveolar pressure had little effect on the shape of the curves (Fig. 11).[15] An increase in alveolar pressure caused a slight decrease in the slope of the pressure-flow curve at pulmonary venous pressures close to the level of the pulmonary arterial pressure, but the major effect was merely a displacement of the curves in the direction of the change in alveolar pressure, and the shift was essentially equal to the change in alveolar pressure.

When Jack Howell and I were still working together at Hopkins, he told me how Moran Campbell had put a condom in a cigar box, which he pressurized to create a special type of load against which human subjects breathed, now called a threshold load. Jack and I always referred to such a system as a Campbell resistor. Shortly before my presentation of the waterfall model at the spring meetings of the American Physiological Society in 1961, I was explaining to John Clements how the pressure-flow relations of a Campbell resistor were like those of a waterfall. He was shocked at my ignorance and informed me that such a system was called a Starling resistor, which Starling had used in his heart-lung preparations. My career has relied on Starling resistors, both conceptually and experimentally ever since.*

In June of 1962, at the Fifth Annual

---

*As a major focus of my work I have used the Starling resistor model and the waterfall analogy to analyze the effects of smooth muscle tone on blood vessels and airways. This concept has been applied by many of my colleagues and other workers to analyze the effects of bronchomotor tone and the pressure-flow relations of the coronary, cerebral, renal, and striated muscle circulations. See S. Permutt, and R. L. Riley, Hemodynamics of collapsible vessels with tone: the vascular waterfall. *J. Appl. Physiol.* 18: 924–932, 1963.

Aspen Conference, I presented a model of the pulmonary circulation that consisted of nothing more than one Starling resistor stacked on top of another. I was satisfied that such a model could very nicely, or at least to my satisfaction, explain the data from every study of the effect of lung inflation on the pulmonary circulation of which I was then aware.[15] This model has been used extensively by a number of investigators to simplify what might otherwise appear complicated. The most notable success was by John West and his colleagues, who explained the effect of gravity on the distribution of pulmonary blood flow.[26,27] The opposite effects of lung inflation on the alveolar versus extraalveolar vessels has been used to provide understanding of the effect of lung inflation on fluid balance[7,12] and the vasoconstrictor effects of hypoxia.[1,25] The concepts have also been used to explain how vasoactive agents and pulmonary edema influence hemodynamics.[5,6,28] To me, the greatest success of the model is that it has provided a framework that allows a systematic approach to the mechanics of the pulmonary circulation. At the end of the published paper from the Aspen Conference of 1962[24] this is what we said:

> . . . we feel that the model we have presented allows the integration of a number of hitherto isolated facts concerning the pulmonary circulation into a coherent picture. To the extent that the model fails to give a complete explanation of experimental findings, it is, perhaps, most useful, for one must think in terms of new experiments and improved models.

Anyone who knows me at all must realize that I was not being sincere. I have tenaciously hung on to every detail of the model long after it was decent to do so. Recent studies suggest that the major effects of gravity cannot be explained by the model we proposed.[3] There is evidence from studies of Dawson, Linehan, and coworkers that changes in pulmonary venous pressure continue to have some influence on alveolar vessels that would not be predicted by the waterfall model.[8,21] Linehan and Dawson explain such effects by invoking a variable resistance model rather than a waterfall or Starling resistor model. Of course, I had completely rejected the variable resistance model with the sudden revelation of the waterfall in 1961!

I must admit that I get a little pleasure when people criticize the model. This means that it is still very useful. When you are young, you are always worried about what people are saying about you, but when you grow old, you realize that they are usually saying absolutely nothing. Criticism is a lot better than nothing!

As I look over my work on the pulmonary circulation during the last 35 years, it is fascinating to see the constructive role of complete ignorance at the start. Jack Howell, Don Proctor, and I would have never carried out the flower pot experiments if we had had the slightest awareness of the literature on pulmonary circulation at the time. There had been heated controversies on the effect of inflation of the lungs on the pulmonary circulation for more than 200 years prior to the time of our initial work. Interestingly, nearly all of the controversies were not related to what the experimental results were but, rather, to the interpretation of these results. Initially our interpretation of our experimental results was met with great resistance and skepticism. It is still somewhat painful to read the critical and even harsh comments made of our work by members of the pulmonary circulation establishment in the discussion that followed two major presentations.[16,23] At the time we carried out our initial experiments, anyone who had made even a cursory review of the literature on pulmonary circulation would have realized that when the lung was inflated under conditions where the pressure in the alveoli rose relative to the vascular pressure, so-called positive-pressure inflation, the pulmonary vessels would be squeezed. Anyone who knew anything about the literature on the pulmonary circulation would have been nearly certain that one would have to apply a pressure to the pulmonary vessels to keep their volume constant when the lung was inflated, something we thought would be a great discovery. The level of certainty was so great that no one had ever carried out studies on the effect of inflation on vascular pressure at constant vascular volume. Our ignorance gave us the opportunity of making a novel observation on the pulmonary circulation, that is, positive-pressure inflation causes a decrease in the vascular pressure at constant vascular volume when the vascular volume is low, in spite of the predictable increase when the volume is high.

These experiments forced us to make a comprehensive analysis of the effects of lung inflation on the pulmonary vascular bed that was independent of the special conditions of the inflation. Nearly all of my studies on the pulmonary circulation since that time have focused on improving the comprehensive analysis. The apparently striking differences between the hemodynamic effects of positive- and negative-pressure inflation still give rise to mistaken inferences concerning the effects of inflation on the pulmonary blood vessels. No one has any difficulty understanding how the alveolar vessels are squeezed under conditions of positive-pressure inflation, because one sees a rise in pulmonary arterial pressure and a decrease in pulmonary arterial flow. It is still not so easy to see how a spontaneous increase in lung volume causes the alveolar vessels to be squeezed where the inflation is accompanied by a decrease in pulmonary arterial pressure and an increase in pulmonary arterial flow.[19]

What has happened to me in the more than 35 years that I have been working in this field is that I am no longer ignorant. Some might even consider me a sort of sage. My sagacity compels me to fight the ignorant ideas of my younger colleagues in the same way the sages of my young days fought me. But I wish I were ignorant again. I wish I could come up with some idea that no one with wisdom and knowledge would ever consider. Ignorance is indeed bliss!

# References

1. Brower, R. G., J. Gottlieb, R. A. Wise, S. Permutt, J. T. Sylvester. Locus of hypoxic vasoconstriction in isolated ferret lungs. *J. Appl. Physiol.* 63: 58–65, 1987.
2. Faridy, E. E., and S. Permutt. Surface forces and airway obstruction. *J. Appl. Physiol.* 30: 319–321, 1971.
3. Hakim, T. S., G. W. Dean, and R. Lisbona. Quantification of spatial blood flow distribution in isolated canine lungs. *J. Invest. Rad.* 23: 498–504, 1988.
4. Howell, J. B. L., S. Permutt, D. F. Proctor, and R. L. Riley. Effect of inflation of the lung on different parts of pulmonary vascular bed. *J. Appl. Physiol. 16:* 71, 1961.
5. Hughes, J. M. B., J. B. Glazier, J. E. Maloney, and J. B. West. Effect of extra-alveolar vessels on the distribution of blood flow in the dog lung. *J. Appl. Physiol.* 25: 701–712, 1968.
6. Hughes, J. M. B., J. B. Glazier, J. E. Maloney, and J. B. West. Effect of lung volume on the distribution of pulmonary blood flow in man. *Respir. Physiol.* 4: 58–72, 1968.
7. Iliff, L. D. Extra-alveolar vessels and edema development in excised dog lungs. *Circ. Res.* 28: 524–532, 1971.
8. Linehan, J. H., C. A. Dawson, D. A. Rickaby, and T. A. Bronikowski. Pulmonary vascular compliance and viscoelasticity. *J. Appl. Physiol.* 61: 1802–1814, 1986.
9. Macklin, C. C., Evidence of increase on the capacity of the pulmonary arteries and veins of dogs, cats and rabbits during inflation of the freshly excised lung. *Rev. Can. Biol.* 5: 199–232, 1946.
10. Martin, H. B., and D. S. Proctor. Pressure-

volume measurements on dog bronchi. *J. Appl. Physiol.* 13: 337–343, 1958.

11. Mead, J., and J. L. Wittenberger. Lung inflation and hemodynamics. In: *Handbook of Physiology,* Sect. 3, Vol. 1, *Respiration.* Washington, DC: American Physiological Society, 1964, p. 477–486.

12. Permutt, S. Mechanical influences on water accumulation in the lungs. In: *Pulmonary Edema,* edited by A. P. Fishman. Bethesda, MD: American Physiological Society 1978, chap. 13.

13. Permutt, S., B. Bromberger-Barnea, and H. N. Bane. The effect of lung size on pulmonary circulation *in vivo. The Physiologist* 3: 125, 1960.

14. Permutt, S., B. Bromberger-Barnea, and H. N. Bane. Mechanical factors affecting pulmonary vascular resistance in living dogs. *Fed. Proc.* 20: 105, 1961.

15. Permutt, S., B. Bromberger-Barnea, and H. N. Bane. Alveolar pressure, pulmonary venous pressure, and the vascular waterfall. *Med. Thorac.* 19: 129–260, 1962.

16. Permutt, S., B. Bromberger-Barnea, and H. N. Bane. Alveolar pressure, pulmonary venous pressure, and the vascular waterfall. In *Progress in Research in Emphysema and Chronic Bronchitis.* Vol. 1: *Normal and Abnormal Pulmonary Circulation,* edited by R. F. Grover. Basel: S. Karger, 1963.

17. Permutt, S., and R. G. Brower. Mechanical Support. In: *The Lung: Scientific Foundations,* edited by R. G. Crystal, and J. B. West. New York: Raven, 1991, p. 1077–1085.

18. Permutt, S., and J. B. L. Howell. Reversal by degassing of changes in the pressure-volume characteristics of lungs due to over-inflation. *The Physiologist* 1: 66, 1957.

19. Permutt, S., J. B. L. Howell, D. F. Proctor, and R. L. Riley. Effect of lung inflation on static pressure-volume characteristics of pulmonary vessels. *J. Appl. Physiol.* 16: 64, 1961.

20. Permutt, S., and H. B. Martin. Static pressure-volume characteristics of lungs in normal males. *J. Appl. Physiol.* 15: 819, 1960.

21. Rickaby, D. A., C. A. Dawson, J. H. Linehan, and T. A. Bronikowski. Alveolar vessel behavior in the zone 2 lung inferred from indicator-dilution data. *J. Appl. Physiol.* 63: 778–784, 1987.

22. Riley, R. L. Effect of lung inflation upon the pulmonary vascular bed. *Ciba Foundation Symposium on Pulmonary Structure and Function,* edited by A. V. S. de Reuck and Maeve O'Connor. London: J & A. Churchill, 1961, p. 261–272.

23. Riley, R. L. Effect of lung inflation on pulmonary vascular bed. In: *Pulmonary Circulation,* edited by W. Adams and Y. Veith. New York: Grune & Stratton, 1959, p. 147–153.

24. Staub, N. C., J. A. Clements, S. Permutt, and D. F. Proctor. Charles Clifford Macklin, 1883–1959: an appreciation (Editoral). *Am. Rev. Respir. Dis.* 114: 823–830, 1976.

25. Sylvester, J. T., W. Mitzner, Y. Ngeow, and S. Permutt. Hypoxic constriction of alveolar and extra-alveolar vessels in isolated pig lungs. *J. Appl. Physiol.* 54 *(Respir Environ Exercise Phys)* 1660–1666, 1983.

26. West, J. B., and C. T. Dollery. Distribution of blood flow and the pressure-flow relations of the whole lung. *J. Appl. Physiol.* 20: 175–183, 1964.

27. West, J. B., C. T. Dollery, and A. Naimark. Distribution of blood flow in isolated lung: relation to vascular and alveolar pressures. *J. Appl. Physiol.* 19: 713–724, 1964.

28. West, J. B., C. T. Dollery, and B. E. Heard. Increased pulmonary vascular resistance in the dependent zone of the isolated dog lung caused by perivascular edema. *Circ. Res.* 17: 191–206, 1965.

# 9

# Encounters with the Pulmonary Circulation

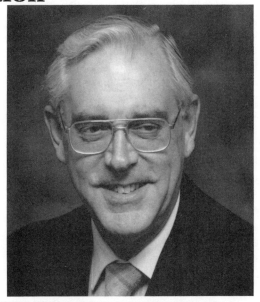

### Thomas C. Lloyd, Jr., M.D.

*Professor, Departments of Medicine, Physiology and Biophysics, Indiana University School of Medicine, Indianapolis, Indiana*

"You don't really believe that hypoxia causes pulmonary vasoconstriction, do you?" That question was put to me by C. J. Lambertsen while I was a medical student at the University of Pennsylvania. Unanswered and forgotten at the time, it ultimately became the basis of my career as an independent investigator. But before getting to that story and to a review of my experiences with the lung circulation, I will review critical points on the path that led to my career and provided, in no organized way, my training for research.

An early interest in technology and science blossomed after being cultivated by my high school physics teacher, who, remarkably, was a young woman in her first and only year of teaching. She enabled me to see that mathematics could be a useful investigative tool and that I could apply physical principles to gain an understanding of natural phenomena. She recognized my curiosity and encouraged my interest with frequent, often demanding, challenges.

As a teenager I had a consuming interest in electronics, and I read avidly about basic circuitry and radio communication, often to the exclusion of school assignments. Although I maintained an active interest in electronics while in college, my undergraduate education was in chemistry. My introduction to biomedical research came during two summers of my undergraduate years when I was able to combine interests in chemistry and electronics through employment under the direction of Britton Chance at the Johnson Foundation for Biophysics at the University of Pennsylvania. This environment

From: Wagner WW, Jr, Weir EK (eds): *The Pulmonary Circulation and Gas Exchange.* ©1994, Futura Publishing Co Inc, Armonk, NY.

provided many lessons on topics in science as well as on the process of scientific investigation. An early lesson about research was that the investigator is obligated to know the characteristics, calibrations, strengths, and weaknesses of his or her instrumentation. Another unforgettable lesson concerned intellectual honesty, and it came about in a painful way. Brit and I were using a hand spectroscope, watching the appearance and disappearance of absorption bands of various cytochromes as oxygen was added to a circulating suspension of yeast. With obvious displeasure at my performance, he insisted that I should be seeing a band at a certain wavelength. I could not see the change and persistently said so. Finally, after inducing considerable discomfort in his employee, he said, "Good. I didn't see it either. Don't ever say you do when you don't." Then he walked away, leaving me to reflect on the experience.

I finished college unsure of whether I wanted to pursue medicine, chemistry, or biophysics, but an early admission to medical school decided the issue, at least temporarily.

Chris Lambertsen's laboratory was a popular spot for medical students to experience research, and it was my good fortune to be able to participate in it during one free summer and several months of senior elective time. My assignment was to build apparatus for continuous recording of pH and for controlling alveolar $P_{CO_2}$ at hypercapnic levels. I also assisted with teaching in the sophomore medical pharmacology laboratory exercises, an experience that gave me a taste of what medical school was like from the "other side." Chris's guidance and personal warmth were intangible assets that I recall fondly. I look on my experience in the pharmacology department at Penn as the determining factor in opting for a career in investigative medicine. Lambertsen's experiments were complicated team efforts in which human subjects were at personal risk. Consequently, experiments were undertaken only after meticulous and detailed planning. I began to appreciate that research must be organized from the start and that inquiry requires an hypothesis and a detailed protocol to test it. Data reduction in Chris's lab was attended to with great care. One of Chris's rules was that everything had to be calculated at least twice, preferably by two different people. His rule made a lasting impression of another fundamental requirement for research: one must be confident in the data and their transformations.

The lung was not a subject of much interest in Cleveland while I was there as an intern and medical resident. However, one dedicated pulmonologist (David Gillespie) at what is now Metropolitan General Hospital introduced me to clinical pulmonary physiology. Through this experience I learned that the lung is an organ whose physiology is susceptible to the methods of physics, mathematics, and engineering, in all of which I had an interest (if not an education), so I decided on a career in pulmonary medicine.

At about that time George Wright had left the Trudeau Foundation at Saranac Lake to assume a position in Cleveland as director of medical research at St. Luke's Hospital, and in 1958 he agreed to serve as my mentor for a fellowship year. I proposed to study the pulmonary circulation, a choice that reflected my interest in both lung and cardiovascular physiology. George apparently believed in the sink-or-swim training method, for he left me on my own to devise and perform my first experiments. His lessons came during the preparations for publication, and he was a stringent editor. One memorable bit of advice he gave me was "to write it as if it was to be published in the Boy Scout Handbook." Like Wiltz Wagner in recent times, George was critical of my unnecessary obfuscation and my use of mathematical expressions where words were a better choice. His tutoring certainly was helpful: my first publication,[29] coauthored with George Wright, was accepted by the *Journal of Applied Physiology* in its initially submitted form. That publication concerned the shape of the perfusion pressure-flow curves of excised dog lobes and demonstrated the roles of venous and alveolar pressures in determining transmural and longitudinal vascular pressure gradients. It was a satisfying piece of work that, in addition to presenting new material, gave me a start toward understanding the physical properties of lung vessels and their perfusion.

Jerome Kleinerman was associated with the research laboratory at St. Luke's during my fellowship. Jerry became my antagonist, protagonist, colleague, and friend. He taught me to think beyond physiology into the areas of anatomy, pathology, and morphometry, and he caused me to consider the relationships between structure and function. Jerry also taught me a lot about the philosophy and politics of science and about the funding of research.

After fellowship I entered the Public Health Service to study the pulmonary effects of air pollutants. One year of service was spent at St. Bartholemew's Hospital in London, where I came upon Donald McDonald and his important book *Blood Flow in Arteries.* I spent many hours chewing on the material in that volume and learning more mathematics so that I could understand what McDonald had written.

After two and a half years I left the Public Health Service for my first faculty position. On returning to Cleveland in 1962 I realized that I had a job but that I had not yet established what I was going to do. I needed a project that would be attractive to granting agencies, and I had to develop my first grant. It was then that I remembered Chris Lambertsen's question and the problem of regulation of the pulmonary circulation in response to hypoxia.

In the following description of the experiments that shaped my perception of the pulmonary circulation I will unashamedly stress my own publications, knowing that in many instances my observations were not unique and that references to antecedent and supporting information are provided in the reports that have been cited.

## Effect of Hypoxia on the Pulmonary Circulation

In 1962 the phenomenon of hypoxic pulmonary vasoconstriction had been known for at least 15 years, but it was not universally accepted. Some investigators had been unable to demonstrate it, and many were uneasy because constriction was opposite to the effects of hypoxia in other organs. Then as now the basic questions included, is hypoxic pulmonary vasoconstriction a direct response of vascular smooth muscle or is it mediated indirectly, either humorally or reflexly? does it occur in the arterial or in the venous bed, or both? and where is the sensor located? In hopes that I might contribute to the confusion, I undertook my first experiments.

The goal of those first experiments was to determine if responses to hypoxia could be demonstrated in excised dog lobes under more rigid control of conditions than in prior investigations and, if so, to attempt to define the anatomical location of the response, the relationship to alveolar and perfusate $PO_2$, and the effects of certain pharmacologic blocking agents. The plan was to excise the left lower lobe of an anesthetized dog, enclose it in a humid, warm environment, ventilate it with chosen gas mixtures, and perfuse it at constant flow with systemic venous blood drawn from, and returned to, the donor dog. Although I had had experience perfusing excised lobes under other conditions in the experiments with

Wright, I was not prepared for the problems that arose when perfusing ventilated lobes with blood for extended periods. It was amazing how quickly lobes would become edematous, and for many months we obtained greater flow out the airway than out the vein. Finally, we learned how to minimize the formation of edema and produce preparations that were usable for several hours. We also were able to dispense with the donor dog and use an external reservoir for perfusion with either blood or a physiological salt-colloid solution.

Some of our findings with those lobes are shown in Figure 1. The percentage of $O_2$ in ventilating gas is indicated above each tracing, but in each case the $CO_2$ composition was 6.5%. The top left tracing illustrates the pressor response of blood-perfused lobes to a bolus of serotonin (5HT) and to reduction of the inspired %$O_2$ from the normal control 14 to 6% and then to 0%. Responses to hypoxia were immediately reversed by raising inspired %$O_2$, as seen in the middle left panel. Responses to 6% $O_2$ would be sustained, but responses to anoxia would spontaneously recede to baseline within 5–7 min. Thereafter, there would be no response to varying inspired $O_2$, although the response to 5HT was unchanged (Fig. 1, top right panel). Sometimes the response to hypoxia would return after many minutes of ventilation with the normoxic mixture. A further finding in all preparations was that responses to hypoxia would disappear after 50–60 min of perfusion, whereas responses to 5HT remained unchanged for several hours. The evanescence of the hypoxic response and its depression by severe hypoxia, in contrast to the sustained responses to 5HT, suggested that the hypoxic response might involve some easily impaired process external to the smooth muscle. Several years later we were to find[5] that preparations would respond to hypoxia for a much longer interval if they were cooled to 25–

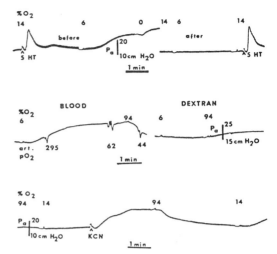

**Figure 1.** Arterial pressure changes in perfused lung lobes during hypoxia and serotonin challenges. Further details for this and subsequent figures are given in the text. From reference 2, by permission.

30°C except for brief periods at 37°C, during which the response to hypoxia was tested. This further supported the idea that there was a relatively fragile active metabolic process involved.

The relation between response and $O_2$ composition of arterial blood and alveolar gas is illustrated in the middle left panel (Fig. 1). Here, the initial ventilating %$O_2$ has been switched from 94 to 6% and then back to 94%. Note that a pressor response began while arterial $P_{O_2}$ was 295 mmHg but that it subsided while arterial $P_{O_2}$ (i.e., $P_{O_2}$ of blood leaving the reservoir) was still falling. This suggested that the response was sensed at either the alveolar or venous level, but not in the arteries. Later, this was followed up in other lobes that were perfused from vein to artery,[3] and we found that the response to hypoxia was again dissociated from input blood $P_{O_2}$, suggesting that the sensory site was not in the veins either. Our conclusion, then, was that the sensor lay somewhere in the alveolar gas environment.

When salt solution was substituted for blood in our earliest experiments, hypoxia usually caused a small depressor effect and never caused constriction, although the responses to 5HT were similar to those seen during blood perfusion. An example of the hypoxic response is shown in the middle right panel of Figure 1. Later, a graduate student, Ben Gorsky, showed that a small amount to plasma potentiates the pressor responses to both hypoxia and serotonin in lobes perfused with artificial perfusates but that small hypoxic responses occurred even in the absence of plasma.[1] Gorsky's results introduced uncertainty into our earlier conclusion that some component of blood was needed for any hypoxic pressor response to occur.

The bottom panel of Figure 1 shows that potassium cyanide also evokes vasoconstriction and that this can be partially reduced by raising alveolar %$O_2$ from 14 to 94%. Note that in the presence of cyanide, changing from 94 to 14% $O_2$ caused constriction, whereas before cyanide this change made no difference. In a later study we found that dinitrophenol caused effects similar to those of cyanide.[3] Thus, a pressor response could be produced by both cytotoxic and hypoxic hypoxia.

Arterial wedge pressures were measured with a 1-mm outside diameter catheter in several lobes of the initial study. Wedge pressure was approximately halfway between arterial and venous pressures and showed characteristics consistent with pressure in small veins. Wedge pressure did not rise during hypoxia, and on a few occasions it fell to zero and lost all responsiveness to alveolar and venous outflow pressures, as though it had been occluded during the pressor response. The wedge pressure measurements were taken as evidence that the pressor response to hypoxia occurred in the arterial bed.

We were unsuccessful in blocking the hypoxic response with hexamethonium, atropine, and brom-lysergic acid diethylamide, thereby provisionally excluding mediation by autonomic ganglia, acetylcholine, or serotonin. Phenoxybenzam-ine, however, significantly reduced the response. Although this could be interpreted as mediation of the response by alpha adrenergic stimulation, we thought it more likely that phenoxybenzamine had merely left unopposed the dilatory beta-adrenergic effect of catecholamines present in the tissue and perfusate at all oxygen tensions.

Several investigators had found that the hypoxic pressor response could be potentiated by acidosis, but this was not universally agreed on. I thought our approach provided better control of perfusion and ventilation parameters, including gas and blood composition, and we studied this problem. We found that the hypoxic response was progressively depressed by alkalosis, whether caused by hypocapnia or by administration of $NaHCO_3$ or tris buffer. Sensitivity to pH was marked—a rise from a baseline pH of 7.3 to 7.5 prevented an hypoxic pressor response. The hypoxic response was pH dependent but not specifically $PCO_2$ dependent. The uppermost trace of Figure 2 shows the arterial pressure response of a perfused lobe when its ventilating gas composition was changed from 6.5% $CO_2$ in $O_2$ to 6.5% $CO_2$ in $N_2$. The second tracing shows that when the lobe was made hypoxic with 100% $N_2$, there was no pressor response. When, however, the lobe was ventilated with room air and the pH of the perfusate was adjusted downward with lactic acid (HCl worked equally well), there was a typical pressor response to 100% $N_2$.

The question of mediation of the hypoxic pressor response by nerve, even in excised lobes, had never been answered. We added the following observations to the controversy.[5] Electrical stimulation at the hilum of the excised perfused lobe caused a pressor response that was somewhat reduced by cooling perfusate from 37 to 25 °C. However, raising perfusate pH 0.16 or ventilating without $O_2$ for 15 min had no significant effect on the response to

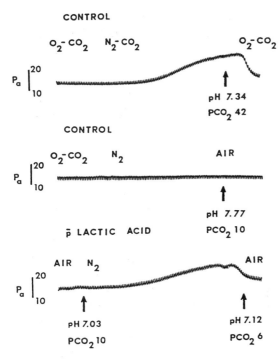

**Figure 2.** Effect of hypocapnic alkalosis on the pressor response to hypoxia in a perfused lung lobe. From reference 4, by permission.

electrical nerve stimulation. Cooling, mild alkalinization, and prolonged anoxia, however, all prevented the pressor response to ventilation with 6% $O_2$. In contrast, procaine at a perfusate concentration of 1 mM or tetracaine at a concentration of 0.1 mM greatly depressed responses to electrical stimulation but had no effect on response to hypoxia. Pressor responses to epinephrine were unaffected by cooling, but the effect of cooling on the serotonin response was interesting. Cooling slightly reduced the serotonin peak response but greatly prolonged the recovery, consistent with temperature sensitivity of the metabolic removal of the agent. Several animals in this series were pretreated with either phenoxybenzamine or reserpine. These treatments did not prevent responses to hypoxia. It was also interesting to note that in lobes from animals given phenoxybenzamine, electrical stimulation during a hypoxic pressor response caused

partial reversal that persisted as long as the stimulation was applied. We thought that these findings allowed us to conclude that the responses to hypoxia and to nerve stimulation were independent events.

An interesting and, I believe, provocative result occurred when we attempted to stabilize vascular smooth muscle membrane potential using high concentrations of procaine and tetracaine.[6] I had expected that this would impair the response of perfused lobes to hypoxia. Instead procaine at concentrations from 2.5 to 10 mM, or tetracaine at one-tenth those concentrations, had pressor effects of their own that resembled the effects of cyanide and dinitrophenol. That is, when given while ventilating with 14% $O_2$ they caused a modest vasoconstriction that was reversed by raising inspired $O_2$ concentration to 94%. In an equivalent fashion, the responses to 6 and 0% $O_2$ were enhanced. But the most remarkable effect was on the tolerance to anoxia and on the useful life of the preparations. Anoxia, which previously caused unsustained vasoconstriction and subsequent unresponsiveness, now caused sustained vasoconstriction. In addition, the life of the preparation during which responses to hypoxia could be demonstrated was extended by several hours. Furthermore, when a lobe previously unexposed to the anesthetics became incapable of responding to hypoxia after the usual 1 hour of perfusion, addition of procaine would restore and enhance hypoxic responsiveness, which then persisted several more hours. I was unable to find a sufficient explanation for those effects, but it seems to me that there may be an important clue here. On which cells did the effect occur? Perhaps an explanation exists that has not been brought to my attention. Until then, I will contend that this phenomenon merits further study.

In 1966 I turned from studies in perfused lobes to studies of excised vessels. Methods were crude by today's standards: although vessels were handled with care, no attempt was made to avoid endothelial injury or to adjust baseline wall stresses to optimum values for development of greatest active changes. In our first study,[7] helical strips were prepared from segmental branches of pulmonary arteries of dogs and rabbits. Strips were immersed in a bath of the same salt solution found earlier to be suitable for perfusion of lobes. Strips were challenged with a number of vasoconstrictor drugs as well as with electrical field stimulation and hyperkalemia. To summarize, no strip, whether precontracted or not, contracted when bath $P_{O_2}$ was lowered progressively from 600 mmHg to near zero. Tensions of untreated strips were unaffected by even severe hypoxia, but tensions of precontracted vessels fell as $O_2$ was reduced. Reduction of strip tension required $O_2$ depletions to near zero, as best shown by responses to electrical stimulation: repeated electrical stimulation caused similar responses when $P_{O_2}$ was reduced from 600 to 100 mmHg and then 40 mmHg, but further reduction to near zero reduced responses by about 30% within 20 min. Strips prepared from perfused dog lobes that moments before were fully responsive to hypoxia and stabilized with procaine behaved like all other strips. Addition of procaine to the baths of previously untreated vessels did not change their responses to hypoxia. In short, there was nothing to suggest that the hypoxic pressor response of perfused lobes resembled the effects of hypoxia on isolated vessels. Instead, everything pointed to a depressor effect of severe hypoxia, similar to the behavior of systemic vessel strips. In retrospect, there probably was endothelial injury in these preparations because acetylcholine usually caused contraction that could be blocked with atropine. This may be important because some investigators now believe that endothelial factors may play a role in the hypoxic pressor response.

Before undertaking the next experiment with excised vessels, I hypothesized that the hypoxic response depended on something released from lung parenchyma. I expected that such a mediator might be diluted to ineffectiveness if studies were made in an aqueous bath. To reduce that possibility, subsequent studies were made in a water-immiscible fluorocarbon that exhibited high solvation for $O_2$ and $CO_2$ but poor solvation of salts and organic chemicals. In the first study,[8] we compared the effects of varying bath $P_{O_2}$ on responses of rabbit lobar arterial strips with responses of similar strips to which a thin layer of lung parenchyma remained attached and to strips of lung parenchyma of a similar size but as devoid of larger vessels and airways as could be achieved. The bath consisted of two phases: a lower (denser) phase of fluorocarbon on which floated a layer of plasma diluted 50% with physiological salt solution. For the first 60–80 min the tissue strips remained in the fluorocarbon phase and were intermittently challenged by lowering bath $P_{O_2}$ from 700 to 45 mmHg. We next attempted to enhance any constrictor effect of hypoxia with procaine as we had been able to do with perfused lobes. Procaine was added to the aqueous phase, and the strips were brought into that phase for 10 min before being returned to the fluorocarbon for further challenges. We found that at no time did strips of isolated artery contract in response to oxygen deprivation, although several relaxed with hypoxia after the procaine treatment, and all contracted vigorously with electrical stimulation. In contrast, arterial strips with attached parenchyma at first relaxed during hypoxia, but, toward the end of the first hour and prior to procaine treatment, about half underwent hypoxic contraction. After procaine treatment 9 of 10 strips contracted as $P_{O_2}$ was lowered. Contraction seemed to begin at a $P_{O_2}$ near 200 mmHg and reached its maximum near 100 mmHg. After about 4 hours of study a subset of strips of artery with parenchyma were removed from the fluorocarbon and immersed in a bath of 10% plasma in salt solution (with procaine) where further challenges with PO$_2$ variations were made. All strips removed from fluorocarbon and placed in the aqueous bath continued to display contractile responses to O$_2$ reduction. This suggested that the washout of materials by an aqueous bath may not have been as important as I first thought. To our surprise, all the parenchymal strips in the fluorocarbon bath contracted with O$_2$ depletion both before and after the procaine treatment. The tension change of the parenchymal strips was almost half that of the artery-parenchyma combination. Figure 3 illustrates the effects described above. In each case tension (T) and bath PO$_2$ were simultaneously recorded. The upper left pair show parenchymal contractions obtained after procaine treatment. The upper right panel shows how the parenchyma-covered arterial strips behaved before they began to show contractions, and the lower curves display a response after procaine treatment. These experiments were interpreted as evidence that something from lung parenchyma could evoke contraction in response to hypoxia and indeed was necessary for vessels to contract.

But my experiences with hypoxia did not end in such a tidy way. There was one more set of experiments.[9]

I wondered how vessels would respond to variations in environmental PO$_2$ if they were suspended in an even more water-free environment. For this I chose first a bath of a more hydrophobic fluorocarbon and then a "bath" of humidified warm gas. This time we used strips of rabbit aorta as well as parenchyma-free rabbit pulmonary artery. The fluorocarbon bath was used to study only pulmonary artery using the same protocol. However, only one strip was treated with procaine or immersed in the aqueous phase above the fluorocarbon. All strips of pulmonary artery contracted reversibly when bath PO$_2$ was reduced from 700 to 100 mmHg and the procaine-treated strip responded similarly to those not so treated. An example is shown at the top of Figure 4. Contractions were modestly well sustained, but after several hours of study, contractions became less well sustained and there was often a rebound contraction when PO$_2$ was raised. When aorta (AO) and pulmonary artery (PA) were studied in the humid gas environment, each contracted as PO$_2$ was lowered. This is illustrated in the bottom traces of Figure 4. In short here was a dilemma: isolated lengths of both

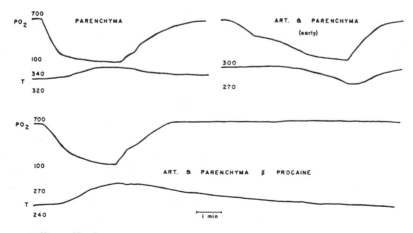

**Figure 3.** Effect of bath PO$_2$ on tensions of strips of pulmonary artery, parenchyma, and artery with parenchyma attached. From reference 8, by permission.

Pulm. Art. Strip in FC 43

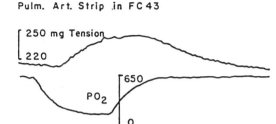

Arterial Strips in Wet Gas Chamber

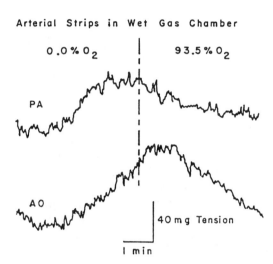

**Figure 4.** Effect of varying bath $P_{O_2}$ on tension of a pulmonary arterial strip immersed in fluorocarbon FC43 and of varying $O_2$ composition of humidified gas in which were suspended strips of aorta and pulmonary artery. From reference 9, by permission.

systemic and pulmonary artery contracted when $P_{O_2}$ was lowered from 700 to 100 mmHg while suspended in humid gas, but both relaxed when $P_{O_2}$ was lowered below 40 mmHg while suspended in an aqueous bath. Note in addition that the in vivo response takes place in the gap between 100 and 20 mmHg $P_{O_2}$, specifically the range found to be without effect on the isolated vessels.

Do my observations with excised vessels provide useful information? I am reluctant to say that I have modeled the in vivo response to hypoxia with any of the isolated vessel techniques. Certainly I am less confident after the second study than

I was after the first. Furthermore, I am not convinced that contemporary studies of more carefully prepared smaller pulmonary vessels, which are reported to show hypoxic contraction in aqueous baths, are suitable models of the excised lobe or whole-animal response to alveolar hypoxia. It seems to me that before venturing much further we need as much proof of the equivalence as can be obtained. One way to start might be to list the typical characteristics of the vascular response that most investigators agree are unique to the effects of hypoxia in situ and then to demonstrate that isolated vessels display each of them. These will probably have to be tested for species dependency. Several characteristics immediately come to mind, including sensitivity to cooling and to alkalosis, potentiation by procaine, evocability by both hypoxic and histotoxic hypoxia, suppression following a period of severe hypoxia without loss of pharmacologic responses, and dependence on calcium movement. For now, I will have to rephrase the question first put to me: "You don't really believe that hypoxia causes pulmonary vasoconstriction as a direct smooth muscle effect, do you?" And it may be my turn to be wrong.

I thought that my studies with hypoxia had come to an impass and that I was unable to answer the question that bothered me most: is the response a direct muscle effect or is it not? The question of neural control of the pulmonary circulation seemed to offer more opportunities for forward movement.

## Reflex Responses of the Pulmonary Vessels

One of the more challenging tasks has been to test the hypothesis that increased pressure in the pulmonary arteries leads to reflex pulmonary arterial constriction. Althought it would seem that such a positive feedback mechanism would lead to a never-demonstrated sustained maximum vasoconstriction, its existence has been postulated, and perhaps demonstrated, several times. The problem lies in the technical difficulty associated with having stimulus and response in the same vessels and in securing certainty that one is in control of the experimental situation. I undertook a study of this problem with Arthur Schneider, an anesthesiology postdoctoral fellow. We believed we had found a way to discriminate between active and passive changes in pulmonary arterial pressure as left atrial pressure was progressively elevated. Experiments were done in anesthetized dogs using biventricular bypass perfusion. We acquired what we thought was convincing evidence that increasing pressure in the pulmonary vascular bed caused pulmonary vasoconstriction and that this was mediated by the sympathetic nerves.[27,28] We were wrong, as I later showed in a subsequent study.[10] What we had observed was related to a purely mechanical effect in the heart, whose activity was indeed affected by the sympathetic nervous system. (I was later informed by Sol Permutt, who served as journal editor for all three manuscripts, that one reviewer was unhappy when two papers he felt to be less than meritorious were published over his objections. When he had to accept a third that disclosed the error, he was incensed. Apparently the publication and subsequent refutation of errors was not the best way to expand my curriculum vita. Sol periodically reminds me of this.)

Several years later I attempted to reevaluate the problem by using balloons to distend portions of the pulmonary arterial bed while monitoring resistance in other portions. Vasoconstrictor responses had been seen by other investigators with this approach, but there were inconsistencies among the results and questions about the methods. Most important, balloons might have caused unseen or unintended passive changes, and changes in pressure might have been caused by changes in flow. Unlike most others, who had chosen to place balloons under indirect observation with chests closed, we opened chests of anesthetized dogs and attempted to place balloons under direct visual guidance. We found that unless they were constrained, balloons in the left pulmonary artery invariably "popped" retrogradely into the main pulmonary artery when they were inflated sufficiently to exert a force on the arterial wall. Ultimately, we tied all lobar branches of the left pulmonary artery and retrogradely placed a balloon in the parent vessel through an opening in the lower lobe branch. This balloon remained in place. Systemic flow was held constant by a left ventricular bypass pump, and gas exchange was provided externally so that lung volume could be held invariant. We were careful to preserve nerves, and we avoided dissection where they were known to be located. Pressure in the main pulmonary artery was recorded as a reflection of perfusion resistance of the right lung. No amount of distension of the left pulmonary artery influenced perfusion pressure of the right lung, although right lung vasoconstriction could be induced by hypoxic ventilation or by stimulating the right stellate ganglion.

Frustrated, and convinced that pressure changes reported by others represented a passive mechanical effect, I wanted to reproduce the findings of Craig Juratsch and his coworkers, who believed they had evoked vasoconstriction by inflating a balloon placed in the main pulmonary artery. The balloon was said not to have altered cardiac output or occluded major branches but instead to have caused the main artery to be distended in accepting cardiac output. Craig and I had met briefly and discussed his findings some years before, and I wrote to him seeking to borrow his balloon. To my surprise, he not only had balloon catheters but said he

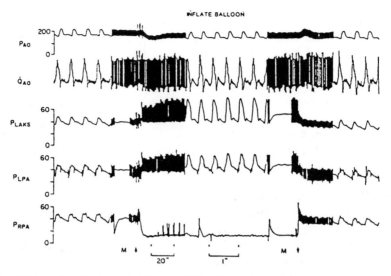

**Figure 5.** Effect of inflating a balloon within the main pulmonary artery on systemic arterial pressure and flow and on pressures measured in right and left pulmonary arteries. From reference 26, by permission.

would like to come do the experiments with me. Craig was, and remains, a delightful individual, enjoyable to work with even though he came fully convinced of the existence of reflex vasoconstriction, while I was convinced otherwise. We worked very hard for one week. On the first day, using fluoroscopy, he passed his balloon from a femoral vein of the anesthetized dog into the pulmonary artery. Sure enough, inflation of the balloon was followed by increased pressure downstream to the balloon in the left pulmonary artery where an extension of the catheter lay. But then we opened the chest and placed catheters in apical lobe arterial branches on each side. Pressures recorded from these during inflation of the balloon in the main pulmonary artery revealed that the right pulmonary artery was completely occluded by the inflated balloon. Every inflation and each subsequent experiment provided the same results. An example is shown in Figure 5. From top down are shown aortic pressure, aortic flow, pressure in the left pulmonary artery measured with the balloon (Laks) catheter, and pressures in the left and right pulmo-

nary arteries measured through apical branches. Bursts at higher chart speed show waveforms, whereas intervals of mean pressure recording can be seen as pulse-free plateaus indicated by "M". The balloon was inflated at the up arrow and deflated at the down arrow. Note that aortic flow and pressure were not significantly changed but that pressure in the left pulmonary artery measured by both devices increased, while pressure in the right fell. Calculated resistance of the left lung actually fell during inflation of the balloon. The changes caused by inflating the balloon were identical to those that followed tightening of a snare around the right pulmonary artery. Throughout this sequence of observations we were careful to test after each step to assure that the original change observed while the chest was closed continued to be present. This experience cast doubt on the interpretation of previous experiments using this particular balloon technique but, of course, did not prove that all prior results were determined entirely passively. We reported the results of this and the preceding study.[20,26]

After several attempts I had found no support for the hypothesis that pulmonary arterial distension would lead to arterial constriction, and I decided to examine other potential initiators of neurogenic pulmonary vasomotion.

Head injury and/or increased intracranial pressure may be associated with pulmonary hypertension and pulmonary edema, and some have proposed that there may be a neurogenic pulmonary vasomotor component. Harvey Cushing had demonstrated that increased intracranial pressure caused proportional systemic arterial vasoconstriction sufficient to raise arterial pressure above intracranial pressure and thereby restore cerebral blood flow. This vasoconstriction was shown to depend on sympathetic efferent activation. Extension of the Cushing experiment to include pulmonary vascular pressures could be expected to provide observations that would bear not only on pulmonary responses to intracranial misadventures but also on the general problem of the role of the sympathetic nerves in control of the pulmonary circulation. Others had used it for that purpose, but results were controversial because it was unclear whether pulmonary vascular pressure changes were determined actively or as a result of changes in the heart and systemic vessels. I believed we had techniques that could better exclude the secondary consequences.

We opened the chests of anesthetized dogs, collected venous systemic and pulmonary venous blood into external reservoirs, and substituted two pulsatile-flow pumps for the ventricles. This allowed control of flow and left atrial pressure while we observed changes in systemic and pulmonary arterial pressures in response to brief intervals of increased intracranial pressure. Intracranial pressure was varied by forcing physiological salt solution into the subarachnoid space through a hollow plug screwed into the skull. Figure 6 shows a typical response. When intracranial pressure (Pic) was increased, sys-

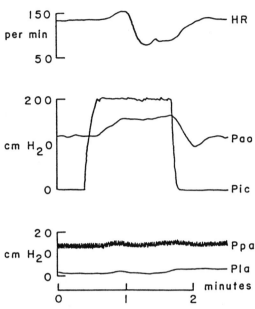

**Figure 6.** Systemic and pulmonary vascular responses in the Cushing reflex. From reference 12, by permission.

temic arterial pressure (Pao) increased. Heart rate (HR) rose transiently with increased Pic but then fell. Atropine eliminated the bradycardia but not the tachycardia. There were very small but statistically significant changes in pulmonary arterial pressure (Ppa), which as a group did not differ significantly from the small changes in left atrial pressure (Pla) that also occurred. The atrial pressure rise probably occurred as a result of a mechanical effect of the bradycardia on discharge rate through the atrial cannula because it was reduced or eliminated by atropine. In spite of the similarity of average arterial and atrial pressure changes, the Ppa-Pla gradient rose an average of 0.36 cmH$_2$O which, though small, was statistically significant. We were unable to find a significant change in pulmonary arterial pulse pressure during the time of increased Pic, suggesting arterial wall stiffness did not change. There was a graded relationship between the magnitude of the imposed increase in Pic and the increase in Pao. During increased Pic we also noted a rise in levels of the external reservoirs. This was not quantified but was believed to reflect the considerable systemic vasoconstriction that was induced. We briefly ventilated the lungs with $N_2$ and found a reversible pulmonary pressor response. This was taken as evidence that pulmonary vessels were capable of constricting under the experimental conditions. These experiments were interpreted as showing that even massive activation of sympathetic efferent activity was incapable of evoking a physiologically significant pulmonary vasomotor response, although there was evidence of a small but statistically significant effect. The systemic vascular changes and the changes in heart rate were in keeping with prior observations.

I was not encouraged by any of the foregoing experiments to believe that there is significant neural control of the adult canine pulmonary vascular bed. My attention was then directed to the possibility that the lung vessels may be an important starting point for reflexes, rather than an important destination.

## Systemic Vasomotor Changes Initiated by High Pulmonary Vascular Pressure

My curiosity was initially drawn to reflex cardiovascular changes that might occur in response to increased left ventricular end-diastolic pressure. There was abundant evidence that reflexes might arise from distension of the left atrium and ventricle, from intraparenchymal pulmonary vessels, and from the major pulmonary arteries. Most information, however, was either in the form of afferent nervous activity in response to pressure changes or hemodynamic variables measured under conditions where primary changes were insufficiently separated from secondary phenomena. I wanted to isolate stimuli

and to control secondary events. Secondary events were to include not only other reflexes, but also changes in systemic flow, lung mechanics, and gas exchange. Furthermore, our efforts were to be directed toward measuring outcome in terms of physiological sequelae rather than as changes in afferent neural activity, for we contended that the former best represents the reflex whereas the latter only represents one form of the input to the controller.

Most work prior to ours had implied that distension of components of the left heart and pulmonary circulation would cause systemic vasodilation and cardiac slowing. Controversy existed. Some investigators were unable to find vasomotor effects of left atrial and/or pulmonary vein distension while others found reflex tachycardia. In other hands distension of the pulmonary arteries had been found to cause systemic vasoconstriction. The hypothesis of our first study was that retrograde pulmonary hypertension brought about by increasing left atrial pressure would cause systemic vasodilation and a fall in heart rate and that these responses would be eliminated by vagotomy and partially suppressed by interaction of systemic arterial baroreflexes. We used biventricular bypass to isolate the stimulus to the left heart and pulmonary vessels and to isolate the response from interacting or secondary effects. This was achieved in anesthetized dogs by opening the chest, stopping the ventricular beat by inducing ventricular fibrillation, draining systemic and pulmonary venous blood from the right ventricle and left atrium, and perfusing the systemic and pulmonary circulations through cannulas in the aorta and left lower lobe pulmonary artery. Pressure in the left heart was controlled by a Starling resistor in the left atrial drain line. The pulmonary perfusion pump ran at constant rate, but provision was made to servocontrol the systemic pump so that blood pressure could be held constant. We measured left atrial pressure, pulmonary and systemic arterial pressures, and systemic arterial flow. Heart rate was acquired from the left atrial pressure pulse. Systemic vascular resistance was continuously computed and recorded. All illustration of effects with ( P = C) and without (Q = C) servocontrol of arterial pressure is shown in Figure 7. When left atrial pressure (Pla) was raised abruptly from 0 to 20–25 cmH$_2$O the typical response was a transient fall of systemic vascular resistance (SVR) averaging 35% that gave way over a period of 40–60 s to a plateau decline of 21%. When systemic arterial pressure (Pao) was not servocontrolled, the respective changes were declines of 26 and 12%, significantly less than with servocontrol. Fall of resistance was accompanied by a fall in heart rate (HR) from tachycardic baseline rates of 150–200 beats/min. In a few instances, increased left atrial pressure brought about a rise in systemic vascular resistance and heart rate. That outcome seemed to occur most often when baseline resistance and blood pressure were unusually and abnormally low. Bilateral cervical vagotomy eliminated all effects of increased left atrial pressure. Use of pulsatile, rather than continuous, pulmonary perfusion did not alter response, although it might have been expected to increase a response if mediated by pulmonary arterial baroreceptors with properties similar to the systemic arterial baroreceptor. We also tested the hypothesis that a change in lung volume would alter the response to increased left atrial pressure. There were three reasons for this hypothesis: (1) lung volume changes can change the effective perivascular pressure and perhaps the vascular strain imposed by a change in intravascular pressure, (2) slowly adapting pulmonary receptors reflexly alter systemic vasomotor tone and may have an influence on further neural modulation, and (3) greater lung volumes may mechanically limit enlargement of the heart and

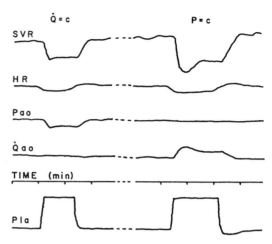

**Figure 7.** Heart rate and systemic vascular changes that occur in response to increased pressure in the left heart and pulmonary circulation. From reference 11, by permission.

any reflex dependent on that strain. And indeed we found that an increase of end-expiratory pressure from 5 to 12 cmH$_2$O significantly reduced the response to increased left atrial pressure.

In the next study[13] of the cardiopulmonary baroreflex, we acquired stimulus-response relationships using both step and sinusoidal input pressures of variable magnitude. In addition we examined the relationship between sinusoidal forcing frequency and response, while using a constant stimulus amplitude. The preparation was the same as that used earlier, although systemic arterial pressure was not servocontrolled. Step pressure changes were applied from a baseline left atrial pressure of 0 cmH$_2$O. The magnitudes of both the transient and sustained falls of systemic vascular resistance were essentially linearly related to left atrial step pressure magnitude over the range 10 to 35 cmH$_2$O. For phasic pressure forcing, we servocontrolled left atrial pressure using a low frequency signal generator and a third pump to impose a back pressure on atrial drainage such that left atrial pressure varied sinusoidally. At frequencies below 0.03 Hz, the systemic arterial pressure output waveform was cyclic but not sinusoidal, whereas from 0.03 Hz to 0.08 Hz the output waveform appeared to be an undistorted sinusoid whose amplitude became progressively less as forcing frequency was raised. Above 0.08 Hz, the response was too small to be detectably cyclic. Over the frequency range 0.03 to 0.08 Hz the input-output characteristics resembled those of a linear second-order system, and on that basis we determined stability characteristics. We found that the system behaved with a natural frequency of 0.05 Hz and that its gain and phase margins assured stability. When left atrial pressure was forced to vary sinusoidally at 0.03 Hz using a range of amplitudes from 5 to 30 $cmH_2O$, the induced systemic arterial pressure variations were linearly related to the magnitudes of the forcing pressure.

In all preceeding experiments with the cardiopulmonary baroreflex the stimulus pressure was imposed equally throughout the lung vessels and left heart chambers. Our next goal was to determine the roles of individual subcompartments. The first of those studies[14] demonstrated responses to pressurization of the pulmonary arterial compartment and pressurization of the left atrium-pulmonary vein compartment. Open-chest anesthetized dogs were provided with external gas exchange and systemic vascular perfusion by draining systemic venous blood from the right atrium and, after gas exchange, returning it to the aorta by a continuous-flow pump. Systemic arterial pressure was sevocontrolled. Valve orifices at the base of the heart were occluded by clamping the fibrillating ventricles with a single large clamp placed just below the atrio-venous groove. A small drain was placed in the left ventricular cavity. Recalling that gas does not traverse capillaries except at high pressure, we were able to distend the arterial and veno-atrial compartments selectively by admitting 5% $CO_2$ in $O_2$ through catheters in the pulmo-

nary artery and atrial appendage. While one compartment was gas pressurized, we opened a drain from the other so that any transcapillary gas passage would not cause a pressure change in the second compartment. Step changes of pressure of various magnitudes were used to determine pressure-response curves. We found that pressurization of the veno-atrial compartment caused systemic vascular resistance to fall in amounts that were essentially linearly proportional to forcing pressure over the range 10 to 30 $cmH_2O$ but that, on average, a plateau was achieved at about 30 $cmH_2O$. Those results were indistinguishable from the earlier experiments in which the entire cardiopulmonary compartment was pressurized as a unit. A similar linear response and plateau were found when pressurizing the pulmonary arterial compartment, but responses were about one-third those obtained from the vein-atrium, and the plateau occurred at 60 $cmH_2O$. The vein-atrial reflex was further characterized to show that responses varied in proportion to rate of rise of pressure if a ramp stimulus was used and that greatest responses would follow a uniform 5 $cmH_2O$ step change if that step was introduced from a baseline pressure of 15 $cmH_2O$.

The gas insufflation experiments did not include pressurization of the pulmonary capillary bed, nor did they separate pulmonary veins from left atrium. Further discrimination was made in preparations using the same basic bypass perfusion technique but in which all pulmonary veins were tied at their atrial junctions so that the pulmonary and left heart chambers could be individually pressurized with blood. Responses to pulmonary vascular pressurization was essentially the same as that found with isolated arterial distension, whereas the response to left heart distension was similar to vein-atrial pressurization.[16] Mild pulmonary edema was induced with sustained pressure in a subset of this study, and more severe edema was caused by alloxan in another subgroup. Edema per se had no detectable effect on systemic vascular resistance or on subsequent responses to pulmonary vascular pressurization.

The experiences with control of systemic vascular resistance by a cardiopulmonary baroreflex indicated that, although vasodilatory responses could occur consequent to increased pressure in the pulmonary arteries, a much larger response followed distension of the left atrium. (We had also shown that distension of the fibrillating ventricle was ineffective over the pressure range used to evoke the atrial response.[15]) I had anticipated that pulmonary congestion would play a bigger role and, anticipating a role for C-fiber reflexes, that capillary congestion would show itself to be important. But this was not so. Furthermore, atrial and pulmonary arterial baroreflexes did not seem to summate when induced together. Although it was apparent that the greatest effect on resistance was transient, this was not detectably different from the time course of the systemic arterial baroreflex, which we often displayed by abruptly increasing set point pressure of the servocontroller. In what seemed appropriate, the optimum baseline pressure from which to acquire the left atrial baroreflex corresponded rather closely with normal transmural pressure and the threshold, and plateau pressures of the pulmonary artery response curve exceeded those of the atrial response by an amount roughly in proportion to the normal mean pressures of those compartments. Teleologically (and to address utility is not without merit), the vasodilatory cardiopulmonary baroreflex would seem destined to respond to acutely higher left ventricular end-diastolic pressures in a way that, at least temporarily, reduces ventricular load and promotes stability. In my experience it has been a robust and reproducible reflex observable under a wide range of conditions. Its effects are dramatically large, most eas-

ily appreciated during servocontrol of systemic arterial pressure wherein it was often necessary to quickly double systemic flow to maintain pressure. One thing not disclosed is whether the left atrium ever "sees" the necessary transmural pressure: in the intact animal, restraints by the pericardium or by mechanical cardiopulmonary interaction may significantly reduce the strain in response to any given change in intraatrial pressure.

## Effects of Cardiac and Pulmonary Vascular Pressures on Breathing

Inspired by reports of cardiodynamic hyperpnea and of the effects of congestion on slowly and rapidly adapting pulmonary receptors and on C-fiber afferent activity, I next addressed the question of the role of cardiac and pulmonary vascular pressures in the control of breathing.

Our first effort made use of the methods described above in which ligation of pulmonary veins and cross-clamping of the ventricles of dogs on cardiopulmonary bypass perfusion enabled independent distension of pulmonary vascular and left atrial compartments. In addition to recording cardiovascular pressures, breathing was monitored by recording the diaphragm electromyogram. Note that in these preparations in which external gas exchange was provided there was no need for lung ventilation. Consequently, lungs were held at a single baseline transpulmonary pressure during the period of perfusion. This approach decoupled breathing activity from lung volume movements and gas exchange and was an important aspect of our experiments on the control of breathing because many secondary effects were prevented in this way. Based on observations of others, I had anticipated that lung congestion would cause tachypnea, but I had no firm preconvictions regarding the effect of atrial distension. We were surprised to find that lung congestion decreased breathing frequency through prolongation of expiratory time. Changes appeared and disappeared immediately on change in vascular pressure. We used vascular pressures ranging from 20 to 70 $cmH_2O$ and found that there was a threshold near 30 $cmH_2O$. Prolongation of expiration varied directly with pressure above that threshold. There were no significant effects on inspiratory time, peak inspiratory magnitude, or the rate of inspiratory activity. An example is shown in Figure 8. Although in 6 of 15 experiments expiration time shortened for two or three breaths at the onset of vascular pressurization, the respiroinhibitory effect of congestion that prevailed in all experiments resembled that of lung inflation, considered to be a response to stimulation of slowly adapting airway receptors. Congestion did not influence breathing after bilateral cervical vagotomy.

The effect of left atrial distension on breathing was inconstant and inconclusive in that early study. However, when there was an effect on breathing it seemed to be weakly excitatory. Subsequent studies[21,24,25] using similar but improved methods have shown that breathing frequency can be stimulated by distension of the left atrium. Shortening of both expiration and inspiration contribute to this change, and, in addition, there may be a small reduction in depth of inspiration. Breathing frequency was, by inspection, a linear function of left atrial pressure above a threshold of 8 $cmH_2O$. An atrial pressure of 30 $cmH_2O$ caused an average change in frequency of 20%. Although the changes were not large, the reflex was robust: it could be demonstrated under a wide range of conditions, it was reproducible, and it could be evoked by changes in left heart loading or by the increased pressure consequent to induction of atrial fibrillation. I concluded that this left atrial reflex could play a role in tachypnea of exercise or left ventricular failure, but it was not clear

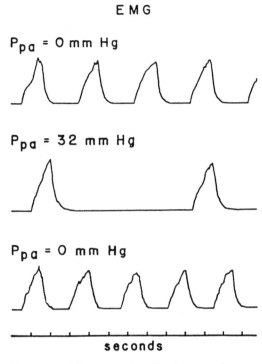

**Figure 8.** Effect on the diaphragm electromyogram of increasing and then lowering pressures in the left atrium and lung vessels, recorded as pulmonary arterial pressure (Ppa). From reference 17, by permission.

how this would interact with the respiroinhibitory effect of lung congestion, which should be simultaneously active under most conditions in the intact animal. We undertook further investigations of the effects of lung vascular congestion and of interaction between lung and cardiac reflexes.

As noted earlier, the anticipated response to lung congestion was tachypnea secondary to stimulation of juxtacapillary C-fiber endings (sometimes referred to as type J receptors). In contrast, our results suggested that slowly adapting receptors had been stimulated. Recall that in those experiments lung volume did not change throughout the breathing cycle. If congestion stimulated or "sensitized" the slowly adapting receptors under normal conditions, where lung volume varies with breathing, congestion may result in tachypnea. The reasoning behind this is that because the slowly adapting receptors may activate the inspiratory off switch, enhancement of their activity will lead to shallow tachypnea if minute ventilation is to be preserved (for example, by the $CO_2$-related chemoreflex). This suggested an experiment to test the hypothesis that congestion enhances the sensitivity of the Hering-Breuer reflex, a reflex attributed to slowly adapting airway receptors.

Anesthetized dogs were prepared by draining systemic venous blood from the right atrium to an external gas exchanger and perfusion pump that returned it to the aorta at constant flow. Ventricular fibrillation was induced, and drains were placed in the right and left ventricular cavities. A second pump perfused the lungs and left heart chambers with blood from the external reservoir admitted through a cannula in the main pulmonary artery. Perfusion flow rate of this second system was intentionally low—about 500 ml/min. Pressure within the lung-heart compartment was adjusted by regulating the resistance of outflow from the left ventricle. During baseline conditions, pressure in the pulmonary artery was approximately 0 $cmH_2O$. Breathing movements of the diaphragm were monitored. The Hering-Breuer reflex was characterized by the relationship between breathing frequency and transpulmonary pressure. Transpulmonary pressure was increased from 2 $cmH_2O$ to 20 $cmH_2O$, or to the point of apnea if that occurred first. Each step was held for 20 s while breathing movements stabilized. After making observations under baseline vascular conditions, the effect of congestion was tested by raising pressure in the pulmonary artery to 60 $cmH_2O$. About 1 min was allowed for stabilization before a Hering-Breuer reflex response relationship was obtained as before. Vascular pressure was then returned to baseline, and another response to inflation was obtained. An example of the results is provided in Figure 9. Note that

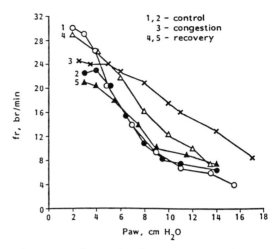

**Figure 9.** Relationship between transpulmonary pressure and breathing frequency before, during, and after congesting the lung vascular bed. From reference 22, by permission.

breathing frequency fell in a nearly linear way as airway pressure (Paw) was raised. Note also that congestion had no significant effect on frequency of respiration (fr) at low airway pressure but that as Paw rose, frequency did not decrease as much as it had while lung vessels and left heart were not distended. Those characteristics pertained to the group as a whole. The failure of frequency to fall as much during congestion implied that the Hering-Breuer reflex was less rather than more effective during congestion. In each of these experiments we also infused a small amount of oleic acid into the lung vessels to cause an acute chemical injury. This was associated with an increased frequency of breathing at low airway pressures, which fell readily with inflation such that at higher airway pressures there was no apparent effect of the acid. The result could be interpreted as enhancement of the Hering-Breuer reflex by lung vascular injury.

In the experiments with the Hering-Breuer reflex we noted that congestion of lungs and left heart did not cause a sustained fall in breathing frequency as it had in the earlier experience with isolated lung vascular congestion, although there was usually a transient dip at the onset of the vascular pressure rise. I wondered if this reflected the combined effects of the depressor pulmonary reflex and the excitor cardiac reflex. Two groups of dogs were prepared using methods for perfusion and stimulus isolation already described. In one group we looked for the effects of isolated pulmonary vascular congestion and in the other the effects of combined lung vessel and left heart distension. In both groups we also attempted to block conduction of myelinated vagal afferent fibers by nerve cooling in an attempt to bring out C-fiber afferent effects. As predicted, congestion of isolated vessels caused marked initial transient depression of breathing followed by a sustained plateau at an intermediate level. Pressurization of combined vessels and left heart, however, caused an initial transient depression followed by an increased frequency significantly above the prestimulus baseline. During vagal block, pressurization of isolated lung vascular or combined lung-heart compartments caused stimulation of breathing. An example of each of these effects is shown in Figure 10.

To complete our studies of the effects on breathing of pressures in the pulmonary circulation, we confined pressure changes to the beating right ventricle and the extraparenchymal pulmonary arteries. Again, bypass perfusion and gas exchange provided control of secondary variables. We found that if outflow resistance from the pulmonary arterial component was raised sufficient to increase arterial pressure to about 65 cmH$_2$O, there would be a small increase in breathing frequency.[19] This result was not seen in all experiments and was not as repeatable as were changes caused by congestion of intraparenchymal vessels or the left heart. Our results conflicted with those of others who have suggested that breathing may be importantly modulated by right heart loading but confirmed studies that showed only a small effect of high arterial pres-

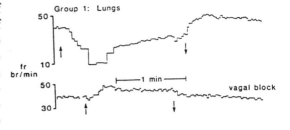

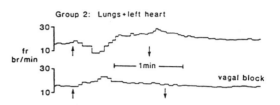

**Figure 10.** Changes in breathing frequency evoked by pressurizing (up arrow) and depressurizing (down arrow) the lung vessels alone or in combination with left heart chambers before and during vagal cold block. From reference 23, by permission.

sures that were confined to the closed extraparenchymal arterial compartment.

My experiences with reflex effects on breathing that arise from the heart and pulmonary vessels have shown that small (5–25%) upward changes in breathing frequency can be generated by increased pressure in the extraparenchymal arterial portion but more particularly by increased pressure in the left atrium. Similar increases can be caused by lung congestion if a dominant and much larger depressor effect is prevented by blocking myelinated afferent fibers. The pressures shown to be effective are within the range of expected pressures in the intact animal, at least at times of stress, and this is particularly true for the left atrial reflex. The lack of uniform direction of change makes it impossible to anticipate the combined effects of these reflexes in the intact situation. Our demonstrations only provide evidence that certain things may happen. They could not test the hypothesis that cardiopulmonary pressure variations are effective in the control of breathing in the intact animal. If nothing else, these experiments serve as useful reminders of the complexity of reflex control systems and the near-futility of creating a valid large-system model without more sophisticated and extensive information. In that regard, performance of these experiments was a rewarding but at the same time a cautionary experience.

## Effect of Lung Vessel and Left Heart Pressures on Airways

Although well established in the experiences of clinicians, cardiac asthma had not been well documented in the physiology laboratory, and I couldn't resist a look to see if left heart and/or lung vascular congestion caused reflex changes in lung mechanics. This was done in two series of experiments, both of which used the now-familiar technique of cardiopulmonary bypass perfusion and external gas exchange. Both studies were combined in a single report.[18] In one study we looked at changes in lung compliance and resistance brought about by increased pressure in the combined chambers of the left heart and pulmonary circulation. In this study, after establishing cardiopulmonary bypass perfusion, the lungs and left heart were perfused with a second pump at low flow admitted through a cannula in one pulmonary arterial branch and drained from cannulas in atrium and ventricle. The lungs were ventilated with 5% $CO_2$ in $O_2$ by a piston respirator connected through a dead space that exceeded tidal volume, incorporated to minimize gas exchange and drying. Airway pressure and flow were continuously monitored, while pressure in the left heart and lung vessels was raised from zero to 45 $cmH_2O$ by partially occluding the outflow of blood. Dynamic lung compliance and resistance were calculated from the airway pressure and flow records. We found that compliance fell and resistance rose whenever pressure was raised in the lung vessels and left heart but that changes of the same direction and size were present after bilateral cervical vagotomy. Induced changes were approximately 20% of baseline values. The effect of vagotomy itself was to increase compliance and reduce resistance. In each experiment we were able to find the expected vagally-mediated change in systemic arterial pressure, confirming the presence of reflex activity secondary to congestion. I inferred from these observations that the changes in lung mechanics brought about by congestion were, in this case, passive and not by reflex.

Because others had found the trachea to undergo reflex contraction typical of smaller airways, I speculated that this may be a more sensitive site from which to detect changes. In a second series of experiments, dogs were once again prepared with cardiopulmonary bypass, but in this group all pulmonary veins were tied at the atrium so that the pulmonary vessels and left heart could be individually pressurized with blood drawn from the external reservoir. Lung ventilation was stopped and an endotracheal tube was passed that had a long compliant cuff. The cuff was inflated to exert a small force on the trachea. Changes in cuff pressure were used to detect changes in tracheal muscle tone. We recorded cuff pressure while pressurizing the left heart and the pulmonary vessels and while imposing different transpulmonary pressures through the endotracheal tube. We found that distension of the left heart consistently caused tracheal contraction. Pulmonary vascular congestion caused contraction in 6 animals but relaxation in 4 others. Lung inflation caused tracheal relaxation in 8 animals but relaxation in 2. Bilateral cervical vagotomy led to tracheal relaxation and loss of changes during lung inflation, vascular congestion, or left heart distension. An example of tracheal contractions with left heart and pulmonary vascular congestion is shown in Figure 11. In this record-

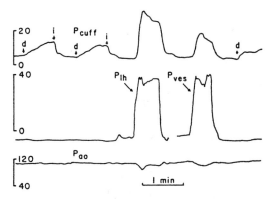

**Figure 11.** Variations in pressure in an endotracheal tube cuff caused by lung inflation and deflation and by distension of the left heart chambers or lung vessels. From reference 18, by permission.

ing the same transducer was used to acquire both the left heart (Plh) and the pulmonary vascular (Pves) pressure by switching from one catheter to the other in the interval between the two episodes of pressurization. Tracheal activity, reflected in the tracheal cuff pressure (Pcuff), can also be seen to vary with lung inflation (i) and deflation (d). Small changes in aortic pressure (Pao) are also apparent.

Unlike the first study, the second provided evidence in support of reflex increase in airway tone consequent to left heart or lung vascular distension. However, we also saw evidence of reflex airway relaxation with lung congestion. This should come as no surprise because congestion has been documented to cause stimulation of each of the several afferent receptor types in the lung. Typically, stimulation of slowly adapting receptors leads to airway relaxation, whereas rapidly adapting receptor or C-fiber ending stimulation results in bronchoconstriction. Note that lung inflation, which also stimulates each receptor group, had a similar divergent effect among the experiments, although the dominant effect seemed to be that attributable to slowly adapting receptors. The appearance of reflex effects of congestion on airways that were appar-

ently dominated by slowly adapting receptors was reminiscent of the effect of congestion on breathing frequency.

# Epilogue

It has been my pleasure for over more than 30 years to explore the lung circulation, lung mechanics, lung-heart interactions, and the control of breathing. Whereas some have preferred to focus more narrowly and to greater depth, I have found satisfaction in covering a range of topics in lung physiology. I am somewhat concerned that a narrow path is tread at some peril, at least to one's students, who may not appreciate the whole from a few of its parts. The whole is too fascinating to let pass by.

Looking back over my experiences, I see the lung circulation as a largely passive system, albeit with complicated physical properties, whose most prominent active regulation comes in response to regional oxygen composition. The lung vessels seem able to play an interesting but as yet uncertain role as the afferent site in several reflexes. None of the above is without controversy, and I am left with more questions than when I began. Looking forward to other topics of personal interest, I see the prospect for demonstrations of control of vascular smooth muscle by a wide range of local and circulating compounds, the regulations of which remain to be explored. I also envision greater interest in an immense vascular surface area that exchanges more with blood than just the respiratory gases and that must be understood in those terms. I look forward to better understanding lung microvascular mechanics and the rheology of pulmonary blood flow, topics about which our knowledge is sketchy and which are in urgent need of further study.

The universe, at least this little part of it, is still expanding.

# References

1. Gorsky, B. H., and T. C. Lloyd, Jr. Effects of perfusate composition on hypoxic vasoconstriction in isolated lung lobes. *J. Appl. Physiol.* 23: 683–686, 1967.
2. Lloyd, T. C., Jr. Effects of alveolar hypoxia on pulmonary vascular resistance. *J. Appl. Physiol.* 19: 1086–1094, 1964.
3. Lloyd, T. C., Jr. Pulmonary vasoconstriction during histotoxic hypoxia. *J. Appl. Physiol.* 20: 488–490, 1965.
4. Lloyd, T. C., Jr. Influence of blood pH on hypoxic pulmonary vasoconstriction. *J. Appl. Physiol.* 21: 358–364, 1966.
5. Lloyd, T. C., Jr. The role of nerve pathways in hypoxic pulmonary vasoconstriction. *J. Appl. Physiol.* 21: 1351–1355, 1966.
6. Lloyd, T. C., Jr. $PO_2$-dependent pulmonary vasoconstriction caused by procaine. *J. Appl. Physiol.* 21: 1439–1443, 1966.
7. Lloyd, T. C., Jr. Influences of $PO_2$ and pH on resting and active tensions of pulmonary arterial strips. *J. Appl. Physiol.* 22: 1101–1109, 1967.
8. Lloyd, T. C., Jr. Hypoxic pulmonary vasoconstriction: role of perivascular tissue. *J. Appl. Physiol.* 25: 560–565, 1968.
9. Lloyd, T. C., Jr. Responses to hypoxia of pulmonary arterial strips in non-aqueous baths. *J. Appl. Physiol.* 28: 566–569, 1970.
10. Lloyd, T. C., Jr. Relation of left ventricular diastolic and lung vascular pressures: atrial effects. *J. Appl. Physiol.* 30: 703–707, 1971.
11. Lloyd, T. C., Jr. Control of systemic vascular resistance by pulmonary and left heart baroreflexes. *Am. J. Physiol.* 222: 1511–1517, 1972.
12. Lloyd, T. C., Jr. Effects of increased intracranial pressure on pulmonary vascular resistance. *J. Appl. Physiol.* 35: 332–335, 1973.
13. Lloyd, T. C., Jr. Cardiopulmonary baroreflexes: integrated responses to sine- and square-wave forcing. *J. Appl. Physiol.* 35: 870–874, 1973.
14. Lloyd, T. C., Jr. Cardiopulmonary baroreflexes: effects of staircase, ramp and square-wave stimulation. *Am. J. Physiol.* 228: 470–476, 1975.
15. Lloyd, T. C., Jr. Cardiopulmonary baroreflexes: left ventricular effects. *Am. J. Physiol.* 232: H634–H638, 1977.
16. Lloyd, T. C., Jr. Cardiopulmonary baroreflexes: effects of pulmonary congestion and edema. *J. Appl. Physiol.* 43: 107–113, 1977.
17. Lloyd, T. C., Jr. Effects of pulmonary congestion and of left atrial distention on breathing in dogs. *J. Appl. Physiol.* 45: 385–391, 1978.
18. Lloyd, T. C., Jr. Reflex effects of left heart and pulmonary vascular distension on airways of dogs. *J. Appl. Physiol.* 49: 620–626, 1980.
19. Lloyd, T. C., Jr. Effect on breathing of acute pressure rise in pulmonary artery and right ventricle. *J. Appl. Physiol.* 57: 110–116, 1984.
20. Lloyd, T. C., Jr. Pulmonary artery distension does not cause pulmonary vasoconstriction. *J. Appl. Physiol.* 61: 741–745, 1986.
21. Lloyd, T. C., Jr. Control of breathing in anesthetized dogs by a left heart baroreflex. *J. Appl. Physiol.* 61: 2095–2101, 1986.
22. Lloyd, T. C., Jr. Effects of lung congestion and oleic acid injury on the Hering-Breuer reflex. *J. Appl. Physiol.* 64: 832–836, 1988.
23. Lloyd, T. C., Jr. Breathing response to lung congestion with and without left heart distension. *J. Appl. Physiol.* 65: 131–136, 1988.
24. Lloyd, T. C., Jr. Effect on breathing of abruptly loading and unloading the canine left heart. *J. Appl. Physiol.* 66: 2216–2222, 1989.
25. Lloyd, T. C., Jr. Effect of increased left atrial pressure on breathing frequency in anesthetized dog. *J. Appl. Physiol.* 69: 1973–1980, 1990.
26. Lloyd, T. C., Jr., and C. E. Juratsch. Pulmonary hypertension induced with an intraarterial balloon: an alternative mechanism. *J. Appl. Physiol.* 61: 746–751, 1986.
27. Lloyd, T. C., Jr., and A. J. L. Schneider. Relation of pulmonary arterial pressure to pressure in the pulmonary venous system. *J. Appl. Physiol.* 27: 489–407, 1969.
28. Lloyd, T. C., Jr., and A. J. L. Schneider. Reflex pulmonary vascular response to distention of lung vessels and left heart. *J. Appl. Physiol.* 29: 318–322, 1970.
29. Lloyd, T. C., Jr., and G. W. Wright. Pulmonary vascular resistance and vascular transmural gradient. *J. Appl. Physiol.* 15: 241–245, 1960.

# 10

# Explorations of an Internal Delta by a Child of Serendip:
## Studies of the Lung Microcirculation

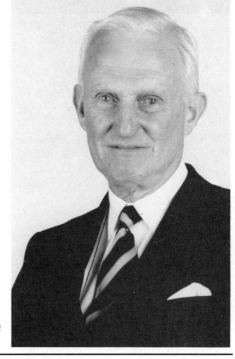

**Grant de J. Lee, M.D.**

*Honary Consulting Physician, John Radcliff Hospital, Oxford, England*

When the story about how Flemming both discovered penicillin and recognized its antibacterial nature was learned, the flurry of scientific commentary that followed indicated his findings were a wonderful example of Serendipity. The word was little used at that time so a subsidiary quest soon followed to rediscover its origin. It led to a man who had not one spark of scientific interest in his makeup. In 1717 Horace Walpole was born in circumstances of privilege and plenty. A reluctant Parliamentarian, he was an ardent writer, prolific correspondent, and avid collector of beautiful objects. In a letter to Sir Thomas Mann, dated January 28, 1754, Walpole wrote the following:

*This discovery indeed is almost of the kind which I call "Serendipity," a very expressive word, which as I have nothing better to tell you, I shall endeavour to explain to you: you will understand it better by the derivation than by the definition. I once read a silly fairy tale, called "The Three Princes of Serendip:" As their highnesses travelled, they were always making discoveries, by accidents and sagacity, of things which they*

From: Wagner WW, Jr, Weir EK (eds): *The Pulmonary Circulation and Gas Exchange.* ©1994, Futura Publishing Co Inc, Armonk, NY.

*were not in quest of: for instance, one of them discovered that a mule blind of the right eye had travelled the same road lately, because the grass was eaten only on the left side, where it was worse than on the right—now do you understand "Serendipity?"*

You will know that Serendip is the ancient name for the island of Ceylon, or Sri Lanka as it is called today. I am fond of this origin because I was born on the island and thus am, by true nature, a Child of Serendip. But genetically my origins derive from a much smaller island— Guernsey, one of the Channel Islands close to the coast of France. This has a proud inheritance, for the Channel Islands were once part of the Duchy of Normandy, whose loyal subjects conquered the Saxons in 1066 and enabled Duke William to become King of England. Thus, to this day we preserve our independent governance within the United Kingdom as loyal subjects of our duke.

Though fertile and beautiful, Guernsey is so tiny that two of its domestic creatures that flourished had to spread far and wide abroad. The most famous today are its dairy cattle and the second are its sons and daughters. In my family's case, my father, who had read Classics at Oxford, found no congenial work in the island. So, when offered a job as a manager of a tea estate in Ceylon, he packed a box of classics and his favorite books in the English language and set off. My mother soon followed him. They found themselves in the foothills of Adam's Peak near Talawakelle in some of the most beautiful hill country in the world.

It was a happy place in which to enter the world and be brought up. We formed a little Guernsey colony of devotion consisting of my two parents, my twin sisters and myself, and Tanner our nanny (a companion for my mother, as much as for us children). The nearest European was 50 or 60 miles away. My father and mother taught us children till I was nearly ten.

Sooner or later the wrench came, for there were no English schools within hundreds of miles of us. So my mother brought us back to Guernsey and left us with her parents. It was a tradition in her family that male children were educated on the mainland at Marlborough College, so each term I traveled by ship across the English Channel to Marlborough. It was a spartan place in those days. Its style of living would best resemble a corrective institution for young offenders today. But the education was good, outside the classroom we had freedom to range independently, and the jungle training course imposed by my fellow inmates was character forming.

For some reason I had always wanted to be a doctor. It is possible that the dim memory from Ceylon of having my appendix out at the age of four and the coincident death of one of the twins from dysentery had something to do with this. At all events, during my last year in the Biology Sixth at Marlborough I came under the influence of a remarkable eccentric named Ashley Gordon Lowndes. He had a passionate research interest in fresh water invertebrates and was a superb observer and taxonomic investigator. I learned all manner of things from him, particularly to be a precise observer as well as to enjoy technical skills. He opened my eyes to biology and exploration.

If one looks at the map of the South Coast of England and the English Channel, one sees that the Channel Islands are very close to the northwest coast of France. In August 1939 I had just left school to go to university and my parents had, at last, retired home to Guernsey from the Far East. But we were destined not to be together there for very long. The 3rd of September was a lovely sunny day, and we all went swimming at the foot of the red granite cliffs of the Gouffre on the south coast of the island. When we got home our neighbor came running in to tell us that Neville Chamberlain had announced that we were at war with Germany. My father reminded us that in the First World War the U-boat blockade had separated Guernsey from the mainland, so we decided that we should all return to the mainland of England at once, as refuges. Within a few months the Channel Islands were invaded and occupied by the German army in its sweep through northern France.

It was exciting to be a medical student at St. Thomas's Hospital across the Thames from the Houses of Parliament in the last world war. The site was a prime target for German air raids. The hospital received its fair share of bombing, so the wards and operating theatres took to the cellars. Even as preclinical students we were involved as apprentices to our seniors. The bulk of the people who taught us were dugouts (like myself now) who were too old for the services and kept one page ahead of us in the book. But they inspired us with their enthusiasm and tantalized us with how little time we had to learn. Four and a half years after entering medical school I was a qualified doctor, had done a short intern job, and found myself in northern Italy as a RMO (Regimental Medical Officer) in a tank regiment in the eighth Army during its final assault across the Senio and Po River when it destroyed the remains of the German army in Italy. Three years later I was finally released from the army. I returned to Britain with an enormous amount of clinical experience of every kind. I had not just treated battle casualties but tropical disease and acute infections of all kinds in Italy, in the Sudan, and in Egypt.

I returned to London to find the place swarming with young doctors who had been demobilized before me but had no jobs. I decided that if I were to get anywhere at all, I would have to do something

different from the others. My first need was to get some scientific training. At that time the only place in Britain where one could learn hard science as a clinician was the Postgraduate (PG) Medical School in London. I had learned another important lesson in the army: always go to the top for an authoritative decision. So I knocked on the door of Sir John McMichael (still plain John then) (Fig. 1). He was professor of medicine at the PG School at Hammersmith and I asked to work for him. He seemed surprised, but a few weeks later I was working for him—as a humble house physician (HP) once more.

During the war McMichael and Sharpey-Schafer had been the first in Europe to study factors affecting cardiac output in man by the direct Fick principle using cardiac catheters.[18] The term of my HP was about to end, when one day McMichael gave me an article to read from

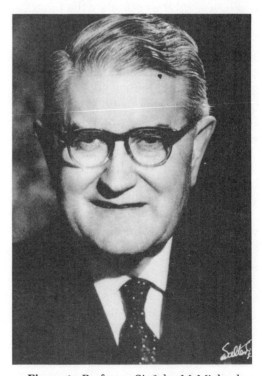

**Figure 1.** Professor Sir John McMichael.

the latest issue of the *American Journal of Physiology*. It was by W. F. Hamilton and his colleagues in Atlanta and André Cournand and his colleagues in New York.[8] They had just published their results comparing simultaneous measurements of cardiac output by the Fick method and the dye dilution method, which Hamilton and his colleagues had devised much earlier.[7]

McMichael was keen that we should set up the dye method, so I did this for him with Harry Kopelman, my registrar and my first lifelong friend made through laboratory work (Fig. 2.). We made simultaneous measurements with McMichael during his studies of the effects of intravenous digoxin on cardiac output in patients with acute congestive heart failure from hypertension and from mitral stenosis.

The dye dilution method not only allowed us to measure cardiac output and to compare it with the Fick method, but it also enabled us to calculate the mean circulation time of the dye through the heart and lungs and thus calculate the intrathoracic blood volume.

We stumbled on a remarkable finding. The patients with hypertensive congestive cardiac failure had a much larger intrathoracic blood volume than those with congestive cardiac failure from mitral stenosis. Yet both groups of patients had approximately the same heart size, measured radiologically. We could only conclude that the patients with hypertensive heart failure had an increased lung blood volume, whereas the patients with mitral stenosis had a lung blood volume that was virtually normal even when in heart failure (Fig. 3).[15] Was this discovery an example of Serendipity? I think so.

Paul Wood was a staff member at Hammersmith at that time. He was a brilliant Australian cardiologist who always seemed to be one step ahead of everyone else. He argued that our finding could best be explained by reflex pulmonary arteriolar vasconstriction in patients with mitral stenosis, which protected their lungs from

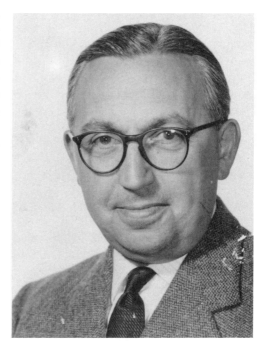

**Figure 2.** Dr. H. Kopelman.

pulmonary oedema. I could not believe this, for lung histology reveals a paucity of vascular smooth muscle in the peripheral pulmonary arteries and veins compared with the systemic circulation.

About this time Peter Sharpey-Schafer left the PG School to take the chair of medicine at my old teaching hospital at St. Thomas's. He was having quite a time of it there trying to persuade his colleagues, particularly the nursing staff at St. Thomas's, that dutifully applied clinical investigation was a gentle science rather than barbaric personal assault. At that time there was no possibility for me to rise up the ladder of academic medicine without having held a junior job in the teaching hospital in which I worked so Peter Schafer invited me to join him as a clinical lecturer and junior investigator. Over the next few years master and pupil became very close friends (Fig. 4).

Sharpey-Schafer had made great strides in understanding how the systemic

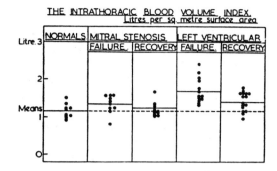

**Figure 3.** Comparisons of the intrathoracic blood volume index (L/sq.M) in normal subjects and in patients with heart failure from mitral stenosis and from hypertension, studied before and after recovery.

baroreceptors reflexly control the blood pressure in man. He recorded the blood pressure directly from the brachial artery and studied the changes brought about by the Valsalva manoeuvre.

You will remember that when a subject blows against an external pressure such as a mercury column, the consequent rise in intrathoracic pressure impedes venous return to the heart. As a result stroke volume falls, manifest by a fall in pulse pressure. This affects the carotid baroreceptors, leading to generalized systemic vasoconstriction. On release of the Valsalva manoeuvre, rapid inflow into the heart is resumed and stroke volume increases, producing a blood pressure overshot affecting both mean and pulse pressure. This activates the carotid baroreceptors, which initiate reflex vasodilatation, and the blood pressure returns to normal. In patients with autonomic failure no such reflex responses take place.

Sharpey-Schafer had also shown that the increase in arterial pressure following the Valsalva manoeuvre was associated with decrease in forearm blood flow except in the sympathectomized limb. In addition, tetraethyl ammonium chloride had just been discovered as a potential blood pressure lowering agent. It worked as a ganglion blocking agent.

We decided to compare the vasomo-

tor responses of the systemic and pulmonary arterial systems simultaneously in response to the Valsalva manoeuvre. If Paul Wood was right and the lung peripheral arterial system was vasoactive, then the pulmonary and systemic arterial responses to Valsalva's manoeuvre would be similar. If, however, the peripheral arterial system of the lungs was insufficiently provided with smooth muscle, then the reflex response would be absent or weak. We therefore studied patients admitted with a variety of cardiovascular conditions but whose blood pressure response to the Valsalva manoeuvre was normal. To make satisfactory measurements we needed to record pressures from the right atrium, pulmonary artery, and pulmonary capillary independent of superimposed intrathoracic pressure changes taking place as a result of the Valsalva manoeuvre and due to effects of respiration. To do this we recorded intrathoracic pressure from a water-filled catheter in the oesophagus at the same time that we also recorded right atrial,

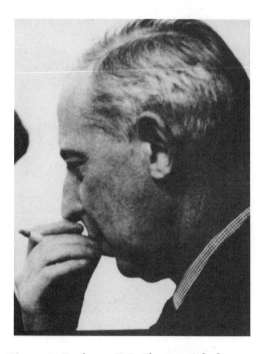

**Figure 4.** Professor E. P. Sharpey-Schafer.

pulmonary arterial, and pulmonary capillary pressures by right heart catheterization. We used Hansen Capacitance manometers and a simple subtractor circuit linking their electrical outputs. In this way we could obtain net right atrial, net pulmonary arterial, and pulmonary capillary pressures independent of superimposed intrathoracic pressure events.

Figure 5 shows what we found. Following the Valsalva manoeuvre there was the usual rise in brachial arterial pressure but little rise in net pulmonary arterial pressure. Moreover, the net pulmonary arterial pressure rises coincided with the inspiratory phases of respiration and fell again with expiration, indicating that the pulmonary arterial pressure was largely dominated by changes in stroke volume as a result of respiration. Following an infusion of intravenous tetraethyl ammonium chloride, the rise in brachial arterial pressure following the Valsalva manoeuvre was abolished due to autonomic blockade by the drug. The response of the pulmonary arterial pressure to the Valsalva remained unaffected. To all intents and purposes the pulmonary arterial system

seemed to respond passively to these changes in pulmonary arterial inflow, secondary to changes in right ventricular stroke volume.

In Britain at that time the only people studying the physiology of the lung were animal physiologists. So when I presented our work at the Medical Research Society it was received with some skepticism, for there was general belief that unless pulmonary arterial inflow was controlled it was impossible to come to the conclusions that we had made. It was plain that if I were to compete I had to learn to be more professional as a human pulmonary vascular applied physiologist as well as clinician. At that time a number of my friends who were becoming the new breed of chest physician were returning from the United States, having worked in the Department of Physiology and Pharmacology at the University of Pennsylvania in Philadelphia under Professor Julius Comroe (Fig. 6). "Uncle Julius," as we all came to know him, had become the guru for aspiring applied lung physiologists in Britain. He enjoyed having young people from our country because we were used to working

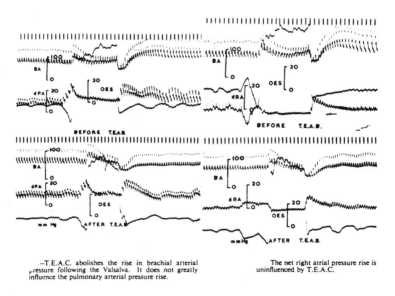

—T.E.A.C. abolishes the rise in brachial arterial pressure following the Valsalva. It does not greatly influence the pulmonary arterial pressure rise.

The net right atrial pressure rise is uninfluenced by T.E.A.C.

**Figure 5.** The effect of the Valsalva maneuver on brachial artery (BA), pulmonary arterial (PA), and right atrial (RA) pressure before and after tetra-ethyl Ammonium Bromide (TEAB).

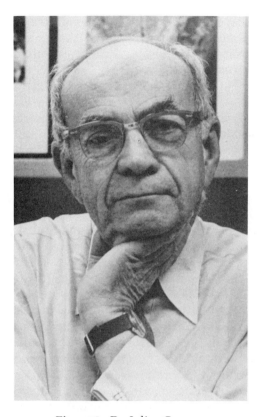

**Figure 6.** Dr. Julius Comroe.

for about half the stipend of any American research follow and therefore worked hard because we had no money to do anything else!

I asked Peter Schafer if I could go and work for Uncle Julius. In no time at all he had found some money from the St. Thomas's Hospital Endowment Trust, and my wife and I set sail for the United States, bound for Philadelphia.

## Terra Nova

We arrived in Philadelphia in April 1953. It was the week of the meetings in Atlantic City of the Federated Society of American Biologists. The whole of Julius Comroe's department was there, with the exception of one man—Arthur Du Bois. Arthur had recently come from the famous stable led by Wallace Fenn in Rochester,

New York, where he had worked with Herman Rahn and Arthur Otis. He had devised a means for studying the lung's airway mechanics in man using a whole body plethysmograph. Julius Comroe built one for him before Du Bois arrived in Philadelphia.

When I arrived I found Arthur working alone in his lab. He asked who I was, apologized for the absence of his colleagues, and, after brief and gentle exchange of pleasantries, asked what my particular interest was. I said I had found that the pulmonary arterial system in man seemed to be largely passive in its response to changes in right heart output due to an absence of any significant reflex vasomotor control. I had come to learn some physiology, as the animal physiologists in Britain had questioned my findings. Arthur has an electric mind. He was silent for perhaps half a minute and then said, "In that case, what do you think happens to lung capillary blood flow?" Without thinking I replied, "It must be pulsatile." At once he replied, "In that case the whole of our physiological understanding of blood-gas exchange in the lungs by steady-state diffusion (Bohr integration) is likely to be wrong. Let's see if lung capillary blood flow really *is* pulsatile!"

Arthur remembered the work of Krogh and Lindhard,[16] who had measured cardiac output in man using nitrous oxide inhaled from a wedge spirometer. So he attached electrocardiograph electrodes to my limbs, gave me a bag of nitrous oxide, and said, "Jump in the box and you can be the first subject." The ambient pressure in the body plethysmograph was measured with a Lilly capacitance manometer, which Arthur turned up to maximum gain. He told me to breathe out maximally, to inhale a full breath of nitrous oxide from the bag, and to hold my breath with my glottis open. He then recorded the pressure in the body plethysmograph as it fell due to the uptake of $N_2O$ from my

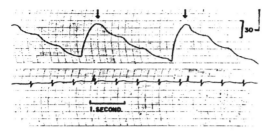

**Figure 7.** Nitrous oxide ($N_2O$) from the lungs in man, measured in the whole body plethysmograph. As the gas is absorbed by the lung capillary blood flow, the plethysmographic pressure falls. The fall is steepest at the time of each ECG *T* wave. The sharp upward deflection of the tracing indicates where the plethysmograph chamber was vented to atmosphere.

lungs. If the blood through my lung capillaries had been flowing at a constant rate, then $N_2O$ uptake would have been constant and the pressure within the plethysmograph would have fallen at a constant rate. But lo and behold, (Fig. 7) the plethysmograph fell in waves, with the steepest fall soon after the *T* wave of the ECG (Fig. 3). We had discovered that lung capillary blood flow was indeed pulsatile with each heart beat. In two and a half months we had all the information we needed to publish a definitive paper on the pulsatile nature of pulmonary capillary blood flow in man.[17]

I had found my own internal delta—the lung alveolar capillary circulation.

## An Oxford Education: Through Its Back Door

I returned to England, excited by what had been possible to find in so short a time. At the time I believed that if I were to dig for gold in the streets I would find it!

So far, my journey from Serendip had shown me that (1) the mean lung volume was not increased in pulmonary venous hypertension from mitral stenosis; (2) this was unlikely to be due to reflex vasomotor control of the lung vascular system; and (3) because of its low peripheral vascular impedence, the lung's capillary blood flow was highly pulsatile during each cardiac cycle.

In Philadelphia, Arthur and I had discussed how the lung's low impedance vascular bed could cope with so pulsatile an ejection of blood from the right ventricle so as to ensure that transcapillary hydrostatic pressure never exceeded plasma oncotic pressure and yet always allowed optimal alveolar-capillary gas exchange. If the capillaries behaved as a fixed volume system then the pulsatile ejection of the blood from the right ventricle would have to be pushed through the capillary bed in squirts. This would be recognized by a linear rise in pulmonary arterial pressure as flow rate increased during systole. Moreover, as blood flow rate increased through the capillaries during systole, there would be a shorter and shorter passage time for individual red cells to traverse alveolar capillaries for gas exchange. If, however, the alveolar capillaries behaved as a series of Starling resistors stacked one above the other, which opened in response to small increments in pressure as blood flow increased, then optimal gas exchange would be maintained and the pulmonary arterial pressure would be down regulated as capillary systems were recruited vertically.

We believed this explanation was correct, for there was intuitive evidence to support it. Cournand and his group in New York had shown that the mean pulmonary arterial pressure did not rise linearly with increases in cardiac output at low levels of exercise, whereas Riley and his colleagues at Johns Hopkins University had shown that the oxygen diffusing capacity initially rose linearly with exercise. These two pieces of information suggested that the lung alveolar capillaries could be acting as vertically stacked Starling resistors and were capable of recruitment.

We had to wait until 1960, when West

and Dollery,[34] using radioactive $C_2O$), found that in erect human subjects blood flow at the lung bases was some eight times greater than at the apexes and that ventilation distribution was also somewhat greater in the lower zones than in the upper zones of the lungs. Intense study of the lung ventilation-perfusion distribution then followed, led particularly by Permutt, Bromberger-Barnea, and Bane[20] in the United States and West, Dollery, and Naimark in Britain.[35] West and his colleagues found that in the vertically suspended, isolated, ventilated, and perfused lung there was no capillary blood flow at hydrostatic levels above which the alveolar pressure exceeded both the pulmonary arterial and venous pressures (West: Zone 1). Flow in the lung capillaries began at a level down the lung where pulmonary arterial pressure exceeded alveolar pressure (West: Zone 2). It continued to rise in a manner determined by the difference between pulmonary arterial and alveolar pressures until a level was reached where the pulmonary venous pressure also exceeded the alveolar pressure. Over the remainder of the dependent lung, blood flow was then governed by the pulmonary arterial-venous pressure difference (West: Zone 3).

These findings postdate the events I have traced in my own life. When I returned to England and St. Thomas's in September 1963 and told my story about the lung capillaries, I found a total lack of interest except from Peter Sharpey-Schafer. I was getting to an age when I needed a more senior position where I could set up my own laboratory. Posts of this kind were scarce, but a senior Beit Fellowship was advertised and I applied for it. The selector was Professor George Pickering from St. Mary's Hospital. He interviewed me kindly but skeptically. No fellowship followed, but about a fortnight later he phoned to ask if I would be interested in being his first assistant in Oxford, as he had just been appointed Regius Professor of Medicine there. He had intended to take Stanley Peart, his first assistant at St. Mary's Hospital, but Peart had gotten Pickering's job at St. Mary's instead! Pickering needed somebody who was competent clinically to run his wards when he was busy with his professorial duties in Oxford, the nation, and overseas. He also wanted someone who could set up a regional cardiovascular diagnostic laboratory to support a new professor of surgery in Oxford who was about to start open heart surgery.

It was not difficult to accept his invitation. The medical school in Oxford has a long and storied history, but until the war it only had a preclinical school. Its graduates went to the London teaching hospitals for their clinical training. As a result of the bombing of London, most London clinical schools were evacuated. Thus the Radcliffe Infirmary in Oxford, which hitherto had been a county hospital, received its first clinical students, and its clinical staff became associate teachers in the university.

Following the war the clinical school remained in Oxford but the general prejudice among the university dons was that it was a second-rate institution compared with the London teaching hospitals. By 1965, when Pickering was invited to be the new clinical Regius Professor in Oxford, the school was at a low ebb. George Pickering was, above all, a great educator. He saw the enormous opportunity Oxford offered him to create an integrated clinical medical school between the basic sciences and bedside medicine. Our job under him was to provide a first-rate clinical service in the hospital, to be available at all times to assist colleagues if they asked for it, to teach clinical students virtually by apprenticeship, and to undertake our own research.

As far as research was concerned, I had one difficulty. Pickering was interested in big research concepts involving the study and relief of major diseases. As a young man he had studied pain. He was now world famous for his research on high blood pressure. He was not a bit interested in the applied physiology of the lung microcirculation, let alone funding me for a whole body plethysmograph!

One or two years after I arrived in Pickering's unit I went into the Red Lion opposite the hospital one evening. In through the door walked Jim Henry, dressed as a colonel in the U.S. Air Force. I had met Jim briefly at the fall meeting of the American Physiological Society at Madison, Wisconsin, in 1953, where he had given a paper immediately before the one I had given with Arthur du Bois on pulsatile capillary blood flow. I was surprised to see him and I asked him what he was doing in Oxford. He told me he was now scientific director in Brussels for the U.S. Air Force Aerospace Research and Development Command. He had come to Oxford to negotiate contracts for research in the university science departments! In no time at all I had asked Jim Henry to come upstairs in the Radcliffe Infirmary to my laboratory to talk about a project for the U.S. Air Force on lung blood flow. After a few glasses of beer a whole body plethysmograph and a small space capsule seemed two very similar devices in which to study the effects of physical and mental stress on cardiac output, measured by nitrous oxide uptake! Henry soon negotiated a research contract with the U.S. Air Force that gave me laboratory independence until 1965.

I was now running a diagnostic cardiac catheter laboratory, and the opportunity to measure the physical characteristics of the pulmonary arterial fluid transmission line in patients was obvious. I could make a beginning by measuring pulmonary arterial pressure and pulmonary capillary blood flow simultaneously during cardiac catheterization using nitrous oxide. A lot of development work had to be done before I could start. I built a body plethysmograph that could be slung from the ceiling and lowered by an electric crane onto the cardiac catheter table. Profiting from my experience in Philadelphia, I made the walls of the plethysmograph circular and of thick perspex to make it rigid. The cardiac catheter table was about two inches thick, so I hoped that this too would be rigid.

In the previous $N_2O$-plethysmograph studies, gas uptake by the lungs was measured by recording the pressure change that occurred in the airtight chamber maintained at constant volume in which changes in chamber pressure due to $N_2O$ uptake were converted to volume by applying Boyle's Law. The immediate challenge was to record the rate of change of gas volume entering the body plethysmograph directly, to replace the volume of $N_2O$ absorbed by lung capillary blood flow. Under such circumstances the baseline for zero gas uptake is a straight horizontal line, and any slow drift due, for example, to temperature change in the plethysmograph or respiratory quotient effects, would be manifest as slight displacements of the baseline. But the main advantage in recording the rate of gas uptake in this manner was that the records produced by pulsatile pulmonary capillary blood flow could be directly compared with simultaneous records of pulmonary vascular pressure.

When I first went back to St. Thomas's to join Sharpey-Schafer I had met a nurse there who had just married a biophysicist who was a brilliant inventor. His name was Frank Stott. He was a member of the MRC Instrument Research Unit, which, amongst other things, had designed the oxygen breathing equipment provided to the British expedition to Everest under the leadership of Sir John Hunt, in which Edmund Hillary and Sherpa Tensing had succeeded in reaching the summit. The unit was subsequently disbanded, and Frank had then been appointed to Sir George Pickering's unit in Oxford.

Frank designed a brilliantly conceived servopneumatic flow meter for use in the body plethysmograph with which to measure the instantaneous rate of $N_2O$ uptake from the lungs. The pneumatic flow meter was a little temperamental, but a greater difficulty was that the flat bed of the catheter table resonated just as the walls of the original plethysmograph had done in Philadelphia. The concrete floor of the laboratory had a terrazzo surface, so we glued a newly designed base for the plethysmograph directly to the floor and were then able to get beautiful curves of gas volume change within the lungs from the pneumatic flow meter.

During this development period we indulged in some amateur respiratory physiology and studied the effect of pulsatile capillary blood flow on oxygen and carbon dioxide exchange within the lungs. We breathed appropriate gas mixtures so as to obtain mixed venous $O_2$ and $CO_2$ tensions within the lungs. This enabled us to measure the alveolar capillary $O_2$ and $CO_2$ exchange individually and to compare them with the pulmonary capillary blood flow. The rate of oxygen uptake was linearly related to capillary blood flow throughout the cardiac cycles, but $CO_2$ elimination occurred at two rates dependent both on the pulmonary capillary blood flow rate during systole and on a more sustained rate of discharge of $CO_2$ stored in solution within the lung tissues[2] (Fig. 8).

It was plain that simultaneous measurements of pulmonary arterial pressure and lung capillary blood flow by cardiac catheterization and $N_2O$ uptake were not going to be ideal if conducted on the floor! Happily for us, at just about this time the hoped-for breakthrough for augmenting the sensitivity of carcinoma of the bronchus to radiotherapy by hyperbaric oxygen had proven ill found. Vickers Research had built a number of single-subject hyperbaric oxygen chambers for this purpose. They were unable to sell them, and the company donated one such

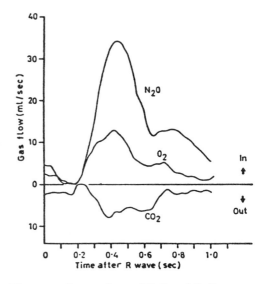

**Figure 8.** Comparison of $N_2O$ and $O_2$ flow rates into the lungs and $CO_2$ flow rate out of the lungs, measured by plethysmographic method. $O_2$ uptake obtained at $P_{\cdot_{AL}} O_2$:100 mmHg and $P_{\cdot_{AL}} CO_2$:49 mmHg. $CO_2$ uptake obtained at P.AL $O_2$:50 mmHg and $P_{\cdot_{AL}} CO_2$:38 mmHg.

chamber to me. The patient could lie on a flat bed, which slid out of the chamber. This enabled me to catheterize the patient in the normal way for diagnostic purposes. With the catheter in situ, including the catheter manometer heads and $N_2O$ supply system all contained within the hyperbaric oxygen chamber bulkhead, it was a simple matter to slide the patient into the hyperbaric chamber and close the bulkhead to make simultaneous measurements of pulmonary arterial pressure and $N_2O$ uptake.

Figure 9 shows our first simultaneous recording of pulmonary arterial pressure and pulmonary capillary blood flow ($N_2O$ uptake) obtained at cardiac catheterization in the Vickers plethysmograph. We found that the $N_2O$ pulsatility closely resembled the pulmonary arterial pressure pulse but was delayed in time. The normal pulmonary arterial–pulmonary capillary flow conduction time averaged approximately 120 ms because of the physical distensibility of the pulmonary arterial transmission line.

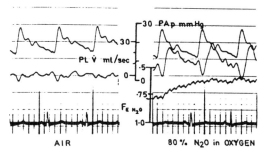

**Figure 9.** The first simultaneous record of pulmonary arterial pressure ($PA_p$) and pulmonary capillary blood flow, measured by $N_2O$ uptake during cardiac catheterization of a patient during routine diagnostic studies. P1V = rate of gas uptake measured in the body plethysmograph. $F_EN_2O$ = $N_2O$ concentration at the mouth. The ECG is also shown.

By now I had been joined by Nicholas Karatzas, a young cardiologist from Athens. He made detailed studies in normal individuals and in patients with pulmonary arterial and venous hypertension secondary to heart disease, particularly mitral stenosis.[13,14] We found that 67% of the stroke volume was required to distend the pulmonary arterial system during systole for onward transmission to the capillaries during diastole. With tachycardia and with pulmonary hypertension the fraction of stroke volume stored in the arterial system during systole became less, indicating that the arterial system was becoming less distensible.

Karatzas then went on to study severe pulmonary hypertension, particularly from mitral stenosis. We expected that in such conditions morphological changes in the small pulmonary arterioles would produce such an increase in precapillary resistance that pulsatile inflow to the capillaries would become damped. We hoped this would allow us to develop a noninvasive method for estimating pulmonary arterial hypertension, simply by measuring how much $N_2O$ uptake pulsatility became damped. But nothing of the kind occurred. In virtually every case of pulmonary arterial hypertension we studied, pulsatile lung capillary blood flow remained unaltered.

It was obvious that empirical comparison of the wave forms of pulmonary arterial pressure and pulmonary arterial blood flow were insufficient to describe the fluid dynamics within the pulmonary arterial system. If we were to develop a method to enable us to measure pulmonary arterial flow as well as pulmonary arterial pressure and pulmonary capillary blood flow simultaneously, we would be able to derive the equations to solve for pulmonary arterial resistance, compliance, and dynamic impedance. The difficulty was that no such flow-measuring device yet existed.

Donald Schultz was an aerodynamic engineer in the Department of Engineering Science. He had first come to Oxford as a Rhodes scholar from New Zealand. After obtaining his doctorate he worked at the National Physical Laboratory in Teddington. He then returned to Oxford as a foundation fellow of St. Catherine's College and university lecturer in mechanical engineering. Soon he was elected to a readership, then a personal chair. He had an international reputation for his research in high-speed fluid dynamics and made important contributions to jet engine turbine design.

Donald and I got to know each other dining at high table in college. One of the joys of an intercollegiate university like Oxford is that much learning comes through recreation and good fellowship. At night after good food and good wine one is able to talk freely and without shyness to individuals of great learning from every discipline under the sun and to share enthusiasms together. From such a chance meeting Donald and I became great friends. Life in Oxford lost some of its fun for me when in April 1987 Donald died suddenly walking the Routburn Track in New Zealand while on holiday with his wife June.

When Donald learned that nothing

was then known about blood velocity distribution within the great vessels of the body, he saw the enormous contribution he could make. So we joined forces to work together for many happy years in the animal laboratory, the cardiac catheter lab, and with my colleague Alf Gunning during open heart surgery. The heated thin film anemometers he used in his aerodynamic research were adapted for this purpose. They consisted of minute platinum films bonded to a ceramic base attached to our catheters and specially designed needles with which to traverse the great vessels of the body. In this way we were able to be the first to map blood velocity profiles in the great vessels entering and leaving the heart in man both in

health and in valve disease, as well as mapping the whole of the velocity distribution of the aorta in the dog. Of relevance here was the important finding that the velocity profile at the root of the aorta and the pulmonary artery is flat. Thus, if one measures the diameter of either these vessels from a transverse chest x-ray, one is able to calculate instantaneous bulk flow within these vessels from a catheter tip velocity device (Fig. 10 a and b).[27,30]

We now had a flourishing, beautifully equipped fluid dynamics laboratory with measuring devices that were unavailable anywhere else in the world at that time. We had needle probes equipped with high frequency velocity sensors, cardiac catheters of every size and description similarly

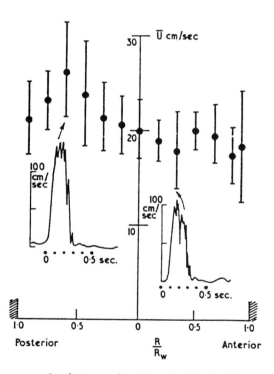

Aortic traverse in adult male with mitral incompetence showing time-averaged velocity at each radial station ± 1 standard deviation. Turbulence at peak systole across aorta. Maximum velocity 130 cm./sec., Re – 7,800.

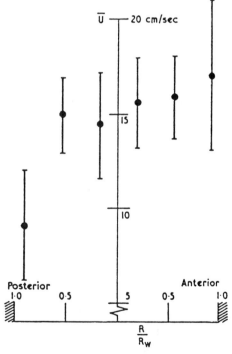

Traverse of pulmonary artery of patient with mitral incompetence; ± 1 standard deviation.

**Figure 10.a.** Aortic traverse in an adult male with mitral incompetence showing time-averaged velocity at each radio station + 1 standard deviation. Turbulence at peak systole across aorta. Maximum velocity 130 cm/s, Re = 7,800. **b.** Traverse of the pulmonary artery of the same patient with mitral incompetence, ± 1 SD.

equipped, as well as microchip ultrasonic methods for measuring the diameter of blood vessels. In addition we had financial security for 10 years from the Medical Research Council in a program grant that enabled us to recruit more people.

Our efforts to diagnose pulmonary arterial hypertension from a damped pulmonary capillary flow pulse had proven fruitless because the pulsatility remained unaltered in virtually all circumstances. It was plain to Donald that the likely explanation for this was that, as pulmonary arterial resistance increased leading to pulmonary hypertension, there was a compensatory decrease in pulmonary arterial compliance.

So Stuart Reuben joined us for this work. He was keen to train as an investigative cardiologist and became the prime mover working on the physics of the pulmonary arterial system that we now embarked on. He was not only a natural experimentalist but also a fine clinician.

Using closed chested dogs in the body plethysmograph and the appropriate devices designed by Donald Schultz, we measured pulmonary arterial pressure and flow in the pulmonary artery simultaneously with pulmonary capillary flow with $N_2O$ from which to derive pulmonary arterial resistance, compliance, and impedance in normal animals in response to hypoxia, serotonin infusion, and stellate ganglion sympathetic stimulation. Similar studies were made in patients with various degrees of pulmonary hypertension from mitral stenosis undergoing routine cardiac catheterization.[26,28,29]

The findings were similar in both dog and man. They provided a satisfactory explanation for the maintained pulsatility of pulmonary capillary blood flow, even in conditions of moderate hypertension in which the mean pulmonary arterial pressure was as high as 45 mmHg (peak systolic pressure 75 mmHg). Figure 11a summarizes these findings in the dog. When the pulmonary arterial pressure rose as a result of increasing pulmonary arterial resistance (R), there was a reciprocal fall in pulmonary arterial compliance (C) proximal to the site of increased resistance. As a result, the time constant of the arterial system as whole remained unaltered (R × C = Kt), thus preserving normal capillary blood flow pulsations even when pulmonary hypertension had developed. The decrease in pulmonary arterial compliance leads to an increase in pulmonary arterial pulse wave velocity (Fig. 11b). Stuart Reuben cleverly exploited this finding to develop a means of calculating pulmonary arterial pressure using nitrous oxide uptake. He measured the opening of the pulmonary valve by means of a phonocardiograph and the arrival of the flow pulse at the capillaries by nitrous oxide uptake. This enabled him to calculate the pulmonary arterial flow conduction time and to derive pulmonary arterial pulse wave velocity and pulmonary arterial pressure.[26]

Having spent so long studying how the fluid dynamics of the pulmonary arterial system regulated inflow into the alveolar capillaries and having learned from others how the alveolar capillaries themselves regulated their own hydrostatic pressure in the lungs at large, it was now time for us to tackle the pulmonary venous system. In the mid-1970s this was virgin territory. The particular question that intrigued me was this: How was it that pulmonary capillary blood flow remained pulsatile in pulmonary *venous* hypertension? The bulk of such cases come from left sided heart disease in which the left atrial pressure is elevated. One would thus expect the elevated pressure pulses emanating from the left atrium to be reflected backward through the pulmonary veins to impede outflow from the lung capillaries, thus altering the wave form of nitrous oxide uptake. But all the evidence showed that the pulmonary capillary flow pulse activity remained unaltered under such circumstances. Presumably the pulmonary venous system must contain a com-

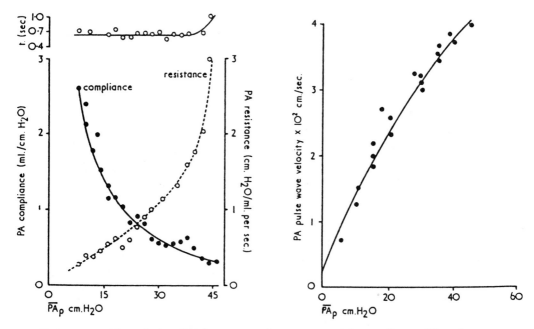

**Figure 11.a.** The relationship between pulmonary arterial compliance (C), pulmonary arterial resistance (R), mean pulmonary arterial pressure (PA$_p$) and pulmonary arterial time constant (t) obtained from the produce of (C × R) in dogs. Combined data from control, hypoxia, and serotonin studies. **b.** The relationship between pulmonary arterial pulse wave velocity and mean pulmonary artery input pressure (PA$_p$). Pulse wave velocity calculated from compliance data using the Bramwell-Hill equation.

ponent that is highly distensible and acts as a *Windkessel* to damp out retrograde pressure pulsations from the left atrium.

Bishma Rajagopalan now joined the group. He had come to Balliol College Oxford as a scholar from India to read medicine. He was keen to study a project in depth and to work toward his doctorate of philosophy. Using the animal body plethysmograph that Stuart Reuben had designed, Bishma undertook meticulous studies in closed chested dogs in which he made simultaneous measurements of pressure and flow in the pulmonary artery, in the pulmonary capillary system, and in the left lower lobe veins external to the lung prior to their entry into the left atrium. The technical challenges were formidable. So Bishma, Stuart Reuben, and I each took a portion of them to get good at. Stuart ran the plethysmographic side of things, I did the surgery, and Bishma de-

veloped the vein techniques to enable him to measure not only pressure and flow simultaneously but also changes in their cross sectional dimension. These were measured ultrasonically using minute crystals glued to the veins.

The first successful studies soon showed that the pulsatile ejection of blood flow from the right ventricle into the main pulmonary artery, which was transmitted as an arterialized pulse through the lung capillaries, had an entirely different wave form in the large pulmonary veins external to the lung prior to their entry into the left atrium. Vein flow, though pulsatile, had a profile that was almost identical to the mirror image of left atrial pressure.

We confirmed identical findings during cardiac catheterization of patients with tight aortic stenosis in whom the left ventricular-aortic pressure gradient had first to be measured for diagnostic purposes. A thin film velocity sensor was placed at the tip of a fine nylon catheter positioned in the mouth of one of the pulmonary veins entering the left atrium, having been inserted via a Brockenborough catheter placed there via the transseptal route. Figure 12 demonstrates findings in both dog and man. It compares simultaneous measurements of left atrial pressure (LA P) and flow in a large pulmonary vein close to the left atrium in a dog (PV Q) and provides a similar comparison of left atrial pressure and pulmonary vein flow velocity (PV Vel) in a patient.

The findings in both dog and man[23] suggested that the large pulmonary veins external to the lung parenchyma must be very compliant to be able to absorb the forward pulse that should have been transmitted from the lung capillary bed to the veins and at the same time prevent retrograde transmission of pressure pulses from the left atrium from reaching the pulmonary capillaries. We tested this hypothesis by undertaking studies in which we could either study the pulmonary vein flow from the lung to the left atrium in continuity (intact mode) or separated from the left atrium by draining the blood from the severed vein into a constant pressure reservoir (divided mode). In the intact mode we saw the normal inverse relationship between pulmonary vein flow velocity and left atrial pressure. In the divided mode we found blood flow through the parenchymatous portion of the pulmonary venous system issued from the lung substance still resembling a lung capillary flow pulse, though somewhat delayed from it in time and attenuated in amplitude.

The flow pulse leaving the lung was very sensitive to changes in transcapillary pressure as a result of changes in intraalveolar pressure due to lung inflation. Blood flow returning from the constant pressure reservoir via the severed pulmonary vein entering the left atrium still had a flow pattern that was dominated by the

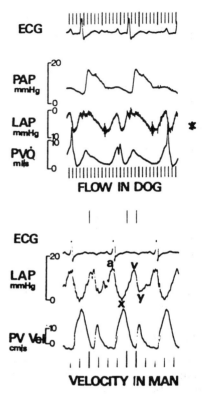

**Figure 12.** Simultaneous measurement of left atrial pressure (LAP), pulmonary vein flow (PVQ) in the dog and pulmonary vein flow velocity (PV Vel) in man. * = Inverted LAP scale.

pressure events taking place within the left atrium. Its flow pattern was still a mirror image of the left atrial pressure.[24] Plainly, the large pulmonary veins external to the lung provided the distensible portion of the system we were seeking.

During this period an enterprising medical student from Chicago named Judy Banks invited herself to the department during a long vacation to undertake a student research project. I am terrified of supervising such projects because they seldom turn out to be fruitful, but in Judy's case I was wrong. We decided that she should measure the distensibility of the large pulmonary veins and compare it with the distensibility of the main pulmonary artery trunk from material collected postmortem from patients who had died from causes from other than lung and heart disease.

We copied the method that Harris and his colleagues had used when they compared the distensibility of the pulmonary artery and aorta in man.[10] Judy made stress-strain measurements on circumferential strips of main pulmonary artery and large pulmonary veins using a simple tension balance. Just as Harris had found, the pulmonary arteries were highly distensible, although their distensibility tended to become less with age. But we were surprised to find out the pulmonary veins were virtually indistensible at all ages. It was as if the pulmonary arteries behaved as elastic tubes, whereas the pulmonary veins behaved as nylon ones.[1] We had found that the pulmonary veins, which acted as capacitance vessels, did so in spite of being virtually indistensible. We therefore postulated that if pulmonary veins were collapsible rather than distensible structures, they could fill or empty over a very narrow transmural pressure range. This would absorb the retrograde pressure pulses from the left atrium and prevent them from traveling backward to the capillaries. The veins would also absorb any forward flow pulse coming from the capillaries toward the left atrium. Once fully filled, the veins could accommodate more blood only by distending. This distension would likely be accompanied by a rapid rise in pulmonary venous pressure.

The first requirement for this hypothesis was that the large pulmonary veins should always assume a collapsed configuration at zero transmural pressure. This was easily proven by taking postmortem pieces of main pulmonary artery and pulmonary vein from both man and dog and examining their shape when immersed in saline within a glass vessel. The pulmonary artery, with its more muscular walls, remained almost circular whereas the pulmonary veins collapsed flat.

Bishma Rajagopalan next compared both left atrial pressure and blood flow within the pulmonary veins with changes in cross sectional dimension of pulmonary veins using minute ultrasonic crystals glued to their walls with biological adhesive. The dimensions of both the major and minor axes of the veins were studied.[25]

When rapid left atrial filling took place during the $y$ descent of pressure early in diastole in the left atrium and again during the $x$ descent in left atrial pressure, there was a concommitant reduction in the dimensions of the minor axis of the pulmonary vein. When pulmonary vein flow into the left atrium was impeded during the left atrial $a$ and $v$ pressure waves, the dimension of the minor axis of the vein increased.

The changes in pulmonary vein dimensions could be correlated with changes in left atrial pressure over a very wide range. The increase in minor axis dimension continued until the intraluminal pressure in the vein reached about 10 mmHg. Thereafter the dimensions of both the major and minor axes increased. This indicated that above a certain pressure within the vein further increase in cross sectional area could take place only by distension. Figure 13 plots the data obtained. The minor axis of the veins is virtually collapsed at zero transmural pressure. Over the normal venous transmural pressure range 0–12 mmHg, the minor axis steadily increases as the vessel changes from a dumbbell to a circular shape. Above 10–12 mmHg both the minor and major axes start to increase together as the vein begins to distend to the limits of its compliance. Thus the pulmonary veins external to the parenchyma of the lung together act as a large variable capacitance. Indeed, we found from silastic casts made of the left atrium and pulmonary veins in both dog and man that the aggregate volume of the distended pulmonary veins could amount to approximately 90% of the average stroke volume from the right ventricle.

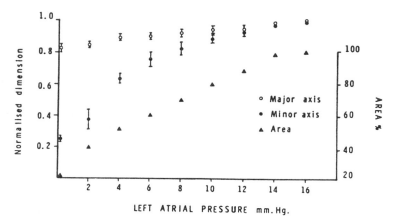

**Figure 13.** Relationship between left atrial pressure ($LA_p$) and the dimensions of major and minor axes of a large pulmonary vein entering external to the lung in a living dog, measured with ultrasonic crystals.

There is still little information about how the pulmonary veins within the lungs themselves behave, but we are confident about the role of the extraparenchymal pulmonary veins. They are collapsible structures that enable blood flow out of the lungs to be accommodated and left atrial supply to be maintained in such a way that the lung capillaries are effectively isolated from left atrial pressures even as high as 15 mmHg. Only when left atrial pressure exceeds the limits of distensibility of the large extraparanchymal pulmonary veins will left atrial pressure events impede blood flow from the lung capillaries. There is another beauty in this system. The large pulmonary veins together act as a collapsible reservoir with which to supply the left atrium to maintain more or less uniform blood supply to the left ventricle despite beat to beat changes in right ventricular output due to alternations in its filling during respiration.

Why is it that the lungs so jealously preserve pulsatile blood flow in their capillaries? I believe there is a very simple explanation. Only during systole does the pressure in the lung capillaries temporarily exceed the equilibration level regulating the net inward direction of water flux

between capillary and interstitium of the lung. So during systole, particularly in the dependent parts of the lung, the transcapillary hydrostatic pressure temporarily exceeds oncotic pressure, and a net flux of water takes place outward from capillaries to interstitium. During diastole, however, the intracapillary pressure falls below oncotic pressure so that the net water flux will be back again from the interstitium to capillary.

During physical rest the diastolic period of the cardiac cycle is longer than the systolic period, so the tendency will always be to keep the alveolar-capillary interstitium dry. During exercise, both heart rate and pulmonary capillary pressure both rise as a result of an increase in cardiac output. Thus with exercise and left sided heart disease, which tend to increase capillary hydrostatic pressure as well as heart rate, the net flux of water will be outward from capillary to interstitium and the alveolar tissues will rapidly become charged with water. Breathlessness will ensue even before clinical pulmonary oedema has occurred. This is because the alveolar interstitial gel loses its compliance once it is charged with water. This stimulates the *J*-receptors of Paintal.[19] These afferent reflex sensors are ideally placed to sense changes in alveolar wall compliance. When the individual stops exercising, the physiological status quo ante is resumed. I believe the loss of inter-alveolar compliance in this way is likely to be a very important pathophysiological trigger initiating the sensation of breath-lessness. Thus, the onset of unexplained breathlessness at rest can be a useful clinical guide to impending lung oedema.

I have one piece of anecdotal evidence to support these views. I once had to study a patient by cardiac catheterization who had aortic stenosis associated with scleroderma. At rest the patient's mean pulmonary arterial wedge pressure was 34 mmHg, her pulse rate was 86 beats/min and the chest x-ray showed Kerley lymph lines at the lung bases, which indicated active lymphatic fluid clearance. There was no overt clinical pulmonary oedema. The patient was not particularly breathless. Unfortunately, she had been ineffectively sedated and became anxious during the cardiac catheterization procedure. Her heart rate increased to 120 beats/min. The mean pulmonary arterial wedge pressure rose to 45 mmHg and she became intensely breathless. A chest x-ray showed florid pulmonary oedema. Rather than give her a diuretic to reduce the oedema, I treated her with intravenous Propanalol to slow the heart rate. The heart rate fell back to 80 beats/min, and she was relieved of her pulmonary oedema and her breathlessness. Her pulmonary oedema was entirely heart rate dependent.

## Walls Do Not a Prison Make

The story so far has dwelt almost entirely on the fluid dynamics of blood flow conduction through the lung vascular system to maintain optimal blood-gas exchange despite major changes from disease leading to pulmonary arterial and pulmonary venous hypertension. But I was still no nearer to understanding precisely how the lungs protect themselves from pulmonary oedema in conditions leading to pulmonary venous hypertension.

Although clinicians were beginning to be aware of the importance of the lung lymphatics in clearing fluid from the lungs in pulmonary oedema, there was a general ignorance of the forces governing net fluid movement across the capillary wall, which Starling had suggested over 80 years previously.[31] Indeed cardiologists in particular never seemed to consider that there could be any other cause but a hydrostatic one leading to pulmonary oedema.

I was getting fed up with the body plethysmograph, so it seemed high time to see if I couldn't find ways of looking at how fluids got *through* the walls of the capillaries rather than *down* their lumen. Just about this time the cardiac department was moved from the old Radcliffe Infirmary into the new John Radcliffe Hospital in Oxford, so I took the opportunity of getting rid of the body plethysmographs from the lab. (One of them is now in my garden acting as a cold frame for young seedlings (Fig. 14). But long before this, I had a strange experience, which I would like to relate in a rather round about way.

Although this tale might suggest a logical sequence of questions and answers, applied physiology involving invasive methods in patients is more haphazard. This is because the measurements needed for research have to be made pari passu with those required for diagnosis—otherwise one would be committing the felony of assault.

Functional pathology is nature's physiological ablation experiment, so the philosophy I had learned from McMichael and Schafer trained me to sharpen clinical skills and to study those common diseases that helped answer particular physiological questions in man. However, I had to wait for patients to turn up with the dis-

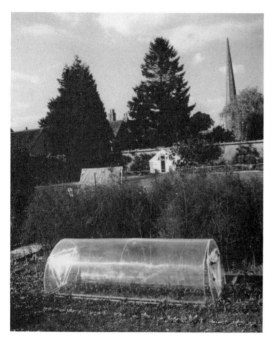

**Figure 14.** Oxford plethysmograph (Mark2) converted for horticulture.

eases whose pathophysiology I needed to precisely perturb the organ function I wished to study. Using such an approach, I benefited from remaining a generalist as a physician so as to trawl for the diseases I needed for my studies. Because of their episodic presentation, it was also wise to be working on a number of interrelated projects.

Yet none of the studies I have described so far had addressed the original problem that had so interested Paul Wood: how the lungs protected themselves from becoming oedematous in mitral stenosis. Clinicians, however, were beginning to recognize the importance of the lymphatic system in this regard.

In 1961 I chanced on an article by Uhley and his colleagues[32] in San Francisco, who had produced experimental evidence on the importance of the lung lymphatics. They measured greatly increased lung lymph flow from the cannulated right lymphatic duct in dogs in whom they had induced high cardiac output heart failure by means of a surgically created chronic aortocaval fistula in the abdomen.

The background to this work was that Drinker and Field[5] had reasoned that the composition of lymph and interstitial fluid was identical. Later Warren and Drinker[33] had shown that lung lymph was removed almost exclusively by the right lymphatic duct. Then in 1949 Courtice and Simmonds[4] had concluded that protein injected into the trachea was absorbed from the terminal respiratory tree by lymphatic pathways alone. It occurred to me that if I were to instill a small bolus of radioiodinated serum albumin (RISA) in saline via a fine catheter into the peripheral airways of the lung in dogs, then the RISA would be cleared from the lung interstitium into the systemic circulation via the lung lymphatics alone. Thus, if I were to count the rate of rise of radioactivity in the blood, I could get an indirect estimate of lung lymph clearance, which I could apply to man if I had first proven by animal experiments the idea was sound.

Bill Gillespie had joined the lab from Arthur Guyton's stable in the other Oxford. Together we attempted the appropriate animal experiments. But our surgery of the right lymphatic duct was not good enough, and we were initially unsuccessful and stopped the experiments. I had to wait until 1963 before I could engineer a sabbatical to go to San Francisco and learn from Uhley. The studies there, though carefully planned, did not work out as we had hoped. Not only was the aortocaval fistula unreliable in inducing heart failure, but also we found that the radioactive albumin readily entered the blood stream across the alveolar capillary endothelium even when right lymphatic duct lymph flow was normal. Thus, there was no hope of developing an indirect means of measuring lung lymph flow by such a method.

I had a couple of weeks left before my sabbatical leave was over when, on September 4, 1965, it was announced that the great Albert Schweitzer—organist, philosopher, theologian, and medical missionary—had died at his leprosarium in Lambaréné, in West Africa. I believe it was in the *San Francisco Chronical* that I read his obituary. The obituary was headed "Reverence for Life." At the time we had two dogs prepared for study who had developed acute pneumonia from distemper, and the animal house veterinarian had informed us that they would have to be put down. The obituary's reference to Albert Schweitzer's dictum for the reverence of life was so compelling that I felt it was wrong to kill those animals just because they had distemper and did not suit our experimental purposes. So we studied them the next day.

Figure 15 shows what we found. We instilled 50 μ Ci Risa in 5 ml saline via a catheter wedged into a peripheral bronchus of the lower lobe in these two animals. Postmortem lung sections later showed extensive staining of alveoli and terminal respiratory bronchioles and peribronchial tissues in the pneumonic areas. The percentage of RISA entering the plasma after its instillation into the pe-

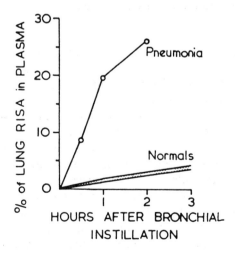

**Figure 15.** Percentage of Iodine-125 albumin entering the plasma after its installation into the lung of a dog with pneumonia, compared with results in 6 normal animals.

ripheral airways in the two dogs with distemper was startlingly different from what we found in our six normal animals. In contrast to the slow absorption of RISA into the plasma in the normal dogs, 26% of the dose instilled into the lungs of the dogs with pneumonia had entered the plasma in under 2 hours. We had stumbled on an extraordinarily simple way of measuring changes in alveolar capillary vascular permeability.[6]

## Consequences, Which Led to Inflammation

I returned to Oxford and got on with my usual clinical and laboratory work, impatient to finish the lung blood flow studies. I had to wait until the mid-1970s before I could find time to start on what turned out to be a new adventure, exploring high permeability lung oedema and, ultimately, inflammatory lung injury.

The wait was worthwhile, for in about 1975 I was joined in the wards by a new senior registrar named John Prichard. The study of lung capillary permeability attracted him enormously as a physiological chemist.

Using the Uhley preparation in open chested anaesthetized dogs, we measured the lung water compartments by sequential intravenous injections of markers labeled with iodine-125. When the markers were fully mixed, we counted the lungs externally with a calibrated scintillation counter simultaneously with counts in peripheral blood samples from which to calculate the distribution volume of each marker. We used (1) RISA-125 from the plasma space, (2) iodine-125 iodide from the extracellular water space, and (3) iodine-125-iodo-antipyrine to label total regional lung water. Prichard then extended the method to calculate the transcapillary flux of RISA from capillary to interstitium in the lung from simultaneous counts of lung radioactivity measured externally and amounts of RISA collected from simultaneous blood samples. This was done using the general flux equation

$$V_I d/dt(C_{I_z}) = K_P \cdot C_P(t) - K_I \cdot C_{I_z}, \quad (1)$$

where $V$ = interstitial volume, $C_P$ and $C_I$ the concentration of tracer (z) in plasma and interstitium, respectively, and $K_P$ and $K_I$ the transfer rate constants of tracer flux from plasma to interstitium and from interstitium to plasma and lymph, respectively. $K_P$ and $K_I$ were calculated from two simultaneous equations generated by integration of the above equation over two periods of time ($t_0 - t_1$; $t_1 - t_2$). Figure 16 shows what we found. Having measured the distribution volumes of plasma and extracellular water in the lung, we continued to count the radioactivity within the lung and compared this with simultaneous blood samples over the same period of time. We were then able to measure the concentrations of RISA in the plasma and in the lung lymph and compare these with the calculated concentrations of RISA in the lung interstitium.

At the end of approximately 90 minutes we found that the concentration of RISA in the lung lymph and the calculated amount present in the lung interstitium were virtually identical. We then went on to study the transfer rate constant for albumin from plasma to interstitium ($K_P$) in experimental pulmonary oedema. We studied the effects of intravenous injections of pseudomonas bacteria, haemorrhagic hypotension, and alloxan. Our measurements were combined with simultaneous measurements of pulmonary capillary pressure (Swan–Ganz method) and plasma oncotic pressure. We found that such a combination of methods enabled us to differentiate successfully among hydrostatic, hypoosmolar, and high permeability pulmonary oedema.[21,22]

In 1980 John was appointed associate professor of clinical medicine at Trinity College, Dublin. His Irish wife, Bernie,

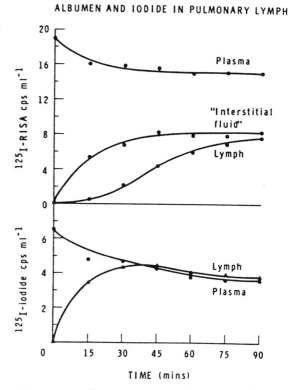

**ALBUMEN AND IODIDE IN PULMONARY LYMPH**

**Figure 16.** Iodine-125 serum albumin and Iodine-125 iodide concentrations in right lymphatic duct lymph, plasma and pulmonary interstitial fluid in a dog. Plasma and lymph concentrations were measured directly. Iodine-125 serum albumin concentration in interstitial fluid was calculated (see text).

was absolutely delighted. I was sad when he left, for John, one of the most creative and generous-hearted of men, had become a lifelong friend.

During the 1970s intensivists the world over had become dismayed by the relentless mortality from acute respiratory failure associated with sudden severe pulmonary oedema, often unassociated with cardiovascular disease, in some of their patients admitted to intensive care wards. The occurrence of this fatal process, originally known as "Shock Lung" or Adult Respiratory Distress Syndrome (ARDS) was unpredictable. Its aetiology was unknown, but it could be anticipated in those subject to violent bodily assault by such events as acute haemorrhagic shock, closed body trauma, anaphylaxis, amniotic fluid embolism, and septicaemia, to name but a few. Studies in animal models had shown that lung injury was the cause[3] and that this was probably associated with granulocyte aggregation in the lungs through the activation of complement.[9,12]

Our method for quantitating increased lung capillary endothelial permeability would be perfect for quantitating similar endothelial injury in patients suspected of developing ARDS—if only we could adapt the method for use in man. The trouble was that after an injection of RISA, some 30% of the radiation detected externally over the chest came from the chest wall itself.

We had to find a trick way to "dissect" the chest wall from the overlying lung. John Prichard thumbed through the periodic tables and determined that iodine-123 would do this. Not only had the isotope a short half-life (13 hours), which would enable us to label our albumin with high intensity as well as to repeat the human studies serially over time without radiation overdose, but it also had two photopeaks, one at 29 KeV and one at 159 KeV. If we used this isotope to label our markers and counted externally over the chest, we could then use the differential absorptions of the two photopeaks by the chest wall to calculate the content of isotope in the lung *independent* of chest wall.

Iodine-123 was not yet commercially available, but Oxford was close to the Atomic Energy Research Establishment (AERE) at Harwell. So we contacted Gary Cunninghame, chief chemist in charge of the variable energy cyclotron at Harwell, who had also spotted the medical potential of iodine-123. He agreed to make the isotope and allow us to test its potential. We used a simple "lung" phantom consisting of a thin-walled perspex container with the dimensions of a human lung filled with a bran/water mixture containing the isotope with the same density as lung tissue. Outside of the phantom lung we placed phantom chest walls consisting of perspex chambers filled with water. External spectral analysis of the counts emanating from the phantom lung after attenuation by the overlying chest wall showed that the photopeak at 29 KeV was much more attenuated than at 159 KeV. The isotope would be ideal for our purposes.

Three or four years of steady battle against government inertia then followed for Gary Cunninghame and myself. AERE Harwell was supposed to undertake research into atomic energy applied to fields *other* than medicine. The government radiochemical centre at Amersham had the latter responsibility, but its cyclotron had insufficient energy to produce iodine-123 isotopically pure enough for medical use. Only Harwell could to this. But bureaucracy won, assisted by clinical inertia in the field of nuclear medicine. When Amersham conducted a market survey of potential users in Britain, not a spark of interest in its medical potential was shown. However, in Europe, particularly in West Germany, there was interest but no ready sources of iodine-123. By this time my research contacts in Europe were extensive and whenever a conference took place in a European city besides London, I visited the British embassy or consulate and called on the scientific attaché. I would bring with me a colleague from the city I was visiting, who kindly expressed interest in getting iodine-123 air freighted from Harwell for research. A foreign office file of inquiries slowly built up in London. A medical working party was set up by the Department of Health, and ultimately a 3-year pilot programme for the manufacture by Harwell of iodine-123 for medical use was approved. We could start at last.

My overseas marketing endeavour had extended to Japan. In 1978 I found myself in Tokyo for the Eighth World Congress of Cardiology. There I met a young respiratory physician named Minoru Kanazawa from Keio University. His boss needed a method for measuring lung vascular permeability in chromium plating workers in the Japanese car industry, some of whom had developed pulmonary oedema. Minoru applied to come and work with me. In due time he arrived in Oxford with his wife and small daughter, having won a Wellcome Research Fellowship from the British Council in Tokyo and having become fluent in English. Not only was he an excellent ambassador for his country but also an example of its superb educational system. He was conversant in the arts and literature of Japan and Europe and used mathematics as a working language.

Calculation of concentration volumes of isotope-labeled fluid markers in the lung independent of chest wall by subtraction analysis using the 29 and 159 KeV photopeaks of iodine-123 counted externally is conceptually easy. It took ability and the ingenuity of Anwar Hussein to make the method reliable for which Anwar obtained his D.Phil.

Figure 17a shows the raw data from a normal subject used to study albumen transfer rate ($K_p$). It compares total counts measured externally over the chest ($R_T$) with simultaneous counts in peripheral blood samples. The calculated counts emanating from the chest wall ($R_W$) and from the lung, attenuated by chest wall ($R_{AL}$), are also shown. Figure 17b shows similar data from a patient with ARDS. Note how the chest counts ($R_T$) rise much more steeply than in the normal subject. This is because of the increased flux of radioactive albumen from lung capillaries to interstitium due to their increased permeability.

Note that the slopes of $R_T$ and $R_W$ run parallel to one another both in the normal subject and the patient with ARDS. We found this to be a constant feature in all the patients we studied, indicating that the proportion of counts emanating from the chest wall remains unchanged throughout the procedure. Thus, for clinical purposes, it is legitimate to eliminate the complicated mathematics required to calculate

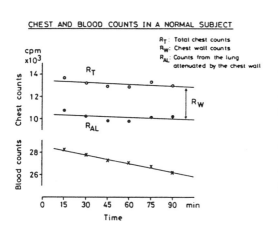
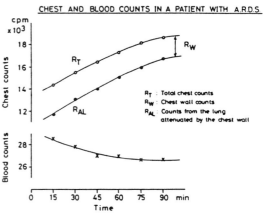

**Figure 17. a.** Comparison of radiation count rates measured from the surface of the chest ($R_T$) and from simultaneous blood samples over time, following the injection of Iodine-123 albumin intravenously in a normal subject. $R_W$ and $R_{AL}$ are the counts emanating from the chest wall and from the lung attenuated by chest wall respectively, calculated from $R_T$ using [29/159] KeV ratio analysis. **b.** Comparison of radiation count rates measured from the surface of the chest ($R_T$) and from simultaneous blood samples over time following the injection of Iodine-123 albumin intravenously in a subject with ARDS. $R_W$ and $R_{AL}$ are the calculated counts emanating from the chest wall and lung attenuated by the chest wall, respectively.

absolute values of counts from the lung independent of chest wall and obtain this same information from measurements of total external counts multiplied by a reduction constant representing the chest wall.

An even simpler method for estimating changes in lung capillary permeability is to measure the percentage changes in externally detected counts from the lung and in peripheral plasma samples over time. At the end of 1 hour the ratio of lung to plasma counts detected externally over the chest in normal subjects rose approximately 5%. In the patients with cardiac oedema due to increased pulmonary capillary hydrostatic pressure this ratio had increased only to 6%. However, in patients with pulmonary oedema from ARDS the percentage ratio of lung to plasma counts had risen to 14% (Fig. 18).

The lung plasma water volume in patients with pulmonary oedema from cardiac causes or from ARDS was statistically no different from the lung plasma water volume in normal subjects. In pneumonia the affected lung had reduced lung plasma volume compared with the healthy lung, indicating a shift of blood flow from the affected lung toward the healthy lung. Interstitial lung water was increased in the patients with pulmonary oedema both from cardiac causes and from ARDS. This increase was similar in both groups, despite their different aetiologies. The increase was over double the interstitial lung water volume found in normal subjects. The patients with pneumonia were not equally affected. In the more severely affected patient, lung interstitial water was grossly increased compared with normal subjects.

As was to be expected, the capillary hydrostatic pressure was significantly elevated in the group with pulmonary oedema from cardiac causes. Most of these patients had chronic mitral stenosis. In contradistinction, the patients with pulmonary oedema from ARDS had normal pulmonary arterial wedge pressures, as did the two patients with pneumonia. Their interstitial fluid oedema was *not* due to an increase in capillary hydrostatic filtration pressure.

Plasma osmolality was normal in all the patients with lung oedema, indicating that plasma hypoosmoality was not an aetiological factor. However, the albumen transfer rate constant ($K_p$) from plasma to interstitium increased in all but one of the patients with ARDS. $K_p$ was also increased in the affected lung of the two patients with pneumonia. Thus, in both ARDS and in pneumonia, pulmonary capillary endothelial injury was responsible for the pulmonary oedema. Note also that in cardiac pulmonary oedema $K_p$ was within the normal range. In one patient with ARDS, $K_p$ rose to $8 \times 10^{-3}$/min. This patient had been inappropriately transfused with fluids, and his capillary hydrostatic pressure had risen to 27 mmHg. The combination of endothelial lung injury and elevation of intracapillary hydrostatic pressure led to intense lung flooding.

I have already mentioned how animal studies by others had suggested that lung capillary endothelial injury in ARDS could be due to the action of inflammatory products released from aggragated granulocytes within the lung. We were therefore interested to see whether this could be the reason patients with pulmonary oedema from ARDS so rarely develop systemic microvascular injury. If the activated granulocytes remain trapped in the lungs, their baleful effects would not be expected to spread to the systemic circulation. So we were delighted to find that transcapillary albumen flux ($K_p$) in the thigh in patients with ARDS was virtually normal. Thus we had strong evidence that granulocyte aggregation in the lungs was responsible for lung capillary endothelial injury in ARDS and the sequestration of granulocytes in the lungs protected the systemic circulation from similar damage.

I was near retirement when in 1984 I

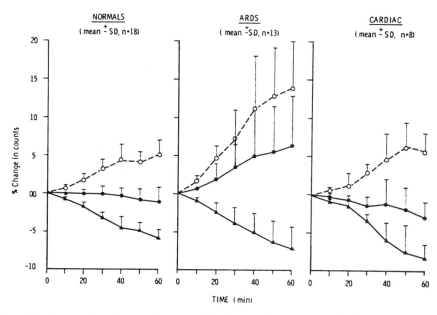

**Figure 18.** Percentage change in externally detected counts from the lung (o----o) and in peripheral plasma samples ( ---- ) after intravenous injection of Iodine-123 albumin in normal subjects, patients with ARDS, and patients with cardiac pulmonary edema (+ 1 SD). Broken lines (o o) represent % change in ratio of lung to plasma counts.

was invited as a McLaughlin Visiting Professor to McMaster University in Hamilton, Ontario. Geoff Coates and Hugh O'Brodovich had proposed that we conduct research together. Geoff had visited me in Oxford some time previously, and we found we had common interests in ARDS. The big question seemed to be this: How does the body protect itself from inappropriate inflammatory responses in the lung rather than invariably developing ARDS?

Geoff Coates and Hugh O'Brodovich were studying experimental inflammatory lung oedema induced by *E. Coli* endotoxaemia in sheep provided with chronically implanted catheters in the pulmonary artery, left atrium, and dorsal lymphatic duct with which to collect lung lymph. The researchers were also interested in finding out why inflammatory lung injury was not the invariable response to injections of bacterial lipopolysaccharide endotoxin (LPS). The usual pathophysiological responses to this in-

sult were well known,[3] but a correlation between these events and changes in systemic blood and lung lymph white blood cell counts had not yet been made. We therefore decided to look at this (Fig. 19).

We infused *E. Coli* endotoxin either into the pulmonary artery or left atrium and observed its effect on the pulmonary arterial pressure, lung lymph flow, and lung lymph protein content (expressed as lung lymph to plasma protein ratio). We followed events for 2 hours and compared them with simultaneous changes in peripheral blood and lung lymph total and differential white blood cell (WBC) counts (lymphocytes, monocytes/macrophages, and granulocytes). Blood and lymph concentrations of thromboxane $B_2$, $PGE_1$, and $PGF_1$ were also measured in some animals.[11] The lung response to lipopolysaccharide (LPS) infusion via the pulmonary artery and left atrium were similar, but much greater when LPS was infused via the left atrium rather than the pulmonary artery. We assumed that this was

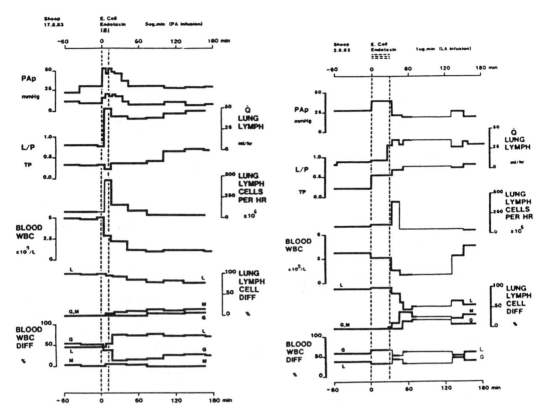

**Figure 19. a.** Effects of 5 gm/min *E.Coli* endotoxin infused for 15 min into the pulmonary artery of a sheep with chronically implanted catheters in the pulmonary artery, dorsal lymphatic duct, and left atrium. $PA_p$ = PA pressure. Q lung lymph = lung lymph flow from dorsal lymphatic duct. L/P = lymph to plasma protein ratio. Blood and lymph total and differential WBC counts also shown (G = granulocytes; M = monocytes/macrophages; L = lymphocytes). **b.** Effects of 1 gm/min *E.Coli* endotoxin infused via the left atrium (LA) for 30 min in a sheep with chronically implanted catheters in PA, LA, and dorsal lymphatic duct. Following endotoxin note increase in lung lymph flow, systemic granulopenia and slow appearance of macrocytes and granulocytes in lung lymph accompanied by a rise in lung lymph protein concentration (rise in lymph to plasma protein ratio). These effects were more marked after LA infusion of endotoxin than when infused into the pulmonary artery.

because the whole systemic system had been challenged in the former case (Figs. 14a and 14b).

We only had time to study six animals when I was unexpectedly called home to England. At the time our findings appeared inconclusive. With hindsight, I believe they tell an important story.

Three of the sheep responded conventionally to LPS. The pulmonary arterial pressure rose, accompanied by a slight fall in left atrial pressure, indicating pulmo-

nary venular constriction and an initial increase in capillary hydrostatic pressure. This was associated with release of thromboxane $B_2$ into the blood. These events led to an immediate rise in lung lymph flow, dilute in protein (reduced lung lymph to plasma protein ratio).

These events were also associated with a granulopaenia and a reversed granulocyte to lymphocyte ratio in the peripheral blood. In addition, we were fascinated by the changes in lung lymph cell counts.

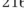
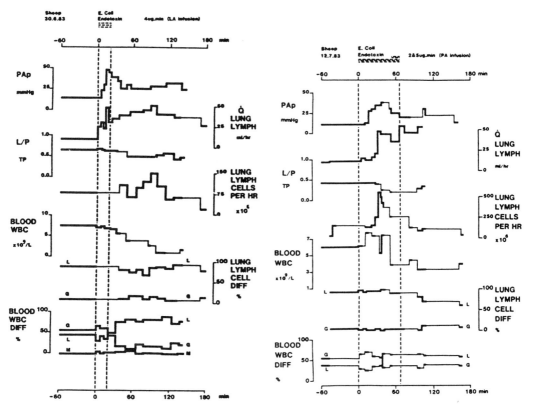

**Figure 20. a.** Effects of 2.0 then 5.0 gm/min *E. Coli* endotoxin infused for 65 min into the pulmonary artery in the same manner as in Figure 14a. **b.** Effects of 4 gm/min *E. Coli* endotoxin infused via left atrium for 20 min as in Figure 14b. Although lung lymph flow increased and systemic granulopenia occurred just as in Figure 14a and 14, no macrophages or granulocytes appeared in the lung lymph nor was there an increase in lung lymph protein concentration (no rise in lymph plasma protein ratio).

After an initial burst of lymphocytes representing those flushed from the system by the surge of increased lymph flow, *the number of monocytes/macrophages steadily rose.* The cells looked sick, with degranulated and vacuolated cytoplasm. *Close behind the macrophages followed granulocytes,* also with the degranulated cytoplasm. *The appearance of these cells was accompanied by a marked rise in lymph protein content.*

The appearance of macrophages in the lung lymph prior to the appearance of granulocytes suggested that it was the local macrophages that had activated the dormant granulocytes sequestered in the lung to release their inflammatory products.

However, an entirely different response was found in the three other sheep we studied, even though they received similar doses of LPS. *There was no migration of macrophages or granulocytes into the lung lymph nor was there an accompanying rise in protein flux into the lymph* (Figs. 20a and 20b). *Endothelial injury did not appear to have taken place,* despite the fact that granulocyte aggregation had still occurred within the lungs (systemic granulopaenia and reversed systemic granulocyte to lymphocyte ratio, as in the previous animals). Yet there was still the same rise in pulmonary arterial pressure, leading to increased lymph flow dilute in protein, just as in the previous three animals.

In summary, granulocyte adherence within the lungs occurred in all of the animals receiving LPS. But in only half of the animals did the granulocytes release their inflammatory mediators to harm the lung capillary endothelium.

Blood levels of thromboxane $B_2$, prostaglandin $E_1$, and prostaglandin $F1_1$ were identical in both groups of animals. This suggested that these autocoids are largely responsible for the vasoactive components of the acute phase response and have little to do with endothelial injury. It was the macrophages activating the granulocytes that was responsible for this.

Could these few amateur observations on the effects of endotoxin on the temporal order of events leading to the acute phase inflammatory response in the lung microcirculation help us understand how the body normally regulates its response to pathogenic material entering the systemic circulation without triggering an inappropriate inflammatory response in the lungs? My hunch is this. The lungs—like the skin, gut, and urinary tract—are equipped to combat microbial invaders entering the body from the external environment. In the case of the lungs, the combat cells alert to these invaders are the fixed macrophages in the bronchial and alveolar epithelium. But the healthy lungs also act as a single-pass filter that removes particulate waste material from the systemic venous circulation (e.g., small venous clots, cellular debris, etc.) to prevent their continued passage as microemboli, which could damage vital organs such as the brain. Our few sheep studies also now lead me to believe that it is likely that normal systemic acute phase inflammatory homeostasis also depends on this same filter to sequestrate those activated granulocytes released in excess of need into the systemic microcirculation. These granulocytes remain dormant in the lung unless something alerts the local alveolar macrophages to "arm" them. When this happens they will harm the alveolar tissues themselves.

Macrophage activity can be triggered by a host of protean pertubations. Acute alveolar hypoxia is one such stimulus. Imagine a small area of lung atelectasis in a patient with severe haemorrhagic shock. The resulting local hypoxia stimulates local macrophages to release their own inflammatory mediators (superoxides, proteases, etc.), as well as the cytokines that now "arm" the sequestered granulocytes adherent in the adjacent capillaries. An overwhelming local inflammatory response results. Oedema fluid floods the local tissues, hypoxia spreads, and the injurious tide of oedema rises. ARDS is the clinical result.

## The Next Crossroads

Some three months before I was due to finish at McMaster my wife Pamela went home to Oxford to make ready for a new grandchild soon to enter the planet. About a month after she left a colleague phoned me to say that he had admitted her to hospital with fever, generalized muscle pains, weakness, inflamed joints, and rapid weight loss. No inflammatory or autoimmune cause had been isolated, and she was responding poorly to steroids. I packed up and went home immediately.

Pamela took months to recover from this strange illness. My new interest in acute inflammation had become altogether too personal for comfort. By the time things had settled down, they seemed to point like a signpost to the next crossroads or *Y* point in life. Why not leave the old road still at a point of mystery and follow where the new road leads? So I did just that.

**Acknowledgments:** I shall always be grateful to the Pulmonary Circulation Foundation for selecting me to be a contributor to this book. This has enabled me to share enthusiasms with those whose vision, work, and friendship have guided me over the years much more than they know. Three special acknowledgments go to Pamela, to John Honour, and to Betty Radburn—for her love and their staunch affection as hidden participants in the work described in this chapter.

## References

1. Banks, J., F. V. McL. Booth, E. H. MacKay, B. Rajagopalan, and G. de J. Lee. The physical properties of human arteries and veins. *Clin. Sci. Mol. Med.* 55: 477–484, 1978.

2. Bosman, A. R., G. de J. Lee, and R. Marshall. The effect of pulsatile capillary blood flow upon gas exchange within the lungs of man. *Clin. Sci.* 28: 295–309, 1965.

3. Brigham, K., R. Bowers, and J. Haynes. Increased sheep lung vascular permeability caused by *E. Coli* endotoxin. *Circ. Res.* 45: 292–297, 1979.

4. Courtice, F. C., and W. J. Simmonds. Absorption from the lungs. *J. Physiol. (London)* 109: 103–116, 1949.

5. Drinker, C. K., and M. E. Field. The protein content of mammalian lymph and the relation of lymph to tissue fluid. *Am. J. Physiol.* 97: 32–39, 1931.

6. Gillespie, W. J., and G. de J. Lee. Vascular and lymphatic absorption of Radioactive Albumin from the lungs. *Cardiovasc. Res.* 1: 42–51, 1967.

7. Hamilton, W. F., J. W. Moore, J. M. Kinsman, and R. G. Spurling. Studies on circulation: further analysis of injection method, and of changes in hemodynamics under physiological and pathological conditions. *Am. J. Physiol.* 99: 534–551, 1932.

8. Hamilton, W. F., R. L. Riley, A. M. Attyah, A. Cournand, D. M. Fowell, A. Himmelstein, R. P. Noble, J. W. Remmington, D. W. Richards, Jr., N. C. Wheeler, and A. C. Witham. Comparison of Fick and dye injection methods of measuring cardiac output in man. *Am. J. Physiol.* 153: 309–321, 1948.

9. Hammerschmidt, D. E., L. J. Weaver, L. D. Hudson, P. R. Craddock, and H. S. Jacob. Association of complement activation and elevated $C5_a$ with ARDS. *Lancet* 1: 947–949, 1980.

10. Harris, P., D. Heath, A. Apostolopoulos. Extensibility of the human pulmonary trunk. *Brit. Heart J.* 27: 651–659, 1965.

11. Hussein, A., J. Loyd, P. Tagari, H. Chapel, G. de J. Lee, M. Buchanan, R. Butt, G. Coates, and H. O'Brodovich. Granulocytes and Slow Reacting Substance (SRS) in higher permeability lung oedema of Adult Respiratory Distress Syndrome (ARDS). *Clin. Sci.* 67: 52P–146, 1984.

12. Jacobs, H. S., P. R. Craddock, D. E. Hammerschmidt, and C. F. Muldow. Complement-induced granulocyte aggregation. *N. Engl. J. Med.* 302: 789–794, 1980.

13. Karatzas, N. B., and G. de J. Lee. Propagation of blood flow pulse in the normal human pulmonary arterial system. *Circ. Res.* 25: 11–21, 1969.

14. Karatzas, N. B., and G. de J. Lee. Instantaneous lung capillary blood flow in patients with heart disease. *Cardiovasc. Res.* 4: 265–273, 1970.

15. Kopelman, H. and G. de J. Lee. The intrathoracic blood volume in mitral stenosis and left ventricular failure. *Clin. Sci.* 10: 383–403, 1951.

16. Krogh, A., and J. Lindhard. Measurements of blood flow through the lungs of man. *Skand. Arch. Physiol.* 27: 100–107, 1912.

17. Lee, G. de J., and A. B. DuBois. Pulmonary capillary blood flow in man. *J. Clin. Invest.* 34: 1380–1390, 1955.

18. McMichael, J., and E. P. Sharpey-Schafer. Cardiac output in man by direct Fick method: effects of posture, venous pressure change, atropine and adrenaline. *Brit. Heart J.* 6: 33–40, 1944.

19. Paintal, A. S. The nature and effect of sensory inputs into the respiratory centres. *Fed. Proc.* 36: 2428–2432, 1977.

20. Permutt, S., B. Bromberger-Barmea, and H. N. Bane. Alveolar pressure, pulmonary venous pressure and the vascular waterfall. *Med. Thorac.* 19: 239–260, 1962.

21. Prichard, J. S., and G. de J. Lee. Measurement of water distribution and transcapillary solute flux in dog lung by external radioactivity counting. *Clin. Sci.* 57: 145–154, 1979.

22. Prichard, J. S., and G. de J. Lee. Transvascular albumin flux and the interstitial water volume in experimental pulmonary oedema in dogs. *Clin. Sci.* 59: 105–113, 1980.

23. Rajagopalan, B., J. A. Friend, T. Stallard, and G. de J. Lee. Blood flow in pulmonary veins. I. Studies in dog and man. *Cardiovasc. Res.* 13: 667–675, 1979.

24. Rajagopalan, B., J. A. Friend, T. Stallard, and G. de J. Lee. Blood flow in pulmonary veins. II. The influence of events transmitted from the right and left sides of the heart. *Cardiovasc. Res.* 13: 677–683, 1979.

25. Rajagopalan, B., J. A. Friend, T. Stallard, and G. de J. Lee. Blood flow in pulmonary veins. III. Simultaneous measurements of their dimensions, intravascular pressure and flow. *Cardiovasc. Res.* 13: 685–693, 1979.

26. Reuben, S. R. Compliance of the human pulmonary arterial system in disease. *Circ. Res.* 29: 40–50, 1971.

27. Reuben, S. R., J. P. Swadling, and G. de J. Lee. Veolocity profiles in the main pulmonary artery of dogs and man, measured with a thin-film resistence anemometer. *Circ. Res.* 27: 995–1001, 1970.

28. Reuben, S. R., B. J. Gersh, J. P. Swadling, and G. de J. Lee. Measurement of pulmonary artery distensibility in the dog. *Cardiovasc. Res.* 4: 473–481, 1970.

29. Reuben, S. R., J. P. Swaddling, B. J. Gersh, and G. de J. Lee. Impedance and transmission properties of the pulmonary arterial system. *Cardiovasc. Res.* 5: 1–9, 1971.

30. Schultz, D. L., D. S. Tunstall-Pedoe, G. de J. Lee, A. J. Gunning, and B. J. Bellhouse. Velocity distribution and transition in the arterial system. In: *Ciba Foundation Symposium on Circulatory and Respiratory Mass Transport,* edited by G. E. Wolsten-holm and J. Knight. London: J. and A. Churchill, 1969, p. 172–199.

31. Starling, E. H. On the absorption of fluids from connective tissue spaces. *J. Physiol (London)* 19: 312–326, 1896.

32. Uhley, H. N., S. E. Leeds, J. J. Sampson, and M. Friedman. Some observations on the role of the lymphatics in experimental acute pulmonary oedema. *Circ. Res.* 9: 688–693, 1961.

33. Warren, M. F., and C. K. Drinker. The flow of lymph from the lungs of the dog. *Amer. J. Physiol.* 136: 207–221, 1942.

34. West, J. B., and C. T. Dollery. Distribution of blood flow and ventilation–perfusion ratio in the lung, measured with radioactive carbon dioxide. *J. Appl. Physiol.* 15: 405–510, 1960.

35. West, J. B., C. T. Dollery, and A. Naimark. Distribution of blood flow in isolated lung: relation to vascular and alveolar pressures. *J. Appl. Physiol.* 19: 713–724, 1964.

# 11

# Adventures in Gas Exchange

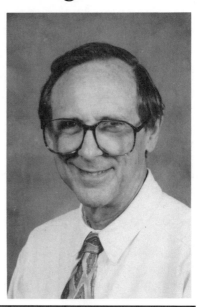

## Robert L. Johnson, Jr., M.D.

*Professor Department of Internal Medicine, The University of Texas, Southwestern Medical Center at Dallas, Dallas, Texas*

Donald W. Seldin was the new chairman of the Department of Medicine at the University of Texas Southwestern Medical School when I arrived as a first-year medicine resident at Parkland Hospital in Dallas in July 1952. I had no plans to enter an academic career nor any concept of what it meant to do so. Seldin was relentless in his demands for excellence from the house staff, and we dreaded the embarrassment of his criticisms. However, he occasionally lowered his gruff facade and allowed the gentler, more human side of his nature to surface. There was the time that, as a volunteer experimental subject, I received an intravenous solution contaminated with pyrogens. I developed chills, high fever, and hypotension as I lay on a floor mattress in the laboratory. Seldin was called by two panicked student research fellows, and I remember him pacing worriedly around me giving orders as I lay prostrate on the floor and saying with genuine concern: "What if this had happened to a *patient*?" Residents, of course, were expendable in those days. But I recovered and became chief resident at the end of that first year. I attained this position not because of my excellence but because I was the only senior resident left. Yet Don Seldin did inspire us to excel and to make the most of our capabilities. One of the student fellows I worked with is presently a dean at Southwestern; the other is chairman of medicine at the University of California at San Francisco.

It was Seldin who convinced me that I could achieve a place in academic medicine and was capable of doing research. I spent a year of pulmonary fellowship with William F. Miller in Dallas before going to the University of Pennsylvania Graduate

From: Wagner WW, Jr, Weir EK (eds): *The Pulmonary Circulation and Gas Exchange.* ©1994, Futura Publishing Co Inc, Armonk, NY.

School of Medicine for further training in Julius Comroe's department. At Pennsylvania, I was placed under the expert tutelage of Robert E. Forster, with whom I had many wonderful and animated discussions. Bob Forster set me to the task of developing a technique for simultaneously measuring pulmonary capillary blood flow ($\dot{Q}c$), tissue volume ($V_t$), and CO diffusing capacity ($DL_{CO}$) during rest and exercise.[16] I spent 2 months in the library; 4 months learning the behavioral idiosyncrasies of the mass spectrometer, infrared analyzers, and Brush recorders; 3 months setting up the technique; and 3 months gathering data. But in that short time I learned vital techniques and had seeds of ideas implanted that were to continually shape my career.

I have often wondered why so many funny things happened in those early days. I think it was because we were all so new to research and to the techniques that we were trying to master. Put more directly, we didn't know what we were doing. For instance, there was the time that John Rankin wanted to show off his Donald Duck voice to the two female technicians in the next laboratory. He took a deep breath of 100% helium and ran into the hall but never made it to their laboratory. He awoke on the floor with the two technicians frantically trying to revive him; John learned that a deep breath of 100% helium couldn't supply enough oxygen to get him to the next lab. Then there was the time Myron Stein and Phil Kimbel were learning how to measure pulmonary blood flow with Arthur Dubois' plethysmographic technique, using Bill Spicer as a subject.[26] The steel whole-body plethysmograph was fit with a speaker for voice communication and a small, round glass porthole for visual communication. Bill Spicer had inhaled an inspiratory capacity of 80% nitrous oxide and was holding his breath for the blood flow measurement. Phil and Myron, struggling with unfamiliar electronic circuitry, kept saying to Bill,

"Hold it. Hold it. Hold it just a little longer!" as Bill Spicer's head slowly slipped beneath the porthole window. The two investigators suddenly remembered that nitrous oxide is an anesthetic. When they opened the plethysmograph door, Bill slipped out onto the floor. Another funny incident illustrating our early problems with handling gases and plumbing occurred after I had returned to Dallas. It involved Harold Lawson,[18] who later would also train under Robert Forster.[17] Harold was filling a "bag-in-a-box system" consisting of a 30-gallon steel drum containing a standard weather balloon. I was in the next laboratory and was startled by a terrific explosion. I rushed next door and found Harold on the floor and the steel drum on the other side of the room with its seam ripped open. Harold had closed the spirometer port too early, thinking that any overpressure would be relieved by the small cork plug in the cylinder head of the drum popping out. The seam of the cylinder head had been ripped out while the cork remained undisturbed. He had forgotten the story of the little Dutch boy who had saved the city of Haarlem by holding back the entire North Sea using his small arm to plug a leak in the dike.

After returning to Dallas, I wanted to set up Bob Forster's method for measuring $\dot{Q}c$ and $DL_{CO}$ at the University of Texas and to determine whether we could use the method to derive useful information about oxygen transport in normal subjects or in patients. Norman Staub, also at the University of Pennsylvania at that time, had measured the kinetics of oxygen uptake by red cells[24] and made it possible to translate measurements of CO diffusing capacity into terms of oxygen transport using the Roughton-Forster equation.[23,25]

Because we wanted to test whether $DL_{CO}$ could predict limits of oxygen exchange by diffusion, we planned to exploit conditions in which oxygen transport in the human lung would be stressed to its limit, i.e., combinations of exercise, pneumonectomy, and high altitude. This approach ultimately led to an examination of how the lung adapted to and compensated for these kinds of stress.

## Pneumonectomy in Humans

Studies began with humans and only later involved animals. Chris DeGraff, then at the University of Texas, knew of a thoracic surgeon in San Antonio who had been doing extensive lung resections on patients with pulmonary tuberculosis.[8] We contacted the surgeon and arranged to study a group of his patients who had undergone from 45 to 66% lung resections. In the spring of 1963, with the help of Carleton B. Chapman and funding from the U.S. Air Force, we moved our laboratory to Willford Hall, the air force hospital in San Antonio, and arranged to use their cardiac cath lab. In Dallas, Jere Mitchell and Carlton Chapman had collected data suggesting that in average humans maximal oxygen consumption is limited by cardiac output and peripheral oxygen extraction, not by gas exchange.[20]

The hypotheses we tested were that, after pneumonectomy: (1) Exercise will become limited by gas exchange because of the loss of capillary bed and alveolar surface area; and (2) We should be able to predict the limitation imposed from measured $DL_{CO}$, membrane diffusing capacity $(DM_{CO})$, and pulmonary capillary blood volume (Vc).

Demographics and maximal oxygen intake of the 8 patients studied after lung resections are shown in Table 1. Six subjects were female. Average age was 34, ranging from 27 to 47, and the average amount of lung remaining was 40.6%, ranging from 55 to 33%. Average time since surgery was 2 years.

Maximal oxygen intake was significantly reduced, almost in proportion to the amount of lung removed; the average was 47% of predicted normal. Contrary to expectations, however, these patients were not limited by gas exchange but, rather, appeared to be limited by a low maximal cardiac output. At peak exercise they reached 83% of their age-predicted maximal heart rate. Yet arterial oxygen saturation fell only from an average of 95% at rest to 90% at peak exercise. Diffusing capacity was not reduced as much as expected from the amount of lung removed (Table 2), suggesting a significant compensatory increase of $DL_{CO}$ in the remaining lung. When this reduction in $DL_{CO}$ was translated into an expected reduction in oxygen transport, it was insuffi-

### Table 1
Demographics and maximal oxygen intake after lung resection in humans

| Patient | Sex | Age years | Height cm | Weight kg | Lung % | Maximal $O_2$ Uptake (ml/min)/kg (% predicted normal) |
|---------|-----|-----------|-----------|-----------|--------|------------------------------------------------------|
| MS   | F | 27   | 166   | 48.4 | 55   | 19.8 (47)   |
| BW   | F | 29   | 163   | 54.4 | 45   | 22.9 (55)   |
| MG   | F | 41   | 150   | 40.9 | 42   | 24.1 (68)   |
| CY   | M | 32   | 170   | 61.8 | 39   | 21.3 (42)   |
| MC   | F | 29   | 159   | 57.3 | 39   | 18.3 (44)   |
| RT   | M | 36   | 172   | 54.5 | 36   | 16.5 (34)   |
| AB   | F | 29   | 167   | 40.4 | 36   | 17.9 (43)   |
| RH   | F | 47   | 153   | 59.5 | 33   | 13.4 (41)   |
| Mean |   | 33.8 | 162.5 | 52.2 | 40.6 | 19.3 (46.8) |

(Reproduced from reference 8.)

| **Table 2**<br>Diffusing capacities and total lung capacities<br>of patients after extensive lung resections<br>as adults | |
|---|---|
| % Lung remaining | $40.6 \pm 6.9$ |
| Single breath $DL_{CO}$ | |
| (% Predicted for 2 lungs) | $52.4 \pm 11.9^*$ |
| Total lung capacity | |
| (% Predicted for 2 Lungs) | $55.1 \pm 11.9^*$ |
| Mean $\pm$ SD. | |
| $^*p < 0.005$ compared to % lung<br>remaining. | |

(Reproduced from reference 8.)

| **Table 3**<br>Diffusing capacities and total lung capacities<br>of adults after pneumonectomy at a mean<br>age of 6.6 years | |
|---|---|
| % lung remaining | $48.8 \pm 5.2$ |
| Single breath $DL_{CO}$ | |
| (% predicted for 2 lungs) | $76.9 \pm 15.1^*$ |
| Total lung capacity | |
| (% Predicted for 2 Lungs) | $85.2 \pm 17.1^*$ |
| Mean $\pm$ SD. | |
| $^*p < 0.01$ compared with % lung<br>remaining. | |

(Reproduced from reference 9.)

cient to explain the low maximal oxygen intake or the significant but modest fall in arterial oxygen saturation.

A similar compensatory increase of $DL_{CO}$ was reported by Giamonna[9] in adults who had undergone pneumonectomy in childhood, which raised the possibility of enhanced alveolar capillary growth in the remaining lung (Table 3).

An alternate and equally plausible possibility, however, is that alveolar distension and increased blood flow in the remaining lung had recruited existing reserves of diffusing capacity. These findings stimulated our interest in the potential that might exist in children and adults for enhancement of lung growth.

## High-Altitude Studies in Humans

It was recognized that diffusing capacity of the lung probably did not limit exercise at sea level but could do so at low alveolar oxygen tensions; thus the question arose whether prolonged residence at high altitude might stimulate lung growth. An adaptive increase in oxygen diffusing capacity had been reported among high-altitude natives in the Andes[27]; however, this increase might reflect genetic selection that had occurred over centuries in this Indian population rather than any induction of lung growth. There was little

opportunity in Texas for satisfying our interest in high-altitude adaptation. However, Carleton B. Chapman, then chief of cardiology in Dallas, learned from Dr. Gilbert Blount, chief of cardiology at the University of Colorado, that a young investigator in his division named Robert Grover was setting up a high-altitude research laboratory in Leadville, Colorado. Leadville is a mining community at 10,200 feet. The resident population is predominantly Caucasian, many of whose families had resided there for one to three generations. Hence, I contacted Bob Grover, who invited me to visit the laboratory and discuss possibilities for a collaborative study.

On my first visit, Bob arranged for me to ride up to Leadville from Denver with a new research fellow working with him from New York. We had to go over Loveland Pass at 12,000 feet because the Eisenhower Tunnel had not yet been built. The New Yorker became increasingly agitated as we left Denver because he was not accustomed to driving in the mountains. It was beginning to snow, and he began to suggest that we turn around or that I drive. At the top of the pass, now in a blizzard with visibility about 20 feet, he stopped the car and asked me to get out and determine which side of a tall red and white pole we should go on. The pole in fact marked the edge of the road and steep precipice, the bottom of which I could not see; it now became my job to lead the car like a balky mule over this section of the pass, all the while reconsidering my commitment to high-altitude research. But we did not make it over the two crossings of the continental divide required to reach Leadville, and my subsequent collaboration with Bob Grover has extended over 26 years in spite of this early test of my fortitude.

We moved our laboratory to St. Vincent's Hospital at Leadville in the summer of 1964 and studied a sample of the Leadville population in collaboration with Bob Grover. Bob and his team had developed an excellent working relationship with Leadville residents, who also had concerns about health problems at high altitude. We studied a young group of lifelong residents of Leadville, 7 males and 6 females, ranging in age from 15 to 31 (mean = 20.8). These data were compared with measurements taken by the same methods at rest and exercise in 8 males and 6 females matched for body size and age raised near sea level and studied in Dallas (mean age = 18.0); prediction equations were derived for the relationships among single breath $DL_{CO}$ at peak inspiration, $D_{MCO}$, Vc, $\dot{Q}c$, and total lung capacity (TLC). The 6 investigators

also were studied in Dallas and after 6 weeks in Leadville to confirm reproducibility of the measurements in both locations. Results for the young Leadville subjects and results for the investigators studied both in Dallas and in Leadville are summarized in Table 4.[7]

$DL_{CO}$ was significantly higher by about 16% in Leadville residents than predicted based on sea level data from our own laboratory. This was due to a significantly higher membrane diffusing capacity ($DM_{CO}$) as well as pulmonary capillary blood volume (Vc). Total lung capacity was significantly larger (by about 11%) than predicted from sea level data, although spirometric data were not significantly different from sea level predictions.

The members of the investigative team from Dallas showed no significant changes in $DL_{CO}$, $DM_{CO}$, or Vc or in lung volumes during the 6 weeks spent in Leadville. We concluded that Caucasians born and raised at 10,000 feet had significantly larger diffusing capacities and total lung capacities than Caucasian natives of sea level. We presumed that the differences were a consequence of enhanced lung growth induced environmentally. But in

**Table 4**
Single breath diffusing capacity and total lung capacity in 6-week sojourners and lifelong residents in Leadville, Colorado (3,100 m)

| | Age (years) | TLC[a] (liters) | $DL_{CO}$ ml/min (torr) | $DM_{CO}$ ml/min (torr) | Vc ml |
|---|---|---|---|---|---|
| Residents (n = 13) | 20.8 | 6.25 (111)[b] | 39.1 (116)[b] | 82.8 (124)[b] | 102.0 (115)[b] |
| Comparison with sea level predictions | | $p < 0.025$ | $p < 0.005$ | $p < 0.025$ | $p < 0.025$ |
| Sojourners (n = 6) | 27.0 | 7.59 (107)[c] | 36.1 (97)[c] | 76.3 (93)[c] | 83.0 (101)[c] |
| Comparison with sea level predictions | | NS | NS | NS | NS |

Mean ± SEM.
[a]TLC estimated by single-breath He dilution.
[b]% of predicted based on matched Dallas resident of similar age and body size.
[c]% of Dallas measurements.
(Reproduced from reference 7.)

the early 1970s Cerny et al.[4] did a similar study in Leadville on newcomers to high altitude, one group that had arrived in Leadville as adolescents and another group that had arrived as adults and lived there for between 1 and 17 years (see Table 5).

The Cerny study was published in 1973.[4] The investigators concluded that lung growth had occurred in adults and adolescents after a period of residence at high altitude. This casts a new light on interpretation of our own Leadville data. Either high altitude stimulates growth of the lung in adults as well as children, or other effects of acclimatization to high altitude independent of growth alters diffusing capacity measured at high altitude. For example, polycythemia and the associated increase in total blood volume might increase both membrane diffusing capacity and pulmonary capillary blood volume. The kinetics of red cell uptake of CO might be affected by acclimatization.

Hence, results in humans after pneumonectomy or after prolonged residence at high altitude had yielded confusing data from which firm conclusions were not possible. Although the data indicate that both lung resection and prolonged

residence at high altitude evoke compensatory increases in lung volumes and diffusing capacities in children and adults, it is not possible to assign the observed changes to growth. In 1976 we decided to use dogs to obtain some answers. We chose beagles. Our questions are listed below:

1. What effect does prolonged residence at high altitude have on lung pressure volume relations, shape of the thorax, lung tissue volume, and diffusing capacity of mature beagles and of puppies?
2. What effect does pneumonectomy have on lung pressure volume relations, shape of the thorax, lung tissue volume, and diffusing capacity of mature beagles and of puppies?

Protocols are summarized below:

A. Intervention as adults
   1. Six beagles, born and bred at sea level, were taken as adults to 10,200 feet and kept there for 3 years.
   2. Six control beagles of the same age were kept at sea level.
   3. Six adult beagles, born and raised at sea level, had a left pneumonectomy at sea level.

B. Intervention as puppies
   1. Six beagle puppies, born at sea level, were taken to 10,200 feet at 2.5 months of age and were raised there until they were 16 months old.
   2. Six control beagles were raised simultaneously at sea level.
   3. Six beagles had a left pneumonectomy performed at 2.5 months of age and then were raised at sea level.

High-altitude data are presented first.[15] Final studies were done after the beagles kept at high altitude had been returned to sea level for 6 to 9 months. This time interval allowed complete reacclimatization to sea level.

---

**Table 5**
Effect of 1 to 17 years' residence at high altitude on $DL_{CO}$ in persons born at sea level

|  | Measured ml/min torr | Predicted ml/min torr |
|---|---|---|
| Arrival as adults ($n = 11$) | 49.0 | 42.6 |
| Comparison with sea level predictions | $p < 0.005$ | |
| Arrival as adolescents ($n = 13$) | 42.8 | 34.1 |
| Comparison with sea level predictions | $p < 0.005$ | |

(Reproduced from reference 4.)

The dogs were anesthetized with pentobarbital and intubated; an esophageal balloon was then placed in the lower 1/3 of the esophagus to take esophageal pressure measurements. A 1,500 ml super syringe was used to inflate the lungs with a volume of 15, 30, 45, 60, or 75 ml/kg of a gas mixture containing 9% helium. After mouth and esophageal pressures had stabilized, pressure measurements were recorded, and the dog was rebreathed with the gas mixture until helium concentration stabilized. Lung air volume was calculated from the inspired volume and helium dilution.

At a separate time, using a gas mixture containing 0.6% $C_2H_2$, 0.3% $C^{18}O$, and 9% helium in a balance of either air or 100% oxygen, pulmonary capillary blood flow, CO diffusing capacity of the lung, and lung volume were measured simultaneously during rebreathing. Measurements were repeated at different lung volumes and at two different oxygen tensions to estimate membrane diffusing capacity and pulmonary capillary blood volume. For brevity, only the data obtained at the lower alveolar oxygen tension are presented here (Fig. 1).

Physiologic studies were done after blood volumes, hemoglobin concentrations, and pulmonary arterial pressure had returned to sea level values.[10,15] The beagles raised at high altitude had significantly larger lung volumes and diffusing capacities at any given transpulmonary inflation pressure. Keeping adult beagles at high altitude for an extended period had no significant lasting effect on either lung volume or diffusing capacity.

At the termination of the study, the beagles were anesthetized with pentobarbital and intubated through a tracheostomy. The abdomen was opened and the lungs collapsed by rupture through the left hemidiaphragm. This was followed by tracheal instillation of 3% gluteraldehyde in phosphate buffer at a hydrostatic pressure of 30 $cmH_2O$. After fixation in situ, the

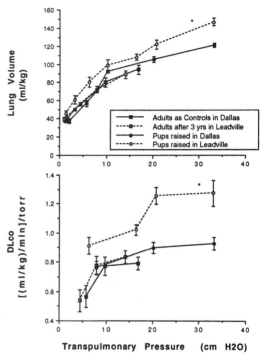

**Figure 1.** Lung volumes and CO diffusing capacities DLCO) are plotted with respect to transpulmonary inflation pressure in four groups of beagles: adult beagles kept at altitude in Leadville, Colorado (3,100 m) for 3 years paired with corresponding controls kept simultaneously at sea level in Dallas (120 m); beagle puppies raised from 2.5 months of age to 16 months of age at altitude and then returned to sea level paired with corresponding controls raised simultaneously at sea level. (Reproduced from reference 15.)

lungs were removed and immersed in Carson's 10% buffered formalin. The volume of each lung was measured by water displacement after fixation. Tissue blocks were taken for light microscopy from six predetermined areas of each lobe, three from the dorsal and three from the ventral aspects; imbedded in methacrylate; and sectioned for morphometric measurements. They are summarized in Table 6 for comparison with corresponding physiologic measurements.

Air space volume, alveolar surface areas, and septal tissue volumes measured by morphometry were significantly larger

**Table 6**

Comparison of morphometric and physiologic data in beagles living at high altitude
for extended intervals with controls near sea level

| Group | Adults | | Puppies | |
|---|---|---|---|---|
| | Controls | High Altitude | Controls | High Altitude |
| Morphometric | | | | |
| Air Vol. (ml/kg) | 54.4 ± 5.5 | 51.9 ± 4.5 | 40.2 ± 4.6 | 58.6 ± 2.8* |
| SA (m²/kg) | 2.92 ± 0.30 | 2.55 ± 0.11 | 2.68 ± 0.19 | 3.52 ± 0.20* |
| $V_t$ (ml/kg) | 14.5 ± 1.5 | 12.3 ± 0.9 | 11.9 ± 1.0 | 16.4 ± 0.6* |
| Physiologic | | | | |
| FRC (ml/kg) | 37.6 ± 3.6 | 36.5 ± 2.6 | 37.3 ± 2.1 | 45.6 ± 3.5** |
| Vt (ml/kg) | 13.8 ± 1.3 | 14.5 ± 1.0 | 13.9 ± 1.2 | 21.2 ± 0.9* |
| Vt-Vc (ml/kg) | 12.4 ± 1.2 | 13.1 ± 0.9 | 11.6 ± 0.6 | 17.9 ± 0.9* |

Mean ± SEM.
Vt = tissue volume of fine parenchyma.
Vc = pulmonary capillary blood volume.
Vt-Vc = extravascular tissue volume.
*$p < 0.05$ in comparison with corresponding controls.
**$0.05 < p < 0.1$ in comparison with corresponding controls.

in the beagles raised from 2.5 months of age at altitude when compared to corresponding controls raised simultaneously at sea level. On the other hand, there were no significant differences in these same measurements between beagles kept for 3 years as adults at altitude compared with corresponding controls kept at sea level. Both morphometric and physiologic measurements indicate enhanced lung growth in the beagles raised at high altitude. These data are consistent with the interpretation that the higher lung volumes and diffusing capacities measured in lifetime residents of Leadville, Colorado, reflect a direct stimulation of lung growth in infancy and childhood. The findings of Cerny and coworkers[4] of increased diffusing capacities in long-term residents who arrived in Leadville as adults may result from secondary effects causing greater recruitment of lung capillary surface, such as expanded blood volumes and increased hematocrits. These effects should be reversible on return to sea level.

The results from the pneumonectomy studies[14] were more difficult to interpret because of the inherent difficulties of separating compensation by recruitment of existing reserves in the remaining lung-by-lung distension or increased blood flow from compensation by growth of new functional lung units.

Diffusing capacity was significantly reduced after pneumonectomy as an adult. After pneumonectomy, both lung volume and diffusing capacity of the remaining right lung were significantly greater than in the right lung of controls. Compensation appears to be greater in puppies than in adults. Morphometric and physiologic data yielded similar conclusions (see Table 7).

This data in Figure 2 and Table 7 indicate significant compensatory increases in lung volume, diffusing capacity, and fine septal tissue volume in the remaining lung of beagles after a left pneumonectomy is performed either as an adult or as a 2.5-month-old puppy; however, compensation is not complete, i.e., functional measurements do not return to normal. Compensation tends to be greater in beagles after pneumonectomy as a

**Table 7**
Comparison of morphometric and physiologic data: right lung of beagles after left
pneumonectomy as adults or as puppies versus the right lung of corresponding controls

| Group | Adults | | Puppies | |
|---|---|---|---|---|
| | Controls | Pneumonectomy | Controls | Pneumonectomy |
| **Morphometric** | | | | |
| Air Vol. (ml/kg) | $30.8 \pm 3.1$ | $45.2 \pm 4.4^*$ | $24.4 \pm 2.8$ | $37.0 \pm 4.3^*$ |
| SA ($m^2$/kg) | $1.75 \pm 0.19$ | $2.30 \pm 0.17^*$ | $1.58 \pm 0.13$ | $2.42 \pm 0.15^*$ |
| $V_t$ (ml/kg) | $8.6 \pm 1.0$ | $13.0 \pm 0.9^*$ | $7.0 \pm 0.7$ | $12.5 \pm 0.7^*$ |
| | | | | |
| **Physiologic** | | | | |
| FRC (ml/kg) | $21.7 \pm 1.7$ | $35.5 \pm 5.3^*$ | $21.6 \pm 1.2$ | $34.5 \pm 4.0^*$ |
| Vt (ml/kg) | $8.3 \pm 0.7$ | $10.3 \pm 1.0^*$ | $8.1 \pm 0.3$ | $13.1 \pm 1.1^*$ |
| Vt-Vc (ml/kg) | $7.0 \pm 0.6$ | $7.7 \pm 0.9$ | $6.8 \pm 0.3$ | $10.6 \pm 0.9^*$ |

Mean ± SEM.
Vt=tissue volume of fine parenchyma in morphometric studies and acetylene tissue volume by physiologi-
calmeasurements.
Vc = pulmonary capillary blood volume.
Vt-Vc = extra vascular tissue volume.
$^*p$ <0.05 in comparison with corresponding controls.
(Reproduced from reference 14.)

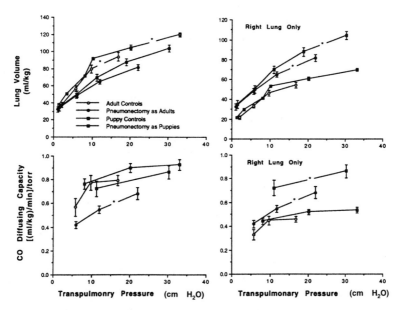

**Figure 2.** Lung volumes (upper panels) and CO diffusing capacities (lower panels) are
plotted with respect to transpulmonary pressure in four groups of beagles. The four
groups include beagles after left pneumonectomy as adults, adult beagles after left
pneumonectomy as 2.5-month-old puppies, and their respective controls.[14] Data from
pneumonectomized animals are compared with respect to both lungs of the controls (left
hand panels) and with respect to the right lung alone (right hand panels). The assumption is that the right lung normally constitutes 58% of the total air volume and
contributes 58% of the total lung diffusing capacity.[19,21,22] Total lung volumes were
significantly reduced after pneumonectomy either as an adult or as a puppy.

puppy, and the significant increase in extravascular tissue volume in the puppies suggests that growth of the lung may have been enhanced. Nevertheless, the relative importance of functional compensation and growth remains uncertain in both immature and mature beagles.

To examine this issue further we developed methods to measure ventilation, oxygen consumption, pulmonary capillary blood flow, and CO diffusing capacity by a rebreathing technique in awake dogs during heavy treadmill exercise.[1,2] We also constructed carotid artery loops in the dogs and inserted flow-directed catheters through the jugular vein into the pulmonary artery for blood sampling and pressure monitoring during heavy exercise.[11,12] Our objectives were to measure maximal oxygen uptake in foxhounds before and after pneumonectomy, to determine the sources of exercise limitation, and to measure the upper limit of diffusing capacity during progressive increments of exercise. Our hypothesis was that we would be able to define an upper limit to the relationship between diffusing capacity and pulmonary blood flow or pulmonary arterial pressure at increasing work loads. A change in this limit might indicate the presence or absence of lung growth after pneumonectomy. Furthermore, if growth of the microvascular bed occurred after pneumonectomy, we should expect to see a change in the pressure flow relationship of the remaining pulmonary vasculature after pneumonectomy such that pressure would be lower than expected for any given flow. Our hypothesis regarding the recruitment of $DL_{CO}$ is schematized in Figure 3.[3]

A similar hypothesis can be developed for the pressure-flow relationship in the right lung before and after left pneumonectomy. What we found before and after left pneumonectomy in three adult foxhounds are shown in Figures 4 and 5.

The data presented in Figure 4 indicates that an upper limit to recruitment of

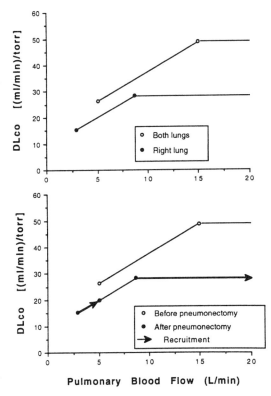

**Figure 3.** Upper panel shows the hypothetical relationship between pulmonary blood flow and $DL_{CO}$ in both lungs (unfilled circles) and in the right lung alone (filled circles) assuming the right lung receives 58% of total blood flow and contributes 58% of total diffusing capacity. In this hypothetical representation, an upper limit of $DL_{CO}$ is reached at a total pulmonary blood flow of 15 L/min and at a blood flow through the right lung of 8.7 L/min beyond which no further increase in $DL_{CO}$ occurs in spite of a continued increase in blood flow. The lower panel shows the expected relationship between pulmonary blood flow and $DL_{CO}$ before and after left pneumonectomy assuming that recruitment of $DL_{CO}$ is unchanged in the remaining right lung after pneumonectomy. Recruitment of $DL_{CO}$ could be impaired if the remaining right lung becomes mechanically distorted after pneumonectomy. If growth of new functional units occurs, the relationship might be shifted back toward that expected for two lungs.

$DL_{CO}$ and presumably of microvascular bed was never reached even after pneumonectomy, when blood flow through the remaining lung reached levels 70%

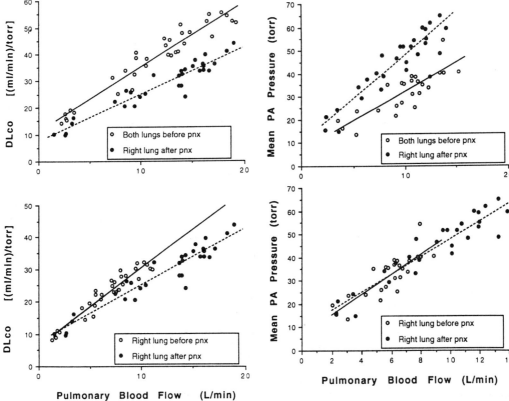

**Figure 4.** In the upper panel DL_CO increased in an almost linear fashion with respect to blood flow before pneumonectomy (unfilled circles, solid line). After pneumonectomy, DL_CO was lower at any given level of pulmonary blood flow, and the slope of the relationship between DL_CO and pulmonary blood flow was significantly less (filled circles, dashed line).[3] An upper limit of DL_CO was not reached either before or after pneumonectomy. In the lower panel the relationship between the DL_CO and pulmonary blood flow to the right lung alone is compared before and after pneumonectomy. Data points after pneumonectomy are superimposed over the normal relationship at lower blood flows but deviate below the normal relationship at higher blood flows, suggesting either that an upper limit of DL_CO was approached or that some structural distortion in the lung after pneumonectomy has impaired normal recruitment.

**Figure 5.** In the left panel, mean pulmonary artery (PA) pressure is plotted with respect to pulmonary blood flow before and after left pneumonectomy.[11] In the right panel, mean pressure-flow relationships in the right lung are examined before and after pneumonectomy. Mean pulmonary arterial pressure is higher at any given blood flow after pneumonectomy than before, although the pressure-flow relationship in the right lung appeared unchanged.

tirely by normal recruitment of existing microvascular bed. Growth of new functional units in the lung need not be invoked to explain our results. These conclusions are reinforced by the lack of change in pressure-flow relationship in the remaining right lung after left pneumonectomy shown in Figure 5.

If new microvascular bed had been added, we would expect a lower PA pressure at any given flow. The lower slope of the relationship between DL_CO and pulmonary blood flow after pneumonectomy

greater than that achieved before pneumonectomy. Furthermore, the compensatory increase in diffusing capacity after pneumonectomy could be explained en-

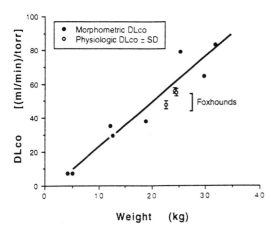

**Figure 6.** A comparison of our physiologic measurements of $\overline{DL}_{CO}$ in foxhounds at heavy exercise with morphometric estimates of $DL_{CO}$ in canids by Weibel et al.[28] plotted with respect to body weight.

suggests that an upper limit of recruitment may be approached at high blood flows through the remaining lung after left pneumonectomy. Left pneumonectomy removes only 42% of the lung in the dog. We are currently testing the hypothesis that the capacity for further recruitment of microvascular reserves might be exceeded after removal of the larger right lung (58% resection).

Previous estimates of $DL_{CO}$ by morphometry in dogs have been reported to be two to three times those measured by physiologic methods under anesthesia in the same dogs.[5,6,28] On the other hand, measurements of $DL_{CO}$ in our foxhounds at heavy exercise before pneumonectomy are very close to those reported by Weibel and his coworkers[28] in canids when normalized with respect to body weight (Figure 6).

Following completion of the physiologic studies in these 3 foxhounds, lungs were fixed by intratracheal instillation of buffered gluteraldehyde for morphometry as in the beagles. Morphometric studies have been performed by Connie C. W. Hsia in collaboration with Ewald Weibel at his laboratory in Bern, Switzerland;

these results are now being prepared for publication. The morphometric data also suggest that the primary effect of left pneumonectomy was overdistension of the remaining lung rather than growth of new lung units. Despite a lack of evidence for structural growth, passive stretching and thinning of the alveolar-capillary membrane, by reducing the resistance to oxygen diffusion, could account for the significant functional compensation observed after pneumonectomy. The magnitudes of functional compensation estimated by physiologic and morphometric methods are similar.[13]

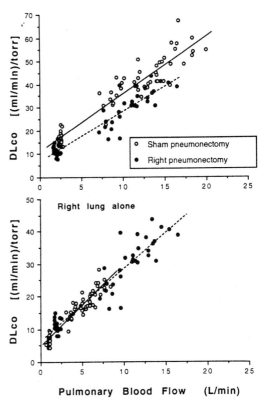

**Figure 7.** The relationship between $DL_{CO}$ and pulmonary blood flow in foxhounds after right pneumonectomy (pnx) compared with that in foxhounds after thoracotomy without lung resection (Sham pnx). In the right panel, the slopes of the two relationships are not significantly different; hence, compensation is more effective after right pneumonectomy than after left.

Connie Hsia and her coworkers in my laboratory have now completed similar physiologic studies in foxhounds after right pneumonectomy, and she is presently working with Ewald Weibel to analyze the morphometric data on the lungs of this latter group of dogs. Contrary to our expectation, an upper limit to $DL_{CO}$ was not reached in the remaining lung at peak exercise after right pneumonectomy, in spite of an increase in blood flow equivalent to over 40 L/min in a normal dog with two lungs (Fig. 7).

Hence, unresolved questions still abound. Where do these apparently inexhaustible reserves of diffusing capacity exist in the lung? What are the mechanisms of recruitment, and can an upper limit ever be reached? Why aren't unrecruited capillaries visible in morphometric studies, or, stated in a different way, why does the whole microvascular bed appear to be fully recruited after tracheal fixation? Are cells just stretched and thinned by overexpansion of the remaining lung, or does hyperplasia also occur in adults after pneumonectomy? Is there a critical level of lung stretch necessary to trigger the growth of cells? Does pneumonectomy enhance growth of the remaining lung in puppies, leading to more functional lung units at maturity?

Not only do the reserves of lung diffusing capacity appear to be inexhaustible, so do the questions derived from that one year I spent in Robert Forster's laboratory, at least for one lifetime. I hope that the questions arising from investigations in my laboratory will also serve as an inexhaustible resource to those who have worked there.

**Acknowledgment:** Particular thanks to Connie C. W. Hsia, who corrected the grammar, organization, and scientific omissions in this manuscript and whose unpublished data I usurped.

## References

1. Ampil, J., J. I. Carlin, and R. L. Johnson Jr. A mouthpiece face mask for the exercising dog. *J. Appl. Physiol.* 64: p 2240–2244, 1988.
2. Carlin, J. I., S. S. Cassidy, U. Rajagopal, P. S. Clifford, and R. L. Johnson, Jr. Noninvasive diffusing capacity and cardiac output in exercising dogs. *J. Appl. Physiol.,* 65: 669–674, 1988.
3. Carlin, J. I., C. C. W. Hsia, S. S. Cassidy, M. Ramanathan, P. S. Clifford, and R. L. Johnson, Jr. Recruitment of lung diffusing capacity with exercise before and after pneumonectomy in dogs. *J. Appl. Physiol.* 70: 135–142, 1991.
4. Cerny, F. C., J. A. Dempsey, and W. G. Reddan. Pulmonary gas exchange in non native residents of high altitude. *J. Clin. Invest.* 52: 2993–2999, 1973.
5. Crapo, J. D., and R. O. Crapo. Comparison of total lung diffusion capacity and the membrane component of diffusion capacity as determined by physiologic and morphometric techniques. *Respir. Physiol.* 51: 183–194, 1983.
6. Crapo, J. D., R. O. Crapo, R. L. Jensen, R. R. Mercer, and E. R. Weibel. Evaluation of lung diffusing capacity by physiological and morphometric techniques [published erratum appears in *J. Appl. Physiol.* 65: following 2800, 1988]. *J. Appl. Physiol.* 64: 2083–2091, 1988.
7. DeGraff, A. C., Jr., R. F. Grover, R. L. Johnson, Jr., J. W. Hammond, Jr., and J. M. Miller. Diffusing capacity of the lung in Caucasians native to 3,100 m. *J. Appl. Physiol.* 29: 71–76, 1970.
8. DeGraff, A. C., Jr., H. F. Taylor, J. W. Ord, T. H. Chuang, and R. L. Johnson, Jr. Exercise limitation following extensive pulmonary resection. *J. Clin. Invest.* 44: 1514–1522, 1965.
9. Giammona, S. T., I. Mandelbaum, J. S. Battersby, and W. J. Daly. The late effects of childhood pneumonectomy. *Pediatrics* 37: 79–88, 1966.
10. Grover, R. F., R. L. Johnson, Jr., R. G. McCullough, R. E. McCullough, S. E. Hofmeister, W. B. Campbell, and R. C. Reynolds. Pulmonary hypertension and pulmonary vascular reactivity in beagles at high altitude. *J. Appl. Physiol.* 65: 2632–2640, 1988.
11. Hsia, C. C. W., J. I. Carlin, S. S. Cassidy, M. Ramanathan, and R. L. Johnson, Jr. Hemodynamic changes after pneumonectomy in the exercising foxhound. *J. Appl. Physiol.* 69: 51–57, 1990.

12. Hsia, C. C. W., J. I. Carlin, P. D. Wagner, S. S. Cassidy, and R. L. Johnson, Jr. Gas exchange abnormalities after pneumonectomy in conditioned foxhounds. *J. Appl. Physiol.* 68: 94–104, 1990.

13. Hsia, C. C. W., R. L. Johnson, Jr., and E. R. Weibel. Lung diffusing capacity after pneumonectomy:physiologic-morphometric correlation. *Clin. Res.* 39: 226A, 1991.

14. Johnson, R. L., Jr., S. S. Cassidy, R. Grover, M. Ramanathan, A. Estrera, R. C. Reynolds, R. Epstein, and J. Schutte. Effect of pneumonectomy on the remaining lung in dogs. *J. Appl. Physiol.* 70: 849–858, 1991.

15. Johnson, R. L., Jr., S. S. Cassidy, R. F. Grover, J. E. Schutte, and R. H. Epstein. Functional capacities of lungs and thorax in beagles after prolonged residence at 3,100 m. *J. Appl. Physiol.* 59: 1773–1782, 1985.

16. Johnson, R. L., Jr., W. S. Spicer, J. M. Bishop, and R. E. Forster. Pulmonary capillary blood volume, flow and diffusing capacity during exercise. *J. Appl. Physiol.* 15: 893–902, 1960.

17. Lawson, W. H., Jr., R. A. B. Holland, and R. E. Forster. Effect of temperature on deoxygenation of human red cells. *J. Appl. Physiol.* 20: 912–918, 1965.

18. Lawson, W. H., and R. L. Johnson, Jr. Gas chromatography in measuring pulmonary blood flow and diffusing capacity. *J. Appl. Physiol.* 17: 143–147, 1962.

19. Massion, W. H., D. R. Caldwell, N. A. Early, and J. A. Schilling. The relationship of dry lung weights to pulmonary function in dogs and humans. *J. Surg. Res.* 2: 287–292, 1962.

20. Mitchell, J. H., B. J. Sproule, and C. B. Chapman. Physiologic meaning of the maximal oxygen intake test. *J. Clin. Invest.* 37: 538–547, 1958.

21. Rahn, H., and B. B. Ross. Bronchial tree casts, lobe weights and anatomical dead space measurements in the dog's lung. *J. Appl. Physiol.* 10: 154–157, 1957.

22. Rahn, H., P. Sadoul, L. E. Farhi, and J. Shapiro, Distribution of ventilation and perfusion in the lobes of the dog's lung in the supine and erect position. *J. Appl. Physiol.* 8: 417–426, 1956.

23. Roughton, F. J. W., and R. E. Forster. Relative importance of diffusion and chemical reaction rates in determining the rate of exchange of gases in the human lung, with special reference to true diffusing capacity of the pulmonary membrane and volume of blood in lung capillaries. *J. Appl. Physiol.* 11: 290–302, 1957.

24. Staub, N. C., J. M. Bishop, and R. E. Forster. Velocity of $O_2$ uptake by human red cells. *J. Appl. Physiol.* 17: 511–516, 1961.

25. Staub, N. C., J. M. Bishop, and R. E. Forster. Importance of diffusion and chemical reaction rates in $O_2$ uptake in the lung. *J. Appl. Physiol.* 17: 21–27, 1962.

26. Stein, M., P. Kimbel, and R. L. Johnson, Jr. Pulmonary function in hyperthyroidism. *J. Clin. Invest.* 40: 348–363, 1961.

27. Velasquez, T., and E. Florentini. Maximal diffusing capacity of the lungs at high altitude. *USAF School of Aviation Medicine Report,* 56: 1–9, 1956.

28. Weibel, E. R., C. R. Taylor, J. J. O'Neil, D. E. Leith, P. Gehr, H. Hoppeler, V. Langman, and R. V. Baudinette. Maximal oxygen consumption and pulmonary diffusing capacity: a direct comparison of physiologic and morphometric measurements in canids. *Respir. Physiol.* 54: 173–188, 1983.

# 12

# An Approach to the Study of the Pulmonary Circulation

## Albert L. Hyman, M.D.

*Professor, Department of Surgery, Medicine, and Pharmacology, Tulane University School of Medicine, New Orleans, Louisiana*

Thou shalt have no false gods before thee! Some of mine have been godlike, some stern, some even cruel, but none have been false. Although, like the great lawgiver, none actually walked upon the Canaan of the pulmonary circulation, whether wittingly or not, they led me step by step in an uninterrupted path to that study. First was my father, a Tulane-educated general practitioner, who was wont to remind me of my great disappointment with kindergarten "because they don't teach no doctor stuff there." Then there was his father, an old-world Hebraic scholar, litterateur, and moralist, who, with my father, had miraculously escaped the Odessa pogroms. He spent most of my childhood attempting to inculcate me with his classical concepts of faith, morality, and justice. Here, I first came to be electrified by ideas and abstractions. In college came a standard platter of American education, food but no feast—some classics, some literature, a bit of science. Then I was off to medical school.

The war with Japan and Germany had just commenced, and the pace of medical education quickened, leaving little time for concepts to germinate. Nonetheless, those 36 uninterrupted months were ample time to elevate new gods. Dr. Richard Ashman, chairman of physiology, delivered the first 20 of the daily physiology lectures. Electrophysiology was his major interest, and one of the several phenomenan he described still bears his name.

From: Wagner WW, Jr, Weir EK (eds): *The Pulmonary Circulation and Gas Exchange.* ©1994, Futura Publishing Co Inc, Armonk, NY.

Sitting in on those lectures were Dr. George Burch, himself soon to become widely published in electrocardiography, and Dr. Sam Levine's nephew, Harold Levine from Boston, a well-known cardiologist in his own right. The curriculum was rushed, and for many reasons these electrophysiology lectures were complex. Moreover, we had not even studied cardiac anatomy. In one of Dr. Ashman's lectures I had failed to identify correctly the electrocardiographic appearance of atrial flutter. In a subsequent discussion, the great electrophysiologist was far more concerned with goading his errant student into formulating a concept that would explain how continuous atrial electrical activity could usurp sinus node function. With my guess that a faster irritable focus depolarizing at 250–300 times a minute could do it, Dr. Ashman was off with a host of experiments he and I could do to further test this widely accepted concept. He suggested that we go off to his laboratory—"Never mind the exam, there will be others and you'll do well." Many years later my wife pointed out that the intensity and dedication I learned as a child had not altered, but I had substituted medical science for theosophy and humanism, and the former had become my new "religion." Electrophysiology, electrocardiology, and cardiac arrhythmias were challenges that came along in rapid succession while working with Dr. Ashman.

Further along, my time at medical school was largely consumed with new icons, each with special cardiovascular skills. Dr. Edgar Hull, the medicine chairman, was an unquestioned master of bedside medicine and cardiac auscultation. At Charity Hospital in New Orleans, patients took to him immediately because he knew their hometown physicians. In fact, he seemed to know every physician who practiced in every parish in Louisiana. He had taught most of them. His was a practical approach. He sought the correct diagnosis to the extent possible but got the patient back to his family and work as quickly as possible. He had an enduring but quiet concern for his house staff members, not only during their training at Charity Hospital, but also throughout their careers. He once postponed an important staff meeting because, as I learned years later, he had gone to northern Louisiana to help reconcile a former cardiac fellow and his wife. His student examinations were always oral, straight from Cecil's textbook, and he enjoyed "helping you out a bit" when you faltered. There was also Dr. Robert Bayley, a former cardiac fellow under Dr. Frank N. Wilson of Ann Arbor. He, like Wilson, had a remarkable talent for mathematics and applied it skillfully and often to electrocardiology. He had devised what has come to be known as the triaxial reference system. Medicine "porch conferences" (porches had ceiling fans) were vibrant with clinical cardiology, electrocardiology, cardiovascular physiology, and the invariable "let's see your data" or "can you give us the mathematical proof." Somehow the other areas of medicine got much less attention.

Undoubtedly the foremost figure in my early progress was Dr. John Samuel La Due. He had done medicine at Harvard, internal medicine at Mayo, and a Ph.D. at Minnesota. He had only recently turned all of his enormous energy to cardiology, joining with Drs. Ashman, Hull, and Bayley. With the fortunes of alphabetic student assignments and a high class failure rate, John La Due was my rounding man all through medical school. One soon came to emulate his penchant for thorough historical inquiry, complete physical exam, and an unabridged write-up. Before case presentation, it was wise to spend the evening in the medical library acquainting oneself with current literature related to the patient's illness. If all went well, the ultimate question was always, "Well, what have you read about this illness lately?" He wasn't one to let you off the hook easily. Two examples are memorable. As a second semester student visiting the wards for the first time, I was asked what the "Robinson-Power-Kelper test" was. "I would have to go to the library; it wasn't yet in Cecil's text." La Due smiled, "Yes, that's a good idea." As we commenced discussion of another patient, he looked up at me rather surprised and shouted "Now!" On another occasion, Dr. La Due prodded a less than ardent medical student to study more and more thoroughly the blood of a patient with unexplained anemia. On the great day, Dr. La Due finally received all the hematologic data and asked for the student's appraisal of the anemia. "I don't know, Dr. La Due, but you've had me take an awful lot of blood out of her." This was one of the few times John La Due was ruffled.

The experience I acquired over three academic years with John La Due left an indelible mark on my approach to medicine and science. "If you don't know and it's not in the library, you have a golden research opportunity," he would say. Although I worked with him on the wards, in the clinics, and in his research laboratory, it was only years later that he expressed any appraisal of my work or productivity. Some seven or eight years later, I saw John in the lobby of the Los Angeles hotel hosting the American College of Cardiology meeting. He insisted that I come immediately to a private reception honoring him upon his election to the presidency of that group. At that reception, I was introduced to the cognoscenti of cardiology and the new specialty of cardiovascular surgery as "one of the best damn medical students I ever contended with." The libations and atherogenic refreshments were lavish, and John had probably partaken heavily of both. With Dr. Ashman and Robert Bayley, La Due perfected the concept of electrocardiographic vector analysis, developed the ventricular gradient of F. N. Wilson, and from the QRS loops identified the effects of anatomic rotation of the heart on the standard ECG. Indeed, my first publi-

cation was with Dr. Ashman, demonstrating that the anatomic axis of the heart, as seen fluoroscopically, could be predicted from the ECG taken in the same position.[1] La Due went on to New York, where, with Wroblewski and Karmen, he was the first to publish the use of the cardiac enzyme (SGOT) in the diagnosis of acute myocardial infarction.

Shortly before I received my medical degree, my father's brother, a colorful gynecologist at Cedars of Lebanon (now Cedars-Sinai), Los Angeles, suggested I learn his specialty and join him in his practice. This digression was short-lived. My professor of obstetrics knew me well, having delivered me about twenty-one years before. He agreed to give me an obstetrics residency if I would first do a rotating internship at Charity Hospital. His conditions were clear: take as many specialty blocks as I could, except obstetrics, and if I still wanted the obstetrics residency at the end of that year, it would be mine. My first assignment was internal medicine, with Drs. Hull, La Due, and Bayley as my clinical staff and Louis Levy, another ardent follower of Dr. Ashman, as my resident physician. Professor Graffagino, Uncle Earl, Cedars, and Los Angeles became a pipe dream (and we used pipe cleaners in those days to project vectorcardiographic loops). It was clear, however, that before embarking on a training program in cardiology, it was necessary to complete that rotating internship and three more years of general internal medicine. My second rotation was onto Dr. Alton Ochsner's surgical ward with a young resident from Philadelphia, Oscar Creech. There was a new surgery, tying off a patent ductus, or turning down a subclavian artery, to the pulmonary artery for Fallot's tetralogy. Oscar was disappointed, seeing that I was much more interested in the cardiovascular and hemodynamic derangements than in the mechanics of surgical repairs. I did the forbidden obstetrics month, for the most part to see first hand how a physiologic volume overload affects healthy people as well as those with rheumatic and congenital heart disease. Alcohol was the only pharmacologic diuretic known then.

The next year was spent at the University of Cincinnati. Dr. La Due had urged me to spend a year with Professor Marion Blankenhorn to learn a more disciplined approach to internal medicine. Dr. Blankenhorn had made many early observations on beriberi heart disease. His son, David, was an excellent fourth-year student on our wards, and we have been friends over the years. He went to the University of Southern California and became interested in atherosclerosis. About halfway through the first-year residency, I was invited to give a cardiology seminar on this new business of vectorcardiography. During the year-end holidays in New Orleans, Richard Ashman took me into his laboratory and his home and amply prepared me for the seminar. Noble Fowler, a senior resident, attended and showed interest. We talked many times during that year. Indeed, after a short visit to Bellevue, he started this "new thing," cardiac catheterization in the heart station at the General. Soon I had learned what little was known about it in 1946. I returned to Charity Hospital for two more years of internal medicine residency. Shortly into that second year, a patient thought to have bacterial endocarditis on the pulmonary valve appeared. It seemed best in those days (1947) to culture blood drawn from the pulmonary artery. A cardiac catheter somehow appeared quickly. Since the only horizontal fluoroscope available was in the tuberculosis hospital unit, the catheterization procedure was done there. There were no strain gauges in those days. One of Dr. Ashman's jerry-rigged smoked-kymographs with a calibrated rubber tambour measured pressures as the fluoroscope guided the catheter up. This was the first heart catheterization at Charity Hos-

pital! The cultures were negative, but we established the diagnosis of pulmonary stenosis with the catheter and kymograph.

Somehow this seemingly minor event did not pass unnoticed in the staid community of Charity Hospital. I got a strain gauge! What's more, on his retirement, Dr. Ashman gave me his prized double-channel Cambridge string galvanometer with the two quartz spare strings and rapidly moving photographic paper. He had had it uniquely designed to take not one, but two ECG leads concurrently. One channel was converted to use with the strain gauge, permitting measurement of one pressure change concurrently with one ECG lead. One channel was standardized against a column of mercury and the other with a DC voltmeter each day. It was large, about the size of the fluoroscopic table, but was a distinct improvement over the smoked kymographic drum and rubber tambour. On the other hand, its quartz strings broke easily, were difficult to insert between the magnet heads, and were expensive. My assignment in the internal medicine residency program somehow became concentrated on the cardiology clinic with the new bright-line fluoroscope (only 5.0 m.a.!), the ECG reading room with Dr. Ashman, and, of course, the catheterization procedure on selected patients seen in cardiac consultations or clinics. Dr. George Burch became interested, and soon we were occasionally studying Tulane patients as well. Dr. Nelson Ordway joined the Louisiana State University's pediatrics service and introduced the Roughton-Scholander glass pipette to measure blood-oxygen content. Pediatric patients from both schools came along, and we grew busy. There were no standards, no procedural texts, no ECG oscilloscope, no defibrillation, no surgery standby. We flew by the seat of our pants, but fortune smiled, and no one was injured. Perhaps the exception was the hair on my hands, which was lost. I was able to get a "bright-line" fluoroscopic screen. Still 5 m.a. T.V. screens, remote or otherwise were unknown!

In the heart station there were new and exciting sessions. Dr. Frank N. Wilson, who first described the precordial electrocardiogram, began coming quarterly to visit his daughter in New Orleans. Dr. Franklin Johnson, his close associate, sometimes accompanied him. Wilson's student, Dr. Demetrius Sodi-Pallares, now chief of electrocardiography at the National Institute of Cardiology, Mexico City, also came. Sodi's *New Basis of Electrocardiography* in 1956 was a classic. He was later to advocate glucose, potassium, and insulin for acute myocardial infarction. With Dr. Ashman reading ECG's in the Charity Heart Station and Drs. Wilson, Johnson, Sodi-Pallares, Bayley, La Due and Hull doing commentary, those were some heady sessions for a medicine resident. Nonetheless, the new potential for hemodynamic studies began to occupy more and more time. Dr. George Burch, who had also embarked on a notable career in electrocardiography, invited me to the Tulane cardiology functions, and I came to know his cardiology staff. On the Tulane surgery service, Dr. Michael De Bakey and his resident Oscar Creech showed great interest in these cardiovascular conferences. The Taussig-Blalock procedure for Fallot's tetralogy had been described at Hopkins, and eventually the first edition of Helen Taussig's book on congenital heart disease appeared. Maude Abbott's book was largely a pathologic anatomy treatise. Cournaud's short book hadn't appeared yet.

I came to know Dr. Burch even more in the third year of the LSU internal medicine residency. Once his secretary called me from Charity Hospital to see to him in his Tulane medicine department office. Something was surely wrong! He explained to me that a young instructor in English had transferred from the School of Arts and Science at Michigan to the one at Tulane. His wife, who had Fallot's tetralogy, was under the care of Franklin Johnson and F. N. Wilson at Ann Arbor. Dr. Burch showed me the rather complete letter he had received from Ann Arbor and asked me to examine his patient in the elite doctor's infirmary at Charity. I was impressed with this attractive young blonde, lying in bed, sparsely clothed, reading Tolstoy's book. After my examination, I returned to Dr. Burch's office armed with Taussig's new text. I confidently assured him I would put a catheter retrogradely through a patent ductus. "A tetralogy has equal distribution of extremity cyanosis, but this young woman has differential cyanosis with pink fingers and blue toes." Burch cautioned that x-ray documentation of the catheter in the ductus would be required. "But Dr. Burch, I've never seen such an attractive young blonde so scantily clothed in Charity Hospital." The Catholic nuns have always maintained strict decorum. "What's more, she was lying there reading *Peace and War*." "Al," he replied, "Tolstoy's book is called *War and Peace*." I paled, but his consummate smile told me a new icon would arise from an unlikely source, Tulane. The x-ray was dutifully brought to his office; he thanked me and kept it. Years later I came to learn that he had sent the film to Ann Arbor and gently chided the doctors there about bedside examination and the need for a university catheterization lab! Years after that I came to truly understand that the judge and the executioner never dine together.

After the rotating internship and three years of "internal medicine," I was now preparing to undertake a cardiology fellowship. Dr. Ashman had me placed with Dr. Louis Katz at Michael Reese Hospital, Chicago, but he wanted most that I set up a catheterization laboratory, not a new experience for me. Drs. Langendorf and Pick were superb students of arrhythmia, but that didn't seem right. Dr. Hull wanted me to go with his friend Sodi-Pallaris in Mexico City, but there was a language barrier. I'd only learned Cajun French at Charity. Dr. Burch had another idea. He had a great interest in systemic veins, because "that's where most of the blood is." He'd written one of his famous primers on venous function, which had been well received. I had studied some of Professor John McMichael's papers dealing with the concepts of digitalis affecting primarily the systemic veins but knew little about how veins controlled heart function. I asked Dr. Burch about this work, and he immediately suggested I go to London and study with Professor McMichael. In June 1948, Dr. Burch and I composed letters to him. About November, I had taken a week to cruise to Havana, and, while there, visited Dr. Castillano's new angiocardiographic laboratory, one of the earliest in this hemisphere. As my boat moored on the bank of the Mississippi River, Dr. Burch's secretary pulled me off and into his office. Professor McMichael had come to Tulane to deliver the John Musser Memorial Lecture and was sitting at Dr. Burch's desk waiting to interview me. He explained that he had place for one American, and Dr. Epstein from Yale had been appointed. A problem arose regarding American Board of Internal Medicine credits for studying in London, and Dr. Epstein was going to stay in the States to complete those requirements. If I had no such constraints, he would accept me. Dr. Burch arranged one of the first NIH Traveling Fellowships for me. I was on my way to London in June 1949.

London may be part of the Old World to Americans, but to me Hammersmith Hospital was an exciting new world. Professor McMichael was surely an icon who strived to reach a balance between man and his instruments, who leaned heavily on experience and less on statistics, and who had the skill to use bedside medicine and keep advanced technology in proper perspective. He was eager for me to visit his own Edinburgh and other British and continental hospitals. "One doesn't come to Europe every day," he was fond of saying. At 8:00 a.m. on the first day, I went to the hospital, only to learn that the British start their laboratory at about 10 a.m. and carry on until 8 p.m. Professor McMichael took me from firm to firm (subspeciality sections) introducing me to the people with whom I'd be working, a remarkably talented group, each of whom was destined for greater tasks. Professor Paul Wood, an Australian, was the rounding man on the largest cardiac ward at Hammersmith. He was an excellent clinical cardiologist, a good teacher, somewhat dogmatic, and very self-assured. He was friendly from the outset and showed me the chapter dealing with electrocardiography in his forthcoming book *Diseases of the Heart and Circulation.* He was well acquainted with the work of F. N. Wilson, Richard Ashman, Robert Bailey, and the other vectorcardiology group. John Goodwin came the same year I did. He was interested in cardiomyopathy and devised a manual compression system to deliver radio-opaque material down a cardiac catheter. His publications on cardiomyopathy are widely known. He and Paul Yu edited an annual *Progress in Cardiology,* for many years. John grew in stature and became one of Britain's renowned senior cardiologists. He was often an invited international speaker at the American Heart Association and the American College meetings. Professor E. P. Sharpey-Schafer was one of the most clever and at times the most acerbic member of the Hammersmith group. He and Professor McMichael had studied heart failure, cor pulmonale, and the effects of ouabain during the late war years.

Richard Bayliss, with whom I worked closely, was a very able clinician and close to the professor. One of Hammersmith's greatest raconteurs, he was fond of the apocryphal tale of Sharpey and the chair in medicine at Thomas's. He was short-listed, but a second round was announced. The story has it that Sharpey and Richard were at a pub on Duncane Road near the White Castle, having a beer before going home. Richard suggested that if Sharpey would obtain a fresh new suit and shirt and present himself as a candidate the second time, he would get the chair. Richard suggested a suit like the blue serge the man next to them was wearing. Sharpey, always direct, commenced a conversation with the man. Soon the two went upstairs and Sharpey emerged with the suit. Some say he bought it; others say he convinced the man to enter Hammersmith Hospital for treatment of his cough. No one will ever know how the transaction occurred, but a few days later, *Lancet* had an announcement that Professor E. P. Sharpey-Schafer had assumed the chair at Thomas's.

Sheila Sherlock was one of the most colorful, clever young women at Hammersmith. She was interested in liver disease and studied hepatic metabolism each afternoon using a catheter passed into a hepatic vein. She always commenced her catheter lab studies promptly at 2 p.m. If Professor McMichaels's firm—which included Dick Bayliss, Morris Ethridge, from Adelaide, and me—hadn't finished in the catheterization laboratory by that time, we experienced the full spectrum of Sheila's colorful nature. She has revised her book *Liver Disease* for many editions. She became a Dame, and Professor Mc-Michael and Dick Bayliss were eventually knighted by the British queen. Sheila is now chairperson at the Royal Free. She is married to Jerry James, a pulmonary physician who was with Professor John Scadding at Hammersmith. Working with Sheila was Alex Bearn, who later studied copper metabolism in Wilson's disease while at the Rockefeller in New York. He had the medicine chair at Cornell in later years. Sam Kaplan was a South African working in cardiology at Hammersmith.

He was interested in going to the United States to do pediatric cardiology and eventually in setting up such a subsection. I urged him to look at Cincinnati, which offered many academic and intellectual advantages, including a marvelous children's hospital, heavily supported by Proctor and Gamble. Besides, the meals there were superb. As a junior house-officer at the General, I arranged to read their ECG's in the lunch hour because of the food differential. In later years, I was to interview quite a few candidates for the pediatric cardiology job at Tulane and two for the Established Investigatorship award of the AHA who had trained with Sam at Cincinnati Childrens. More recently, Bill Friedman, who joined the AHA Research Committee as my term was ending, told me he had lured Sam out to the pediatric department at UCLA. The professor was rightfully proud of the bright young people he brought together at the Hammersmith—not only British physicians, but also those from the provinces, South Africa, Australia, India, New Zealand, and Canada. (In spite of reminding him about a certain melee in 1776, I was always introduced as being from the American province!)

Finally I was conducted to a laboratory where thoracic blood volume was being measured by the blue-dye technique. There I met Harry Kopelman and a tall young physician who was introduced as "Grant Lee." I smiled at the professor, who had me explain, "In my country, nobody is called both Grant and Lee." There began a long and still cherished friendship that has lasted even through this most recent pulmonary conference outside of Denver.

Hammersmith Hospital was always frenetic with excitement—new ideas, new research initiatives, cardinal seminars, and penetrating, and at times, acerbic grand rounds. The professor was the obvious leader and the arbitrator among sharply circumscribed opinions from the diverse firms. Hammersmith had newly been designated the Postgraduate Medical School of the University of London and was considered by British medicine to be a heterodox, not one that taught the skilled orthodox British tradition of clinical excellence. At Hammersmith, the position was that one had acquired those skills before coming. Nonetheless, as late as 1949 the other great teaching hospitals were not sure about this Hammersmith place.

This was only four years after the second Great War, and London had only begun to rebuild. The single catheterization laboratory was in a galvanized hut jerry-built onto the end of the hall. Dick Bayliss, Morris Ethridge, and I used it to study the effects of digoxin on the heart and circulation in different types of heart failure. Sheila and her group were studying liver function, and John Goodwin and his group were doing angiocardiography, looking at various forms of cardiomyopathy. When the London fog turned quite green, Hammersmith went out of control. The professor, Sharpey, Sheila Howath, and our group were looking at the effects of ouabain on acute cor pulmonale induced by that thick, soupy green fog. Because of the urgency and large number of patients, these catheters were floated in at the bedside with the help of a water manometer. Some nearby residents of East Acton actually came in to have the "arm-tube with the digitalis." Watching the pressure level and the oscillations of the tip of the column of water was all that was needed. A mixed venous sample, a quick arterial sample, and, where possible, 3 min of collected exhaled air. A rapid Haldane blood oxygen analysis and an $O_2$ meter and we had pressure and flow—no balloons, no thermodilution, not even dye dilution. We were not sure of the salutary effects of ouabain in acute cor pulmonale, as opposed to other types of failure, but it often produced a remarkable pulmonary hypertension. We reported our data but were not sure of the mechanism of the enhanced pulmonary hypertension. The hypertension didn't seem to be due to enhanced flow, and the patient's oxygenation improved. I've concerned myself with it for many years and am still not sure. Ironically, last year in my laboratory we spent much time characterizing the electrogenic Na-K-ATPase pump in the pulmonary vascular bed of healthy cats. There is no doubt that, at elevated tone, activation of the pump induces vasodilation. When the pump is blocked with ouabain, a sizeable pulmonary hypertension quickly appears. When we go about writing up those experiments, we'll quote that 1950 paper describing this strange aggravation of pulmonary hypertension by ouabain in cor pulmonale.

Many stimulating visitors came to Hammersmith. Werner Forsmann came from his small hospital practice in southern Germany. He had been a thoracic surgeon who had studied with Adolph Fick. He had searched for Fick's mixed venous sample with the zeal of Jason searching for the Golden Fleece. Alas, his one publication on right heart catheterization for obtaining the sample was telling. He had used a ureteral catheter, which he had passed upon himself with a system of mirrors and a fluoroscope. But the x-ray he published clearly indicated that the catheter was too short and had stopped at the superior vena cava—right atrial junction. Nonetheless, he had come up with the idea, and he, with Cournaud and Dickinson Richards, who did get the mixed venous sample, were awarded the Nobel prize. Forsmann had apparently done no research since that x-ray was taken. He had had problems with other surgeons at their hospital and seemed to have gone to a small practice in a small German hospital during and after the war. He told us that newspaper reporters had found him in this small city and asked him how he felt having just received the Nobel prize. He said he thought for a moment and replied,

"Like a village priest who had just been elected pope." Visiting the clinical research facilities at Hammersmith, he was indeed a village priest. With the advent of dye dilution, and now thermodilution, one wonders, like Jason, about the value of the Golden Fleece after it served its purpose. Indeed, no one knows its ultimate disposition.

Dr. Sam Levine came from the Brigham. At grand rounds he demonstrated his legendary auscultatory skill, correctly predicting the length of the PR interval by listening to the intensity of the first heart sound. I was elated at this demonstration that American physicians, too, had great clinical skills and could reach a balance between the bedside and the laboratory. Sitting in the back of the room with Paul Wood, I heard his quip, "Let him try that again." Well he didn't but he'd shown it could be done. Von Euler from Stockholm lectured on sympathetic control of cardiac inotrophy and attempted to relate that to Starling curves. The family of curves came later, as did Von Euler's Nobel prize. Lenegre came from France and described fibrosis in the cardiac conducting tissue and heart block. Somehow he was rumored to have obtained his normal control specimens at the guillotine. I erred badly, with my weak command of the Cajun-French patois, when the French cardiologist Professor Heim de Balzac, a nephew of Honore de Balzac visited us. Thinking in English but speaking the patois, I referred to Lenegre as "l'homme guillotiné."

Then Sheba came from the new medical school at Jerusalem and invited us to visit him. He had just been appointed Israeli minister of health. Some of us took him up on his invitation. The Hebrew University Hospital in 1950 was not the Hadassah Hospital of today. Nonetheless, it was fascinating to read the patient charts in a language untarnished by 3,000 years of history but suddenly transformed and transliterated into scientific medical English. And one who had helped modernize Hebrew had been my father's teacher Chiam Naham Bialik in Odessa. Several Russian delegations came to Hammersmith from time to time but left fairly promptly. The professor, like his prime minister, never trusted the Russians and their brand of communism. Borst came from the Netherlands and showed the ability of licorice to increase blood volume by a DOCA-like salt-retaining property. The value of the jugular venous pressure in accurately measuring right atrial pressure at the bedside was demonstrated, even if a tilt table was needed for low pressure. C. Heymanns came from Ghent and lectured on the carotid sinus function. He also received a Nobel prize. Andre Cournaud gave a superb lecture on the pulmonary blood flow and ventilation-perfusion matching. Bill Briscoe, who was in our Hammersmith group, eventually went to work with him at Bellevue. He spent much of his time calculating the distribution of ventilation and ventilation-perfusion ratios. Bill was a heavy smoker, but these were the days before smoking became an anathema.

One other perk appeared in London when postwar rationing was still necessary. The first month, my NIH check hadn't arrived, so I went to our embassy at Grovsner Square. No one had heard of this new NIH, but "if it has anything to do with the Public Health Service, you're in luck because the European chief is here." He hadn't heard of the NIH either, but somehow I ended up with an embassy passport and Navy ship-store privileges. Like being at Macy's in a ration-ridden London! The professor always enjoyed a wee bit of whisky (Scotch). To earn dollars, the Scotch was made in the U.K., shipped to New York, and back to the U.S. Navy ship stores in London by return flight. For errant young sailors preparing to visit the continent, ladies' stockings were packed in special boxes, a single stocking each.

The professor was quite correct in his

appraisal of the remarkable effect of that digitalis on systemic vessels. Much later it was shown to be related to its blocking action on the electrogenic pump. We were all convinced that much, if not most, of its effect was on the heart, but the two are closely intertwined, and sorting out the differences was difficult in intact man. Nonetheless, it fell to me to present the group paper at the First World Heart Congress in Paris, September 1950. It was to be presented in French; I protested that others spoke fluent French. They explained that the English and the French speak each other's languages but won't. But my patois was insular and far from contemporary French; even my university cheering-song was "Geaux Tigers." Sure enough, before I had completed the presentation, my first ever, Dr. Cournaud was on his feet presenting a response in his staccato native French. I suggested that, because he was now an American, he would be good enough to repeat his comments in English. Only later did English become the lingua franca of science. At the meeting, I had an interesting discussion with Bill Milnor from Johns Hopkins and Tom Mattingly. Bill was interested in the electrocardiographic criteria for the diagnosis of ventricular hypertrophy. Tom, a general in the U.S. Army Medical Corp, was studying trauma to the heart.

Working back at Charity Hospital, I told Dr. Burch that we had finally convinced Professor McMichael that the primary effect of digitalis was on the heart. Without a hesitation, Burch replied "Well, I'm not so sure anymore!" He said that Tulane was undergoing changes. The esteemed Dr. Ochsner was about to retire as chairman of surgery, and Tulane wanted the cardiovascular surgeon Dr. Michael DeBakey to succeed him. Mike was a Tulane graduate and had been Dr. Ochsner's finest before going to Baylor. But Mike suggested that Tulane invite Oscar Creech instead. He had done a superb job with Dr. DeBakey at Baylor and should make an

excellent successor to their mentor, Dr. Ochsner. Soon after Oscar assumed the surgery chair, he busied himself setting up a combined cardiology-cardiovascular surgery service. Dr. Burch asked me to come over to Tulane, set up the cardiology-surgery catheterization laboratory in the surgery department, and work closely with the surgeons. Dr. Burch, who never quite trusted surgeons, felt that a well-trained cardiologist in their midst would reduce their mortality rate. Neither he nor any in his group had the time or penchant for that work. The job carried a major hazard. I would be working directly with the chairman of the surgery department, but my own chairman, Dr. Burch, had very little interest in surgery, much less cardiovascular surgery. At later conferences, he was wont to point out that the major cause of death from ventricular septal defect was surgery. Nonetheless, he assured me that the need was great and my uneasiness ill-founded.

When Oscar walked into his newly activated catheterization lab and saw me, he decried, "Lord, not you again!" Oscar was one of the most princely men I've ever had the pleasure to know. He was an accomplished cardiovascular physiologist who happened to be a master surgeon. Work went well; new brooms sweep well. There were daily cardiac catheterizations, attendance at surgery and the intensive care unit, and presenting or standing in for Dr. Burch at cardiology conferences and at his student rounds during his important visits to the NIH, to other universities, and to Europe. The research seminars were replete with promising young people. Tom James was studying coronary arterial supply to specialized conducting tissue and electronmicroscopy of the sinoatrial and atrioventricular node, Ralph Lazarro was doing early electrophysiologic experiments, Lewis Thomas was involved in cardiac pathology, Thorpe Ray was studying sodium and tagged rubidium excretion induced with the new mercury diuretics.

Leo Horan was looking at mechanisms in atrial fibrillation. Victor Ferrans was finishing clinical cardiology training on my ward and doing his Ph.D. in cardiac electronmicroscopy, and Bill Love was estimating coronary blood volume by dye dilution. In physiology, Dr. Hyman Mayerson and Karlman Wasserman were measuring pulmonary lymph protein.

The ivory-towered top floor of the medical school was Burch's Berchtesgaden. Here his hemetically sealed temperature- and humidity-controlled rooms had been constructed. In them, I did bedside cardiac catheterizations to measure pulmonary vascular pressures and Fick outputs. We were studying the effects of temperature and humidity on human cardiovascular function. New Orleans could get hot in the summer, and hospitals weren't yet air-conditioned. Moving quickly to make measurements and keep the instruments functioning in those rooms often caused incapacitating weakness within 15 to 20 minutes. Dr. Burch himself had once experienced a syncopal episode in one of the rooms. Strangely, the volunteer, who lay quietly on a couch, sweated but had no real discomfort. Cardiac outputs were measured 35–40 L/min at the most humid and hottest temperatures.

Work had proceeded quite well until an unlikely incident changed all that. I had visited John Ross at the NIH and received instructions in his newly introduced transseptal catheterization technique. The transbronchial approach we previously used to cross the mitral valve was difficult for the patient, and twice the PE–50 tubing had knotted inside the left atrium before it could be passed through the mitral valve. Fortunately, both were in patients with severe mitral stenosis. In each, the PE–50 was drawn tautly against the patient's lips, and Oscar Creech caught the errant loop during a finger fracture, closed valvulotomy. Back at the Tulane lab after the NIH visit, I was doing a transseptal catheterization on one of Oscar Creech's patients. The catheter had gone across the atrial septum but entered the left inferior pulmonary vein. A plastic 3F was then passed out the transseptal catheter into a peripheral pulmonary vein, and pressures in the left atrium and large and small pulmonary veins were recorded concurrently as the patient lay comfortably on the catheterization table. This approach simulated to a great extent the continuous measurements of systemic venous pressure that Dr. Burch had studied. He had described the spontaneous fluctuations in pressure in these vessels.

At that moment Dr. Burch, who generally wanted little to do with cardiac catheterization, walked in and asked about the progress of the procedure. When I explained how readily one could measure pulmonary venous pressure in a man resting quietly, he was enthusiastic. He watched the pressure tracings carefully as he asked the patient to undertake complex mental tasks. After the diagnostic procedure was complete, he announced with great conviction, that I was to study pulmonary circulation. There was no need for me to do all of these diagnostic catheterizations; other people could be brought to Tulane to do that, but to study the intact pulmonary vessels was a more important undertaking. Responding to my reluctance to undertake the study of a circulatory system about which so little was known, he smiled again and said, "Can't think of a better reason to do it." After many years of clinical cardiology, electrophysiology, and about twenty-five hundred diagnostic heart catheterizations, I was now into the pulmonary circulation.

Many months of long evenings were consumed in the medical library, reading what was not quite "so little." The relation of vascular flow to pressure, interstitial lung pressure to lung volume, hypoxia, gravitational effects, distention and recruitment, pulmonary capillary blood flow, pulmonary venous pressure, and pulmonary reflexes were among the major topics of interest. Rewarding weekends were spent with Bill Milnor at Hopkins learning from his work on pulmonary venous and arterial pressures in open chest dogs. Bill had recently transferred from cardiology to physiology at Hopkins and was even then formulating plans for his unique book, *Hemodynamics,* published in 1982. It wasn't that far from New Orleans, and my sister was there with her husband, who was on the child psychiatry faculty.

Dr. Burch advised me to make simple, direct measurements in intact dogs. I contrasted the spontaneous changes in large and small vein pressures, after taking elaborate pains to ensure that this was not pulmonary venous wedge pressure. Output and pulmonary blood volume were measured by dye dilution. We then looked at the effects of transfusion, of a cold environment, and of balloon occlusion. A pressure gradient between the large pulmonary vein and the left atrium was never identified. We found no support for the concept of large vein throttling pulmonary venous flow in the left atrium. Interpreting the data provoked interesting discussions. Measurements dealing with pulmonary hemodynamics are not interpretable in terms commonly used in the systemic circulation. I urged those near Dr. Burch who were reviewing my data with me to remember that this is a high flow, low pressure bed, modulated by Starling-type resistors not seen in the systemic bed; that flow and pressure are not always nearly linear; and that calculated resistance values must be interpreted with great caution. Moreover, although changes in small vein pressure are valid, the more the vein constricted, the more likely the size of the catheter was to interfere with exact calculations of absolute venous resistance.

Nonetheless, papers began to be published, and Oscar Creech urged me to apply for my own NIH grant. By then I was looking at pulmonary embolism and the possibility that sudden distention of a pulmonary vessel could induce reflex bradycardia and hypotension, with possibly reflex pulmonary arterial and venous constriction. Dr. Greene, from the NIH, was visiting Tulane, and Oscar arranged a meeting, where I learned for the first time how to apply and write a grant application. The application was submitted under Oscar's aegis, and, to my complete surprise, the study section funded my project. Oscar was delighted, there was joy in Mudville, the first of this growing junior faculty had gained independent support. There was, however, an unforeseen problem, and my Icarian wings experienced the first rays of the sun's heat. A member of the medicine faculty only applies for grant support from the medicine department, not surgery. The careful instructions from the NIH hadn't covered this point. They saw my laboratory in surgery, my close clinical and laboratory relationship with the surgeons, and said that's the way to go. In spite of the progress of the research, I could not bring any of these studies to readily provide for a definitive experiment. One had to differentiate between passively induced pulmonary hypertension from mechanical obstruction with embolization and actively induced vasoconstriction. Paul Yu from Rochester was chairing the American Heart Association session at which Abe Rudolph was presenting a paper suggesting that the pulmonary hypertension resulting from embolus was mechanically induced, and I followed with data suggesting reflex contribution. I had known Paul for many years. He was working in the American Heart Association and was soon to be its president. He spoke to us before the session and developed an excellent discussion during the session based on prior knowledge of the presentations. Abstracts were not published until later, if at all, in those days.

The implications of all these studies were becoming increasingly obvious. The pulmonary vascular bed could not be studied by methods used in the systemic bed. Techniques were available to perfuse an excised lung or to perfuse it in situ at constant pressure or constant flow, or even in the intact chest to look at three points on a pressure-flow curve. However, what was needed was a technique permitting the study of a hemodynamically isolated lung lobe perfused at constant flow, and constant left atrial pressure, in an intact, spontaneously breathing animal. With such a preparation, the pharmacologic responses of pulmonary blood vessels could be more closely studied with respect to dose response curves, receptor sites blocking agents, and, later, transduction mechanisms. Moreover, reflex responses of the pulmonary vessels are better examined in intact chest animals. In the clinical árena, this was the time of a great thrust toward surgical pulmonary embolectomy. Working with Oscar Creech and his surgical group, we had done some but saw the unfortunate complication of a successful embolectomy followed rapidly by adult respiratory distress syndrome. Indeed, the sanguinous froth appeared in the endotracheal tube less than an hour after embolectomy in one memorable patient. The concept of reperfusion injury was not yet developed. Along with many others, I was trying to devise a large cardiac catheter method to extract larger emboli without thoracotomy and bypass, and then later to use thrombolysis with streptokinase. I soon learned that, with suction on the catheter, the pulmonary arterial wall quickly obstructed large catheters and that technique was not going to be effective.

Serendipitously, I was surprised to learn how large a catheter one could put into a dog's pulmonary artery without causing any evidence of hemodynamic alteration, as long as one didn't apply negative pressure. I could put a balloon on that large catheter, isolate the left lower lobe artery by balloon distension, and perfuse the lobe with blood through the large

catheter with an extracorporal pump. I had the transseptal technique for lobar vein pressures. In those days, one simply went to Glens Fall, New York, and showed U.S. Catheter and Instrument Company what was needed for research, and they developed the catheter. Marketability or patent rights were not issues. The company directed me to an unusual balloon designer in New Jersey, just outside New York City. He devised the balloon and showed me how to attach it and a length of PE–50 tubing to the catheter with thread and a quick-drying glue.

After introducing this catheter with the attached balloon and side PE–50 catheter into the dog's left external jugular vein, one could guide it, under fluoroscopy, through the tricuspid and pulmonary valves by altering the distal catheter curve, simply changing the tension of the PE-50 on the distal curve. The left lobar artery was entered with the standard 0.035-inch guide wire. The left lobar vein was easily entered transseptally with a Ross needle and sheath from the right external jugular vein via the left atrium. The Cope adaptor permitted concurrent measurement of pressure in a large and small pulmonary vein in left lower lobe. The surgeons had now abandoned isolated coronary perfusion in favor of hypothermia for bypass surgery. Those pumps served well (and still do) for pumping femoral arterial blood through the catheter to the left lower lobe. The lobar artery was hemodynamically isolated from the pulmonary artery by balloon distension. The transseptal technique was developed with much trial and error. In man, the transseptal catheterization is done from the right femoral vein, but in the lower animals, the plane of the atrial septum is such that one must approach it from the external jugular vein. Fortunately, in these animals the external jugulars are very large and accommodate these catheters easily. Moreover, for those trained in cardiac catheterization before the percutaneous transvenous technique appeared, catherterizing the pulmonary artery from the superior cava was easier than from the inferior cava. Positive pressure ventilation during catheter insertion prevented air embolus.

The catheters and needles were improved and miniaturized for smaller animals as time went on. The cat is the sturdiest animal, remaining hemodynamically stable for 6–8 hours of experimentation. The dog is not as stable for long periods, often has heart worms (with or without a negative microfilaria blood test), is expensive, and requires large catheters. The sheep is too large, and its atrial septum is often very difficult to find fluoroscopically. The rabbit is a flower than wilts easily. It readily develops shock with pulmonary hypertension, both of which we found to be easily corrected with cyclooxygenase blockers. Its septum is soft and often tricky to puncture. We have used pigs and occasionally monkeys with some success.

The organizers of the Eighth National Symposium on the Pulmonary Circulation had invited a number of prominent investigators of this vascular bed to the Philadelphia meeting. Bill Rashkind had been interested in congenital anomalies of pulmonary veins, and he somehow asked me to show my data at the meeting. The concept of active changes in pulmonary venous tone was not readily accepted in those early days. Aviado's group and Milnors' group had data in open chest isolated perfused lungs, and now I had data in intact dogs with constant lobar flow. That afternoon session had three speakers. The first speaker, an internationally known authority, spoke about the physiology of the pulmonary circulation. I was chagrined to see his first slide, a comparison of the histology of a pulmonary artery and a pulmonary vein. He stressed the musculature of the pulmonary artery and by comparison the sparse musculature of a pulmonary vein. He also ex-

pressed wonder at "what Al Hyman was going to talk about for forty-five minutes." Bloodied but unbowed, I expressed the angst of a relative novice in this subject but proceeded to present 45 minutes of data. A lively exchange followed (the first of many over the years), which was finally interrupted by introduction of the third speaker, Domingo Aviado. He was to speak on the pharmacology of the pulmonary system but spoke to the vascoactivity of pulmonary veins, measurements he had made in his laboratory. Domingo was obviously in pain, hobbling about the podium because the colchicine hadn't relieved his acute gout. His comments directed toward the first speaker were more trenchant, indicating pedagogically to the lead speaker that "he hadn't done his homework."

Among the speakers the next day was Gil Blount from Denver, who spoke presciently on an interesting topic, "High Altitude Effects on the Pulmonary Circulation in Cattle and Man." Bob Grover and Jack Reeves worked in his cardiac catheterization laboratory, and their later contributions to our understanding of pulmonary hypertension are well known. Gil was superb and showed us how things are done in Denver. In the freezing Philadelphia night, Gil came to Bookbinders with us wearing a light jacket, no vest, sweater, or top coat! Others in the group, Jesse Edwards, Art Sahshara, Ray Truex, Al Fishman, and Van Mierop, were more conventionally attired.

Having finally experienced relief the next day, Domingo was more placid and spent the afternoon with me in his laboratory. Soon after that session, he moved on to do toxicology for the army, a loss to the pulmonary circulation group. We waited many years until Chris Dawson, John Linehan, and their group in Milwaukee developed a better technique to assess pulmonary venous reactivity and in large measure showed more clearly what we were trying to demonstrate. Only recently Chris was kind enough to have me to his laboratory. Their work is unique.

It seemed clear that a more detailed study of the pharmacology of the pulmonary vessels was a fruitful area of study. First the endogenous peptides. Bradykinin actually constricted the dog's pulmonary veins at resting tone, a finding recently reported at the New York Academy of Science by Paul Guth. I was able to find him and discuss the data when I learned he was a professor of pharmacology at Tulane. I began working more closely with the basic science groups, especially pharmacology. The pharmacology of pulmonary vessels was apparently not a topical research area. Although the grant renewal was funded, one of the pink sheets contained the query, "How many ways does this fellow intend to make the lung cry ouch!" A cartoon framed in my lab shows a lung with a megaphone and the inscription "ouch." Many years later, a prominent pulmonary vascular investigator visited my laboratory, saw the cartoon, and laughed. "You know, years ago, I put that same remark on someone's NIH grant critique," but he couldn't recall who the applicant was. Well enough. He didn't believe in pulmonary veins either.

The Schuller Memorial Lecture is sponsored annually by the pharmacology department at Tulane. Sol Langer from Paris delivered a remarkable lecture dealing with subtypes of adrenoceptors and their pre- and postjunctional activities in the systemic vascular bed. But the pulmonary vascular bed functions at a lower level of tone, and virtually none of this data is available in the pulmonary bed. Following his lead, we looked at the neural control of the pulmonary bed as a short-term project. We found that the problem was more complex in the lung vessels because of altered response at various levels of tone. At low tone, stellate stimulation induces pulmonary vasoconstriction, but when tone is increased, stimulation produces a transient alpha-1–induced vasoconstrictor response followed by a longer vasodilator response, induced by beta-2 adrenoceptor stimulation. We also found the beta-2 adrenoceptor activity was enhanced at elevated tone. Moreover, agents such as epinephrine and phenylephrine, which have both alpha and beta adrenoceptor activity, reverse from vasoconstrictors to vasodilators as tone is increased. Several years later, I was giving a seminar on this topic at Sol Langer's laboratory in Paris. I pointed out that the pulmonary bed was unusual, because in that bed, phenylephrine, which is the paradigm of alpha-1 adrenoceptor agonists, has clear beta-2 activity in the lung vessels. Both Sol and Icilio Cavero beamed as they pointed out that they had published similar data using right atrial muscle preparation several years before.

Our studies of hypoxia in the dog revealed only a modest vasoconstrictor response, quite similar to that reported earlier by Al Fishman's group. The sheep gave a somewhat more vigorous response, and we studied hypoxia in this species. Bob Grover and Jack Reeves had reported a far more vigorous response in their dogs. We thought it might have been related to acclimatization to high altitude and exchanged a group of dogs via air freight to and from Denver. Sure enough, the first two of his dogs were vigorous responders in my laboratory, and the first of mine gave the weakest response they had ever encountered. The next was more responsive, and Bob asked me to check where the vendor got the dog. Probably a high-altitude area. "No, the only place flatter than New Orleans is Mobile." That theory faded. We are still not sure of the reason, but the difference was real.

In clinical cardiology, Tulane was handicapped in those days. We used the huge and academically rewarding Charity Hospital, but there was no private Tulane

Medical Center, which only came later. More and more patients were being referred directly to Oscar Creech and placed in two large private hospitals. These hospitals now had catheterization laboratories, and Oscar asked me to study and follow them outside the Tulane-Charity system. Only those referred patients with more complex problems were admitted by special arrangement to Charity for diagnosis and treatment. As the university medical and surgical groups became more and more disunited, the inevitable happened. A departmental reorganization resulted in my faculty appointment being placed entirely in the surgery department, with the catheterization laboratory. My Icarian wings had now completely melted, and I was now at sea, treading research alone. Friends, advisors, and coworkers came from time to time, but, alas, the last icon had departed, and my approach to the pulmonary circulation became a complete immersion in my own research laboratory, with my own model.

I miniaturized the apparatus to study the cat, an animal almost free of heart worms (a nemesis in New Orleans). To do so, we lost the small pulmonary vein measurements because the lung is too small. We gained in sturdiness, reproducibility of responses, and ease of catheterization. My coworkers and I have devised experiments to study pulmonary vascular regulation by the sympathetic and parasympathetic nervous system, by the prostaglandins, by acid-base alterations, by hypoxic sensors in the arteries upstream to gas-exchange vessels, and by adrenergic and purinergic receptors. Most recently, a unique opportunity was presented to look at central regulation of the pulmonary bed. About twenty years earlier, Donald Richardson, a young academic neurosurgeon, had been studying pain and temperature fibers in cats in his laboratory next door to me. He grew in stature and eventually assumed the chair in neurosurgery. He was now implanting electrodes in man to stimulate opoid receptors to relieve chronic intractable pain. In the faculty parking garage we exchanged pleasantries, and he suddenly asked me how to treat ventricular tachycardia. He had inserted this electrode and stimulated; in lieu of producing relief of pain, the response was hypertension and ventricular tachycardia. "Don, there are 15 people in the cardiology department who can help you treat tachycardia as well as I, but where did you put that electrode?" He showed me in his cat model, in the supraoptical diagonal band of Broca. I spent the summer months that year relearning the neuroanatomy I'd forgotten since 1942. Function had been added to the bland memorization of sites and tracts. We combined techniques in my laboratory, using stereotactic electrode insertion and cardiac fluoroscopy for pulmonary catheter insertion. Alas, the stimulation induced the systemic effects he had already shown but no pulmonary responses.

For many years, I had been concerned with the effects of pulmonary vascular tone on responses. I had devised a technique infusing a thromboxane $A_2$ simulator U46619 which raised lobar pressure from 12 to 35 mmHg at constant flow with a stable baseline. We repeated the stimulation, and now we saw a vigorous biphasic response, a vasoconstrictor that commenced with 5–10 s of stimulation followed shortly by a vasodilator response that persisted 3–4 min. We were excited. Aubrey Taylor in Mobile suggested that the vasodilator response should be looked at more thoroughly. How did we know it wasn't mediated by a circulating vasodilator rather than directly by a neurogenic mechanism? Well, we didn't, but the introduction of a 4-min trap in the femoral artery–lobar artery pump clearly identified two separate vasodilator responses, one before the perfused blood from the femoral artery reached the lung, and one 4 minutes later, when that blood arrived. Although the earlier constrictor and dilator responses were not affected by standard blocking agents, the late dilator response was clearly blocked by ICI 118551, a specific beta-2 adrenoceptor blocker, and by propranolol. Moreover, the serum epinephrine levels rose 5- to 10-fold with the stimulus. Our earlier work had demonstrated the tone dependency of responses to some phenylethylamines. At low resting tone, epinephrine is a vasoconstrictor, but a very active dilator with even small increases in pulmonary vascular tone. Jack Reeves was one of the referees selected by the journal editor. He wrote that he checked it out with the Colorado neurology department, and we were quite on target—he even signed his name to the reviewer's comments.

The effects of tone on the pulmonary vascular responses have continued to fascinate and perplex us. At low resting tone, epinephrine, acetylcholine, serotonin, phenylephrine, adenosine, ADP, ATP, and bradykinin, to name a few, are vasoconstrictors, but at high tone, induced by U46619, hypoxia or selected vasoconstrictors, these agents become vasodilators. On the other hand, alpha-2 adrenoceptor agonists are greatly potentiated at high tone but prostaglandin F2 alpha, Bay K 8644, and angiotensin II are not potentiated as vasoconstrictors at high tone. This remains one of our areas of intense study. In the past three and a half years, since being joined by my young colleague, Howard Lippton, a pulmonologist, we have returned to looking at vasoactive peptides and their tone responses. Indeed, endothelins are also vasodilators at high tone!

Presently, I remain pleasantly at sea, paddling around in the pulmonary circulation. I still do my own experiments at the bench, an old curmudgeon myself now, but steadfastly refuse to be anyone's icon, false or true. Moreover, I maintain an active interest in clinical cardiology, doing consultations and invasive procedures in the cardiac catheterization laboratory in the early morning hours, before going to my research laboratory.

## References

1. Hyman, A., R. B. Failey, and R. Ashman. Can the longitudinal anatomical axis of the ventricles be estimated from the electrocardiogram? *Am. Heart J.* 36:906–910, 1948.

# 13

# The Pulmonary Artery Seen as a Convergent Tree

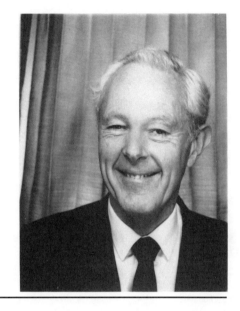

**Keith Horsfield, M.D.**

*Halton, Lancaster, United Kingdom*

Research is about answering questions, questions about problems that intrigue you and challenge you, questions that must be capable of being answered. It is therefore all about asking the right questions.

My first research was stimulated by working in a hospital in an industrial town in northern England, where the effects of atmospheric pollution and cigarette smoking combined resulted in large numbers of patients with respiratory failure. I did not at that time know the right questions, but I was helped by Jack Howell, who suggested that I study alveolar $CO_2$ by the rebreathing method. Although there was nothing in it for him, he gave me his time, instruction, and advice freely and started me off on a long and exciting road.

## Birmingham

Later, while I was still not sure what I wanted to do, I applied for a job in Birmingham with professor Melville Arnott. I am sure that my brief experience with research into respiratory physiology helped me get that post. The move was entirely unplanned and serendipitous and landed me in a very active department that included Peter Harris. John Butler had recently left, and Donald Heath was in the nearby Department of Pathology. Though a little overawed, I was thrilled at being in such an atmosphere, with constant discussions of ideas, physiological problems, and research techniques. It was a whole new wonderful experience for me. I was given a project—studying the circulatory

From: Wagner WW, Jr, Weir EK (eds): *The Pulmonary Circulation and Gas Exchange.* ©1994, Futura Publishing Co Inc, Armonk, NY.

dynamics in chronic bronchitis. Although I didn't particularly enjoy doing cardiac catheterisations, this was an excellent opportunity to learn about the techniques of gas collection and analysis and the measurement of intravascular pressure and cardiac output. Subsequently I was taught how to do the routine pulmonary function tests for the clinical service and ran this operation for two or three years. In addition I helped run a clinical service and teach medical students.

The point of doing routine clinical and research work is that you gradually learn what the problems really are, and from this base you start to ask the right questions. For clinical research I believe that a basis in routine work is most important in stimulating appropriate questions and in helping place the problems in context.

A little while after I had started in Birmingham someone whom I had not met before turned up at coffee time one morning. He was Gordon Cumming, and he had just returned from working for two years in New York with Gomez. He was talking excitedly about a concept of centrilobular emphysema being a dilatation on the respiratory bronchioles, a critical position for interfering with the movement of gas in and out of the alveoli. He wanted to demonstrate the anatomy of this lesion so that he could study its possible effects but did not know how to do it. I was captivated by his stimulating ideas and intellectual approach and suggested that he make a cast of the airways in emphysema. He replied, "Why don't *you* do it?" And so I did. The direction of my future research was sealed at that instant by his best possible of replies.

We made polyester resin casts of the airways in various types of emphysema[11] partly answering the question as to the geometry of the lesions but posing many more questions as to their pathogenesis and physiological effects. It soon became clear that we had no hope of understanding the processes by which gas molecules reach the alveoli in the pathological lung

until we understand them in the normal. We decided to switch to studying the normal airways, and I was fortunate to obtain the lungs of a 25-year-old man who had died from nonrespiratory causes. Partly by good fortune and partly by following Tompsett's[26] advice carefully, we produced a near-perfect cast first time.

Gordon's continuing advice, discussion, criticism, and refusal to accept the received wisdom as necessarily true saw me through this exciting time and enabled me to develop my own ideas. He was a great facilitator, letting you get on with your own ideas if you had them and stimulating you to think up new ones if you had run out. He always preferred to think about a problem afresh and advised those working with him to read the literature *after* doing the experiment so as not to be biased by what had been done before.

About this time Gordon bought a copy of a marvelous book, one that was to have a profound effect on my approach to analysing the airway and vascular trees in the lung. The book was *Morphometry of the Human Lung*, by Ewald Weibel.[29] The demonstration (to me, discovery) that anatomy could be analysed and represented in mathematical terms, by concise formulae and equations, was exciting indeed. I almost devoured the book in my excitement. Like all good intellectual stimuli, it posed exciting questions. What did these mathematical relations mean? How did they come to be there? What other equations were hidden in these structures? I stared at my cast for a long time. There did not seem to be any point in repeating Weibel's work. Surely these findings must be related to function? While looking at the cast I realised that the size of an airway related in some way to the flow of air it carried.

## Generations and Divisions Up

But Weibel's method of counting generations downward classed together branches of widely differing diameter and did not seem to relate well to probable function. I hit on the idea of counting upwards instead of downwards, and devised a new (to anatomy) method of classifying the branches (Fig. 1a). Counting starts at the most peripheral branches, which are numbered order 1, and two of these meet to form an order 2 branch. (Originally orders were termed "divisions up"). Two order 2 branches form an order 3 branch, and so on up the tree. When branches of differing orders meet, the order number continues from the higher of the two meeting branches.[8] Thus the longest pathway contains a branch of every order, while the shorter pathways miss some orders.

With great excitement I did a preliminary study of one bronchopulmonary segment, laboriously recording all my data on punch cards. Finally the cards were sorted, the numbers added together, and the plots made. Mean diameter, mean length, and number of branches were all more or less linear on a logarithmic scale against order. This was a new discovery, one that later would prove to be applicable to many different structures.

I continued the work of measuring and counting the airways down to 0.7 mm diameter in all the bronchopulmonary segments and a large sample of peripheral airways from 0.7 mm diameter down to the most distal respiratory bronchioles. This took me 14 months, including many evenings and weekends. It was a labour of love, the prime motivation being that it was to form the basis of my thesis for the M.D. degree (in England this is awarded for research). Without that personal motivation I doubt whether I would have completed the task. The results confirmed the preliminary study, although the plots of log dimension against order were not perfectly linear (Fig. 2). The data could be divided into three zones, within each of which the plots were much more linear.

By counting all of the third generation respiratory bronchioles (RB3) in each sample distal to 0.7 mm diameter branches, an average number of RB3 subtended by branches of 0.4, 0.5, 0.6, and 0.7 mm in diameter was calculated. Having attributed these numbers to each terminal branch on the cast according to size, we could then add the numbers of RB3 all the way up the tree to the trachea. Finally the mean number of RB3 supplied by branches in each order was calculated. This is plotted on a logarithmic scale against order in Figure 3

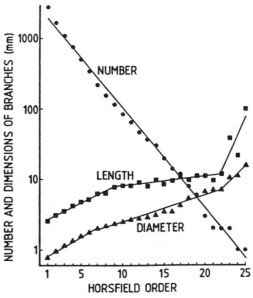

**Figure 2.** Horsfield ordered data for a cast of the human bronchial tree, pruned at 0.7 mm diameter.[8] Mean diameter (mm), mean length (mm), and number of branches in each order are shown on a logarithmic scale.

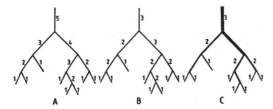

**Figure 1.** Two methods of ordering a dichotomously branching tree: (a) Horsfield's method, (b) Strahler's method, stage 1, and (c) Strahler's method, stage 2.

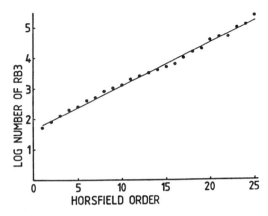

**Figure 3.** Logarithm mean number of third generation (distal) respiratory bronchioles supplied by branches of each order in the same tree as in Figure 2.

and shows a linear relation. Thus the mean number of RB3 increases in constant proportion in successive orders up the tree. If the number of RB3 can be taken as an indication of the quantity of air flowing through a branch, then order is closely related to function.[8,9]

### Pulmonary Artery Cast

Following the success of the bronchial tree analysis, we decided to try to do the same for the pulmonary arterial tree. An Indian research fellow, Siam Singhal, who also wished to work for an M.D. thesis, agreed to try to tackle the job. He was able to produce an arterial cast from a pair of normal human lungs, and this was pruned at 0.8 mm diameter branches, samples of smaller branches down to 0.1 mm diameter being saved for measurement. These samples were photographed, and the measurements were made from the plates by another research fellow, Robert Henderson, from Canada.[25]

These methods were similar to those used for the airways cast, but this turned out to present serious unforeseen difficulties, throwing doubt on the use of orders in the pulmonary arterial tree. There were two main problems. First, a significant number of arteries branch into three or four daughter branches, and, second, many tiny daughter branches are given off that do not appear to affect the direction or magnitude of the parent branch. If a new order were attributed at each such minor branchings, there would be hundreds of orders in the arterial tree. With some misgivings, I agreed to an arbitrary rule, to ignore branching points where a daughter of less than 0.8 mm diameter was formed. This resulted in loss of information and probably invalidated the ordering.

### Denver

At about this stage in the project I left to work in Denver for a year with Professor Giles Filley. Also there were Robert Grover and Wiltz Wagner. Giles gave me a desk to sit at in a room with two American students who were doing research jobs during the summer vacation before going on to study medicine. He provided any facilities I needed but otherwise left me to get on with it. His wisdom and kindness were of great help to me, and my first son was later named for him as a tribute. (We did also like the name!) It was Giles Filley who suggested that "divisions up" should be known as "Horsfield orders." When our paper was submitted for publication I received some stern criticism from referees for suggesting my own name for this method of ordering. But several other methods of ordering existed, and the eponymous terminology is the simplest way of distinguishing between them.[12]

I was keen to further the analysis of the airway data that I had brought with me and was able to do this with time to think, free from clinical and teaching interruptions. This was a valuable opportunity that all clinical research workers should try to come by at some stage in their careers.

One of the students with whom I shared the room was Dan Olson, a graduate student in fluid mechanics engineering and a great enthusiast. We had many discussions relating to British and American society, and Dan subsequently came over to England to do his Ph.D. at Imperial College in London. With him began my education in hydraulics. I was also to reciprocate with medical and physiological knowledge. I believe it to be of the utmost importance that engineers and physicists starting work in physiological research are carefully monitored and tutored to make sure that their work relates to real physiology and not just to a convenient computer model.

In Denver I worked on the problem of how to represent asymmetry in a dichotomously branching tree. The solution, as is so often the case, was simple. After all the branches of a tree have been attributed an order number, the asymmetry at each bifurcation can be quantitatively stated as the difference in order (delta) between the two daughter branches.[12] Where the two orders are the same (delta = 0) the branching is symmetrical with respect to orders (Fig. 4). It is then possible to make a histogram of the distribution of delta for parent branches of each order in the bronchial tree and to find a representative value, which turns out to be 3. A complete model tree (apart from the terminations) can be made using this one value, which gives an average degree of asymmetry, but better models using this principle have different values of delta at different levels in the tree. Various workers have used this method to form asymmetrical bronchial tree models,[3,4,12,22,24,28,36] which have the advantage of being easy to use for calculations because the connectivity is defined.

Much more recently I realised that a tree with a constant value of delta is a fractal, each more peripheral part of the tree being a miniature of the more central branches. Thus the airways do have features suggestive of fractals and can be represented mathematically in this form.[7,31]

While I was working in Denver, unbeknown to me an American geographer from Harvard (later Buffalo) had come across our work with the help of Ewald Weibel and arranged a visit to England with Gordon Cumming. A tall, friendly, garrulous, hard-working, enthusiastic man, Mike Woldenberg had been studying the drainage patterns of rivers and had noted the similarities with lung airway and vascular patterns. He suggested using the Strahler method of ordering for pulmonary structures, a method well known in the world of geomorphology (Fig. 1). In this method too the order numbering starts peripherally and carries on up the tree, but order number increases only when two like-numbered branches meet. If two branches of differing order meet, then the next branch up takes the same order as the higher ordered of the two meeting branches (stage 1, Fig. 1b). When all the branches have been thus ordered, contiguous branches of the same order are considered to constitute just one branch (stage 2, Fig. 1c). Thus a branch of a given order may consist of one or of several segments. There are some well marked and important differences between trees ordered by the two methods. A Strahler ordered tree has fewer orders and fewer branches than the same tree when Horsfield ordered, the only exception being a tree with perfectly symmetrical branching (i.e., when delta = 0 throughout) when both methods give the same result.

The great advantage of Strahler's

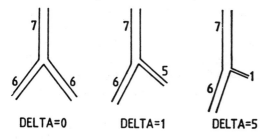

**Figure 4.** Expression of asymmetrical branching by use of orders. Delta is the difference in order between the two daughter branches at a bifurcation.

method is that the minor branches of the pulmonary vessels, just like the minor streams that join rivers, do not affect the order number of their parent branch. Thus, at a stroke, the main worry that I had had about ordering our pulmonary artery data was removed—in my absence and without my knowledge! Mike and another fellow at Birmingham, Keith Harding, re-labeled and reanalysed all the data in terms of Strahler orders. The results were plotted using a logarithmic scale for mean diameter, mean length, and number of branches in each order against order number (Figs. 5 and 6).

Because the plots for diameter and length are much more linear with Strahler orders than with Horsfield orders, a slope to the line can be more confidently attributed. These slopes, expressed as positive numbers, are known as the diameter ratio, the length ratio, and the branching ratio, respectively, for the diameter, length, and number plots. These ratios are the factors

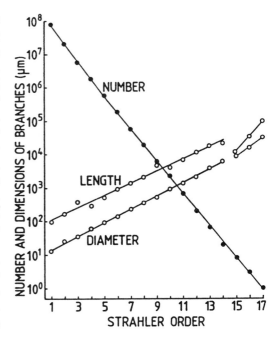

**Figure 6.** Strahler ordered data for a cast of the human pulmonary arterial tree.[6,25] Mean diameter (μm), mean length (μm), and number of branches in each order are shown on a logarithmic scale.

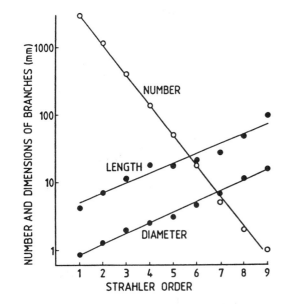

**Figure 5.** Strahler ordered data for the same tree as in Figure 2, represented in the same way. Note that there are fewer orders and fewer branches than when the tree is Horsfield ordered, and the data plots are more linear (cf. Fig. 2.)

by which mean diameter, mean length, and number of branches increase in successive orders in the tree.[10]

Strahler ordered trees of many kinds, such as rivers, glaciers, bile ducts, arteries, veins, Purkinje cells, and botanical trees[1,32] show similar features when plotted in this way. Because of this, Strahler orders have been used to compare trees between species[15,16] and within species[10] and to study growth.[5,14] However, much information is lost in the simplification involved in Strahler ordering, especially the connectivity, that is, the way in which the various branches join together. Because of this, Strahler ordered trees are not good for making physiological calculations.

This is an appropriate point to consider where generations, as used by Ewald Weibel, fit into this scheme. The counting of generations starts at the main stem, trachea, or pulmonary artery and continues outward. The generation number is thus a statement of the position of a branch within the tree with respect to the stem. Applied to pathways, it is a measure of their lengths, and a plot of the distribution of generations to terminal branches is an expression of the asymmetry of the system. This approach looks at the tree as a divergent system and is particularly helpful in describing its structure.[30] In contrast, the methods of ordering look at trees as convergent structures, most obviously thought of in these terms are rivers and venous trees in which flow is toward the main stem. The order number is not a statement of position in the tree, for branches of a given order can be found at various distances from the stem. The number is, however, much more closely related to function, as branches of a given order supply similar subtrees and have smaller ranges of diameters than do branches within a generation. Thus the two methods are simply looking at different aspects of the same thing and are not in conflict with each other.

## Return to Birmingham

By the time I had returned to Birmingham from Denver, Mike Woldenberg had left, and I had to await his next visit before meeting him. He returned most years after that, sometimes twice a year, during the university vacations to work with us on the properties of branching trees and the flow fluid in them. I am not aware of any other instance of a geographer and a physician cooperating on basic research in the lung. Our association has lasted 21 years, has been full of interest, and has resulted in a number of published papers.[17–20,33,34,35] However, a proportion of my published work has been based on, or has incorporated, ideas originating from Mike without his name being included among the authors. This has been an unintentional injustice, and I would like to take this opportunity to acknowledge his great contribution to my research efforts and to state that it would have been proper for his name to have appeared on several papers I wrote without him.

This brings to mind a point on authorship of papers. I have never found it disadvantageous to include someone's name on a paper when that person has made any contribution toward it. Several times I have asked someone to be a coauthor who has declined; this is fine and no one is offended. But if you leave off the name of someone when that person thinks that they should be included, then unnecessary resentment and bitterness may ensue.

## The Midhurst Medical Research Institute

A little while after my return from the United States we heard that an anonymous donor had given the sum of 5 million pounds to set up a new research institute at the King Edward VII Hospital at Midhurst in Sussex. Subsequently, Gordon Cumming was appointed medical director, and he asked my to be deputy medical director. Many members of the medical establishment were strongly opposed to siting a major institute outside of London in the beautiful countryside of Sussex. But the donor insisted that his institute should go there or nowhere. At the time he was a patient of the hospital, and I believe he hoped that putting a research institute there would improve the hospital's standing and help put it in the front line of British hospitals. We had the wonderful experience of helping design, seeing built, and equipping the Midhurst Medical Research Institute to our own specifications. Her Majesty the Queen officially opened the building on November 2, 1973.

However, there were many difficulties. One was trying to meld the staff member of the hospital, who had no experience of the academic world and were therefore highly suspicious of it, with the academic staff of the institute. In my view, this was never achieved. Another problem was the geography. King Edward VII Hospital had been founded as a tuberculosis sanatorium, a function it performed with worldwide distinction. But it was isolated, well away from all teaching hospitals, and difficult for patients to get to. The donor died, and the chairman of the Board of Governors negotiated our takeover by the Cardiothoracic Institute in London. Three years later the Midhurst Medical Research Institute closed, 14 years after it had opened, and our foundation passed to the Cardiothoracic Institute, now the National Heart and Lung Institute. In retrospect, I believe we were doomed from the start. The donor had, with the very best of motives, ignored the advice of the medical profession regarding the siting of the institute. Once he had died, only those who worked there thought that it should continue at Midhurst. Gordon Cumming, who had wanted to leave a viable institute behind when he retired, had to witness its closing as he left. It was an unhappy end to his career and to what had been a promising new project.

At Midhurst we produced a steady flow of papers, predominantly in the cardiac and respiratory fields. Only a few of them were clinically oriented. I finished the work I started in Birmingham of measuring branches of the pulmonary artery from 100 μm down to 13 μm diameter, thereby completing a sample of Strahler ordered data for the full range of diameters. From these data a complete Strahler ordered model of the pulmonary arterial tree was developed, shown in Figure 6.[6]

I was lucky in that I had made an almost complete cast of the tree, using the "anatomical resin" described by Tompsett.[26] Following a political disruption of our oil supplies (oil being used in the manufacture of polyester resins), the manufacturers ceased making this resin. No other has proved to be as satisfactory for making anatomical casts, and I am certain that I would not have had as good a cast to study had I not made it when I did.

## Venous Cast

At a later date it was decided to make a study of the human pulmonary venous tree. This turned out to be a much more complicated business. For the cast to remain in one piece, it must include the left atrium, which can be cannulated via the left ventricle. Our anatomical resin had run out, and the substitute was decidedly inferior. The quality of the venous casts in no way approached that of our arterial cast but was just sufficient to make measurements down to 0.2 mm diameter. From these data we constructed a dimensional model of the venous tree, shown in Figure 7.[13]

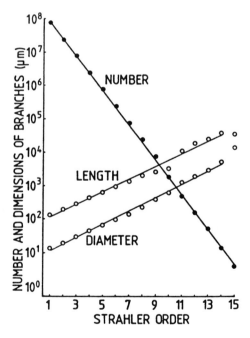

**Figure 7.** Strahler ordered data for a cast of the human pulmonary venous tree,[13] represented in the same way as in Figure 6. Note that there are two fewer orders than in the arterial tree, as four pulmonary veins join the left atrium, which thus represents two orders. From branches of 0.2 mm downward, the points were obtained by both extrapolation and interpolation.

## Murray and Optimization

It was Mike Woldenberg who introduced me to the work of Murray, published in 1926.[23] Murray had looked at optimization of arterial diameters to minimize power (work per unit time) using the following approach. To minimize the resistance to flow, the arterial diameters should be maximized. But to minimize the metabolic work of maintaining the tissues of the arterial wall and the blood within them, the diameters should be also be minimized. To minimize total power output, the diameter should have some optimal value, probably related to the flow it has to carry, as vessels carrying larger flows are likely to have greater diameters. Murray showed that in an ideal situation, where perfect laminar flow occurs and Poisseuille's equation holds, flow is proportional to diameter cubed when the total power output is minimum. This idea was taken further by Uylings,[27] who showed that if turbulent flow were fully developed, for power to be minimum, flow would have to be proportional to diameter to the power of 2.3. The exponent, that is, the value 3.0 in the first case and 2.3 in the second, we called z.

What value of z is found in the arterial trees in the body? Mayrovitz and Roy[21] measured flow and diameter in directly observed peripheral systemic arteries and found that z = 3.01, a remarkable confirmation of the efficient "design" of the arteries predicted 57 years earlier. Mike and I decided that it would be fascinating to find the value of z in the pulmonary arterial tree. We could not have flow measurements in individual arteries, but, fortunately, if the diameters of the three vessels meeting at a bifurcation are known, than z can be calculated for that junction.[19] We measured the diameters at 1,937 bifurcations on the two casts we had previously used for arterial studies and found that z = 2.3 ± 0.1.[19] The immediate implication seemed to be that pulmonary arterial diameters are optimized for fully developed turbulent flow. But further study of the subject denied this. Although the main pulmonary artery has a Reynolds number (which gives information as to the type of flow) of over 2,000, this rapidly diminishes in the smaller vessels, and turbulent flow, even in the main arterial trunk is unlikely.[2]

This value of z, which we had found in a previous smaller study,[34] is intriguing and tells us that the pulmonary arterial tree is optimized for other factors in addition to straightforward minimum power. If the diameters of the higher ordered branches are increased, the calculated value of z falls. Larger diameters in the higher orders could be advantageous in reducing acceleration of the blood during systole, reducing turbulent flow, and giving a reservoir function to the vessels. The latter allows much of the blood expelled from the right ventricle during systole to be accommodated in the larger elastic vessels and to be expelled gradually during the remainder of the cardiac cycle, maintaining a fairly steady flow. These functions are not required in the small systemic arteries in which z was found to be close to 3.0.

Using the same data, we plotted the summed cross sectional area of the two daughter branches at each bifurcation against the cross sectional area of the parent branch on logarithmic scales (Fig. 8). The linear relation, parallel to and slightly above the line of identity, indicates that the cross sectional area of the arterial tree increases by an average value of 1.0879 at each bifurcation and that this value is independent of the position of the bifurcation in the tree.[19]

How is the diameter of a branch adjusted to meet these requirements? First, a genetic factor must control diameters to be somewhere near the ideal. But just as muscle and bone can respond to applied stress by growth, so can the branches of the arterial tree adjust their diameters in re-

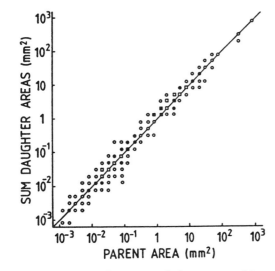

**Figure 8.** Data from 1937 bifurcations of human pulmonary arteries.[19] The summed cross sectional area of the two daughter branches is plotted against the cross sectional area of the parent branch (mm² on logarithmic scales). The line of best fit lies just above the line of identity, which cannot be separately shown. Data are grouped at log intervals of 0.2. ○, 1–10 data points; ●, 11–30 data points; □, 31–100 data points; ■, more than 100 data points.

sponse to pressure and flow within them. The mechanism by which this is achieved has not been worked out, but it may be in the following manner. It now seems that the vessel wall is sensitive to shear stress and can respond to it by producing chemical stimulators. Thus, if a vessel is too small for the flow it carries, flow velocity, and hence wall shear, is increased, causing the release of growth-stimulating factors. The growth of the vessel wall increases vessel diameter, which reaches the optimal value such that diameter is proportional to the 2.3 root of flow. If there were laminar flow with $z = 3$, shear stress would be equal throughout the tree.[21]

## Optimality and Branching Angles

Mike and I also looked at optimality in relation to angles of branching. Consider a triangle ABC (Fig. 9). If a branch originates at A and bifurcates at D so that the two daughter branches go to B and C respectively, then the minimum sum of length of the three branches occurs when the branching angle is 120° between each pair of branches. This is true whatever the shape of the triangle. In our analysis a "cost" is attributed to each branch, and this cost has to be minimized. In the above example the cost is the length of the line. More realistically, suppose the cost is volume that has to be minimized and that the branches each have different diameters. Then at the minimum the larger of the two daughter branches will deviate from the line of the parent with the smaller angle and from the smaller branch with the larger angle (Fig. 10). This pattern of branching is observed in the majority of bifurcations in the bronchial, venous, and arterial trees and confirms that optimization of angles of branching of some kind is operating.

Other cost principles have been studied, including surface area, drag, and power dissipation.[35] The latter two are not

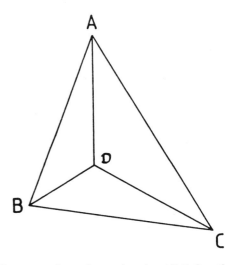

**Figure 9.** Location triangle ABC for three branches (roads, routes, etc.) arising from the points A, B, and C and meeting somewhere in the middle. The position of the meeting point can be optimized to minimize a cost function, such as line length or branch volume.

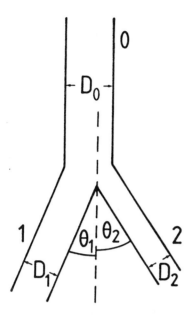

**Figure 10.** General form of a typical bifurcation. Parent branch O gives rise to the two daughter branches 1 and 2. $D_0 > D_1 > D_2$ and $\theta_2 > \theta_1$, where D = diameter and $\theta$ = branching angle.

ters and branching angles and their relation to flow may seem esoteric and theoretical. But they give great insight into the "design" of the airways and blood vessels and the relation between structure and function in these trees. They also provide a basis for future haemodynamic studies. The word "design" is in quotes. Given that the lung evolved, each evolutionary change in structure that gave a biological advantage to its owner was more likely to survive. Thus, over many years the lung became a more efficient organ for gas exchange. But this does not mean that the most efficient possible design has evolved, only that of those tried so far, the most efficient are probably those that have survived.

only a function of diameter but also of the value of z. Knowing the diameters of the three branches at a bifurcation from which z can be calculated, one can calculate an ideal branching angle for each cost function and compare it with that observed. These techniques were developed to provide a methodology for studying optimality in branching angles; they have not yet yielded any clear answers.

These studies of optimality of diame-

## Conclusion

A glance at a cast of the airways or blood vessels of the lung shows that these structures are well adapted for distributing and bringing together air and blood in the capillary network so that gas exchange may occur. The way in which these structures are adapted to their task has proved to be a fascination for me for nearly 30 years, and studying them has been a great pleasure. The people with whom I have worked have both allowed and helped me get on with the research that I wanted to do. In this I recognise that I have been extremely lucky, and to those who have facilitated my path I am most grateful.

## References

1. Barker, S. B., G. Cumming, and K. Horsfield. Quantitative morphometry of the branching structure of trees. *J. Theor. Biol.* 40: 33–43, 1973.
2. Caro, C. G., T. J. Pedley, R. C. Schroter, and W. A. Seed. *The Mechanics of the Circulation.* Oxford, UK: Oxford University, 1978, p. 504.
3. Dawson, S. V., and K. E. Finucane. A prediction of the distribution of oscillatory flow in human airways. *Bull. Physio-Pathol. Respir.* 8: 293–304, 1972.

4. Fredberg, J. J., and A. Hoenig. Mechanical response of the lungs at high frequencies. *J. Biomech. Eng.* 100: 57–66, 1978.
5. Horsfield, K. Postnatal growth of the dog's bronchial tree. *Respir. Physiol.* 29: 185–191, 1977.
6. Horsfield, K. Morphometry of the small pulmonary arteries in man. *Circ. Res.* 42: 593–597, 1978.
7. Horsfield, K. Diameters, generations, and orders of branches in the bronchial tree. *J. Appl. Physiol.* 68: 457–461, 1990.
8. Horsfield, K., and G. Cumming. Morphol-

ogy of the bronchial tree in man. *J. Appl. Physiol.* 24: 373–383, 1968.

9. Horsfield, K., and G. Cumming. Functional consequences of airway morphology. *J. Appl. Physiol.* 24: 384–390, 1968.

10. Horsfield, K., and G. Cumming. Morphology of the bronchial tree in the dog. *Respir. Physiol.* 26: 173–182, 1976.

11. Horsfield, K., G. Cumming, and P. Hicken. A morphologic study of airway disease using bronchial casts. *Am. Rev. Respir. Disease* 93: 900–906, 1966.

12. Horsfield, K., G. Dart, D. E. Olson, G. F. Filley, and G. Cumming. Models of the human bronchial tree. *J. Appl. Physiol.* 31: 207–217, 1971.

13. Horsfield, K., and W. I. Gordon. Morphometry of pulmonary veins in man. *Lung* 159: 211–218, 1981.

14. Horsfield, K., W. I. Gordon, W. Kemp, and S. Phillips. Growth of the bronchial tree in man. *Thorax* 42: 383–388, 1987.

15. Horsfield, K., and A. Thurlbeck. Volume of the conducting airways calculated from morphometric parameters. *Bull. Math. Biol.* 43: 101–109, 1981.

16. Horsfield, K., and A. Thurlbeck. Relation between diameter and flow in branches of the bronchial tree. *Bull. Math. Biol.* 43: 681–691, 1981.

17. Horsfield, K., and M. J. Woldenberg. Branching ratio and growth of tree-like structures. *Respir. Physiol.* 63: 97–107, 1986.

18. Horsfield, K., and M. J. Woldenberg. Comparison of vertex analysis and branching ratio in the study of trees. *Respir. Physiol.* 65: 245–256, 1986.

19. Horsfield, K., and M. J. Woldenberg. Diameters and cross-sectional areas in the human pulmonary arterial tree. *Anat. Rec.* 223: 245–251, 1989.

20. Horsfield, K., M. J. Woldenberg, and C. L. Bowes. Sequential and synchronous growth models related to vertex analysis and branching ratios. *Bull. Math. Biol.* 49: 413–429, 1987.

21. Mayrovitz, H. N., and J. Roy. Microvascular blood flow: evidence indicating a cubic dependence on arteriolar diameter. *Am. J. Physiol.* 245 (*Heart Circ. Physiol.* 14): H1031–H1038.

22. Mon, E., and J. S. Ultman. Monte Carlo simulation of simultaneous gas flow and diffusion in an asymmetric distal pulmonary airway model. *Bull. Math. Biol.* 38: 161–192, 1976.

23. Murray, C. D. The physiological principle of minimum work. I. The vascular system and the cost of blood volume. *Proc. Nat. Acad. Sci. USA* 12: 207–214, 1926.

24. Sidell, R. S., and J. J. Fredberg. Noninvasive inference of airway network geometry from broadband lung reflection data. *J. Biomech. Eng.* 100: 131–138, 1978.

25. Singhal, S., R. Henderson, K. Horsfield, K. Harding, and G. Cumming. Morphometry of the human pulmonary arterial tree. *Circ. Res.* 33: 190–197, 1973.

26. Tompsett, D. H. *Anatomical Techniques.* London: Livingstone, 1956.

27. Uylings, H. B. M. Optimization of diameters and bifurcation angles in lung and vascular tree structures. *Bull. Math. Biol.* 39: 509–520, 1977.

28. Watson, J. W., and A. C. Jackson. $CO_2$ elimination as predicted by augmented dispersion and convection in an asymmetrical dog airway model. *Comput. Biomed. Res.* 18: 233–243, 1985.

29. Weibel, E. R. *Morphometry of the Human Lung.* Berlin: Springer, 1963.

30. Weibel, E. R. Design of airways and blood vessels considered as branching trees. In: *The Lung: Scientific Foundations,* edited by R. G. Crystal and J. B. West. New York: Raven, 1991, Vol. 1, p. 711–720.

31. West, B. J., V. Bhargava, and A. L. Goldberger. Beyond the principle of similitude: renormalization in the bronchial tree. *J. Appl. Physiol.* 60: 1089–1097, 1986.

32. Woldenberg, M. J. *Hierarchical Systems: Cities, Rivers, Alpine Glaciers, Bovine Livers, and Trees* (Dissertation). New York: Columbia University, 1968.

33. Woldenberg, M. J., G. Cumming, K. Harding, K. Horsfield, K. Prowse, and S. Singhal. *Law and Order in the Human Lung,* Off. Nav. Res. Rept. (AD.709602). NTIS, U.S. Department of Commerce, Springfield, VA 22151, 1970.

34. Woldenberg, M. J., and K. Horsfield. Finding the optimal lengths for three branches at a junction. *J. Theor. Biol.* 104: 301–318, 1983.

35. Woldenberg, M. J., and K. Horsfield. Relation of branching angles to optimally for four cost principles. *J. Theor. Biol.* 122: 187–204, 1986.

36. Yeats, D. B., and N. Aspin. A mathematical description of the airways of the human lung. *Respir. Physiol.* 32: 91–104, 1978.

# 14

# Pulmonary Vascular Disease in Sheffield, the Andes, Tibet, and Tanzania

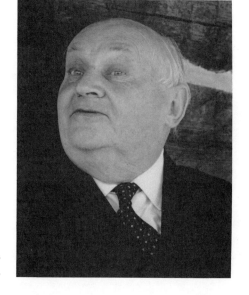

## Donald Heath, D.Sc., M.D., Ph.D.

*The George Holt Professor of Pathology, Royal Liverpool Hospital, Liverpool, England*

When I graduated from medical school in 1952, I determined to train as a cardiologist and was fortunate to obtain a junior clinical post at the Regional Cardiovascular Centre at Sheffield in the north of England, which was just being set up as part of the new British National Health Service. At the time I did not realize just how good that fortune was, for the first cardiologist to head the new unit was Dr. James W. Brown (Fig. 1). He was a physician from the fishing port of Grimsby who had a special interest in congenital heart disease in infants and children. In 1939 he had published a book, *Congenital Heart Disease,*[3] long before the widespread use of cardiac catheterization or angiocardi-

ography in cardiological investigation. In it he described the diagnosis of various forms of congenital cardiac anomaly by purely clinical means by fingers and stethoscope at the bedside.

### I Remember "J.W."

He brought to his appointment great clinical expertise and a clientele of young patients with every conceivable form of congenital cardiac anomaly who could now seek help from the rapidly developing cardiac surgery. He always regarded them as part of his family rather than as patients. At Christmas every child re-

From: Wagner WW, Jr, Weir EK (eds): *The Pulmonary Circulation and Gas Exchange.* ©1994, Futura Publishing Co Inc, Armonk, NY.

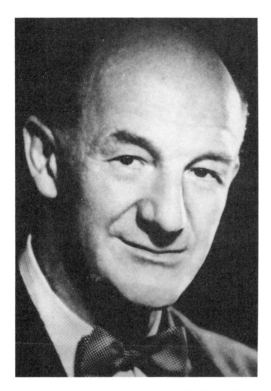

**Figure 1.** Dr. James Brown, cardiologist from Grimsby who published a book on the clinical diagnosis of congenital heart disease in 1939.

ceived a signed card from him and was invited to a party with games for which prizes were awarded. J.W. cheated outrageously during these exercises so that the most cyanotic and breathless little child in his arms was able to win. He arrived for his ward rounds in a Rolls in which he took an inordinate pride. A quarter of an hour before the anticipated arrival, little faces were pressed against the windows to get the first sight. Suddenly a cheer would go up: "It's Doctor Brown!" On his instruction no special preparations were made for his visits, and the beds were incredibly untidy and littered with toys. He would carry out his ward round on these complex cases holding the hands of two small patients who had gained the honour for that day. Commonly his clinical examination began by his drawing a rabbit on the arms of the patient, a symbol

to be treasured and remain unwashed. In this atmosphere the children cooperated fully in cardiac catheterization and angiocardiography, which were just being introduced. There were no tears or difficulties, and it was only in later years that I came to realize what a remarkable example of clinical medicine I had witnessed as a young man. J.W. was soon joined by Dr. William Whitaker from the National Heart Hospital in London, where Whitaker had been an assistant to Dr. Paul Wood, the renowned cardiologist. He brought with him the latest techniques available at that time for the investigation of cases of congenital heart disease and an enthusiasm for a full scientific study of the various anomalies. J. W. and Whitaker had a deep liking for one another and thus formed a formidable team to start off the unit.

The children occupied halves of two wards, the other sides being occupied by men who came to be known as "blue bloaters." In those days the steel industry and coal mines of Sheffield produced a large number of cyanosed and breathless patients with pulmonary emphysema. The physician caring for them was Professor (later Sir) Charles Stuart-Harris. Thus I found myself in a world of cyanotic and breathless patients with pulmonary hypertension but of very different types, either young children with congenital heart disease or middle-aged blue bloaters.

## Hypertensive Pulmonary Vascular Disease

It began to dawn on us that the pulmonary circulation, particularly a raised pressure within it, was playing an important role in determining the clinical picture and prognosis in these patients. It appeared that there was a hitherto unexplored pathology of the pulmonary vasculature to be investigated here. From the outset it seemed probable that there were two major forms of pulmonary vascular disease, one involving congenital cardiac shunts and the other sustained alveolar hypoxia. By 1956 Whitaker and I had come to the conclusion that the clinical picture in congenital heart disease is often dominated by symptoms and signs characteristic of pulmonary hypertension that often mask the underlying cardiac anomaly and are often associated with definitive pathological changes in the pulmonary vasculature.[21] We suggested that the term "hypertensive pulmonary vascular disease" be given to this condition in a paper we submitted to a British clinical journal. The paper was rejected on the grounds that the subject was of little medical interest or importance. When the paper was subsequently published by *Circulation,* we were gratified by receiving several hundreds of requests for reprints. After this, as the most junior member of the unit, I was charged with developing the study of the pathology of pulmonary hypertension. The only training I had received in histopathology was that of a medical student, so I applied for a temporary junior lectureship for one year in pathology at the University of Birmingham. This proved to be a one-way ticket, and I never found my way back to cardiology.

Soon after the commencement of my new post, two events took place that were to influence greatly my studies. I was awarded a Rockefeller Traveling Fellowship by the Medical Research Council in London to enable me to carry out research for one year at the Mayo Clinic in Rochester, Minnesota, under the supervision of Dr. Jesse Edwards, on the pulmonary vascular disease associated with congenital cardiac anomalies.[12,14,15] The other event was a chance remark made to me over tea one afternoon by a physician, Peter Harris, who had recently been appointed to the faculty at Birmingham. He suggested that we study the effects of alveolar hypoxia on the pulmonary circulation in subjects free of heart or lung disease.

This would necessitate our going to work on the top of high mountains. Without taking the suggestion seriously I told him that he should go ahead and arrange the funding so that we could be off. Some months later as my aircraft, boarded at Heathrow, was making its descent over the Andes to Lima at 2 a.m., I could not believe this Peruvian adventure was really happening to me. My involvement with the pathology of high altitude began chronologically after my stay at the Mayo Clinic, but I start my consideration of pulmonary vascular pathology with the hypoxic form of hypertensive pulmonary vascular disease found in native highlanders and in blue bloaters.

## Pulmonary Vascular Remodeling in Native Andean Highlanders and Blue Bloaters

It has been known for 40 years that the Quechua Indians of the Peruvian Andes (Fig. 2) have pulmonary arterial hypertension that is mild in adults[36] but more apparent in children.[38] From the beginning there was evidence that this elevation of pulmonary vascular resistance was associated with structural changes in the pulmonary arterial tree. Quantitative studies[2] showed that in Quechua Indians from the region of Cerro de Pasco (4,330 m), there was muscularization of a considerable number of the peripherally situated pulmonary arterioles without appreciable medial hypertrophy in the parent arteries. This was a notable contribution, for it showed that significant structural remodeling occurs in the terminal portion of the pulmonary arterial tree in the face of sustained hypobaric hypoxia in the alveolar spaces. However, this classic paper had an unfortunate title that implied that the remodeling was confined to arterial vessels and was found in all people native to high altitudes. We carried out two studies, a

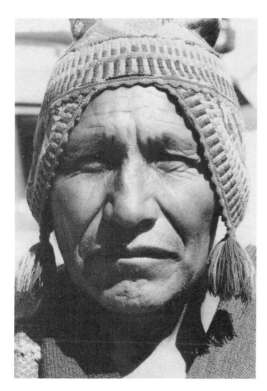

**Figure 2.** Quechua Indian from Cuzco (3,400 m) in the Peruvian Andes.

decade apart[19,25] of the pulmonary vascular remodeling that occurs in citizens of La Paz, Bolivia (3,800 m).

We found that the changes involved are far more complex than the simple peripheral muscularization of the pulmonary arterial tree envisaged by Arias-Stella and Saldaña.[2] It was easy to confirm that in the Aymara Indians hypobaric hypoxia brings about muscularization of the most peripheral portion of the pulmonary arterial tree so that muscularized pulmonary arterioles as small as 30 μm in diameter are commonplace.[19] There is extension of smooth muscle even into precapillary vessels, consequently even minute arteriolar vessels of a diameter comparable to that of macrophages have a distinct muscular coat. These very small muscular vessels appear to be brought about by a hyperplasia of vascular smooth muscle cells rather than by a constriction of parent arteries.

Hence they have a thick outer elastic lamina corresponding to the original single elastic fibril of the arteriole, a coat of circularly oriented smooth muscle, and a much thinner, newly formed elastic lamina.[25]

An additional striking feature of the pulmonary arteries and arterioles of the Aymara is the development of longitudinally oriented smooth muscle in the intima. At first these nodules are purely muscular, but later elastic fibrils develop between the individual muscle cells, and finally the nodules and layers become increasingly sclerotic, with the muscle cells widely separated by collagen. Classically, such intimal longitudinal muscle in states of chronic hypoxia is found in association with pulmonary emphysema and has been ascribed to longitudinal stretch around abnormal air spaces such as the distended respiratory bronchioles, which occur in centrilobular emphysema. However, its development in young Aymaras, free of heart or lung disease, suggests that it is more likely due, in both high-altitude Indians and emphysematous patients, to the effects of alveolar hypoxia per se.

Another typical feature of the remodeling of the pulmonary arterial tree in chronic hypoxia is the development of inner tubes of circular smooth muscle, which come to line the intimal longitudinal muscle in pulmonary arteries and arterioles and extend into the precapillaries.[25] Sometimes two or three muscular tubes are found in one pulmonary artery. In the older lesions elastin develops between the muscular tubes within the confines of the thick elastic lamina comprising the wall of the pulmonary arteriole.

The pulmonary veins and venules are also involved in the remodeling that occurs in response to the hypobaric hypoxia in the Aymara. Vascular smooth muscle cells appear in the intima, but they are widely separated by collagen. Thus it would appear that the form of the muscular proliferation in the pulmonary vasculature in response to hypoxia is greatly modified by haemodynamic forces within the class of vessel in question. Overt muscular hyperplasia in the pulmonary arteries may be a response to arterial pulsation, whereas in the pulmonary veins the myofibroblasts develop more their fibroblastic features. The widespread extent of the structural changes suggests that one should conceive of the field effects of hypoxia as on individual muscle cells in small pulmonary arteries, arterioles, and venules lying adjacent to alveolar spaces rather than on only the terminal portion of the pulmonary arterial tree.

The original observations of Arias-Stella and Saldaña[2] were made on a pure Quechua population in the Andes, and not surprisingly the muscularization of the pulmonary arterioles was found throughout the community. Our studies on the heterogeneous population of La Paz yielded different results.[25] We found muscularization of pulmonary arterioles in 5 of 25 Aymaras and mestizos and the development of intimal longitudinal muscle in 4 of 13 Aymaras and in 5 of 12 mestizos. Inner muscular tubes were recognised in only one of the Aymaras and in none of the mestizos. We have not found hypoxic hypertensive pulmonary vascular disease in Caucasians resident at high altitude. Personal communications from Inder Anand suggest that remodeling of the pulmonary vasculature is not to be found in the native highlanders of Ladakh (3,600 m). This may be a reflection of their different genetic background from that of Andean highlanders, or it may be simply an expression of the fact that they live at lower altitudes.

Our studies on the lungs of patients with chronic obstructive lung disease, included in the study of the British Medical Research Council on the effects of long-term oxygen therapy in this condition, reveal that an identical form of remodeling with the same triad of changes (Fig. 3) occurs in emphysematous patients and to a

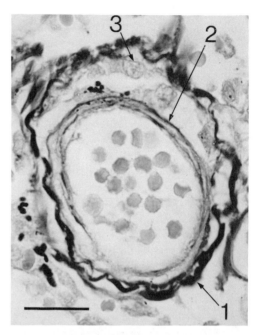

**Figure 3.** Transverse section of a pulmonary arteriole from a man of 64 years with centrilobular emphysema. The elastic lamina comprising the wall of the arteriole is thick (arrow 1). There is an inner muscular tube consisting of a circular muscle coat sandwiched between thin inner and outer elastic laminae (arrow 2). Smooth muscle cells that have migrated from the media lie between the inner muscular tube and the arteriolar wall (arrow 3). (Elastic Van Gieson). Scale line = 26 μm.

more advanced stage than is found in Andean highlanders.[46] This supports the view that sustained alveolar hypoxia is the basic cause of this remodeling of the pulmonary vasculature. Recent studies in my department of the ultrastructure of pulmonary arteries and arterioles in cases of pulmonary emphysema have shown that the intimal longitudinal muscle arises from the migration of smooth muscle cells from the media through gaps in the inner elastic lamina. These muscle cells closely resemble adult vascular smooth muscle cells and are unlike the migrating muscle cells found in plexogenic pulmonary arteriopathy, which are electron dense and have lost their tesselated outline. The similarity of the migrating muscle cells to adult myocytes of the media may be reflected in the restriction of these cells to the intima of pulmonary arteries and the mild, benign pulmonary hypertension in patients with chronic obstructive lung disease and in native highlanders. The inner muscular tubes found in both Aymara Indians and emphysematous subjects are formed by a thickening of the layer of circumferentially situated attenuated smooth muscle cells normally found immediately beneath the endothelium. These cells secrete elastin around themselves, which forms thin inner and outer elastic laminae around the layer of circular muscle. This is the basis for the development of the inner muscular tubes of the pulmonary arteries and arterioles in states of chronic alveolar hypoxia.

## Chinese Infants at High Altitude in Tibet

Our studies in Bolivia demonstrated the histological changes in the pulmonary vasculature that occur in a fully acclimatized population of adult Aymara Indians living at high altitude in the Andes. We have found it important to distinguish in high-altitude studies between subjects who are acclimatized and those who are genetically adapted to the hypobaric hypoxia.[22] At present, increasing numbers of lowlanders of Han origin are being introduced as residents of the Tibetan capital as part of Chinese governmental policy. This has resulted in a mix of population at high altitude of native Tibetan highlanders and lowlanders freshly arrived from low altitude. When infants of Han origin are taken up by their parents to reside in Lhasa (3,600 m), many die within months of congestive cardiac failure.

This condition was brought to the attention of Western medical circles by my colleagues Peter Harris, formerly of the National Heart and Lung Institute, London, and Inder Anand, of Chandigarh, India. They designated this condition "subacute infantile mountain sickness."[43] It ap-

pears to represent a failure to achieve initial acclimatization to hypobaric hypoxia and may thus be compared with brisket disease in calves being taken up for spring grazing in the Wasatch Mountains in Utah. I was privileged to examine specimens of lung brought back from Tibet by Peter Harris. The small pulmonary arteries showed severe medial hypertrophy, and there was muscularization of pulmonary arterioles. Of considerable interest was the migration of vascular smooth muscle cells from the media of the pulmonary arterioles into their lumens. This pulmonary vascular disease appeared to increase pulmonary vascular resistance, for at necropsy the infants showed hypertrophy of the right ventricle and dilatation of the right atrium and pulmonary trunk (Fig. 4),

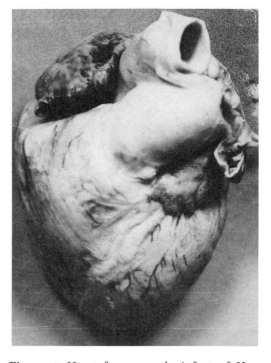

**Figure 4.** Heart from a male infant of Han origin, aged 16 months, who died from subacute infantile mountain sickness 3 months after being taken up to live in Lhasa, Tibet (3,600 m). The initial clinical diagnosis was one of measles bronchopneumonia. There is pronounced right ventricular hypertrophy and dilatation of the right atrium and pulmonary trunk.

features consistent with the development of severe pulmonary hypertension.

## Pulmonary Vasculature in Indigenous Mountain Species

During my studies of the human pulmonary vasculature at high altitude, I took the opportunity to study pulmonary arteries of indigenous mountain species in the Andes and in the Himalaya. These are mammals showing genetic adaptation to the adverse environment. Adaptation, as contrasted to acclimatization, is the development of biochemical, physiological, and anatomical features that are heritable and of genetic basis that enable the species to explore the environment of high altitude to its best advantage. Most of these studies have been carried out over the years with David Williams. In all of the species we have studied, the small pulmonary arteries have been thin walled, with a meagre amount of smooth muscle in the media and pulmonary arterioles devoid of a muscle coat. Such vessels offer a low resistance to blood flow, and consequently these indigenous mountain species do not show a significant elevation of pulmonary arterial pressure but maintain a low ratio of right-to-left cardiac ventricular weight.

We found that animals that show these microanatomical features are the high-altitude camelids of the Andes, such as the llama, the alpaca, and the guanaco.[10] Care must be taken in interpreting these findings in camelids, for the camel family is characterized by a thin-walled pulmonary vasculature even at sea level. More reliable are similar findings in the mountain viscacha *(Lagidium peruanum),*[24] for in general rodents respond to sustained alveolar hypoxia by muscularization of the peripheral pulmonary arterial tree. A noted example of a species adapted to the hypobaric hypoxia of high altitude is the yak *(Bos grunniens),* for the other members of the cattle family at low altitudes have a muscular pulmonary vasculature. Indeed in the mountains around Salt Lake City, calves may not achieve initial acclimatization to high altitude and then develop the potentially fatal condition of brisket disease, as noted above. In the Himalayan yak, however, the pulmonary arteries are exceedingly thin walled and the pulmonary arterioles devoid of smooth muscle.[23] This results in a low pulmonary arterial pressure and a diminished propensity to high-altitude pulmonary hypertension.[1]

We found that cardiac catheterization in the yak is not without its interests and complications. Prior to our expedition to the Himalaya, Peter Harris and David Williams carried out a reconnoitre to Whipsnade Zoo in the United Kingdom. They found the yaks in their paddock very muscular and aggressive. Their keepers volunteered the information that they would be unwilling to enter the paddock to feed them, let alone carry out a cardiac catheterization. A major surprise awaited us on our arrival in Ladakh, for here the yaks under the scrutiny of the village head man were tranquil and cooperative. It was clear to us that, if one wished to see wild yaks, the place for it was England rather than the Himalaya. An exotic example of an indigenous high-altitude species that we have studied is the Tibetan snow-pig *(Marmota himalayana)* (Fig. 5).[44] It also

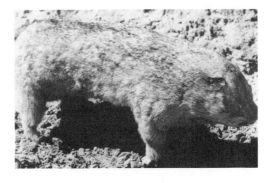

**Figure 5.** Tibetan snow-pig (*Marmota himalayana*).

has thin-walled pulmonary arteries and a low pulmonary arterial pressure.

## Plexogenic Pulmonary Arteriopathy

When I carried out research under Jesse Edwards at the Mayo Clinic in the year from the autumn of 1957, we studied the histopathology of the pulmonary circulation and devised a grading system for the changes we saw.[12] This has pleased some but not others. The central feature of the pathology was a striking lesion combining vascular and cellular proliferation that Jesse had termed the "plexiform lesion". This proved to be of physiological and clinical importance as well as of histopathological interest. Its presence was found to be an indicator of pulmonary blood flow falling below the normal range and a rapidly rising pulmonary arterial pressure.[14] It appeared to be a useful histological marker in lung tissue of a shift in the nature of pulmonary vascular resistance from one determined largely by functional factors to one of fixed organic basis. This in turn suggested an immediately irreversible pulmonary hypertension that would not be susceptible to benefit from closure of a congenital cardiac septal defect. The implication was that the plexiform lesion was of importance in indicating whether a patient with a congenital cardiac anomaly and associated pulmonary hypertension should be referred for corrective heart surgery.[15]

In 1973 I was attending a World Health Organization meeting on primary pulmonary hypertension in Geneva with Kees Wagenvoort. This meeting had been called in response to the epidemic of the disease that broke out in Western Europe during the period of 1967–70. At the end of one of the morning sessions the chairman charged the two of us with producing a name for the pulmonary vascular pathology underlying the clinical syndrome of primary pulmonary hypertension. It was to be ready by the opening of the afternoon session, we were told. Professor Wagenvoort and his wife, Noek, and I repaired to the restaurant, and over lunch with red wine had an urgent discussion to come up with an appropriate term. We concluded that the designation must indicate that the essential feature of the disease was the plexiform lesion, which need not, however, be present in every case. In other words, the condition was "plexogenic" rather than "plexiform". The term was accepted by the meeting in the afternoon, and the disease became known as "plexogenic pulmonary arteriopathy."[11] That is how the term was born, and it has not been loved by all clinicians, who, once having read this account, may conclude that the drinking of wine should be banned on such occasions.

## Vascular Smooth Muscle Migration

Early studies of the pathogenesis of plexogenic pulmonary arteriopathy suggested that constriction of small pulmonary arteries was of central importance, particularly in the formation of the plexiform lesion.[45] However, our studies over the years have demonstrated that tissue proliferation is also of considerable importance, and this is demonstrated well by electron microscopy.[41] Thus the pulmonary arteriopathy of primary pulmonary hypertension, congenital cardiac shunts, and rare examples of cirrhosis of the liver or portal vein thrombosis should be regarded as not entirely vasoconstrictive in nature but in part a manifestation of abnormal cell growth. This concept has considerable relevance to the use of pulmonary vasodilators in primary pulmonary hypertension, which cannot be expected to reverse overgrowth of cellular tissues.

In our original description of the grading system[12] we paid scant attention to

Grade 2, and at that time we did not appreciate its significance. We referred to it as a "cellular intimal reaction" and suggested it might be due to endothelial cells. Further studies over the years by light and electron microscopy have revealed that it is due to migration of smooth muscle cells from the media into the intima, where there is a transformation into myofibroblasts, which proliferate in the vascular lumen obstructing it. Subsequent investigation of the ultrastructure of plexogenic pulmonary arteriopathy has shown that, early in the disease, the muscle cells in the inner half of the media show increased electron density[18] (Fig. 6). They lose their tesselated outline, become smooth, and can be detected in the act of passing through gaps in the inner elastic lamina to reach the intima.

Such migration of smooth muscle cells from the media into the intima through gaps in the inner elastic lamina is reminiscent of the process that occurs in patients with emphysema or in native highlanders and leads to the characteristic layers of intimal longitudinal muscle in states of chronic alveolar hypoxia. However, in plexogenic pulmonary arteriopathy the process is different in ways that have great pathological and clinical implications. Here the muscle cells are electron dense and have smooth outlines. Having reached the intima the myocytes become transformed into myofibroblasts which replicate vigorously in the intima and give rise to other changes such as fibrosis and elastosis. They then proliferate in the lumens of arteries and arterioles, occluding them and elevating pulmonary arterial resistance. This leads to a severe pulmonary hypertension, which may prove rapidly fatal. This is a very different outcome from the mild, benign pulmonary hypertension of the native highlander. It is as though in plexogenic pulmonary arteriopathy the smooth muscle cells have had their nature and behaviour changed by something like a growth factor permeating the inner half

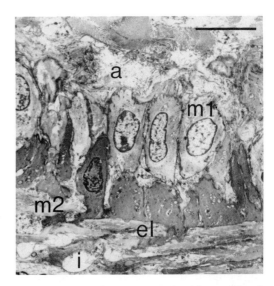

**Figure 6.** Electron micrograph of longitudinal section of a muscular pulmonary artery from a woman of 23 years with primary pulmonary hypertension. The adventitia (a) consists of a discontinuous external elastic lamina and a loose collection of collagen fibrils. The media contains smooth muscle cells sectioned transversely. Those in the outer media (ml) are pale with numerous peripheral attachment points between which the cytoplasm bulges outward. Smooth muscle cells in the inner media (m2) are denser and lack a ruffled border. Two of them can be seen in the process of sending out cytoplasmic extensions between gaps in the internal elastic lamina (el) into the intima (i). Here they are associated with elongated cytoplasmic processes from other smooth muscle cells (arrow). Scale line = 13 μ*m*.

of the media, perhaps from the vascular lumen or the endothelium.

## Pulmonary Endocrine Cells, Peptides, and Pulmonary Vascular Disease

Further investigation of this migration of smooth muscle cells from the media of pulmonary arteries has shown an interesting association with pulmonary endocrine cells and the peptides they contain. Through the kindness of Professor Magdi Yacoub, we gained access to specimens of lung he removed at combined heart-lung operations at Harefield Hospital in London. The two major peptides found in human pulmonary endocrine cells are calcitonin and bombesin, and their functions are unknown. We found that pulmonary endocrine cells increased in number and prominence in only one form of hypertensive pulmonary vascular disease, namely, plexogenic pulmonary arteriopathy, be it primary or secondary (Fig. 7).

The peptide concerned was gastrin-releasing peptide, the human counterpart of that of amphibian skin, bombesin. There is, moreover, an interesting association between the proliferation of neuroen-docrine cells containing this peptide and the stage of plexogenic pulmonary arteriopathy that has been reached. Thus they are numerous when classic cellular plexiform lesions are present, and their numbers fall off when these dilatation lesions become mature with wider vascular channels. The most interesting feature is that they are most numerous in the preplexiform stage, before the plexiform lesions have developed, when the major component of the pathology is migration of vascular smooth muscle cells from media to intima.[7,27] The basis for this association remains obscure. Increased prominence of pulmonary endocrine cells containing bombesin is also found in cases of subacute infantile mountain sickness in Tibet.[13]

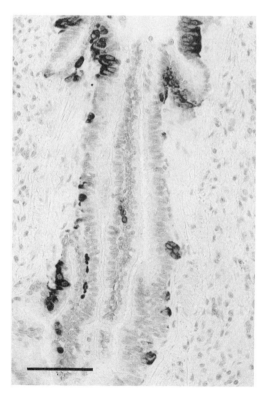

**Figure 7.** Pulmonary endocrine cells showing strong immunoreactivity for gastrin-releasing peptide in the terminal bronchiole of a boy of 6 years with Eisenmenger's syndrome secondary to common atrioventricular canal complicating plexogenic pulmonary arteriopathy. Scale line = 53 μm.

## Muscular Evaginations

When smooth muscle cells constrict, they do not simply become shorter and thicker but become covered in bulbous extrusions.[6] This was originally shown by scanning electron microscopy of the smooth muscle cells of the stomach wall of *Bufo marinus*. We wondered if these extrusions could be demonstrated by transmission electron microscopy, for if they could, they would indicate a very early stage of constriction in pulmonary hypertension, long before the migration of smooth muscle cells from the media or their proliferation in the intima. Our investigations confirmed that they could indeed be found in the pulmonary trunk and small pulmonary arteries of rats exposed to hypoxia[40] and in the pulmonary arteries and arterioles in this species following the administration of pyrrolizidine alkaloids.[39] Such prominences were found to be due to evaginations of the cytoplasm of the smooth muscle cells between attachment points in the plasmalemma, which act as points of anchorage for the intracellular fibrils of actin and myosin. The clear cytoplasm of the evaginations is devoid of myofilaments and organelles (Fig. 8).

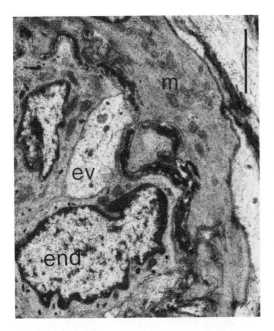

**Figure 8.** Electron micrograph of lung from a Wistar albino rat subjected to a reduced barometric pressure of 490 mmHg simulating an altitude of 3,550 m. Part of the wall of a muscularized pulmonary arteriole is shown. A distinct media (m) consisting of circularly oriented vascular smooth muscle cells is sandwiched between inner and outer elastic laminae. A muscular evagination (ev) has formed and is pressing on the undersurface of endothelial cells (end). It has passed through a gap in the inner lamina. Scale line = 2 μm.

When vascular smooth muscle cells constrict, the evaginations squeeze through deficiencies in the adjacent inner or outer elastic lamina of the wall of the blood vessel to extend into the intima or adventitia, respectively. Because deficiencies in the pulmonary arteries occur naturally in the outer lamina, muscular evaginations in these vessels tend to be into the adventitia. In contrast, deficiencies in pulmonary veins occur mainly in the inner elastic lamina so that in these vessels the evaginations are found in the intima. In this situation the surface of the muscular evagination presses on the undersurface of the endothelial cells. Because the cytoplasm of muscle and endothelial cell comes into such intimate contact, substances may pass between these two cells, which raises interesting physiological possibilities. Only lungs that have been fixed in distension are satisfactory for a search for muscular evaginations, for they are also readily produced by collapse. These evaginations are the earliest structural changes detectable at ultrastructural level in animals that indicate pulmonary vasoconstriction.

In a recent experiment we subjected Wistar albino rats to a reduced barometric pressure of 490 mmHg to simulate an altitude of 3,550 m. They developed numerous muscular evaginations in muscularized pulmonary arterioles, but, when some of the rats were allowed to recover in room air, the evaginations disappeared within a week. Clearly they represent an acute vasoconstrictive response soon lost after removal of the hypoxic stimulus. As far as I am aware muscular evaginations of pulmonary arteries have not been described in man.

## Venous and Parenchymal Changes in Plexogenic Pulmonary Arteriopathy

Studies of plexogenic pulmonary arteriopathy have largely been restricted to the histopathology and ultrastructure of the pulmonary arterial tree. In 1987 I began receiving considerable tissue from Harefield Hospital transplantation cases, which included cases of plexogenic pulmonary arteriopathy, both primary and secondary to congenital cardiac septal defects. As a result of this experience, my concept of the pathology of this disease has been modified. It has become apparent to me that in plexogenic pulmonary arteriopathy changes occur in the pulmonary veins and venules and in the lung parenchyma, together with a considerable accumulation of lung mast cells.

In a study of the histopathology of 36

cases of plexogenic pulmonary arteriopathy,[5] we found intimal proliferations in pulmonary veins in all but 5 cases, 4 of the exceptions being children 6 years of age or less. However, three children of 5 to 7 years of age showed widespread intimal fibrosis of pulmonary veins, one of whom had a luminal obstruction of 18.8%, defined as the average thickness of the intima expressed as a percentage of the internal diameter of the vein. Three adults with primary arteriopathy who had luminal venous obstructions of greater than 28% had an appreciably more cellular type of intimal thickening. Embedded within the collagenous matrix of the thickened venous intima, cells were identified that closely resembled myofibroblasts, and in some areas bundles of mature smooth muscle were seen. Similar changes were found in 5 cases of secondary plexogenic pulmonary arteriopathy. Electron microscopy confirmed the identity of the cells within the intima as myofibroblasts.

Some of the intimal fibrosis in pulmonary veins in plexogenic pulmonary arteriopathy may be an expression of age change or a consequence of the increased levels of pulmonary blood flow found early in the life history of pre- and posttricuspid congenital cardiac shunts. In some instances, however, the myofibroblasts in the pulmonary venous intima appeared to be transformed smooth muscle cells that had migrated from the media, thus resembling the migration of myocytes in the pulmonary arteries that occurs in plexogenic pulmonary arteriopathy. This recalls the remodeling of pulmonary veins of the Aymara Indians. Associated with this intimal proliferation in pulmonary veins and venules, one finds a whole range of parenchymal changes in the lung in plexogenic pulmonary arteriopathy. These include focal haemorrhages, proliferation of granular pneumonocytes, accumulations of alveolar macrophages, dystrophic calcification, small osseous nodules, periarterial accumulations of lymphocytes, and even groups of cells resembling meningocytes around pulmonary venules.[5]

In view of the venous and parenchymal lesions in plexogenic pulmonary arteriopathy, we were prompted to study the population of lung mast cells in this disease.[26] Mast cells were found to abound in the lung parenchyma, with perhaps a greater tendency to accumulate in the adventitia of pulmonary arteries. They occurred equally commonly in the primary and secondary forms of the arteriopathy, and their numbers did not appear to be closely related to the stage of the disease reached. If anything, they were somewhat more numerous in association with cellular plexiform lesions and even more so in the preplexiform stage, when muscle cells were migrating into the intima. They were less common with mature plexiform lesions. When Ehrlich discovered mast cells in the last century, he noted at the outset that they were abundant in the lung in the brown induration of mitral stenosis.[37] We were subsequently able to confirm this finding in mitral stenosis and chronic left ventricular failure[20] and in association with the similar parenchymal changes induced in the lung by metabolites of monocrotaline.[28] It is probable that in plexogenic pulmonary arteriopathy the accumulation of lung mast cells is also part of the parenchymal changes found in the lung substance. An intriguing possibility is that the periarterial mast cells are secreting histamine, which in man appears to have a dilating effect on pulmonary arteries in which H-2 receptors seem to be dominant.

## Dietary Pulmonary Hypertension

In the 1960s Michael Kay and I became aware that dietary factors could lead to severe pulmonary hypertension in animals. Lalich and Merkow[34] and Lalich and

Ehrhart[33] had observed that prolonged oral administration of *Crotalaria spectabilis* seeds or their active principle, the pyrrolizidine alkaloid monocrotaline, to rats induces in them medial hypertrophy and arteritis in the pulmonary arteries with associated cardiac hypertrophy. Initially we confirmed that the seeds of this plant, which originated in India and came to be used as a cover crop in the southern states of the United States, were capable of inducing pulmonary hypertension in rats.[29] The elevation of pulmonary arterial pressure was found to have an organic basis in pulmonary vascular disease characterized by medial hypertrophy of small pulmonary arteries, which in a minority of cases progressed to necrotising arteritis.[30] There was associated muscularization of the pulmonary arterioles and of the pulmonary trunk.[16] There was, however, no migration of muscle cells from the media to lead to any form of intimal proliferation, and no plexiform lesions developed. An important aspect of monocrotaline pulmonary vascular disease was hypertrophy of the intimal muscular pads of pulmonary veins.[30] This venous obstruction became associated with a wide variety of exudative lesions in the lung parenchyma, ranging from pulmonary haemorrhage, osseous nodules, aggregations of pulmonary macrophages, and proliferation of granular pneumonocytes,[42] to accumulations of mast cells.[28]

It soon became apparent that other members of the genus *Crotalaria* and its alkaloids were capable of inducing pulmonary hypertension in animals. Fulvine is a pyrrolizidine alkaloid contained in the foliage and seeds of *Crotalaria fulva*. This leguminous plant is one of several that was used in the West Indies for the preparation of bush teas, consumed by the indigenous population for medicinal and social purposes. Fulvine and the other alkaloids contained in bush tea were known to cause veno-occlusive disease of the liver in the Caribbean, but there was no suggestion that their ingestion led to pulmonary veno-occlusive disease. Fulvine is closely related chemically to monocrotaline, and Professor Bras was so kind as to send us some of the alkaloid from Jamaica. We were able to show that fulvine produces in rats hypertensive pulmonary vascular disease identical to that produced by *Crotalaria spectabilis*.[31]

We found that the genus *Senecio* was also effective in inducing pulmonary hypertension and associated pulmonary vascular disease in animals. There is a common belief in the United Kingdom that any natural substance is "good for you," an idea encouraged by commercial television. Ragwort, sometimes called "stinking nanny," (*Senecio jacobaea*) is a common herb of the English countryside and preparations of it are freely available from herbalists and so-called health stores in Britain, where they are recommended for the treatment of various ailments (Fig. 9). In fact, the seeds and foliage of *Senecio jacobaea* contain at least six pyrrolizidine alkaloids. Dr. Burns, on our staff, visited a store to buy a bagful of this health food. It was given to rats in their diet, and within the month all had died of congestive cardiac failure secondary to hypertensive pulmonary vascular disease of a type similar to that produced by *Crotalaria spectabilis* seeds.[4]

An important question left to be answered was whether pyrrolizidine alkaloids could induce hypertensive pulmonary vascular disease in man. For some years I acted as external examiner for medical students in Tanzania. On one occasion I was shown lung sections from a young man of 19 years, who had died from congestive cardiac failure in Muhimbili Hospital in Dar-es-Salaam. They showed the typical features of plexogenic pulmonary arteriopathy. The patient came from Kilwa, an area where witch doctors practised, administering herbal concoctions to their customers. Growing in profusion around Kilwa was a leguminous plant,

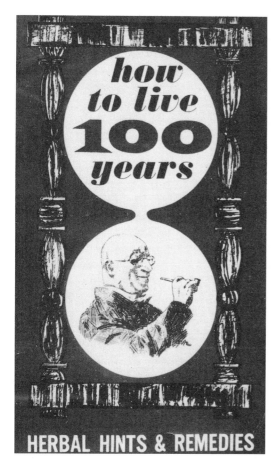

**Figure 9.** Advertising material supplied with a packet of ragwort obtained at a "health store". Said to be efficacious for gouty and arthritic joint pains, the plant led to the death from hypertensive pulmonary vascular disease of Wistar albino rats when added to their diet.

*Crotalaria laburnoides,* which has a widespread distribution in East Africa, occurring in Tanzania, Kenya, and Uganda (Fig. 10). It is sometimes called *C. bagamoyo-ënsis* because it grows in the coastal area around the small township of Bagamoyo, an important centre of the African slave trade in the last century and well known to the missionary-explorer David Livingstone. We were unable to establish that this boy had been given any herbal infusion containing this plant species. Nevertheless, I collected its seeds and brought them back to Liverpool where they were

administered over a period of 2 months to Wistar albino rats. A proportion died in congestive cardiac failure secondary to hypertensive pulmonary vascular disease of the type associated with pyrrolizidine alkaloids.[17]

All of these studies confirmed that the pyrrolizidine alkaloids contained in the genera *Crotalaria* or *Senecio* were capable of inducing pulmonary hypertension and associated pulmonary vascular disease in a variety of animals. There was no proof that dietary factors were involved in the aetiology of pulmonary hypertension in man. The concept of dietary pulmonary hypertension had been born, but at that time it did not seem to have a clinical application. These investigations appeared to be a classic example of "ivory tower" research, for the amusement and indulgence of professors protected behind the walls of their academic institution.

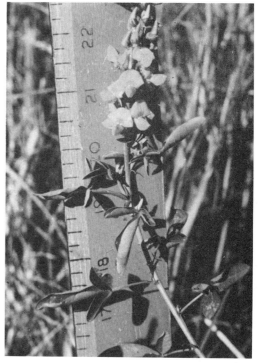

**Figure 10.** *Crotalaria laburnoides,* growing in swampy ground near the coast of Tanzania.

## Menocil Pulmonary Hypertension

In 1967 the attitude toward such experiments changed dramatically, and the concept of dietary pulmonary hypertension to humans was considered seriously when a sudden 20-fold increase in the incidence of primary pulmonary hypertension was observed in a Swiss medical clinic.[9] A considerable number of the patients concerned had taken the appetite-suppressing drug aminorex, 2-amino-5 phenyl-2-oxazoline, with the commercial name of Menocil, which was available in Switzerland from November 1965 to October 1968. A similar increase in the incidence of this disease occurred in Austria and West Germany, where the drug was available. I found myself involved in this epidemic in two ways. First, I was called on to visit various centres in the three countries seeking to establish the nature of the pulmonary vascular disease emerging in Europe. The pathology proved to be that of plexogenic pulmonary arteriopathy, indistinguishable histologically from that found in classic primary pulmonary hypertension. Second, with colleagues in my department I undertook experimental studies to ascertain whether the drug could induce pulmonary vascular disease in animals. In fact, high oral dosage of aminorex for 43 weeks in rats, as we have seen above, a species susceptible to dietary pulmonary hypertension, and for 20 weeks in dogs failed to reveal any evidence of hypertensive pulmonary vascular disease.[32] Grover and Byrne-Quinn failed to produce pulmonary hypertension by injecting aminorex daily for a month into calves in which the pulmonary vasculature was sensitized by chronic hypoxia induced by living at an altitude where the barometric pressure was 625 mmHg.[8]

Twenty years after these events there appears to have been a general acceptance of an association between the ingestion of aminorex fumarate and the development of plexogenic pulmonary arteriopathy to an extent that the diagnosis "menocil pulmonary hypertension" has entered medical parlance. Yet the present position with regard to aminorex is that, although statistical epidemiological evidence linked this drug to pulmonary hypertension in humans there was no direct proof by animal experimentation that aminorex causes plexogenic pulmonary arteriopathy in patients. The caveat remains that failure to produce pulmonary vascular disease in animals by the drug may merely reflect a species difference in the reactivity of the pulmonary arteries.

## An Animal Model for Primary Pulmonary Hypertension

Many workers have sought an animal model for primary pulmonary hypertension, but our studies over the years convince us that none is satisfactory. A widely used model is the administration of monocrotaline to rats, either by injection of the alkaloid or administration of *Crotalaria spectabilis* seeds to the diet. Fatal pulmonary vascular disease is induced readily enough, but it differs in important respects from that found in humans. Thus it readily induces hyperplasia of vascular smooth muscle cells, and in about 30% of cases leads to fibrinoid necrosis and an acute inflammatory reaction. However, it does not bring about migration of myocytes into the intima so that there is no intimal fibrosis or elastosis, concentric laminar intimal proliferation, or development of plexiform lesions, the hallmarks of plexogenic pulmonary arteriopathy in man. Our later studies have revealed that in rats showing medial hypertrophy or fibrinoid necrosis in their pulmonary arteries induced by monocrotaline, bombesin cannot be demonstrated in the pulmonary endocrine cells.[35] This is in striking contrast to what occurs in humans, where the migration of muscle cells from the media into the intima and the formation of plexiform lesions are associated with an increase in the numbers and prominence of bombesin-containing cells in the terminal bronchioles. Apparently the rat is not capable of developing intimal proliferation in the pulmonary arteries, and in some way this may be related to absence of bombesin-containing pulmonary endocrine cells.

The pulmonary vascular remodeling brought about by exposing rats to hypobaric hypoxia in a decompression chamber also forms a disappointing animal model for what occurs in humans. In rats, many of the muscular evaginations referred to above develop in the pulmonary arteries. They indicate intense vasoconstriction in response to the hypoxic stimulus and remain for about a week. Such evaginations have not been reported in human lung specimens. In rats, expo-

sure to hypobaric hypoxia and the development of pulmonary vasoconstriction with muscular evaginations and right ventricular hypertrophy is rapidly fatal.

In humans the remodeling of the pulmonary arterial tree in response to hypoxia comprises the formation of intimal longitudinal muscle and tubes of circular muscle internal to it. Such complex remodeling of longitudinal and circular muscle is not seen in rats. In native highlanders and emphysematous patients, such remodeling is hardly more than a marker of chronic hypoxia; it appears to be benign and not to reduce longevity. Clearly the rat provides a poor animal model for pulmonary hypertension and vascular disease in man.

**Acknowledgements:** I am indebted to the following publishers and journal editors for permission to reproduce the illustrations indicated: Fig. 1 *(Br Heart J.)* Fig. 2 (Springer Verlag), Fig. 3 *(Q.J. Med)*, Fig. 4 *(Respir. Med)*, Fig. 6 and 7 *(Histopathology)*.

## References

1. Anand, I., D. Heath, D. Williams, M. Deen, R. Ferrari, D. Bergel, and P. Harris. The pulmonary circulation of some domestic animals at high altitude. *Int. J. Biometeorol.* 32:56–64, 1988.

2. Arias-Stella, J., and M. Saldaña. The terminal portion of the pulmonary arterial tree in people native to high altitudes. *Circulation* 28:915–925, 1963.

3. Brown, J. W. *Congenital Heart Disease.* London: Staples, 1939 (1st ed.), 1951 (2nd ed.).

4. Burns, J. The heart and pulmonary arteries in rats fed on *Senecio jacobaea. J. Pathol.* 106:187–194, 1972.

5. Caslin, A. W., D. Heath, B. Madden, M. Yacoub, J. R. Gosney, and P. Smith The histopathology of 36 cases of plexogenic pulmonary arteriopathy. *Histopathology* 16:9–19, 1990.

6. Fay, F. S., and C. M. Delise. Contraction of isolated smooth muscle cells: structural changes. *Proc. Nat. Acad. Sci. USA* 70: 641–645, 1973.

7. Gosney, J. D. Heath, P. Smith, P. Harris, and M. Yacoub. Pulmonary endocrine cells in pulmonary arterial disease. *Arch. Pathol. Lab. Med.* 113: 337–341, 1989.

8. Grover, R. F., and E. Byrne-Quinn. Attempted induction of pulmonary hypertension in the calf with anorexigens. Presented at the Symposium on Obesity, Circulation and Anorexigens, Lucerne, Switzerland, May 15 and 16, 1970.

9. Gurtner, H. P., M. Gertsch, C. Salzmann, M. Scherrer, P. Stucki, and F. Wyss. Haufen sich die primär vasculären: formen des chronischen Cor pulmonale. *Schweiz. med. Wschr.* 98: 1579, 1695, 1968.

10. Harris, P., D. Heath, P. Smith, D. R. Williams, A. Ramirez, H. Krüger, and D. M. Jones. Pulmonary circulation of the llama at high and low altitudes. *Thorax* 37: 38–45, 1982.

11. Hatano, S., and T. Strasser. Primary pulmonary hypertension. Report on a WHO meeting. World Health Organization, Geneva, October 15–17, 1973.

12. Heath, D., and J. E. Edwards. The pathology of hypertensive pulmonary vascular disease: a description of six grades of structural changes in the pulmonary arteries with special reference to congenital cardiac septal defects. *Circulation* 18: 533–547, 1958.

13. Heath, D., P. Harris, G. J. Sui, Y. H. Liu, J. Gosney, E. Harris, and I. S. Anand. Pulmonary blood vessels and endocrine cells in

subacute infantile mountain sickness. *Respir. Med.* 83: 77–81, 1989.

14. Heath, D., F. Helmholz, H. B. Burchell, J. W. DuShane, and J. E. Edwards. Graded pulmonary vascular changes and hemodynamic findings in cases of atrial and ventricular septal defect and patent ductus arteriosus. *Circulation* 18: 1155–1166, 1958.

15. Heath, D., H. F. Helmholz, H. B. Burchell, J. W. DuShane, J. W. Kirklin, and J. E. Edwards. Relation between structural changes in the small pulmonary arteries and the immediate reversibility of pulmonary hypertension following closure of ventricular and atrial septal defects. *Circulation* 18: 1167–1174, 1958.

16. Heath D. and J. M. Kay. Medial thickness of pulmonary trunk in rats with cor pulmonale induced by ingestion of Crotalaria spectabilis seeds. *Cardiovasc. Res.* 1: 74–79, 1967.

17. Heath, D., J. Shaba, A. Williams, P. Smith, and A. Kombe. A pulmonary hypertension producing plant from Tanzania. *Thorax* 30: 399–404, 1975.

18. Heath, D., P. Smith, and J. Gosney. Ultrastructure of early plexogenic pulmonary arteriopathy. *Histopathology* 12: 41–52, 1988.

19. Heath, D., P. Smith, J. Rios Dalenz, D. Williams, and P. Harris. Small pulmonary arteries in some natives of La Paz, Bolivia. *Thorax* 36: 599–604, 1981.

20. Heath, D., T. Trueman, and P. Sukonthamarn. Pulmonary mast cells in mitral stenosis. *Cardiovasc. Res.* 3: 467–471, 1969.

21. Heath D., and W. Whitaker. Hypertensive pulmonary vascular disease. *Circulation* 14: 323–343, 1956.

22. Heath, D., and D. R. Williams. Life at high altitude. In: *High-Altitude Medicine and Pathology.* London: Butterworths, 1989, p. 327, 331.

23. Heath, D., D. Williams, and J. Dickinson. The pulmonary arteries of the yak. *Cardiovasc. Res.* 18: 133–139, 1984.

24. Heath, D., D. Williams, P. Harris, P. Smith, H. Krüger, and A. Ramirez. The pulmonary vasculature of the mountain-viscacha *(Lagidium peruanum):* the concept of adapted and acclimatized vascular smooth muscle. *J. Comp. Pathol.* 91: 293–301, 1981.

25. Heath, D., D. Williams, J. Rios-Dalenz, M. Calderon, and J. Gosney. Small pulmonary arterial vessels of Aymara Indians from the Bolivian Andes. *Histopathology* 16: 565–571, 1990.

26. Heath, D., And M. Yacoub. Lung mast cells in plexogenic pulmonary arteriopathy. *J. Clin. Pathol.* 44: 1003–1006, 1991.

27. Heath, D., M. Yacoub, J. R. Gosney, B. Madden, A. W. Caslin, and P. Smith. Pulmonary endocrine cells in hypertensive pulmonary vascular disease. *Histopathology* 16: 21–28, 1990.

28. Kay, J. M., T. D. Gillund, and D. Heath. Mast cells in the lungs of rats fed on Crotalaria spectabilis seeds. *Am. J. Pathol.* 51: 1031–1044, 1967.

29. Kay, J. M., P. Harris and D. Heath. Pulmonary hypertension produced in rats by ingestion of Crotalaria spectabilis seeds. *Thorax* 22: 176–179, 1967.

30. Kay, J. M., and D. Heath. Observations on the pulmonary arteries and heart weight of rats fed on Crotalaria spectabilis seeds. *J. Pathol. Bacteriol.* 92: 385–394, 1966.

31. Kay, J. M., D. Heath, P. Smith, G. Bras, and J. Summerell. Fulvine and the pulmonary circulation. *Thorax* 26: 249–261, 1971.

32. Kay, J. M., P. Smith, and D. Heath. Aminorex and the pulmonary circulation. *Thorax* 26: 262–270, 1971.

33. Lalich, J. J., and L. A. Ehrhart. Monocrotaline-induced pulmonary arteritis in rats. *J. Ath. Res.* 2: 482–492, 1962.

34. Lalich, J. J., and L. Merkow. Pulmonary arteritis produced in rats by feeding *Crotalaria spectabilis. Lab. Invest.* 10: 744–750, 1961.

35. O'Neill, D., R. Ferrari, C. Ceconi, A. Rodella, P. Smith, P. Harris, and D. Heath. Pulmonary peptides, norepinephrine and endocrine cells in monocrotaline pulmonary hypertension. *Cardioscience* 2: 27–33, 1991.

36. Peñaloza, D., F. Sime, N. Banchero, and R. Gamboa. Pulmonary hypertension in healthy man born and living at high altitudes. *Med. Thorac.* 19: 449–460, 1962.

37. Riley, J. F. *The Mast Cells.* Edinburgh: Livingstone, 1959.

38. Sime, F., N. Banchero, D. Peñaloza, R. Gamboa, J. Cruz and E. Marticorena. Pulmonary hypertension in children born and living at high altitudes. *Am. J. Cardiol.* 11: 143–157, 1963.

39. Smith, P., and D. Heath. Evagination of vascular smooth muscle cells during the early stages of Crotalaria pulmonary hypertension. *J. Pathol.* 124: 177–183, 1978.

40. Smith, P., D. Heath, and F. Padula. Evagination of smooth muscle cells in the hypoxic pulmonary trunk. *Thorax* 33: 31–42, 1978.

41. Smith, P., D. Heath, M. Yacoub, B. Mad-

den, A, Caslin, and J. Gosney. The ultra-structure of plexogenic pulmonary arteriopathy. *J. Pathol.* 160: 111–121, 1990.

42. Smith, P., J. M. Kay, and D. Heath. Hypertensive pulmonary vascular disease in rats after prolonged feeding with Crotalaria spectabilis seeds. *J. Pathol.* 102: 97–106, 1970.

43. Sui, G. J., Y. H. Liu, I. S. Anand, E. Harris, P. Harris, and D. Heath. Subacute infantile mountain sickness. *J. Pathol.* 155: 161–170, 1988.

44. Sun, S. F., G. J. Sui, Y. H. Liu, X. S. Cheng, I. S. Anand, P. Harris, and D. Heath. The pulmonary circulation of the Tibetan snow pig *(Marmota himalayana). J. Zool. (London)* 217: 85–91, 1989.

45. Wagenvoort, C. A. The morphology of certain vascular lesions in pulmonary hypertension. *J. Pathol. Bacteriol.* 78: 503–511, 1959.

46. Wilkinson, M., C. A. Langhorne, D. Heath, G. R. Barer, and Howard, P. A pathophysiological study of 10 cases of hypoxic cor pulmonale. *Q. J. Med.* new series 66 (249): 65–85, 1988.

# 15

# The Pulmonary Circulation of Some Domestic Animals at High Altitude:
## The Real Story

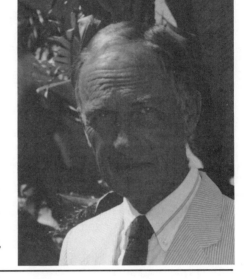

**Peter Harris, M.D., Ph.D.**

*Editor, Cardioscience, Canal Press, Venice, Italy*

## June 3

Roberto had flown in yesterday from Italy and we were up early this morning, waiting for Gigi Anand to take us to Heathrow in her battered old VW beetle. At the airport, she pressed a ten-pound note into my hand.

"That's to buy film for Inder when you meet him in Srinagar."

It was eight o'clock. But, from all our past journeys together, I would have expected Donald Heath to have checked in hours before. So I was surprised to see him and David Williams at the counter.

"They didn't confirm our seats," he shouted across. "Thank God we got here early to sort them out."

He was right. The agency had messed it up.

"We're incredibly over weight," I muttered, as we humped our bags off the trolley.

"Don't worry! They're all too confused over the seats to notice."

And that's how we got through without paying.

I pulled Roberto over. Donald caught him by the shoulder.

"And what do you think bombesin is

From: Wagner WW, Jr, Weir EK (eds): *The Pulmonary Circulation and Gas Exchange.* ©1994, Futura Publishing Co Inc, Armonk, NY.

doing in the lung?'' was the opening sentence of what would be a life-long friendship.

It was 2 a.m. when we arrived in Delhi, and the air was as warm as milk. A new airport but old old customs. We all had something to hide: Donald's terrifying postmortem knives, David's little tubes of white powder, Roberto's test tubes and balance, my batteries and cardiac output computer and Swan Ganz catheters. I was the one who got caught and spent the next half hour signing documents.

## June 4

We took two rickety taxis to the India International Centre, the IIC, luggage protruding from the boots. A stupid race between the drivers almost wrecked the mission before it had started. Inder rang at five, before he took the plane from Chandigarh to Srinagar to get things ready there for our first stop. At nine, our tickets to Srinagar arrived, and I found Donald and David finishing a hearty breakfast.

We awakened Roberto and took a taxi into town. Cows, tricycles, and beggars hindered our way as we hooted down a labyrinth of malodorous side streets. Donald, as always, in dark suit and tie, and carrying his brief case, was already sweating. He turned from the front seat, his eyes lit up.

"And what do you think of all those meningeallike excrescences are doing in the pulmonary veins in pulmonary embolism?'' he asked a bewildered Roberto.

There was trouble at the Jama Mashid mosque. Donald was prepared to take off his well-polished leather shoes but didn't like trusting them outside.

"They're my only pair,'' he explained.

"Same here,'' I lied. "But they are quite safe.''

For a moment he was satisfied. But, as he reached the other side of the mosque, he had doubts and sent David back to fetch them. My guess is that David had problems with the guardian. He didn't return, and soon Donald made a beeline across the oven-hot stones of the quadrangle, treading as lightly as a saint on trial by fire.

Sweat cascaded down my old friend's neck as we elbowed our way down side streets. He put on his hat to protect against the sun, looking more than ever like a mirage direct from Liverpool. Heads turned, veils dropped. And then began his initiation into an Indian soft drink industry protected from American imports— Thumbs Up and Limca and Kampa Cola. Every other stall received our custom, and during the succeeding two hours he must have consumed twenty bottles.

Returned to the IIC, I tried to ring Mr. Liddell. He was commander-in-chief of the Indo-Tibetan Border Police. This paramilitary force, known universally as the ITBP, had been set up to monitor the sensitive border between India and China. Mr. Liddell had been immensely helpful on previous expeditions and had offered to help us again this time. Quite unlike the military prototype, he was a man of great culture and sensitivity, devoted to his garden and insisting on the provision of indoor plants in the various camps under his command. Unfortunately his sister was in hospital, his PA explained, so he was not there. I had a pocket calculator I had smuggled in as a present and wanted to take it over. But I could not get a clear idea from the PA where the headquarters were.

"Just next door,'' he said. But that was patently not so. Various people in the IIC gave me conflicting directions. Outside was an afternoon oven and I had no intention of walking down the road, turning right or left at the first crossroads (according to my various sources) and hunting around for a building without a name, on the fourth (or was it third?) floor of which would be an office from which, by the time I got there, the PA would surely have left for tea. So I gave up and went into the Lodhi Gardens and sketched a tomb instead (Fig. 1).

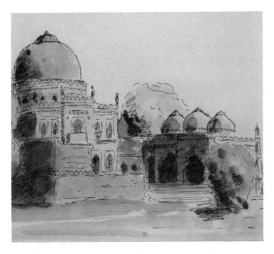

**Figure 1.** The Lodhi Gardens, Delhi.

Beer in the bar before supper seemed a good idea. But, within minutes, Roberto, in a distraught state, rushed from the room, returning in a heavy sweater.

"Bloody air conditioning," he explained, trembling. "It has given me a cold."

"But, Roberto!"

"I know you think I'm crazy. But, I tell you, it has given me a cold." He shivered.

And I am remembering last year when Roberto turned up in tropical Chandigarh wearing the same sweater. It must have been 40°C. And we had all laughed. And he had said, "I tell you, air conditioning always gives me a cold." When, a few days later, I developed a cold, it was generally agreed that he was right.

I fell asleep as the storm broke. First of the monsoons?

## June 5

It was baking at the airport, where Roberto was exerting his invaluable Italian skills getting us at the head of the right queue at the right time. We had first been approached by a Kashmiri posing as a fellow traveler. His main interest soon turned out to be fixing us up in his uncle's houseboat, where we would be unforgettably welcome.

"But unforgettably. Definitely."

As soon as he heard that we were already fixed up at the university, he lost interest and told us with great authority to wait at precisely the wrong place. Our first contact with Kashmiris.

Inder was waiting for us at Srinagar Airport, a great smile of welcome on his face. And, from the back of the crowded hall, a little man rushed to throw his arms around Roberto. He turned out to be Hassan, who owned a stall on the airport and who had, generously and without any thought of repayment, helped Roberto when he had been in difficulties there a year before. Our second contact with Kashmiris.

Brushing aside the undergrowth of clutching hands, we humped our luggage into an old ambulance that Inder had commandeered. It was good to catch up with the news. From London, Srinagar had been the weakest link in the chain. This was where the first stage of the experiments was to be done: a combination of haemodynamics and histology of the pulmonary circulation of the local breeds of sheep and goats and cows so that we could compare them with similar breeds at the higher altitudes of Ladakh. But, within twenty-four hours, Inder had organised everything. We were to stay at the staff quarters of the Medical Institute; contact had been made with Animal Husbandry and the Sheep Institute, where laboratories had been made available.

We had the run of two concrete houses in a compound, where we were looked after by an off-hand villain with his half-witted assistant. It was not long before we would realise that most of the food they bought on our behalf found its way into their own cook pots. Placing a grimy dish of half-cooked gristle in front of us, they would retire to the cushioned splendour of an adjacent room where they entertained their guests with delicacies.

I put my luggage into the bedroom, splashed across the bathroom floor to the inevitably leaking WC and back and joined the rest. We went straight to the "laboratories." Inder had found an ideal place, a low brick building with a corrugated iron roof. Inside it consisted of a corridor, from which opened, through bolted, wooden-slatted doors, some five or six rooms. They had been designed as pigsties, the floors of rough concrete with deep gullies round the edge, filled now with dust and rubble. Glassless windows looked out on to a small farmyard, on one side of which were more stables. Nobody had been there in years.

The place was a turmoil. Men were sweeping and sprinkling the floors at the same time, pushing everything into the already blocked-up gullies. Someone was trying to fix up a wooden pole for a drip stand. The chief problem seemed to be the electricity supply, for which no provision had evidently been necessary in the original building. The solution was to tap the bare supply cables that ran at roof height in the road in front of the building. From a rickety pair of steps, two men were engaged in hooking two wires from the cables, gingerly manipulating the bare ends of the wires with long, crooked sticks. The piratical supply of electricity was led into the first room, where a crude patchboard of sockets had been constructed. This was to be the haemodynamics lab in which we deployed our apparatus—the pressure transducer taped to the drip stand, alongside it the manometer system and the cardiac output computer. On the other side of the room was Roberto's arrangement of centrifuge, homogeniser, and pressure cooker.

Up the corridor a smell of formalin started to escape from the room where Donald and David were organizing themselves for histology. David's hands had already acquired the lurid yellow colour from the Bouin's fluid that would distinguish him for the rest of the expedition.

The transport of picric acid for the Bouin's fluid had proved a problem. As it may be explosive, airlines do not look favourably on it. In the end, Inder had smuggled it in on his flight from Chandigarh without saying anything—a Sikh carrying explosives across terrorist-ridden Punjab.

Now we were invited into the farmyard for tea and sweet cakes. It was the first occasion to sit and relax with our new friends. A cuckoo called across the roof tops; but the rest of the birdsong was exotic, with sudden outbursts of pure Messiaen. While we were sitting, the gates opened and a boy drove in a group of sheep and goats—our sheep, our goats!

Happy with the day's preparations and full of enthusiasm for tomorrow, we piled into the institute car to go out to the Shalimar Moghul Gardens. Indian buses and trains are famous for overcrowding; we were now to find that private cars were susceptible to the same problems. But the gardens were delightful—the "abode of love," created by the Emperor Jahangir for his queen, Nur Jahan, under the purple shadow of the foothills of the Himalayas. We strolled up through flower beds of roses lining each side of a long straight waterway, pausing at each pavilion to enjoy the waterfall and the ever-expanding view. Away from the watercourse, the gardens extended into a less formal parkland where long-nosed Kashmiri families were picnicking in the evening shadows of the enormous cynar trees.

It was already getting dark when we returned to the car and its waiting chauffeur. He was upsmoothing his gray military moustache.

"Yes, Sahib. Yes, Sahib," as he opened each door.

A little later and we were drinking Indian whiskey and watching the sun go down over the pearl-pink waters of the lake from which three tall poplars appeared to be supporting the darkening sky.

The male-voiced choir from the local mosque was in full throat when we returned home. It seemed as if they were singing all through the night, their chanting filtering through into my consciousness every time I stirred from sleep. They were singing for the Eid, as we were to discover.

## June 6

And here we are in the outhouse, waiting to start. Brilliant shafts of sunlight through the window holes pierce the gloom of the room. Inder is checking the pressure recorders and the cardiac output equipment. Roberto is in the opposite corner fiddling with the wiring for the homogeniser and centrifuge, lifting the lid of the liquid nitrogen container to allow a few reassuring wisps of smoke to escape, starting up the boiler-steriliser we stole from the Animal Husbandry Unit. I am opening the lurid purple and pink notebook that I bought in Rymans back in London and into which would go all the haemodynamic data. I am thinking at this all-too-late moment about the numbering and coding system for the animals. Important to standardise. I decide on Animal, followed by Place, followed by Sequential Number. And at that moment in walks Sheep Kashmir One. (Afterward Inder will point out that Ladakh is also part of Kashmir. But that's how it has to stay. "We're biologists, not geographers," I tell myself.)

Sheep Kashmir One is content. I see her now through the first page of that lurid notebook and, behind the scribble that tells me she had a mean pulmonary arterial pressure of 16 mmHg and a cardiac output of 3.1 L/min and weighed 15.9 kg, her gentle, trusting face looks through to me. So, throughout the ages, she has fulfilled her sacrificial role.

"And Isaac spoke to Abraham his father and said, 'My father!' And he said, 'Here I am, my son.' And he said, 'Behold the fire and the wood, but where is the lamb for the burnt offering?'"

But now her disconnected head looks up vacantly from the bloody floor down the corridor and on a table covered with American cloth her heart and lungs are being taken out of her body. Donald is standing back, his transparent green plastic tear-off apron tied tightly round his abdomen. His shirt sleeves are rolled up, and his rubber-gloved hands are holding a lobe of lung into which David pours fixative through a brown plastic funnel that we found just in time in a stall in Delhi.

In a month or two she will undergo a further transfiguration, and Donald will meet her again as a lacework pattern of pink and blue, as he looks down the microscope in the sitting room of a Liverpool home carefully protected from any interruption from the telephone. And the final transformation will be into numbers— numbers of cells, thickness of arteries. And that is how Sheep Kashmir One will pass into history in the statistical tables of a seldom-read learned journal. It is because of this, because the black and white numbers will never give any idea of the colour and smell of the real experience, that I am sitting in my bedroom, trying to write it all down.

But will she? A few hours later we are sitting in the farmyard, with not very adequately washed hands, drinking tea and eating the cake and bread provided by our Kashmiri friends. There has been one alarm in the haemodynamics stable, when there was an intermittent failure of the current. After a few moments of panic, we found a bird outside trying to dislodge one of the wires from the overhead cable with his beak. But, apart from this, everything has gone smoothly. So everybody is happy in the sun. Sheep and goats with the mark of the vampire on the left side of their necks are wandering round among the party, sharing some of the cake. On the back of one goat is perched an enormous raven, trying to reach down to peck at the dried clot of blood.

And, at this moment, we find that we

have been studying the wrong sheep. Sheep Kashmir One, all for Hecuba. There is a long and serious talk with the men from the Sheep Institute who promise to provide us, the next day, with the same breed as the breed we shall be comparing at high altitude in Ladakh.

Meantime, we have to tidy up and clean ourselves up for a formal invitation to attend the speech given by Mr. Mukwalla, a member of the cabinet, to the Medical Institute. I have let us in for this and am not too popular.

## June 7

I woke at dawn and checked that the battery had recharged during the night. Through the hole in the wall of the shower, the sky outside was powder blue. Beyond the pebble-dash residences of the compound and over the concrete water reservoir was a distant glimpse of snow-topped mountains.

We managed only one goat before it was time to go and lecture to the Sheep Husbandry Unit. Scanty curtains had been drawn halfway across the windows through which streamed the sunshine. A dusty hand-operated projector was brought and various complicated systems of wiring and junction boxes were tried out before a dull red light appeared on its side and it was pointed toward a large blackboard. After consultation, it was agreed that the blackboard would serve better to cover one of the windows, and the projector could now be seen to produce a dim yellow patch on the soup-coloured wall. Focusing revealed the faint outlines of my first slide, and we were off, only an hour late. Donald's slides must have been thicker than mine, and David had great difficulty getting them in and out. Time was running out, and we were getting dangerously close to our midday lecture at the Medical Institute, so Donald drastically abbreviated his talk. David

would break a couple of fingernails getting one slide out and take ages putting the next one in.

"We'll leave that one out," Donald would say, as its faint outline appeared on the wall.

So, after another minute and one more yellow fingernail broken, the next image would appear, probably to be rejected also. Payment for the lectures—the promise of four cows.

Things at the Medical Institute went better. The meeting was in the hall where Mr. Mukwalla had spoken the evening before. The same two high-backed, leather-covered chairs stood on the podium, as if for royalty. The audience was keen, asking many real questions as well as the usual rhetorical ones. Lunch in Dr. Khuroo's office afterward was attended by the director. He had been rather obtrusively called out of the beginning of our meeting and was apologising.

"Oh, we all use that trick," I felt able to say and he laughed.

On the centre of the dinner table rested a fly swat. Every now and then, one of the diners would reach for it and deal some mercifully ineffective blow at a fly on the food. Often the fly would have moved off by the time the diner had the swat in his hand, whereupon he would stay holding the swat poised in the air, waiting for the next target to settle within range. So frustrating had been the marksmanship that Inder, on impulse, snatched the swat out of the hand of one of our hosts and took a great swipe at Dr. Khuroo's chest.

After the laughter, the director told the story of his professor who was "becoming a bit thin on top."

"He was bald as a coot," interjected Khuroo.

"You may put it that way. In any event, on one occasion, he felt a fly on his head while he was wearing sterile gloves, and asked the nurse to swat it. The poor girl was terrified, but the professor was getting frantic with the tickle. So she took a swipe, which hit him on the ear. Nobody remembered whether this dislodged the fly."

Five goats after lunch. Toward the end there was a power cut. My first reaction was to run outside to see if there was another bird on the line but, this time, it was a genuine failure. Luckily our emergency batteries allowed us to finish the haemodynamics. The pathologists were unaffected but Roberto needed electricity to finish processing his specimens, so we took them back to the residence.

There was another blow for Roberto. The liquid nitrogen container, which Inder had filled in Chandigarh, had given up. All the nitrogen had evaporated, and the specimens for measuring catecholamines had thawed. There was no more liquid nitrogen to be found in Srinagar, so we had to give up this part of the project. Luckily, the lung extracts for peptides could be salvaged by keeping them on ice. So a thermos flask was put on the shopping list for tomorrow.

We left late in the afternoon for another black-hole-of-Calcutta ride to the memorial of Sheikh Abdullah. As we arrived, the lake was turning an iridescent purple, lighter than the sky. Two or three shikara fishing boats were etched in black and on the far shore stood a huddle of brown village houses. From the verandah of an adjacent house came the voice of Ritchie Benaud on the radio. India was ten runs behind England, with two wickets in hand. We dined at the new conference centre. Exquisite food but, beyond all, the enchanting music of the Santoor.

## June 8

David and Inder were up early filming the animals. The men broke off branches from the acacia trees in the farmyard, enticing the sheep and goats to come into view of the cameras. Always, of course, the wrong animal got there first.

Mericfully, the correct breed of sheep had now been found, and we started in earnest. We were in a hurry, since all our plans had been upset by the unforeseen arrival of the Eid.

Kashmir is predominantly Muslim and the Eid Festival is the end of the period of Ramadan, during which the faithful neither eat nor drink from sunrise to sunset. So Eid is a day to look forward to. There will be feasting, fireworks, and a general holiday for two days. It was a break in our tight programme we had not expected, made worse by the extraordinary uncertainty of the actual date of the Eid. The festival is pronounced by the Imam after two reliable men tell him that they have seen the new moon. The world of Islam is also the birthplace of an astronomy surely capable of predicting the precise phases of the moon for millennia to come. And yet all commercial and social life will hover in uncertainty, waiting for the day on which the Imam decides. Eid is already over in Mecca, they say, and the Pakistanis are searching for the new moon from helicopters.

Our original plans had been to leave Srinagar on the tenth and travel by road to Leh, a two-day journey over the mountains. But, as we left London, we learned that the passes were still blocked with snow, and so, instead, Inder had managed to get us on a flight into Leh, leaving on the twelfth. These extra two days would now be valuable. On the other hand, we had already lost one day doing the wrong sheep, and we still had no definite news about the cattle. They also posed a problem. Although Kashmir is almost entirely Muslim, the holiness of the cow is a matter of national sensitivity, and we were not at all sure whether we would get permission for histology.

I suppose all these uncertainties lent a tension to the morning's work. Also it was hot, the flies had found us, it was difficult to get fresh buckets of water, and dust was everywhere. Sheep Kashmir Five came in baaing loudly in answer to calls from her sister in the farmyard outside. This shouted conversation between them continued while we were trying to make our measurements and was wrecking the results. The only solution was to bring the sister in, so a man was sent out to invite her to join us. I suppose it was inevitable that he picked up the first sheep he laid hands on and the two sisters continued their conversation through the window. Finally the real sister was brought in, nuzzled up to the Kashmir Five with a short baa, and then all was quiet.

Turning round in a room strewn with unswept sheep shit to rinse my hands in a bowl of blood-stained water matted with dirty sheep shearings, I looked for a precious box of Kleenex brought with foresight from London.

"Where on earth's my . . .? Roberto, have you got my Kleenex?"

"No, not me. Donald, he took it."

"Bloody hell!"

"I'm sorry. I tell him he can have it." And then, "He needed it for the toilet. Diarrhoea, I think." And Roberto turned back to his water bath.

Sheep Kashmir Six had now come in, treading with indifference through the shit and blood of her predecessor. Abandoning the conversation, I knelt down to put a finger on the bottom of its jugular to make it visible for Inder's needle and trying, at the same time, to keep the workbook out of the mess.

"What's its age?"

The man holding it pulls its lips apart and, looking at its teeth in a knowing sort of a way says, "Two years."

I know that he is guessing and write it down. Two years.

"Weight?"

"We do after."

The catheter is now in the pulmonary artery and Inder is shouting out numbers.

"Pulmonary artery twenty-three, sixteen, eighteen. Twenty-four, sixteen,

eighteen. Twenty-four, fifteen, seventeen."

I try to get it down before the sound of the words dies from my ears. "OK. Give me the wedge."

Inder inflates the balloon on the catheter, and we both watch the pressure tracing as it falls.

"There. What about that?"

"That looks OK. Wedge eleven?"

"Wedge eleven. No, ten. No, eleven."

I write eleven, smudging across the page the drop of saline that has fallen on to it from the drip stand.

"Ready for the cardiac output?" Inder asks.

I switch on the computer and check it, then draw up 10 ml of glucose-saline into a syringe from the bag on the drip stand and hand it to Inder. I press the start button of the computer and shout, "Start!"

Inder opens the three-way tap and injects the glucose-saline as fast as he can. We wait for the value of the cardiac output to come up on the computer, while Inder hands me back the empty syringe.

"Two point nine," I say and draw up another syringe full, expel the bubbles, and hand it back to him.

I press the button again, shout "Start!" and hurriedly write 2.9 in the book while Inder is injecting.

The ritual of pressures and cardiac outputs is repeated twice more, by which time my fingers and the pen and the page are sticky with the glucose solution. As Sheep Kashmir Six trots out, Sheep Kashmir Seven passes it in the doorway.

I blow up.

"No more animals in here until the floor is cleaned and I have the weight."

"Wait?"

"No! Weight."

I mime a pair of balances and get a blank look. And then the right word comes:

"Kilograms. Kayjee."

"Ah! Kayjee." And off he goes.

"And, please, somebody clean the floor."

Somebody comes in with a piece of corrugated cardboard and scrapes the droppings into the gully. I turn with hands sticky with glucose and blood to find a shallow layer of something like soup in the plastic wash-hand bowl. Still no Kleenex.

White with anger, I shout, "No more experiments until we've got some clean water," and stride down the corridor to the pathologist's room.

"Where's my Kleenex?"

Donald looks up from the lung he is holding.

"We've used it all," he says and points to the buckets of formalin, in which his specimens are wrapped in tissue, and to the empty Kleenex box.

I explode.

"We had to have it," he says. "We just had to have it."

But we all felt better after lunch. All the physiological studies on the sheep and goats were done. Donald and David had all their specimens ready for trimming next morning. There was growing confidence that tomorrow would be Eid, and Dr. Khuroo was making arrangements for us to stay the two days of holiday on a houseboat. This could still leave a day to study the cows before flying to Leh.

This afternoon Donald and David were anxious to do some background filming in Srinagar. Roberto and I wanted to look at the shops, and Roberto was desperate for nose drops for his maturing cold. So we all crammed into the Sheep Institute Ambassador and went into town.

The Ambassador has become one of the symbols of India. It is a copy of the old Morris Oxford, which had been produced in England just after the war. The Indian reincarnation lives forever, rattling over the continent in a state of geriatric bliss, kept going by the devoted care of human attendants who are content to make spare parts by hand.

I took to Srinagar. Wooden houses with corrugated iron roofs sprawl round the lakes. If you can cast off Western associations of corrugated iron, you find the effect light and elegant, the fresh metallic sheen of the iron shading off into rust. The local architects seemed to be going through a vogue of making the top of one side of the roof overlap the other. At the same time, they put a gentle upward curve to the lower edge, which gives the roof an attractive lambda shape, seen end-on.

The driver had just extricated us from some impossible traffic jam through the market and was honking his way across a low bridge dense with humanity and clapped-out automobiles when Donald and David decided they needed to get out. The driver threw up his hands in despair when Inder explained. He stopped just beyond the policeman the other side of the bridge, more to argue the toss than to let Donald and David down. But he had underestimated the Liverpuddlians; they knew absolutely that that was the place for them.

As David opened the rear door to extricate Donald from the front seat, the policeman arrived. He was not pleased. This immediately put the driver in the opposite camp and more than ever on his mettle. How could the police possibly stand in the way of so distinguished a scientist and his film crew making an important film of the city?

While the battle of words was building up, Inder quietly told Donald and David to get lost but to be sure to be back in the same spot by six. We watched them disappear along the edge of the river. As the driver-policeman battle died down, the driver returned to his seat, the policeman shrugged his shoulders, and we moved on to the shops.

First things first; we found drops to unclog Roberto's dripping nose. While he sat in the back of the shop, dropping in massive quantities. Inder and I pored over the small print of boxes of cold remedies. Our final choice was Actifed, which Roberto took gratefully and with touching trust.

Having sorted out the urgent medical problems to the best of our ability, we wandered off in search of a thermos flask down alleys strewn with tied up chickens. A friend of Roberto's who owned a shop in Bologna had asked him to bring back some Pashmina shawls to sell. The important thing was that they could be pulled through a ring. That is what the Italian ladies wanted, and that is what every Kashmiri in town wanted to demonstrate to us.

Escaping down some narrow alley, we found ourselves in the carpet zone and amidst captivating Kashmiri carpets with patterns of flowers and animals. We went for the animals, refusing to be interested if anything else was shown.

"No flowers. Where are your animals?"

And a look of despair filmed over a pair of crafty Kashmiri eyes as their owner foraged through arm-aching, dusty piles to find the animals. "Stupid buggers. Why don't they take flowers like everybody else. Animals!"

At last we found what we wanted, covered with primitive child-embroidered lions and birds and snakes and elephants, none of which had ever been seen in Kashmir. One for Roberto and one for me. Except that Roberto knew that he wanted one and I didn't think I did. My skepticism beat down the price until we reached titration point—175 rupees—at which the merchant turned his back on us. Roberto, sitting on a pile of carpets, responded with equal eloquence to this gesture by tilting his head back and ever so deliberately instilling two more drops into his nose. For the moment we left them and bought a dusty thermos flask and some ripe mangoes before getting back to the Ambassador.

It was past time to pick up Donald and David, and the driver swung the Ambassador round and headed for the bridge at full throttle, which approximated thirty miles per hour. By now the traffic had thinned and our turbaned policeman advanced to meet us all smiles. But no sign of the professor, he said. And, of course, we could wait. Just pull in a little way from the end of the bridge.

We sat waiting, watching the darkening sky. Every so often our policeman friend (as he now was) would stroll back from the bridge to try and work out the complex family relation, which, it now appeared, existed between him and the driver. Impatience gave way to anxiety and back to impatience and we turned for home. The driver was in a hurry, short tempered. Perhaps also the family link with the policeman had not proved as profitable as he had hoped. Pedestrians scattered before him as he did a Monte Carlo through crowded streets half lit in the twilight. A child's elbow was struck a glancing blow but neither that nor our shouting could stop him until he got back to the residence.

And there, of course, were Donald and David, halfway through their third bottle of beer.

## June 9

Was it Eid? Or wasn't it?

Had the chief Mullah seen the moon last night as he climbed to his turret? Or hadn't he?

Our only sources of information were the telephone, which was in one of its recurrent phases of nonoperation, or the houseboy.

Me: Is today Eid?
HB: Id? What ees?
Me: Eeeeeed. We're not Jungians.
HB: Yes, Sir.
Me: Is it Eeeeeed today?
HB: Mullah look at moon.

Me: Yes, but did he see the moon?

HB: No Sir.

Five minutes later:

Roberto: Is it Eid today?

HB: Yes Sir.

Roberto: Not tomorrow?

HB: Yes Sir.

Me: Do you support Arsenal or Tottenham?

HB: Yes Sir.

But it was. HB went to find a taxi to take Donald and David to trim their specimens but came back with a more than usually hopeless look. "No taxi, Sahib."

So we went out into the street and found a rickshaw for one rupee. They returned soon with Inder in a military jeep that he had somehow commandeered. We packed enough small things for two or three days and escaped to Nagin Lake (Fig. 2).

Where boatmen are resting beside their shikaras.

The body of a shikara is long and slender, turning up to a point at each end, a little like a gondola. A large straw or canvas canopy supported by four curtained posts curves across the boat, sloping downward from prow to stern (Fig. 3).

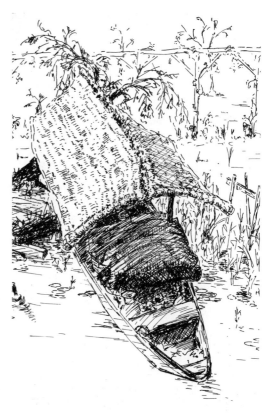

**Figure 3.** Old shikara beached beside our houseboat.

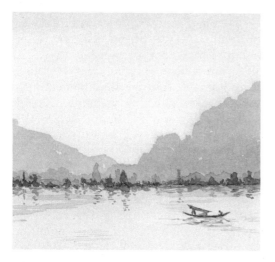

**Figure 2.** View across Nagin Lake from the houseboat.

Inside is a mass of luxurious gaudy cushions. We decide on two. The boatmen take a last puff of their hookahs and pull us with their heart-shaped oars across the blue lake. Inder isn't sure which houseboat was ours. We are taken first to one close by, and we enter astonished up wooden steps and across an elaborately carved verandah. We pass on through palatial sitting and dining rooms to a long corridor from which open four luxurious bedrooms.

Yes, please. We wanted this one. But Inder took us back to the boats. "It is not for us," he said.

Then, from the boat, he began bargaining. The owner shook his head in anger and disbelief. "Go!" shouted Inder to the oarsmen, and we were gliding once more across the lake toward a group of four palaces, no less imposing than the one we were regretting. We climbed the steps into a clone of the first and took tea and doughnuts while waiting for the owner.

A miracle. He was expecting us.

We sorted ourselves out in elaborately carved cedar wood bedrooms smelling like cigar boxes, cleaned up in our private bathrooms, and emerged to find the table laid by the houseboy who had decorated it with patterns of petals and WELLCOME traced in coloured rice grains. The magical insight behind the misspelling did not go unnoticed, and we wondered whether we should send a photo back to our sponsors at the Wellcome Trust.

## June 10

I woke early and went up onto the flat roof of the houseboat. The lake was covered by a sheet of mist through which emerged the massive chinar and poplars on the far shore. Beyond them the eastern hills floated in midair, and beyond again diamonds of snow sparkled high up in the first sun. From across the valley floated the sound of waking voices and the cuckoo.

I sat sketching in a rush before it all changed. It was a landscape from which all colour had been drained, a Chinese painting in grey and white. But, within minutes, the sun had topped the mountains, dissolving the mists and pouring the day's colours into the darkness of the valley. At which point I lay back in the growing warmth and dozed off until the heat forced me down to the shade of the verandah.

Throughout the day shikaras floated across the lake bringing Coca Cola, carpets, fruit, lacquered papier-maché. We read or chattered or talked about the great mystery of hypoxia or worked out the results of the previous days. Donald sat hours in his room watching a kingfisher that used his window sill as an observa-

tion and jumping-off post. The samovar was in constant use.

Throughout the afternoon there had been intensive preparations in the adjacent house on shore and in the dining room of the houseboat for the great traditional Kashmiri meal, the Wazwan, which was planned for that evening. As the sun was setting, we were joined by the proprietor, his father and brother, and by Dr. Khuroo. Out of the tiny kitchen the first of the thirty courses of the Wazwan started to be brought out—gushtaba lamb meatballs stuffed with paté, grilled tabaqmazh reeking of coriander, and karam spinach. So anxious were the sweating serving boys that the courses began to appear too fast to be eaten, and a pause had to be called before the feast could continue into the night. When the eating was done, hours later, we lay back on our cushions while the proprietor's brother and a group of friends sang Kashmiri songs, accompanied by a portable harmonium ventilated by lifting the lid up and down and by a lutelike stringed instrument, the rababa, played brilliantly by the houseboy.

## June 11

Leaving paradise, we returned to clear up the mess at the Sheep Institute. Inder had at last gotten permission to study cattle but autopsies would not be done until September, when they were necessary for the veterinary students. Donald and David stayed in Srinagar while the rest of us went out with a cattle doctor to the farm. We traveled nearly an hour through valleys spread with rice fields, each surrounded by a thin mud wall about a foot high and flooded with water. The young rice shoots were bright green, about four inches high. It was transplantation time, our Kashmiri colleague explained. Men and women waded barefoot in the water, planting the young seedlings in tufts a few inches apart. In other fields pairs of oxen, joined together by a wooden yoke, pulled wooden ploughs through the water. The whole effect was as if the countryside were a weirdly fragmented or cloissonéed mirror on which green dust had settled. Or a microscopic view of some scaly, metallic martian with his day's growth of green beard yet unshaven.

We skirted the Lake Manasbal before reaching the farm. The massive iron gates were shut. A notice bore the name of the institution, under which was written, "Exotic cattle breeding." While I was pondering whether, in this construction, it was the cattle or the breeding that was exotic, two men had appeared in answer to our motor horn and were trying with their fingers to undo the padlock and chain that seemed to hold the gates shut.

"Why don't they use the key?" I asked.

"Oh no!" the driver said. "You see, there is no key. The lock is there just to look good."

Then he got out of the car, motioned the men aside, and with firm and decisive movements of his fingers pulled the whole arrangement apart.

We drove round a large corrugated iron hay barn to a two-roomed concrete building beside which was a metal cattle restrainer. Inder was for working inside, but I persuaded him that it would be better to use the restrainer. Our first subject confirmed that decision. He was a two-year-old bull who was more scared than angry and kept trying to leap or charge out of the restrainer. Inder sat at his head, cool as cool, trying to protect his precious catheter from being mangled.

"Its only your jugular," he was explaining to the bull.

The rest of the animals were ladies. They submitted willingly to the procedure, even seeming to enjoy it, their heads on Inder's knee, getting a stroking from time to time. The size of the animals got progressively smaller as the farm hands tried to choose the easiest to handle. But the third had to be rejected because she was too small and we broke off for ten minutes while the unhappy men went off to find a bigger one.

According to my workbook we had started at 12:41. At first the sun had been covered by thin cloud, but soon it came out at full strength. Flies swarmed in from nowhere at the smell of blood and sweat. And then the cardiac output machine started to play up, with a succession of crazy results. The sun had warmed the injectate up to over 27°C, so we cooled off another bottle in a bucket of water. But still the trouble persisted. Then the machine started to tell us that it was not connected to the catheter (but it was). We tried two other catheters before deciding that the instrument had sunstroke. Perhaps working outside was not so clever; so we took the instrument inside, with the wires attaching it to the catheter trailing out through the glassless window. Roberto stayed inside to control it, while we shouted to him through the window when we were ready. But it still didn't work. Heat, flies, shouting, bad results all contributed to the tension of the afternoon. Then a large, fat cow upped its tail and produced a jet of urine a fireman would have been proud of that turned our operating floor into a wash of mud. Roberto heard the noise, stopped honking his nose, looked out through the window and burst into a laugh that sent us all into convulsions; and tension was broken.

By five o'clock we had finished six cattle and tidied up and were on our way back, passing groups of slim Kashmiri girls on the road, also returning from their day's work, carrying pitchers or baskets of rice plants on their heads. Here the river Sind snakes its way through rice fields and cherry orchards and plantations of willows. Kashmir is the world's source of cricket bats, and, only that morning, the

296 • THE PULMONARY CIRCULATION AND GAS EXCHANGE

news had reached us that India had beaten England by five wickets for the first time at Lord's *Sic transit gloria . . .* When Lord Curzon had word that the English had taken the Sind territory, he telegraphed his famous Latin pun back to the India Office in Whitehall: *Pecavi,* I have sinned.

Throughout the day Roberto had been tormented by the growing conviction that he wanted one of those animal rugs we had turned down the day before in Srinagar. So, as soon as we reached the residence, we went back into town.

"We're back," Roberto announced as we entered the shop.

The merchant shook his head. "You here before?"

"Yes. We saw two carpets with animals on."

"Carpets with animals?"

It was clear that we had come to the wrong shop. We looked at each other, edging back toward the street.

"How much were they?" the merchant shouted.

"A hundred and fifty rupees," Roberto lied.

"No. One hundred and seventy-five." And that is what we paid.

## June 12

Low morning clouds brought apprehensions that our plane might be unable to land at Leh, always a tricky landing in a route that was handled by only a few pilots. (Rajiv Ghandi had been one.) By 7:30 we were all packed, batteries charged overnight and equipment in good order. Our luggage filled the ambulance that Dr. Khuroo had sent, leaving room only for David to act as guard. Donald, Roberto, and I went ahead in an Ambassador. Calling for Inder, we got our first intimation of troubles ahead.

"Plane delayed twenty minutes," he said. "There's no hurry. I'll follow in ten minutes."

By the time we got to the airport the delay had extended to midday—"or after." Rumour was that it was raining so hard in Chandigarh, where the incoming plane had to make a stop, that the pilot had turned back to Delhi. As we lined up our seventeen pieces of luggage, Derek and Peggy Bergel joined us. Inder moved off through the crowd. By the time he returned he had given two cardiac consultations, on the strength of which we would be allowed to take all our equipment in the cabin. Our gross excess weight was tactfully ignored at the check-in desk, and the boarding cards in our hands gave hope.

I sat calculating the results from the cattle. Rumours floated in the air around me. The plane had just left Delhi. The plane was still on the ground. They had decided to fly straight to Srinagar, leaving out the passengers for Chandigarh. The pilot was ill. Kashmir Cow Number Four, pulmonary artery mean pressure 35 mmHg. Weather conditions at Leh were impossible. The airport computer had broken down. Milky sweet tea came and went.

As the morning dragged on, the rumours became increasingly hysterical. It was almost a relief when the cancellation was announced. Inder was first in the queue at the ticket counter, then he let me take over there while he went quickly into town to the Indian Air office to see what could be done about tomorrow's flight. Elbowed from back and sides, I stood firm while the clerk laboriously made out vouchers for accommodation overnight and returned our tickets, ignoring the mass of other tickets waved in front of him or placed on his desk. Meanwhile the others had been collecting back all our luggage.

We stood waiting outside for the bus that would take us to our hotel. A fight between two taxi drivers relieved the monotony. A crowd gathered. Sides were taken. Police in red turbans arrived and also took sides. A war was beginning. Derek was telling us horror stories of the violence after the British left. There was this white family up the Kulu Valley who hid a group of Muslims in the cellar of their house. . . . And then the war was suddenly over.

After the first hour, our periodic enquiries were met with the reassurance that the bus was on its way. After the second hour we ducked under the check-in counter and pushed into the manager's office. We were not alone. A crowd of angry tourists was menacing Peter Sellers, who sat at the manager's desk promising this and that. His assistant was on the phone shouting, "Hallo." Eventually Sellers told us that the bus was coming and we had better be quick if we were to catch it, and we hurried out.

A half an hour later we were back in the office.

"I promise you," Sellers shouted. "I promise you. If bus not come in ten minutes, we put you in taxis. We are working only for you. Only for you, you must understand."

All those Olympic watches registered the exact second, and precisely ten minutes later we were back.

"I promise you," shrieked Sellers, his hands flying in all directions. "If bus not come in five minutes, I order taxis. We are working only for you."

"Bloody hell!"

"Look, mister!"

By some miracle of persuasion we found ourselves outside again.

Five minutes further on all hell broke loose in the manager's office.

"I promise you sincerely. Sincerely I promise you. If bus not here in ten minutes, you have my own bus. I work only for you, sincerely."

The fact that no private bus could be seen on the airport was not even an issue. Another war, this time of international proportions was about to break out.

The situation was saved by the arrival of the bus. Rain sweeping in from the south also helped to cool tempers. Within half an hour we were at the Broadway Hotel.

We hated it at first sight. The dining room was rendered uninhabitable by the hyperamplification system of a grotty group playing Western music, and I yearned for a pair of wire cutters. Outside, the rain dripped into a swimming pool beside a shack on which had been written the enigmatic sign, "Unndres Coffee House."

Most of the day was taken up by convoluted discussions about travel. Inder's contacts with the Indo-Tibetan Border Police were helpful. He had gotten the promise of the two official seats reserved for the ITBP on tomorrow's flight. There might be other government seats free, and we were first on the waiting list for them. The alternative to flying was to go over land. This had been our original plan. It normally takes two days, with an overnight stop in Kargil. The problem was the Zoji La Pass. This is normally open from the end of May; but the winter had been particularly severe and a hundred and ten feet of snow had fallen. Some of it had been recent, to which the mountains round Srinagar bore testimony. Whether the pass was clear was another source of conflicting rumours. We decided to try first for tomorrow's flight, and get all the equipment and as many people as possible on it. The rest would either wait for the next flight or take their chance by road. The trouble was that the next flight was in four days, and time was getting short. During our expedition in Leh the year before we had met people who had had to wait two weeks for a flight in.

We waited until the Broadway Quartet took its break and dashed into the dining room for a quick supper, but got waylaid by the manager who wanted to discuss his right bundle branch block. Finally we escaped carrying our puddings.

## June 13

The day's start was inauspicious.

"No breakfast," David said as Roberto and I struggled down with our baggage, watched by the porters. "Breakfast starts at 7:30."

"But the Broadway Manifesto says 7:00."

"We told them that. They said it's a mistake."

"Well, well."

The cashier came up with a pink scrap of paper.

"Twenty-four rupees for Limca in room," he said.

"Where's our breakfast?"

"Breakfast at 7:30."

"No, 7:00." Derek reached to a pile of handouts and showed him the official meal timetable. The cashier shrugged.

"OK. We'll take the Limca in lieu of breakfast."

An ITBP truck took us to the airport, where were were first in the queue. Donald and David were checked in. Then a large group of German tourists turned up.

"Not much hope," said Inder. "On Indian Airlines you lose your money if you don't show up."

But, eventually, around the time that the flight should have closed, we heard that we would also get on. But why didn't they check us in? A fat Sikh came stumbling in with a battered suitcase, desperately agitated that he might miss the plane, but he couldn't attract any attention. Nobody seemed at all interested any more.

Looking back, we should have known. Within an hour a delay had been announced. By eleven o'clock the pilot told Inder that there was no hope and left for his hotel. We had a quick council of war, decided to take the overland route, and left just as they were announcing the cancellation of the flight.

Inder and I went by jeep with an ITBP

captain to cash in our air tickets and find something to take us over land to Leh, while the others had lunch at the ITBP headquarters. The Indian Airlines office was swarming with discontented travelers through which Inder cut a characteristically direct path to the manager's office. The manager's advice was clear. There was no prospect of a flight for two to three days, and he said we should take the road. By this time the captain had found out the going rate for transport by road, so that we were in a position to bargain. Jeeps were scarce, it seemed. We decided on two Ambassadors for the passengers and a jeep to carry the luggage and be ready to help in the likely event that the Ambassadors got stuck. In the centre of town we found a parking lot, at one end of which was a taxi office. In the middle was parked a good-looking jeep with its Ladakhi driver beside it. And, yes, he was interested. But not at the price we were offering. We moved over to a group of Ambassadors, but word of our interest had already gotten there. Forward stepped a young Kashmiri with the eyes of a goat, offering his Ambassador and that of a friend. We went to inspect his battered property. The tread on the front wheels was less than a micrometer thick. We took it, on condition he changed the front tyres. His friend's Ambassador was in tip-top condition, he promised us. But tip top. No problems. Meanwhile the Ladakhi jeep driver had come round to our price and we went over to the shack to work out the finances with the boss.

The office was empty.

"Boss busy some place," said goat-eyes.

Opening an inner door, we found him stretched out on a couch and not too happy to be woken up in the middle of the day. But every detail was finally agreed upon, and Inder handed over a sum of money, receiving in return a complicated document. The drivers went off to get their belongings for the journey, promising to be at the ITBP headquarters at three o'clock.

By some miracle they were. And in next to no time we were on the road. And in next to no time later goat-eyes' friend's Ambassador had had its first puncture. One denuded wheel was exchanged for another, and we were off again. It was clear that this Ambassador, carrying Donald and David, was the least road-worthy; so it was decided that it should lead the convoy, goat-eyes carrying me and Inder in the middle and the jeep coming up behind with Roberto. In this way we could be reasonably sure to keep together, and the jeep would always be available if one of the Ambassadors broke down. The decision proved unpopular with the two drivers behind, who had to be restrained from overtaking the leading Ambassador and hareing off into the distance.

We journeyed in the afternoon sun along the valley of the Sind, first through rice fields and then through apple orchards. White roses flowered wild by the roadside. From time to time we would meet a truck or bus coming in to Srinagar covered with its garish and ornate decorations and slogans. "Rust in God" still haunts me. But none of them seemed likely to have come all the way from Ladakh.

It was difficult to tell whether our first stop, in the village of Kangan, was by design or whether it just happened that the leading Ambassador had its second flat tyre there. It was on Donald's side, and, after the wheel had been changed, the driver blamed it on Donald's unacceptable weight, pointing out that the car was tilting heavily over toward Donald's side. Friendship as well as the search for truth would not allow us to accept this hypothesis. David was unconscious. The rumour was that he had taken four dramamines to knock himself out for the jour-

ney. Goat-eyes' Ambassador was also in trouble and out from some mud brick hovel arrived a mechanic to solder up the radiator, which was flopping loose.

Meanwhile we could explore Kangan. It consisted of a cluster of houses around a triangular green through which trickled a stream into which everybody seemed to have thrown their garbage. Two small bridges of planks crossed the stream. Hindi movie music blared from a shop where we found bottles of Limca for Donald. A little further up was Kangan International Haircut. To my surprise, there was also a little post office, in the darkness of which the officials broke off playing cards to serve stamps for postcards.

After everything had been put in order, we moved on up the valley, which became increasingly narrower. Forests of walnut trees gave way to pines and the wild roses changed from white to pink. After another hour the valley widened again into the broad highland pastures of Sonamarg, just beyond which would be the Zoji La Pass.

This would be a critical point. The Zoji La is only 3,500 metres high, but is on the Kashmiri side of the route, where there is abundant snowfall. The higher passes of the Ladakh side have little snow. So whether the route is open depends on the Zoji La. Bulldozers and snowploughs cut a way through the deep glacial snow of the tenuous route across the mountains, and each year portions of the road are swept away.

The first sign of the checkpoint was the tail end of a long line of trucks waiting to go through. We carried on past them and, after a further half mile, saw the barrier of the checkpoint. Jeeps, trucks, and people were strewn in the fields around. As we drew up, a massive German came up gesticulating.

"You think you are going through? We been waiting here ten hours."

Roberto wasn't impressed. He had done it before last year.

"You'll see. We'll start moving in five minutes. We wait till the convoy comes through from Dras, the other side. Then they will let us through."

The barrier was controlled by an army unit. On the verandah of a wooden shack straight out of a Western movie sat an officer and a sergeant at a rickety table. Inder went over.

"There's an army convoy coming through," he said when he came back. "But they think that one of the trucks has broken down. As soon as they are through we can move."

We put the cars in the wasteland opposite the shack and alongside two rival stores housed in broken-down sheds. They were called the Arzoo and the Zoji La. Both had the same collection of frowzy Indian biscuits and served tepid tea. After exploring the shopping centre, there was little else to do except stare up the road that would round the side of the hill toward the pass. Every now and then the sergeant would lift the receiver and wind up the phone and shout "Hallo" into it, whereupon there would be a stir of interest from the tea-stained trestles of the Arzoo and the Zoji La. After an hour a small herd of cows appeared round the bend, raising false hopes. The sun dipped down under the rim of mountains, and suddenly it was cold. We piled on woolens and waited.

Inder returned from another talk with the military. They had no idea what was going on. By now it was clear that, even if the convoy did get through, we would have to face a journey over the pass in darkness. The drivers were surprisingly confident and keen, and Inder went back to the checkpoint. We stood watching his silhouette leaning over the captain in the light of a hurricane lamp. The captain could not give permission for civilians to cross at night.

"I'll speak to the Commandant," said Inder.

Much winding of the phone and shouting "Hallo," and then the commandant was on the line, God knows where. The sergeant stood to attention as he spoke, saluting at the end of every sentence.

"Teeka Sahib."

"Teeka Sahib."

"Atcha Sahib."

"Teeka Sahib."

"Atcha Sahib."

"Atchacha Sahib."

Inder took the phone and laid it on thick to the commandant. Important foreign scientists. Vital medical research. ITBP support.

"Then, if you can't give me permission, get me the General," he shouted.

But the general was not obtainable. Some ludicrous rumour reached us that he was playing golf. By moonlight?

At that moment, the lights of the first jeep swept round the bend and halted at the barrier. The sergeant ran out to lift the pole, but the jeep was already so surrounded by the travelers that it couldn't move.

The driver leaned out of the window.

"It's OK," he said. "You have to get out and push from time to time, but you can make it." One of the army trucks had gotten stuck in the snow, and this had held everybody up.

But still the captain was adamant.

"Not tonight. Definitely. Definitely."

And there was a sudden rush back to Sonamarg to find a place to sleep. We were slow off the mark, and, when we got to the village, Inder and I cut off quickly in the darkness to a group of bungalows up the mountainside.

All beds except one had been taken, but there was room on the floor. For the moment, we accepted the exorbitant price and started to move everything, stumbling over the frosty rough grass in the darkness. Inside was electric light but no heat. Most of us had sleeping bags. Donald found himself some not too wholesome blankets and spread himself on the floor, flat on his back in suit, collar, and tie, as always.

I offered him a sleeping tablet.

"I've never taken such a thing," he said, and was snoring away before the rest of us had found our corners and the lights were out.

## June 14

The alarm woke us at three. Roberto stumbled across the room in the darkness and found the light switch. What he saw when he switched it on sent him into an attack of the giggles that lasted half an hour. Whether it was the grotesque sight of everybody strewn over the floor, or whether some particular person had prompted the flood of irrepressible laughter, we never found out. The icy air outside helped cool it. A crescent moon hung over the valley, and, below the bungalow, the cars were revving up. The Ladakhi driver had been threatened by the Kashmiris during the night, and that needed sorting out. Inder was shouting at the proprietor over the exorbitant price.

"Hilton rates for floor space. My God!"

We arrived at the checkpoint just as the sky was lighting up over the eastern ridge. The guard, shivering beside a dying hurricane lamp, lifted the barrier and we were off. We felt lucky. Normally, traffic over the pass was restricted to east–west in the morning but we had been allowed to make a dash before the convoy left Dras on the eastern side at seven.

At any time this road must be one of the loneliest in the world, but the early morning lent an extra dimension of remoteness. Until the Chinese invasion in 1959, it had been a simple track for Yak and Dzo trains over the Great Himalaya range into and out of Ladakh. Since then it has been maintained as a supply line to the forward areas. A never-ending succession of hairpin bends took us soon well above the grass line through a kaleidoscope of brown and grey and black that became progressively occupied by vast drifts and glaciers of snow. The track itself, seldom more than ten feet wide, and often much less, alternated between rock and mud rutted with the tracks of the trucks. These last held the wheels of the Ambassadors like tram lines, forcing them from time to time against boulders or ice that had avalanched down during the night. A number of times we had to get out and clear the way and lift or push the leading Ambassador. In many places the snow had been cut deeply away, so that we skidded between walls of snow and ice thirty feet high. At one such point Roberto replenished the ice in his thermos flask, which had leaked disastrously into his sleeping bag. He came back delighted with having scratched "The Heath was here" on the side of the glacier.

The pass itself was an anticlimax, a wide valley dreary with snow and rubble of stones and rock. But here we saw a group of distant figures crossing the snow—our first yaks. Down from the pass we chugged and slithered a further twenty or thirty miles along the Drass Valley to the village of Drass.

The Ambassadors tore through the village at full throttle and were turning the first hairpin the other side when we saw a man leaping up the hillside from the village at an incredible rate to intercept us on the road above. He proved to be a policeman and flagged us down with calm authority while colleagues from the village arrived in a jeep. The Kashmiri drivers were jittery. Passbooks and documents were produced, and long explanations were given requiring the support of a great deal of body language. The upshot was that the Kashmiris had no authority to carry passengers to Leh. They were supposed to report to the police as they passed through the village. That explained why they had been so keen to travel by night. Arriving in daylight, they had tried to run for it. Only they had not reckoned on the chamoislike agility of the police. They were required to attend the magistrate's court at Srinagar next week, and our much subdued convoy at last moved on. I even felt sorry for goat-eyes.

Although technically we had entered Buddhist Ladakh, the people of this "Little Baltistan" area were Muslim. Many of the women still wore the veil, and each little village had its mosque. The road continued to follow the Dras River as it flowed toward the Indus but now the landscape became increasingly precipitous. At midday we approached Kargil, set in a confluence of valleys in the middle of orchards and cultivated fields. In centuries past it had been an important crossroads of the caravans moving east into China or north into Russia and, last century, a centre of espionage in the "Great Game" between the British in India, the Russians, the Tibetans, and the Chinese. Now it is little more than a one-night stop between Srinagar and Leh.

The drivers were tired (and the Kashmiris depressed) but anxious to move on as quickly as possible to reach Leh by nightfall. By moving rapidly in the middle of the day, they said, we would avoid the many hours of delays behind the slow convoys of army trucks. Roberto said they were right. Last year he had had to stand in a queue behind a military convoy for four hours over the Namika Pass. The hurry also suited us, although it meant that we could not spare time on the remote treasures of religious art past which the route would take us. So we sped past the mud-brick houses of Kargil and were soon climbing out of the valley.

Now we were entering Tibetan Ladakh. Long-faded prayer flags fluttered from the corners of flat roofs made of osiers over mud-brick dwellings. Women were working in the fields in Ladakhi clothing. Here and there a Gompa shrine. With the strict limitation on sightseeing, we passed by the old monastery at Mul-

bekh but stopped a little further on at the Chamba statue, a gigantic four-armed effigy of the Maitreiya, the future Buddha, carved two thousand years ago in the rock by the wayside. We sat sipping bottles of Limca under the shade of a curious tree, which the monk said was a Bali tree. From a trunk of thick-crusted black bark sprouted side branches white as silver birch from which hung clusters of small green fruits like catkins.

We left the enormous statue, its eyes cast down impassively on each new century's travelers along the ancient road, and moved on up to the Namika La, the first of the two passes over the Zanskar Range and 3,700 meters high. "La" means a pass, and the name "Ladakh" itself signifies a country of passes.

Shortly after, the drivers stopped in the little village of Khangral. While we were debating why we had stopped in such an insignificant place, four boys ran out from the huddle of houses with old army cans full of petrol, which they poured into the tanks using broken bottle tops as funnels.

"Everybody knows this is the place for petrol," the drivers said. They were also worried that the engines of the Ambassadors were heating up. Goat-eyes was continually blaming me for insisting that he stay behind the leading Ambassador, complaining that the engine was overheating, and every so often, if he thought I had nodded off, he would try to make a dash for it, only to be pulled back. Now, at Khangral, they packed a mixture of straw and wet mud round the petrol pump to keep it cool.

We had to stop twice on the way up to the next pass, the Fatu La, at 4,100 metres. Each time the Kashmiris baled water out of a stream and soaked the mud packs round the petrol pumps.

"Why can't I go on?" complained goat-eyes, on one of the many occasions I stopped him from making a dash past the leader.

"You just do as I tell you."

The reply was brief and in Kashmiri.

Now we were looking east down the valley of the Indus, which would lead us to Leh. As far as the eye could see in any direction, there stretched a wilderness of mountains. To the north the Ladakh range and to the south the Zanskar. Although we were now at the highest point of the route, and much higher than the Zoji La, there was no snow. We had passed eastward, out of reach of the monsoons and into the arid climate of the world of rock and sand that is Ladakh.

After a further ten miles of hairpin bends and more water on the mud-packed petrol pumps, we stopped on a cornice; there below, halfway up the mountainside, were the roof's and chortens of the Yungdrung Monastery at Lamayuru. This gompa had been established in the tenth century, and the main building still dates from that time. Because of its great holiness, it was declared a sanctuary for criminals in the sixteenth century, and perhaps that is what goat-eyes was remembering as he led us along a ridge from which we could sit and look down on the four or five-storied central building perched on a dizzy outcropping of rock and the jumble of lower buildings and massive chortens that spilled down the side of the mountain. Prayer flags fluttered at all corners and hung from long lines joining roof to roof like broken spiders' webs. A winding track led down from the ridge past lines of chortens into a deserted courtyard. Nothing moved. Yet the little cultivated walled fields further down the mountain showed that it was still inhabited.

Soon the road swooped like a roller coaster down to the Indus, and we stopped in the little village of Khalsi, full of almond trees just to the north side of the river. We drank tea under a gigantic walnut tree, unable to face the rice and dahl that had been proffered.

This was the last lap of the journey. It was still only mid-afternoon, and we knew we would make Leh in good time. Soon we were passing a Sikh Gurudwara to which Inder and I had been taken two years before. In the temple is a large rock with an indentation in the shape of a crouching man. The holy man had been saying his prayers when the devil came up behind and hurled the rock at him. But the bionic holy man continued praying, and it was the rock that got dented. Last time we were there it had been mid-winter and the place had seemed deserted. Then, by magic, out of valleys and distant villages, a crowd of turbaned sikhs could be seen converging on the shrine.

Other familiar sights were telling us that the journey was nearly over. Spitok Monastery stood on its little mountain to our right. My daughter, Libbie, and I had watched the monks making a mandala out of coloured sands there a year before. Then there were the military camps that now spread all round Leh, principal centre of frontier defense against China. We skirted the airfield and could see the gaunt outline of the palace over the town. At the Lha-Ri-Mo Hotel we found food, beer, cold running water, and beds—which were all we needed.

## June 16

The ITBP jeep pulled up in front of the hotel shortly before nine. Donald and David had been sitting outside with their packages of equipment since eight, while cows and dzos and people wandered past on their way to and from the vegetable market on the other side of the road. A broad grin of greeting spread over the face of the jeep driver, who had been with us the previous year. We were loading the jeep when Mohammed Deen's jeep arrived carrying Inder. Roberto and Peggy and Derek and I were taking our belongings and sleeping bags, intending to stay up at Sakti. The hour and a half journey in the back of a jeep over rough tracks is romantic enough at first but becomes tedious twice a day, and the tranquility of each dawn and dusk at Sakti would more than compensate for sleeping on the floor and the lack of toilet facilities.

This year we had, once again, been generously provided with the commandant's jeep. Viewed from the outside, it was a brightly shone specimen ready for the veteran car market. The driver flicked specks of dust from the flag-holder on the front of the battered and gleaming bonnet. Inside, you entered Arabian nights. Floors and seats and walls were covered with oriental carpets; lace curtains were neatly tied back at the side and rear windows. In the front ashtray was smoking, as always, a joss stick.

We crowded into the two jeeps and set off down Leh's high street, honking imperiously at animals and humans, neither species taking much notice of the military presence. At the right angle at the bottom of the high street the elaborately turbaned policeman blew his whistle as he saw us approaching and held up impatient hordes of nonexistent traffic to let us pass. We left the town, passing the man-high prayer wheel installed since last year and the quarter-of-a-mile-long mani wall built to commemorate Queen Skalzang Dolma in the seventeenth century and covered with hundreds and thousands of smooth stones, each engraved with the mantra: "Om mani padme hum," Hail, jewel of the lotus.

The valley of the Indus, the Sengze Kha-bab, along which our route ran is a wide expanse of sand and rock. Here, the river runs from east to west, with the Ladakh range to the north. The modern road keeps to the north side of the river, but a more ancient track follows the south bank to the old monastery of Hemis. The south side of the valley is flanked by the Stok range and, behind that, the massive peaks of the Zanskar range, which separate it from the remoter Zanskar Valley. The names of the old regions are from fairy tales: to the east is Stod, to the west Sham, to the north Nubra.

It had been mid-winter when I had first come here with Inder two years before to make our plans for the expeditions. The whole valley had been yellow-grey-brown, the ground hard with frost, and the streams solid with ice. Now the intense rays of the unfiltered sun poured heat across the valley, the streams were fringed with willows and poplars, and the fields along the river green with young barley. But, at any short distance from flowing water, the sand took over, piling in immense drifts up the mountainsides. This is, paradoxically, one of the driest regions of the world, a high-altitude desert with no snow and less rain than the Sahara. Only the distant fringe of remote peaks was capped with snow.

Just past the ITBP camp, where we made a brief visit to pick up the generator, a side road leads down to a bridge that crosses the Indus to the palace of Stok. The old royal palace, standing in the shadow of the Stok Mountains, is occupied by the Rani of Stok, widow of the last king of Ladakh, Raja Kunsang Namgyal, who died in 1974. Further along the valley, in a piece of level land on the north banks of the Indus, a modern shrine records the visit of the Dalai Lama. To the north of the road at this point is a small monastery from the roof of which each evening the monks blow six-foot-long horns away from the setting sun. A little further on, we stopped at the old Royal Summer Place of Shey. It had been the castle of the first king of Ladakh, Lhachen Palgyigon, and contains a thirty-foot gilded copper statue of the Lord Buddha constructed in 1633 as a memorial to King Singyi Namgyal by his son. Behind the palace and its associated gompa, lines of chortens stretched up into the foothills. From the roof and the blackened ruined apartments of the palace, friend or foe would long be visible in either direction along the valley.

Further east, we passed the Thikse gompa, perched on its hilltop overlooking the valley. It is the largest monastery in the area. The present buildings are five hundred years old. But, centuries before that, Thikse had been an important religious centre of the ancient region of Naris, which comprised western Tibet, and the great scholar Lotsawa Rinchen Zangpo had translated the Buddhist texts from Sanskrit into Tibetan there, in an extensive monastery, the ruins of which lie scattered beside the present gompa.

At Karu there is a division of the ways. One road turns off south across the river to Hemis gompa, where the festival was in full swing. The main route continues ultimately to Manali through a zone so close to the Chinese border that it is forbidden to foreigners. We took the track leading north up the valley leading to our village of Sakti. Ruined hilltop fortresses guarded the approaches and, high up the west side, was the white monastery of Chemre. Children appeared from nowhere out of the fields and shouted and waved and tried to chase the jeeps. Soon we were bumping over the streams and rocks that had defied all attempts to make a road and into the little collection of low mud-brick houses of Sakti. For me the name had a magic long before I came to associate it with the name of the goddess, wife of Siva the destroyer.

Now we were climbing more steeply round the hillside, and there, past a line of chortens (Fig. 4) and mani walls, was our white-washed bungalow beneath the buildings and chortens and prayer flags of Tak Tok gompa stuck high up above on the cliff side.

The jeeps drew up in the circle of dry-stone walls, which formed a sort of courtyard to the bungalow and from which steps led up to the entrance and terrace. Waiting on top of them was our old friend Mohammed Singh, the ITBP cook delegated to look after us. His joy at seeing Roberto and me quite overcame all

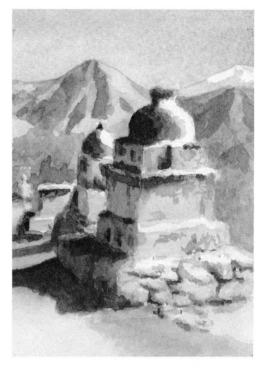

**Figure 4.** Chortens at Sakti.

military protocol, and we each received a long embrace accompanied by much patting on the back. In seconds we had learned that he was now "Assistant Inspector." After being introduced to the new arrivals, he turned to me and asked,

"And where is sister? Sahib."

It gave me great pleasure to report this back to my daughter.

The bungalow was chaotic. Built some years ago, it had somehow been forgotten and lay empty until a few weeks before. We had camped out in it last year, when a priest from the gompa had given a permission that was doubtless more correct ecclesiastically than legally. Now its existence had somehow come to the notice of the officials in Leh, who had decided that it should immediately be made habitable. A group of workmen was encamped in one of the rooms. Carpenters clambered through glassless windows. The workmen reexplored the original system of drains with archeological precision only to find that the drains ended blindly underground two feet from the building. Electricians hammered wires into the ceilings. Dust choked every room. In the lean-to at the back, the three ITBP men were boiling tea on a kerosene stove.

The "sitting room," which last year had been so useful as a laboratory, was piled high with rickety furniture. We set about stacking it up at one end, leaving enough room for the carpenters to finish their sawing and for us to get started on the goats that we were told were waiting down in the village. Dust and wood shavings were swept up, and Inder and I set up the tables for the haemodynamic equipment, slinging the drip bottles precariously from some of the electricians' new wiring tacked up high on the wall. In one corner Roberto organised his equipment, and, in the window, Derek was preparing his apparatus.

Outside there were problems. Nirankari, Inder's technician from Chandigarh, who had arrived ahead with heavy equipment, had put the generator on a low wall in front of the main entrance. Cables led from it through one of the many holes in the windows to a makeshift patchboard from which leads ran to manometers, the cardiac output computer, the centrifuges and a spare light bulb. Nirankari had pulled his right arm out trying to start the generator but had eventually succeeded with the help of the "Assistant Inspector." Now he was running backward and forward to check the voltage on the voltmeter on the patchboard, which was fluctuating wildly, judging by the lamp, the light from which swung from a dull glow to a sun-tanning intensity. At this point Derek took over. A lifetime's experience fiddling with electrical circuits bore down on the problem, calculated resistance, put in bits of missing wiring, adjusted the generator, and eventually some sort of respectable current flowed and we could start.

In the meantime, Donald and David had established themselves in a little room provided with an ample table, the sole item that they had insisted was necessary. Pots of formaldehyde and Bouin's fluid were arranged on a side table, together with plastic boxes for specimens and a range of spine-chilling dissecting instruments neatly spread out. Donald sat with his sleeves rolled up in one of his green plastic aprons and waited. David sat on one side and waited.

And waited. The physiologists were in trouble. After the delays of setting up the equipment and getting the generator to work, two Sakti goats had been brought up from the village by Dr. Deen's assistant, and Inder and I had studied them, expecting that they would then be turned over to Donald and David. But, at that moment, the farmer decided that he did not want them slaughtered. After some delays, Deen's assistant brought in two more whose owners had agreed to sell them for slaughter. But, by the time we had studied them, it was one o'clock in the afternoon and the slaughterman had disappeared somewhere up the valley for his midday meal.

The physiologists broke off for lunch of dahl and rice, but the pathologists sat waiting, eager to get started. At this point Roberto felt ill and febrile. I took his temperature and found it high, dissuading him from taking antibiotics until there was some clearer idea of the cause of the fever.

There was still no sign of the slaughterman, so Inder and I went back and continued with the remaining goats. Eventually the slaughterman returned from his long lunch break, singing happily. But Donald and David weren't. It was then too late, they judged, to start their work. So everybody was angry with everybody else. Inder was eager to finish as many haemodynamic studies as possible, so we continued working on the goats until six in the evening.

After Inder, Donald, and David had left to return to Leh, Roberto revealed the contents of his carrybag. And no wonder it was so heavy, crammed as it was with every variety of pasta, tins of tomatoes, beans, tuna fish. For Roberto, last year's daily menu of dahl and chappatis was an indelible source of anxiety. Even then he had managed to relieve the monotony with a packet of bouillon cubes he happened to have on him and that he taught an astonished group of army cooks how to dissolve in boiling water. This time he was prepared. The only thing missing was an enormous tin of olive oil, which, to Roberto's disgust, I had left behind at Srinagar Airport. But, all things considered, he was content, despite his fever. He and Peggy selected penne con tonno and went into the kitchen to cook it under the admiring eyes of the Assistant Inspector and his two men, who had been persuaded to get some onions from the village. It was a memorable candlelit meal; only Roberto couldn't do it justice. As I blew out the candles, the moonlight slanted in through the empty window, and all the dogs of the village were barking.

## June 17

I woke early, but the sun was already beaming across the valley. In the kitchen the boys were up and the water boiling in a cauldron. I took some and went out onto the terrace to wash and shave.

Dawn in London is a threat, a needle in the side of the night. Dawn in Chandigarh had been maternal. You stirred happy as a fetus in the warmth. Dawn at Sakti was different again, neither threatening nor mothering but indifferent. A transcendental statement. A bell sounds from the gompa. Distant voices carry from far across the valley. And, suddenly, you are aware that there are people in all the fields, as if by witchcraft.

Back in our room, Roberto was still sleeping, propped up to prevent breathlessness. I sat using the solar calculator that I had bought as a present for Phuntsog, an ITBP corporal who had worked with us on previous visits. It looked as if the pulmonary arterial pressure was higher in the Srinagar goats than in the indigenous Sakti breed, and I was pleased.

Soon Roberto woke, miraculously cured. We joined Derek and Peggy for breakfast of dried egg omelette and ITBP ration vitamin pills. Inder had decided to go to the Hemis Festival, which I had seen last year. So Derek and I made an early start. Or tried to. We found the room occupied by painters who were rolling distemper over the walls. But, by the time Donald and David arrived, the walls were finished and everyone started in earnest.

The pathologists were happy now, their room rapidly converted into a butcher's shop. Derek and I started on the remaining goats. The windows were full of children's faces, and they kept infiltrating into the rooms, from which they were ejected complaining. The adult villagers wandered in and out freely or sat outside on the terrace chatting or spinning their hand prayer wheels.

Soon specimens were arriving from the pathology room: bits of lung for Roberto, bits of pulmonary artery for Derek. So Derek moved to his table in the window while Nirankari helped me with the goats. Roberto, recovered from his illness, was busy in the corner. David would bring pieces of lung on an enamel tray. Roberto would cut and weigh samples, some of which would go immediately into the liquid nitrogen container to be taken to Brescia for catecholamine analysis, while others were taken out to the kitchen and boiled in dilute acetic acid in a pressure cooker for peptide analysis. The pressure cooker had been brought from Inder's home and was needed because the low pressure at high altitude reduces the boiling point of water. After boiling these specimens, Roberto returned to his corner to homogenise and centrifuge them.

Beside him, at a table by the window, Derek had set up his homemade apparatus, the design of which Heath Robinson would have been proud. To the rest of us it was a mystery. The overall appearance was that of one of those antique clocks whose brass mechanism is open to view under a glass dome. Glass dome there was, resting on a greased glass plate. From it emerged a sphygmomanometer, converted so that Derek could increase the pressure under the dome and, thus, the partial pressure of oxygen. The mechanism under the dome was a complex assembly of bits of wire, string, and cardboard in which plasticine seemed to play a dual role of adhesive and counterweight. In the middle of the mechanism was an old-fashioned clock hand, which traveled round a scale inscribed by hand on a piece of card. Somewhere into this assembly was inserted a tiny piece of pulmonary artery, the contraction of which Derek was studying at different partial pressures of oxygen and in the presence or absence of noradrenaline.

He was blissfully taken up with this in the midst of all the hubbub around him: goats bleating, goats defaecating and urinating, me shouting out numbers to Nirankari or shouting to the children to get out, Roberto making whirring noises with his homogeniser and centrifuge, and the general chatter and laughter of the villagers who crowded in to enjoy this heavensent diversion. Every so often the Assistant Inspector arrived with a tray of cups of tea, at which blood-stained hands would reach out.

Halfway up the cliffside above us, a different ceremony was taking place near the gompa. The sound of horns and drums and chanting floated down from groups of monks and children who seemed to be engaged in some rite concerned with a bunch of branches and prayer flags that had been roughly put together on a precariously projecting piece of rock. The children were running along paths that were not visible to us below and seemed to be moving weightlessly on air across the vertical rock face.

Inder returned at lunch, and, by the time we had finished the day's work, everybody was satisfied. As Inder and Donald and David rattled off down the valley, I took a stroll toward the main river, which flowed down the valley, full of melted snow. Up toward the pass at the top of the valley, a Y-shape of silver marked the waterfall to which we had walked last year together with Phuntsog. To our disappointment, he was unable to join us this year as he was down in Delhi collecting a medal for having climbed one of the major Himalayan peaks. But Phuntsog's brother-in-law had been helping us, and I hoped to go with him later to visit his wife and children in their little house way up the valley.

And now I have to describe a mysterious and intimate happening. This morning I had wandered toward the river, in roughly the same direction as I was now taking, in search of a suitable place to defaecate. Perhaps it was this quest that, as I commented in my earlier note, had made me aware of suddenly how full the fields were of people. I had eventually found a discrete spot in which the dry-stone walls formed the shape of a horseshoe. It had evidently appealed to others, probably also from the party at the bungalow, for there were several other deposits in various stages of aging. Now it happened that my path this evening took me past the same spot. When I glanced into the horseshoe, I was astounded to find that my deposit had gone. The others were there as before; mine alone had been removed in broad daylight. I went down to the river's edge pondering over this happening. Had some animal devoured it? But why single out mine? Or had it been removed by some human hand? Did the excrement of a Professor of Medicine from a far-off land have, itself, healing properties? Was it being used in some form of magic against me? Perhaps because I had sanctioned the killing of the animals?

As I returned to the bungalow the smell of yet another delicious past supper reached my nostrils from the kitchen where Peggy and Roberto were busy over the stove, watched, as always, by the ITBP boys.

## June 18

It is half past six in the morning. I am sitting calculating yesterday's results on the present for Phuntsog. Roberto is asleep. And suddenly there is the noise of a jeep outside and in bursts Inder. A radio message has been received by the ITBP at Leh. Roberto's wife Sandra is ill in Italy, and it seems that she will need an operation. Inder shows me the ambiguous note. A white-faced Roberto has just time to gather his things and take the jeep back to Leh in the hope of catching the morning flight to Chandigarh and Delhi and the night flight to Rome. He leaves behind a touching parcel of four packets of spaghetti, one packet of penne, four tins of tuna, one tin of beans and two tins of tomatoes, together with presents for various people.

## June 19

Within three days we had catheterised fourteen sheep and fifteen goats. Four each of the sheep and goats had been autopsied, but the problem of permission to kill the low-altitude goats and, especially, the cows had not be solved. Inder, who was normally in charge of haemodynamics, had stayed behind in Leh to see the District Commissioner, while Derek and I made an early start on the four remaining Merino sheep. Permission had been granted to slaughter two of those because of their poor health. One poor old sheep was crawling with fearsome ticks, which Derek delicately removed with fine

scissors and placed in a bowl of methylated spirit.

Usually the jugular vein was easy to find, but occasionally it was obscure, confused with bands of muscle or folds of skin or remaining wool.

"If you can see it, you can see it," Derek said.

But, if you couldn't the village men were eager to give their advice. Everybody put a finger at the base of the neck and felt for the swollen vein. In fact the villagers were adept at finding the vein, and, after a time, a consensus of opinion would emerge.

While we were occupied with the sheep, Donald and David were taking stills and cine films of the dzo and two stolls, which had arrived the evening before, Donald sitting on a stone wall, as always, impeccable in city suit, collar, and tie, issuing precise instructions to David as to which animal, which angle, which background. The dzo is the offspring of a cow and a yak. The stoll is the offspring of a female dzo and a bull yak.

After lunch of the inevitable rice and dahl, we moved the equipment outside, choosing a piece of level ground shaded by a wall of the bungalow. Shade was important both to prevent the glucose-saline from getting too hot and to protect the investigators from the sun.

The fist dzo was a bull, and thus referred to as a dzobi, the female being a dzomo. Few of the dzobis survive infancy, but this one had thrived to a massive size. With the upswept horns and shaggy hair that he had inherited from his yak father, he had a fearsome aspect, but, like all the domestic dzos and yaks, was entirely docile, quite different from the aggressive wild yaks that Inder had investigated a few years before at Whipsnade Zoo, where, on one occasion, he had come close to disaster. As I sat beside the dzobi to feel his neck, he turned a slimy nose against my cheek and seemed satisfied with the contact. The jugular was big as a garden hose. He didn't even feel the needle of the local anaesthetic, and I am sure that it wasn't necessary. They are much more apprehensive of sudden movements or the unnecessary gripping of the handlers at critical moments. The dzobi stood placidly while first the introducer, then the catheter went into his jugular. His left eye, soft brown with large black pupil, looked straight into mine. Tears flowed continuously from its corner down the side of his face to join the salivary edge of his mouth. What was he thinking? He had a high pulmonary arterial pressure.

## June 20

The last morning in Sakti was set aside for filming. Two yaks had come down from the pass, roped together. They were brothers and had lived all their lives roped like this. But only one would return that morning to his high pastures.

At lunch the cooks had excelled themselves with a delicious dish of local turnips. In Leh, women in high hats sit by the roadside with piles of turnips on the ground, defending them vehemently against the sly cows that wander freely down the street, nosing through the rubble with one innocent eye on the vegetables. After lunch I went with Rintzen, Phuntsog's bother-in-law, to visit Phuntsog's wife about a mile up the valley. The path led up across a sandy waste strewn with granite boulders. We passed the new gompa, dedicated by the Dalai Lama and placed facing China as a sort of spiritual radar station against communism. Groups of ruined chortens and mani walls littered the mountain side. At each chorten or mani wall, the path divided, beaten by feet that walked round holy objects correctly, keeping the holy place on the right. The sun was pitiless, and, when we reached the Phuntsogs' house, we were thirsty. Mrs. Phuntsog was surprised and delighted. She ushered us into the living room, where we sat on the floor and quenched our thirst with spring water. And there, in a crude gilt frame, were the photographs Libbie had sent after last year's expedition. It was clear that Mrs. Phuntsog would not come and sit with the men in the sitting room, so I moved into the kitchen where we had all been entertained last year. One small window in the mud-brick wall cast a feeble light on the wooden table, the cast iron stove with its pot always boiling over a wood fire and the low bench covered with carpet. Mrs. Phuntsog went automatically to the Gur-Gur, the traditional wooden cylinder about a yard long and four inches wide, bound in brass in which yak butter tea is made. The mixture consists of rancid yak butter, strong black tea, and salt. It is all put into the Gur-Gur and emulsified by rapid up and down movements of a wooden plunger. Two best cups and the only saucer were brought out, and there were exclamations of delight each time we accepted a refill.

I brought out the little presents for the family. Each time I pulled something new out of the bag, Mrs. Phuntsog's face lit up and she stuck out her tongue to an enormous extent with the pleasure of it. We took some polaroids, mostly for her to keep, and started back down the valley.

There was time for a brief visit to the gompa before leaving. I went with Rintzen, who found a twelve-year-old monk to show us round. We climbed the stone steps in the side of the cliff, entering a series of courtyards. We went first into the "chapel." Here the brightly coloured wall paintings were lit from a hole in the centre of the ceiling. Long parallel banks of cushions would seat some seventy monks at prayer but I doubt whether there are so many now. The original shrine was built well into the side of the cliff, under an overhanging ledge of rock. Inside was dark. Images of the Lord Buddha, hanging drums, and goats' horns were dimly visible. And there, hanging from the ceiling, was the bell that Libbie had left last year. Behind the sanctuary was the cave in which the holy mahasiddha had meditated for seventeen years, a boy bringing him food up the cliffside each day. The cold sucked the warmth from our bodies, and the lights of our candles flickered against the blackened walls.

"And what was his name?" I asked.

"Kunga Phuntsog," was the reply.

As we returned to the main courtyard, the boy monk asked shyly if I would take a photo of the ornaments made out of yak butter in the sanctuary for him. After days of pestering for self-portraits, the request was refreshing.

"Why does he want it?" I asked Rintzen.

"He is allowed in the sanctuary only a short time each day for prayers, and he wants to study the ornaments carefully so that he will know how to make them himself."

We went back into the sanctuary, where the ornaments ("offerings," he called them) were in a glass case. The boy struggled desperately with the flimsy lock and eventually handed over to Rintzen, who broke it open with brute force. I had two shots left, one for him and one for me.

"Please don't show it to anybody else," he said.

Neither the boy nor Rintzen knew how old the gompa was.

"I'll ask the chief lama," Rintzen said.

We found him in a little garden consisting of a few willows surrounded by a dry-stone wall at the bottom of the cliff. Three or four senior lamas were seated on rusty steel tubing chairs around a plastic-topped table. Rintzen leaned over the wall and asked the age of the monastery. But the voice that answered did not come from any of the monks round the table. Peering over the wall, I could then see the chief lama lying on his back on a sort of wooden

stretcher, rubbing his abdomen and chest up and down with both hands. He continued this soothing motion, looking straight up into the sky, while he gave a long reply to Rintzen's question.

"One thousand seven hundred years old," Rintzen said as we turned to go.

## June 21

I was sitting writing in the garden of our hotel in Leh when Inder called for me in the ITBP jeep. Our first stop was the Army Agricultural Development laboratories where Inder had met a veterinarian major who said that he was having difficulties with the high-altitude "Brisket Disease" in his cows. We went first to meet the colonel in charge, a Sikh who made us politely and cautiously welcome. As soon as Major Chandon arrived it was clear that the two men disliked each other, and Inder explained later that the major had been in charge of the unit until the colonel arrived. We went to see the two sick cows. The path, lined with painted ammunition boxes planted with sweet williams and antirrhinums, led us between experimental plots of wheat and barley, various vegetables and hops for high-altitude beer. Afterward we were taken to a curious octagonal dining room, where we studied details of the obstetric history and milking charts. We were not convinced of the diagnosis but decided, in any case, to study the two cows together with two controls in the afternoon (when we found that they had no great pulmonary hypertension).

Our next call was the Indian Airlines office to try and wangle seats on the flight to Chandigarh in two days' time. All the seats reserved for the army and administration had been taken up, and Inder's string-pulling had, so far, been without effect. The trouble was that the manager of the airline office was a locum for a week. Nobody knew him and he was under no obligation to anybody—a frustrating and unusual state of affairs. Even the district commissioner was powerless. The locum looked entirely healthy, and our preliminary enquires had revealed no medical, let alone cardiac, problem. He talked long and seriously with Inder, whom he finally handed over to a man with protruding eyes at the back of the office. From where I was sitting, the conversation appeared jovial and encouraging. Our tickets were handed over and something done to them.

"See you Monday at the airport," I heard him say.

But when Inder returned the news was bad. We would have to wait and see.

We were already late for our next appointment at the cattle farm nearby, where we hoped to study the indigenous high altitude cows. We went in Mohammed Deen's jeep past the airstrip and across some wasteland and beds of dried-up streams to a group of mud-brick huts near the river. Seated behind a plate of half-finished saffron rice on the desk of an office was a bearded man with large spectacles who was introduced as the assistant district commissioner. By the wall to his left sat the manager of the farm. We shook hands, and all sat down except Inder, who went back to the jeep to fetch something.

Mohammed Deen was explaining our mission to the manager. Indian conversations, part in Hindi and part in Indian English, are confusing, and it was a little while before I realised that things were going badly.

"These are precious animals," emerged from the taught lips of the manager. He was now clearly angry.

Inder came in at that moment and sat beside me.

"What's going on?" he asked me.

"I don't know," I said. "Something's wrong."

We sat listening to the rising voices of the two men. The assistant district commissioner was sorting out papers on the desk.

"What's wrong?" Inder put the question to both of them.

"I am manager of this farm," the manager shouted back.

"So?"

"I am responsible for these cows. This is a dangerous procedure."

Mohammed Deen said, "But you have seen it done last year in Sakti. You know it's not dangerous."

"You open the jugular vein. Is that not dangerous? You put things in the heart. Is that not dangerous? These animals are precious. I have to account for them."

"It is not dangerous. We have had similar procedures carried out on ourselves."

"The milk also is precious. They will stop milking. And many of them are pregnant. They will abort. And . . ."

Inder interrupted. "We are not interested in pregnant animals. We don't want to study them."

"And they are milking. This stuff is valuable. I cannot be responsible for. . . ."

Despite the tension, Inder and I grinned at each other. We were remembering how, last year, the villagers at Sakti had been reluctant to let us study their yaks. Then the head man had persuaded his daughter to let us have one of her yaks. Next morning she had come running up from the village in her excitement. Never had her yak produced so much milk. From that moment, there was no shortage of supply of yaks at Sakti.

"We can assure you that it won't interfere with milking," I said.

"And many of them are pregnant. I cannot, certainly not, give permission. . . ."

And so the argument ran on, simultaneously through different channels, like a stream searching for a new path every time you block it with a stone. And, at last, when everybody had repeated many times what they had to say and the voices died down, the real problem revealed itself. Nobody had told the manager.

We had descended on him with all our demands. How was he to know what authority we had? There followed a long and complicated discussion about who had been told, who had agreed, when who had said what. Bigger and bigger names were coming out. But the manager insisted that this was the first he had heard of it. We sympathised, but he was not to be placated. Only direct permission from the cattle vet from Animal Husbandry would do the trick. Luckily the vet was due to join us, so we sat waiting in the office while the assistant district commissioner and the manager continued another acrimonious conversation, which we had interrupted. It wasn't the Manager's morning.

The cattle vet, a friend of Mohammed Deen, was a gentle person—"Too gentle," Inder had said—and I followed his placatory and kindly expression as he spoke to the tightlipped manager. And, eventually, the manager would allow us to study one cow, provided that the vet assured him that the animal was not pregnant.

"How will he do that?" I asked Deen.

"Rectal examination of the uterus."

"But. A cow. How do you do it? The whole hand?"

"Come and see."

We went out to the cattle pen. The intense sun was pouring down on the sand, throwing back heat. The vet had rolled up his left shirt sleeve to the elbow and a boy was pouring yellow savlon over his left hand. One man held the cow's head, another lifted the tail, and in went the vet's arm up to the elbow. The cow was entirely indifferent to what was going on. Sweat poured down the vet's face as he felt for the two horns of the uterus through the rectal wall.

"That bastard of a manager," I said to Inder. "He's making him do this just to pay him back."

"It's not pregnant," the vet said at last. He withdrew his arm, covered with yellow-brown cow shit up to above the elbow. (And he had not rolled his sleeve high enough.)

As he was washing his arm and the edge of his shirt in a bucket of water, the manager slouched up.

"That's not the one I meant," he said. Just like that.

I shall not easily forget, and cannot easily describe, the look on the vet's face.

At that moment Inder blew his top.

"We're not going to be buggered about like this," he shouted. The phraseology was effective and, in an obscure way, apt.

"I tell you. I will take this matter to the highest authority. You are deliberately interfering with an official scientific programme. You will certainly hear about it." He towered over the manager.

It was absolutely the right thing to do. In next to no time we were studying two cows.

## June 25

And, of course, the flight didn't even come in. Instead, we got seats on a plane to Srinagar the next day, and now we are once more waiting on Srinagar airport, hoping to get on the flight to Delhi. To our surprise and suspicion, we have been checked in straight away, and now we are waiting three hours for the plane to arrive. I bury my head in the workbook with the aid of David's calculator. Ladakh Goat Number Twelve. Average systolic pulmonary arterial pressure so many millimetres of mercury. On my left the Limca bottles come and go. Hassan's stall has just opened up.

And, by some miracle, the plane does arrive and we are being called to go through Security where our baggage attracts the usual attention. Donald and David have packed their bags with hundreds of little specimens of lung in plastic boxes. That takes a little explaining. As David opens his personal belongings, the official notices a box of paracetamol tablets.

"What's in there?"

"Headache tablets."

"Let me see."

David opens the lid.

"They good for headaches?"

"Yes."

"I got headache."

"Take two. They'll make it better."

"Both at once?"

Now he is searching through my sponge bag and abstractly wiping his hands on my face cloth.

In the body search room I empty my pockets and raise my arms.

"Where you from?"

"England."

"What you do?"

"I'm a doctor."

"What sort doctor?"

"A heart doctor."

"You feel my pulse. I want see my heart OK."

I take a sticky wrist, half a mind to tell him he'll drop dead.

"You're fine. You'll live to be a hundred."

And at last we are on the plane, and Donald is telling us of the cactus that Professor Wagenvoort gave him five years ago in full bloom. Each year since he has waited in vain for another bloom. But this year, just before he left for India, an all-promising bud appeared. He put it under the stairs hoping that some trace of the blossom would be left when he got back. And I am dreaming of the roses in my garden.

## June 26

Delhi had cooled off. We left in the early hours of the morning by Thai Airlines. Our only problem was the nitrogen

cylinder. It looked for all the world like a bomb. We put it though the x-rays but the operator insisted on our opening it. As Inder took off the top, a cloud of deadly looking gas poured out.

The operator took a step back.

"It's OK," said Inder, with less than his normal conviction. "It was specially designed for air travel. Look here on the labels. It says so."

"I'll get the boss," the man muttered, and beat a hasty retreat, looking over his shoulder.

The boss wore a macho moustache. He lifted the lid once more.

"That's OK. It's dry ice." He said.

It stayed between my legs all the way home.

## Postscript

The results were not spectacular. OK, but not spectacular. The year before, when we had not been able to get outside funding, had produced results that were so much more exciting. I guess that is why we got the funding this time. Maybe the funders are usually one step behind. We wrote a dull article.[1]

Some time later, Donald was rung up by an administrator from the Wellcome Trust, asking for copies of all of the papers that had come out of their support (which had been generous) over the years.

"Of course," said Donald. "And would you also like a pile of those which came from projects that you turned down?"

"They would be of even greater interest," laughed the man from Wellcome.

He was probably right.

## Personalia

Prof. Inder Anand, Postgraduate Institute of Medical Education and Research, Chandigarh.

Dr. Derek Bergel, University of Oxford

Prof. Roberto Ferrari, University of Brescia

Prof. Donald Heath, University of Liverpool

Dr. David Williams, University of Liverpool

## Reference

1. Anand, I., D. Heath, D. Williams, M. Deen, R. Ferrari, D. Bergel, and P. Harris. the pulmonary circulation of some domestic animals at high altitude. *Int. J. Biometeorol.* 32:56–64, 1988.

# 16

# Pulmonary Hypertension:
## The Price of High Living

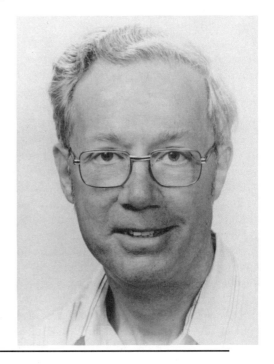

**Robert F. Grover, M.D., Ph.D.**

*Emeritus Professor of Medicine, University of Colorado Medical School, Arroyo Grande, California*

I began life in Rochester, New York. My earliest companion was a big old English Setter named Sport. You see, we always had bird dogs at home because my father was an avid pheasant hunter. I still have fond childhood memories of succulent roast pheasant, and my cap was often adorned with the colorful sweep of their long tail fathers. One of my father's hunting companions was James Sherman Houck, a surgeon who removed my appendix and then gave me the preserved specimen in a jar of formaldehyde; I displayed it proudly, to the distress of my parents' guests. Dr. Houck was probably my first role model, and when he died his wife gave me one of his college textbooks in chemistry.[31] To this day, that badly worn volume still holds a special place in my library.

That it was a chemistry textbook is significant, because while my teenage friends were discovering the biology of the opposite sex, I was exploring the mysteries of chemistry in a laboratory I built in the basement. The orderliness of chemical reactions fascinated me. You could write simple equations that described the behavior of the elements and then observe the reaction in a flask. Of course the consequences were inevitable. I drove my parents out of the house with clouds of smoke

From: Wagner WW, Jr, Weir EK (eds): *The Pulmonary Circulation and Gas Exchange.* ©1994, Futura Publishing Co Inc, Armonk, NY.

and noxious gases, shook the windows with violent explosions, and blew out the electrical circuits with my attempts at electrolysis. People today don't know the meaning of "hazardous chemicals"! It's a wonder I didn't injure myself.

Based on my interests in chemistry, physics, and mathematics, my parents decided I was destined to become a chemical engineer. So the autumn of 1940 found me high above Cayuga's waters, enrolled at Cornell University. Among my belongings was the 1940 edition of *The Merck Index,* because I had discovered it contained tantalizing bits of information. For example, I read that acetophenone was not only used in the perfume industry for its orange blossom scent, but also acted as a narcotic and hypnotic. This I had to explore. So I "borrowed" some acetophenone from the organic chemistry laboratory, lured one of the neighborhood cats (the feline variety) to my room, and proceeded to inject 1 ml subcutaneously. The cat became drowsy, went to sleep, and became unconscious. Next morning, the cat was still breathing heavily but couldn't be roused, so I went off to class. That afternoon, my landlady asked me if that were a dead cat in my room. I rushed up and was relieved to find my cat still sleeping soundly. By the next morning, after 36 hours, the cat awakened, and when he could stand, I put him outside. When he staggered home, I'm sure his owners wondered why he reeked of orange blossoms. Was I really destined to become an engineer?

## The Road to Denver

December 7, 1941, and our lives would never be the same again. I was only 17 at the time and still at Cornell, but when I became 18, I enlisted in the army and was called to active duty early in 1943. The next three years were spent in the military, half of that time overseas. Three significant events occurred during that period. First, I met my future wife Estelle, and we were married in 1944. Thus began a partnership that lasted nearly 50 years. Three months after our wedding, I was shipped to Europe. I served as a radio operator in the Signal Corps, and my unit was part of the Seventh Army pushing from France through southern Germany to Austria. Our radio relay stations required high locations, and one of these was in a permanent weather station atop the Zugspitze at 10,000 feet in the Alps. It was a magnificent location, surrounded by jagged peaks and massive glaciers. Living in that spectacular high-altitude environment made a deep impression on me, and I resolved that when the war was over, Estelle and I were going to live in or near mountains. This alpine experience was the second major event in my life.

The third event took place at sea. Following the end of hostilities in Europe, our Signal Corps unit was sent to the port of Marseilles and loaded on a troop ship. For the next 6 weeks we sailed across the Atlantic, through the Panama Canal, and then across the Pacific to the Philippines. For 6 weeks we were packed on a crowded ship, sleeping on deck trying to avoid that heat, day after day surrounded by nothing but water; it was no picnic. I met a fellow named Ben Cogan who, it turned out, had a Ph.D. in physiology. In the course of many conversations, I learned about physiology as a discipline and realized that at last I had found my direction. Hence, I decided that when this war was over, I would become a physiologist.

Hiroshima. Nagasaki. Japan surrendered. Estelle had been working at Oak Ridge on the Manhattan Project after losing her brother, a marine lieutenant, on Guadalcanal. Thus, she had played a role in bringing an early end to World War II, saving thousands of lives, perhaps even mine. Our unit was sent to Japan as part of the occupation forces, and after several months, once again we boarded a troop ship, recrossed the Pacific, and were finally home. At the Separation Center, I was invited to join the reserves. No thank you! Conformity has never been my strong suit, and in 3 years, I had seen enough of the military to know beyond a doubt that such a life was not for me.

Now to get on with our lives. Before I could begin graduate work in physiology, I had to complete my bachelor's degree. Returning to Cornell would have involved a delay of 8 months. However, thanks to friends at home, I was able to enter the University of Rochester within 2 months of leaving the army, enabling me to graduate with a B.A. in chemistry in June 1947. In selecting my course work, I told my advisor of my plans for graduate school. He recommended a course called Physiological Chemistry taught by E. S. Nasset. This turned out to be a course in nutrition for home economics students. Never did he mention Wallace Fenn, Herman Rahn, Arthur Otis, or their former trainee Alberto Hurtado. What if I had been put in contact with them? We can only speculate on the impact that might have had on my career. The hand of fate moves in strange ways.

As I have indicated, my decision was to study physiology near the mountains. One look at a map of the United States reveals only two locations where that is possible: Salt Lake City and Denver. We chose Denver. When we announced our decision, the reaction was "Nobody goes to Denver to live. That's only a place for vacations." Undaunted, I applied for admission to the University of Colorado and was elated by a telegram of acceptance from Richard Whitehead, head of what was then the joint Department of Physiology and Pharmacology.

There was just one problem. We had no money for moving expenses or the train fare from Rochester to Denver. So for the summers of 1946 and 1947, I was hired as a "hod carrier," even though I had no idea what a "hod" was. I simply knew I would be assisting brick layers. It turns out that a hod is a sort of box on a pole used to carry bricks. Of course I never actually carried a hod, because all bricks and mortar were hauled about in wheel barrows. During those summers, I learned much about mixing mortar and laying bricks. This experience was to pay off handsomely a few years later when Estelle and I built our mountain cabin high in the Rockies. We became proficient stone masons, and the stonework of our walls, fireplace, and chimney was indeed admirable. I repeat, the hand of fate moves in strange ways.

## Graduate School

August 1947, and we stepped off the train at Union Station in Denver. The mountains were just west of the city, seemingly within walking distance, and the air was so clear at that time. At the medical school, Dr. Whitehead introduced me to Clarence A. Maaske, Ph.D. (Fig. 1), head of the physiology section of the Department of Physiology and Pharmacology. I learned that Maaske had worked with Earl Wood at Wright–Patterson Air Force Base during World War II testing pilots on the human centrifuge. That work required monitoring intravascular arterial and venous pressures employing strain gauge pressure transducers. Maaske brought that technology with him to Denver, and from him I learned the physics of dynamic pressure transducers. Together we constructed a recording system using string galvanometers that required a one-meter optical arm for amplification of the oscillations of the tiny mirrors, the light beams falling on the lens of a slit camera. A heavy black drape enclosed the system to exclude external light. Mounted on a wheeled table, it was cumbersome, but it produced beautiful photographic recordings.

Colorado General Hospital decided to enter the emerging field of cardiac surgery

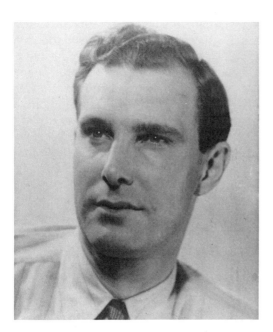

**Figure 1.** Clarence A. Maaske, ca. 1950, first chairman of the Department of Physiology, University of Colorado School of Medicine.

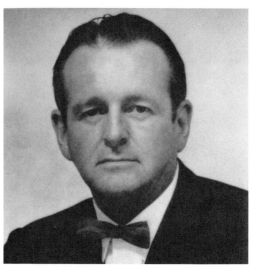

**Figure 2.** Henry Swan II, ca. 1950, chairman of the Department of Surgery, University of Colorado School of Medicine, first director of the Cardiovascular Pulmonary (CVP) Laboratory.

and recruited a young surgeon, Henry Swan II (Fig. 2), in 1947. For the first time in the history of cardiology, it was now possible to consider surgical correction of congenital cardiac defects. Accurate diagnosis of the anatomical lesion together with an assessment of the hemodynamic derangement became prerequisites. This required a cardiac catheterization laboratory, so naturally Swan turned to Maaske for that technology. Soon I became involved, not only in performing the pressure recordings, but also in assisting in their interpretation. Ultimately, this work became the basis for my doctoral thesis.[13]

## My Introduction to Pulmonary Hypertension

In those early days, the late 1940s, the cardiac surgery program began modestly with the correction of such extracardiac defects as coarctation of the aorta and patent ductus arteriosus. We soon learned

that in young children a patent ductus was sometimes associated with pulmonary hypertension and the left-to-right shunt was not always large. Naturally we wondered if resection of the ductus would relieve the pulmonary hypertension in such cases. To find out, we decided to make direct recordings of pulmonary arterial and aortic pressures in the operating room both before and immediately after resection of the ductus. This called for my bulky table with its pressure-recording galvanometers and slit camera, all covered with the very nonsterile heavy black drape. The operating room supervisor protested mightily, but Swan prevailed, and I was relegated to a far corner of the operating room and became the subject of many harsh glances. I was unperturbed, and surgery proceeded: the chest was opened, and the great vessels were exposed. Swan called for the pressure transducer. A meter length of semirigid Saran tubing, sterilized in preparation, was filled with saline, and one end was passed to me to attach to the transducer. Swan then attached a hypodermic needle, I zeroed the system, he

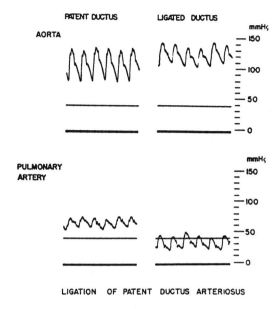

PATENT DUCTUS   LIGATED DUCTUS

AORTA

LIGATION OF PATENT DUCTUS ARTERIOSUS

**Figure 3.** Intravascular pressure recordings made by the author in 1948 during surgical resection of a patent ductus arteriosus by Henry Swan. Note only partial relief of pulmonary hypertension.[21]

punctured the pulmonary artery and aorta in succession, while I, head under my black drape off in the corner, recorded the pressures. Swan then proceeded to resect the ductus, after which the pressure recordings were repeated. Over the next few months we made similar recordings in seven additional patients.

This was 1948, only 3 years after Cournand made the first recordings of pulmonary arterial pressure in man, a patient with mitral stenosis and pulmonary hypertension.[7] Our pressure tracings also showed pulmonary hypertension as well as the wide pulse pressure in the aorta. Following closure of the ductus, the pulmonary arterial pressure was less, while the diastolic pressure in the aorta was now higher (Fig. 3). I presented these findings from our series of patients at the FASEB meeting in 1949 with Swan and Maaske as

my coauthors.[21] I had made my debut into the field of the pulmonary circulation; that was 42 years ago.

## Medical School

For cardiac surgery to advance, a trained cardiologist was needed. In 1950, Swan recruited S. Gilbert Blount, Jr. (Fig. 4), from Johns Hopkins to fill that role. Soon construction began on an addition to the hospital to be known as the Cardiovascular Pulmonary (CVP) Laboratory, which came to house the cardiac catheterization laboratory. Swan was the first director of the CVP, while Blount became director of the cath lab.* Swan went on to become chairman of the Department of Surgery. Under the team of Swan and Blount, cardiology became a major discipline, leading to the creation of a new Division of Cardiology headed by Blount. Meanwhile, the Department of Physiology and Pharmacology was split into its two components, and Maaske became the first chairman of the new Department of Physiology.

When Blount established the permanent cath lab in the CVP, I continued to do the pressure recording. Thus began our association, which has continued for over 40 years. Blount became my mentor and urged me to go on for an M.D. degree. In fact, I had decided that was the proper course if I intended to conduct cardiovascular research involving humans. So after I received my Ph.D. in 1951, my ever-supportive wife continued working in cytology[28,29] while I went through medical school. Following my internship, Blount invited me to take a cardiology fellowship with him, after which he obtained for me a faculty appointment and asked me to run the cath lab, although he retained the title of director. That was 1957.

*Other members of the original CVP staff who occupied the new laboratory area were Jerry Aikawa, Leighton Anderson, John Berry, Giles Filley, Joseph Holmes, Dalton Jenkins, Fred Kern, Morris Levine, Clarence Maaske, Frank Princi, John Singleton, and Kurt and Edith VonKaulla.

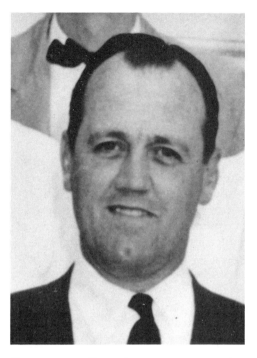

**Figure 4.** S. Gilbert Blount, Jr., ca. 1956, founder and first head of the Division of Cardiology, University of Colorado School of Medicine.

## The Beginnings of Research

In the summer of 1957, Blount brought to the cath lab one of his new cardiology fellows, a lanky, good-natured guy from Kentucky named Jack Reeves. I was to teach him the art of cardiac catheterization. From the first, Jack and I hit it off, and now, 34 years later, we're still working together (Fig. 5).

One afternoon, Giles Filley told us that the veterinarians from Fort Collins were doing some work he thought would interest us. Giles said those fellows were up in South Park, a broad valley at 9,000–10,000-feet elevation, attempting to measure pulmonary arterial pressures in cattle with a condition known as "brisket disease." Something about pulmonary hypertension. Not ones to pass up a lead, we drove the 80 miles to South Park, located the Hartsel Ranch, and walked into a cold

barn. There were Arch Alexander and Rue Jensen at the neck of a 1,000-pound steer standing in a restraining "squeeze chute." They had made an incision over the jugular vein and were threading in a length of rubber urethral catheter filled with saline and attached to a U-tube mercury manometer. Heart catheterization was by then our business, but we had never seen anything like this! We were utterly fascinated. As the catheter tip entered the right ventricle, the mercury in the U-tube began to oscillate vigorously. Advancing further, a sustained displacement of the mercury appeared, with superimposed smaller oscillations. By measuring the difference in height of the mercury in the two arms of the U-tube, it became apparent that the pulmonary arterial mean pressure was about 60 mmHg.

We got to talking and pointed out that we had somewhat more elegant techniques for measuring intracardiac pres-

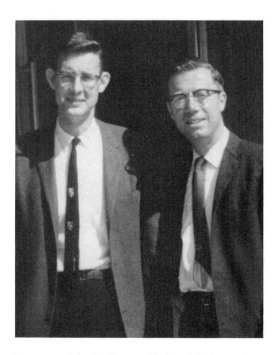

**Figure 5.** John T. Reeves (left) with the author in the early 1960s, collaborators for nearly 35 years.

sures. Would they be interested? Yes, indeed. Thus began the association between the CVP Laboratory and the Physiology Department of the College of Veterinary Medicine at Colorado State University in Fort Collins, an association that continues to this day.

Many medical conditions bear the names of those who first described them, so we like to tell the unsuspecting that Brisket disease was named for Oswald K. Brisket in 1897. That's nonsense, of course. The term "brisket disease" is used by ranchers to describe an illness in cattle characterized by dependent edema. Because cattle have tight fascia surrounding their legs, the legs do not swell. Rather, the edema accumulates in the ventral regions of the torso. In particular, edema distends the normally loose fold of skin at the base of the neck over the parasternal muscles, the so-called brisket of beef. It is as if the brisket itself were grotesquely swollen.

George H. Glover and Isaac E. Newsome, two veterinarians on the faculty of what was then Colorado Agricultural College (now Colorado State University) in Fort Collins, published the first description of brisket disease, "dropsy of high altitude," in 1915.[12] They recognized the importance of altitudes in excess of 7,000 ft in the etiology of this condition and that the edema was a manifestation of heart failure. Speculation was that "exertion before acclimatization at high altitudes, or in the case of calves, inherited cardiac weakness . . . caused exhaustion of the heart muscle." This theory was remarkably accurate, especially regarding inherited susceptibility, considering this was 30 years before U. S. von Euler and G. Liljestrand discovered hypoxic pulmonary hypertension.[11] Not until the 1950s was atmospheric hypoxia of high altitude suspected as the primary etiologic factor in brisket disease, and the pathogenesis considered hypoxic pulmonary hypertension leading to right heart failure. So it was

this hypothesis that Jensen and Alexander were exploring that cold day in South Park.[1]

## Cowboys

From Arch Alexander and Don Will, Jack Reeves and I learned in 1958 the techniques cattlemen used to handle steers.[2,52] We were mightily impressed by the cattle's remarkable pulmonary hypertension, apparently caused by hypoxia, and intrigued by the possibility of using this species in research. Could a couple of young guys who had never worked with cattle before become cowboys? Why not? So Jack and I began formulating our own project. If cattle developed moderate to severe pulmonary hypertension over several months at 10,000 feet, would the phenomenon be accelerated at a higher altitude? Why did some steers develop much more severe pulmonary hypertension than others? If hypoxic pulmonary vasoconstriction were the cause, could it be reversed by oxygen administration? And if airway hypoxia were the culprit, what might be the added stress of hypoxemia on the cardiovascular system? Pursuing that question, how would sheep react to high altitude, considering their unusual hemoglobin with its low affinity for oxygen? Would sheep also develop pulmonary hypertension?

To explore these questions we needed an experimental site at high altitude but within easy commuting distance from Denver because Jack and I had to maintain the heart catheterization schedule for the clinical program in cardiology. Look west, and there rises Mt. Evans, with a paved road to the summit at 14,143 feet. Furthermore, there was the Inter-University High Altitude Laboratory on Mt. Evans at Summit Lake, elevation 10,600 feet, which could serve as a base of operations. Above timberline near Summit Lake at 12,700 feet was a broad, level area called Summit Lake Flats, easily accessible from the road; we obtained permission to work there. But how do you study cattle and sheep when there is nothing but open tundra? Somehow we had to construct a field laboratory on the site.

Local experts on the care and feeding of livestock were found at Denver Union Stockyards. We sat down with them, explained our needs, and they proceeded to sketch out a pair of corrals joined by a feed storage area. The entire structure would be both portable and self-supporting, assembled from 6 ft x 16 ft panels constructed from 2 x 6 lumber bolted into channel iron. Fine. So in the spring of 1960, each morning at 5:30 a.m., Jack and I met at the stockyards to construct the panels for our future corral. A fine pair we were in our coveralls with skill saw and power drill, sawing, drilling, and bolting until 7:30, when we had to return to the CVP cath lab, change our "hats," and become "people doctors." Our project was underway.

Once we had completed construction of the corrals, we disarticulated the 16-foot panels and loaded them on a rented truck, which I then drove up Mt. Evans to Summit Lake Flats. There we transferred the panels, two at a time, to a 4-wheel-drive Jeep to get them from the pavement over the rough terrain to the actual site. Here Jack, Estelle, and I reassembled our creation, and thus we had our field laboratory. Our animals would need a continuous supply of water, so we ran 1,200 feet of plastic pipe to Summit Lake and established a siphon. For electrical power, we hauled in an old generator from the Echo Lake laboratory. At last, all was in readiness.[17]

Six weeks earlier, we had purchased ten 6-month-old steers (average weight 230 kg;—that's big!) and twelve 3-month-old lambs. We were impressed at how fast lambs grow; their average weight was already 37 kg. These animals became acquainted with our intentions during the baseline studies carried out at the Denver Union Stockyards. To transport them to the mountain, we hired a livestock trucker who loaded his semitrailer truck with 4 tons of hay, straw, and feed, the 10 steers, and the 12 lambs. Somehow he maneuvered that long rig up the twisting mountain road without mishap, but when he arrived at 12,700 feet it was clear he was suffering from the altitude. Again with our 4-wheel-drive Jeep, we shuttled the great load of hay and feed, and our animals, from the big rig over to our corrals. Meanwhile, our truck driver was all too eager to get the hell off that mountain with his long and now empty rig. Jack proposed driving ahead of the semi to stop approaching traffic on the tight curves and give the truck more room. The descent began that way, but the impatient and hypoxic driver soon passed Jack and went careening down that narrow road, scaring the wits out of every white-knuckled tourist who had the misfortune of driving up Mt. Evans that day. Several had to leave the road to make way for this madman, but miraculously he got off the mountain without demolishing his rig or any tourists' cars. Estelle and I never forgot that day, July 3, 1960, our 16th wedding anniversary. What a way to celebrate!

Nor will I ever forget the months that followed. Apart from conducting serial studies on each of our 22 animals, we had the responsibility of keeping them healthy and well nourished. This meant putting out fresh hay and food concentrate pellets every day, but what goes in must come out. So every Sunday afternoon, Estelle and I drove up to the corrals, broke out the pitch forks and wheel barrow, cleaned out the week's accumulation of manure, and spread it on the surrounding tundra. By the end of the summer that was the greenest plot on the entire mountainside!

On the days of study, we spent the preceding night at Echo Lake, left before daylight, and arrived at the corrals at dawn. Many mornings we would drive up through low-hanging clouds, only to break through to a clear sunrise shining on the sea of clouds now below us. Breathtaking. Literally. Our steers would often greet us bellowing with thirst because their water trough had frozen over during the night. Hence, chopping ice was top priority. Occasionally the siphon had stopped running, usually because some curious tourist had pulled the submerged end of our plastic pipe out of Summit Lake. Get out the step ladder, take it to the lakeshore, pour water into the pipe until it was filled again, and then resubmerge it; we were back in business.

Weather on a mountain at 12,700 feet can get downright interesting. Afternoon thundershowers were common. As heavy, dark clouds would blow overhead, every point of metal would start buzzing with static electricity, and your hair would actually stand on end. Lightening rods were fastened to our structure in hopes they would protect us and our animals from a lightening strike; we never saw one. Wind brought rain, then sleet and hail, covering the ground with that cold, white stuff. Hypoxia was not the only environmental stress up there.

Our hemodynamic and ventilatory studies went well. We even measured arterial blood-gas tensions up there on the mountainside. In 1960, blood-gas electrodes were not widely available, so with Jack's guidance, Estelle mastered the Riley bubble method.[38] This required introducing a gas bubble of known composition into a sample of blood in a Scholander syringe, placing the syringe in a water bath, and measuring the change in the size of the bubble with the aid of a low-power microscope. For this delicate procedure to be carried out, a very small shed was erected to protect Estelle from the elements. Each day you could see this hooded figure huddled in her shelter, squinting down the barrel of the microscope. Thanks to such heroic efforts, we obtained highly reliable blood-gas data.

Undoubtedly, Estelle was the last of the Riley "bubblers".

Each steer was catheterized five or six times and each lamb four times. An enormous amount of data resulted. We didn't stop with physiological measurements. At the end of 2 months, the animals were returned to the Denver Union Stockyards, and thence to a packing house for "anatomical studies." You might think you couldn't become attached to a bunch of steers, but we did. Each of the 10 had a distinct personality. Number 9 would always try to tear down the restraining chute, whereas number 3 was docile and gentle. Lambs? They're not big on personality. Regardless, after you spend that much time and effort caring for your livestock, you have regrets about ending the association. Such were our lives as "cowboys" that memorable summer of 1960. Over subsequent years I worked on other remarkable research projects in many exotic locations, but none ever rivaled this one. It was truly unique.

## We're Not All Alike

As Jack Reeves has often said, "It doesn't matter what you set out to investigate. The important thing is to do the work. You will always learn something." Of course he is absolutely correct. We learned far more than we ever anticipated and made observations that formed the basis for countless further studies. Most impressive were the differences between cattle and sheep in their responses to high altitude. The steers developed moderate to severe pulmonary hypertension,[20] whereas the lambs had virtually no elevation of their pulmonary arterial pressures.[36] We had a beautiful demonstration of species variability in response to the hypoxic stimulus[37] (Fig. 6). Over subsequent years we had the opportunity to expose many other species to chronic hypoxia, searching for clues to explain the

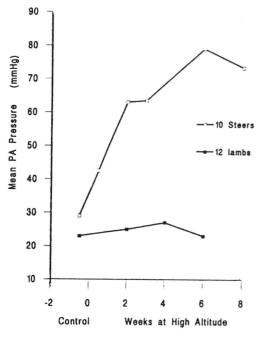

**Figure 6.** Species variability in the development of hypoxic pulmonary hypertension at 12,700 feet altitude on Mt. Evans in 1960. In response to the same hypoxic stimulus, only steers developed pulmonary hypertension, whereas lambs did not.[20,35]

basis for this variable pulmonary vascular response. The bottom line is that we still do not know.

In 1946 von Euler and Liljestrand published the first evidence that when a cat breathes a gas mixture with a low oxygen tension, the pulmonary arterial pressure increases.[11] This acute response results from hypoxic pulmonary vasoconstriction. Ever since then, thousands of investigators have been trying to figure out just how this works. It has become the cornerstone of many research careers, including mine. We believe that when an individual is exposed to sustained hypoxia at high altitude, the initial response is again hypoxic pulmonary vasoconstriction. During prolonged hypoxia, additional factors come into play, such as vascular remodeling, but at first it's just vasoconstriction. Furthermore, we know that the response is dose related; as the airway

$PO_2$ is lowered, there is a curvilinear increase in vascular resistance.[14]

When we see one species with a greater rise in pulmonary arterial pressure than another, we look to see if the hypoxic stimulus might have been greater as a result of differences in ventilation. In the case of our animals, we had direct measurements of arterial (rather than alveolar) $PO_2$ as well as $PCO_2$. On arrival at 12,700 feet, $PaCO_2$ fell from 40 to 35 Torr, indicating an increase in alveolar ventilation. However, with the passage of time, $PaCO_2$ returned to the low altitude value of 40 Torr, indicating that the initial ventilatory response was not sustained. Consequently, $PAO_2$, which was about 50 Torr on arrival, fell further, to 45 Torr in the steers and to 40 Torr in the lambs. Thus, if anything, the hypoxic stimulus was less, not greater, in the steers, and yet this was the species that developed pulmonary hypertension (Fig. 6). Remarkably, owing to species differences in the affinity of hemoglobin for oxygen, the arterial saturation in the steers was 80% compared with only 60% in the lambs.

If differences in the intensity of the hypoxic *stimulus* do not account for the variability among species, then it is reasonable to seek an explanation for the differences in the *response* to the same hypoxic stimulus. We have proposed that the initial response is pulmonary vasoconstriction. Does the pulmonary pressor response to acute hypoxia vary from one species to another? Yes. Then does the acute response correlate with or predict the response to chronic hypoxia? Sometimes,[16,54] but differences in pulmonary vasoreactivity are inadequate to explain the wide variability we observed between our cattle and sheep. Obviously vasoconstriction requires vascular smooth muscle. Hence, we may ask if the quantity of pulmonary arterial smooth muscle, i.e., the thickness of the media, varies among species? Again the answer is yes. So then does medial thickness of small pulmonary arteries in normoxic animals relate to the magnitude of pulmonary hypertension during chronic hypoxia? Overall, yes,[43] but with notable exceptions. For example, Wiltz Wagner has found that one species of coati mundi, *Nasua narica* from Central America, has pulmonary arteries with a remarkably thick media, and yet this species does not develop pulmonary hypertension during chronic hypoxia.[25] Perhaps in addition to species differences in the *quantity* of vascular smooth muscle, there are also differences in its *function,* i.e., vasoreactivity. That's a more difficult question to answer.

In seeking the basis for variability among different species, recall that variability among individuals of the same species also exists. Our steers on Mt. Evans made this point very clear. After 8 weeks at 12,700 feet, the range in individual pulmonary arterial mean pressures was 53 to 102 mmHg (Fig. 7). We had observed similar individual variability among our cattle in 1958.[52] Clearly some individuals were susceptible to hypoxic pulmonary hypertension, whereas other individuals were relatively resistant.

To test the hypothesis that these traits were genetically determined and therefore inherited, Arch Alexander and Don Will undertook a long-range breeding program at Fort Collins using individual bulls and heifers identified to be either *susceptible* or *resistant* on the basis of the severity of their pulmonary hypertension at high altitude.[53] After 6 to 8 years, they had demonstrated that these traits were transmitted intact through two to three generations of offspring. Note that pulmonary hypertension per se was not transmitted. All of the offspring at low altitude had normal pulmonary arterial pressures. Rather, only during exposure to hypoxia were the hyperreactive and hyporeactive traits manifest.[22] This was a landmark study.

Once these two populations of cattle had been established, one susceptible and the other resistant to hypoxic pulmonary

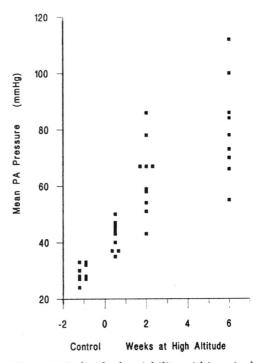

**Figure 7.** Individual variability within a single species (bovine); some steers were very susceptible to hypoxic pulmonary hypertension, whereas others were relatively resistant to it.[17]

hypertension, it became possible to explore the basis for these traits. So it was "back to the fort"—Fort Collins that is—where we from the CVP laboratory again joined forces with the veterinarians at Colorado State University 20 years after our first collaborative effort. Ken Weir and the rest of us found both functional and structural differences between the two groups of cattle.[51] Those that were *susceptible* exhibited greater pulmonary vascular reactivity, not only to acute hypoxia but also to other vasoactive agents, and they also had greater medial hypertrophy of their small muscular pulmonary arteries when biopsied. This provided a link between structure and function; more muscle gives a greater vasoconstrictive response. So it appears that the degree of muscularization of the pulmonary arteries is an inherited trait, both among individuals of a given species as well as among different species.

But why do such differences exist? Why should a steer have thick-walled vessels in his lung whereas a lamb has thin-walled vessels? True, that's a teleological question, but such differences usually serve some purpose.

## From the Bottom to the Top of the Lung

Denver has a long history of interest in the lung, dating back to the days when patients with tuberculosis were sent to "the mountains" as a form of treatment, just as they were in *The Magic Mountain* by Thomas Mann. That was how the National Jewish Hospital in Denver started. In the early 1960s, those of us interested in the lung from throughout Denver formed an informal club that met once a month in the home of one of the members. We formed a sort of think tank where we could throw out ideas to be kicked around by the group. It was great. Sol Permutt and his colleagues from National Jewish were always vocal participants. One evening we were discussing our findings from Mt. Evans and again the question came up, why do cattle develop severe pulmonary hypertension when made hypoxic? Sol tossed out the suggestion that in a very large animal with a deep chest, gravity would distribute more of the pulmonary blood flow to the ventral regions of the lung, whereas the dorsal regions would be relatively underperfused. This of course called to mind John West's zones 1, 2, and 3 of the lung. Such uneven distribution of pulmonary blood flow should make the lung inefficient in oxygenating blood. When the alveolar $P_{O_2}$ is fairly high, as at low altitude, this might not matter, but when the $P_{A_{O_2}}$ is low, as at high altitude, it might be advantageous to have lung perfusion more uniform. Raising pulmonary arterial pressure would accomplish this, and the deeper the chest, the more pressure would need to be raised. Hence,

large steers would need to raise their pressures more than small lambs. (We didn't discuss how hypoxic pulmonary hypertension was "useful" to the rat.) Sol is not one to be shot down easily, so his argument stood for lack of a more rational explanation.

After several years, Sol Permutt's casual thought was put to the test by Jim Will and his associates from the University of Wisconsin. I had become acquainted with Jim in 1967 when he came to Leadville with John Rankin and Jerry Dempsey to study the ventilatory adaptation to high altitude.[10] Those who know Jim realize he is not one to do things halfway. He had a graduate student named Anibol Ruiz who wanted to examine changes in the distribution of pulmonary blood flow in calves taken to high altitude. Once again we had to confront the question of where to work, because our facility on Mt. Evans was for one summer only and had been removed. At the time, Clyde Tucker and I had been studying goats[44] on land owned by American Metals Climax at 11,300 feet, and we appeared to have a long-term arrangement with the mining company. So Jim Will approached the company for permission to erect a more permanent laboratory facility on their property. They agreed, Jim raised the money, and we poured a concrete slab and proceeded to erect a prefabricated steel building, fully insulated, complete with electrical wiring, plumbing, and heating. Adjacent corrals completed the layout. It was really quite elegant.

The Wisconsin team then obtained eight Holstein calves. We studied them in Madison and then trucked them to Climax, where they were followed serially over the next month. As expected, all developed pulmonary hypertension; group mean pulmonary arterial pressure increased from 26 mmHg in Madison to 74 mmHg in Climax. Regional distribution of pulmonary blood flow and alveolar ventilation were measured using radioactive [133]xenon. Recall that in erect humans, hydrostatic forces result in an increase in perfusion from apex to base. In contrast, in the horizontal lung of the standing calf, perfusion *decreases* dorsoventrally, ventilation also decreases, and ventilation perfusion index increases from top to bottom. With the increase in pulmonary perfusion pressure at high altitude, perfusion became virtually uniform while ventilation did not change.[42] So Sol Permutt's prediction proved to be partially correct. Marked pulmonary hypertension in the bovine calf at high altitude did result in regional lung function becoming more uniform. However, in the absence of pulmonary hypertension at low altitude, the distributions of perfusion and ventilation-perfusion ratios were unexpectedly in the opposite direction from that normally found in man. Hence, the direction of the changes in regional perfusion were not as Sol had postulated. As they say, you can't win 'em all.

But wait. Sol Permutt's idea underwent yet another test, this time in humans. My phone rang one day, and Arthur Dawson from the Scripps Clinic in La Jolla was on the line. He too was interested in the distribution of regional lung function and had studied the changes in man during early exposure to high altitude.[8] In the sitting position, the normal increase in perfusion from apex to base became less apparent, and the distribution of ventilation-perfusion ratios became more uniform. He asked, why don't we see what happens in long-term residents at high altitude, meaning Leadville at 10,150 feet, of course? Great idea. Using [133]xenon, we found that in Leadville residents seated at rest, relative regional ventilation-perfusion ratio was again more uniform than at sea level[9] (Fig. 8), presumably as a result of their mild pulmonary hypertension, and exactly as Sol Permutt had predicted.

The question remains whether this

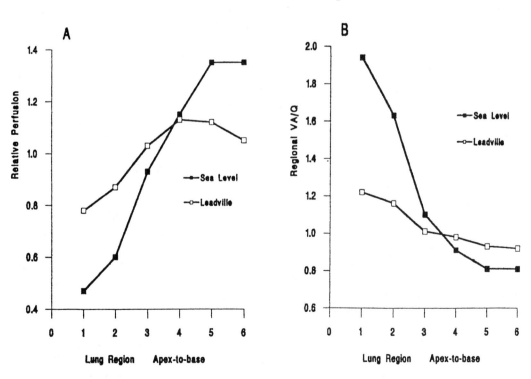

**Figure 8.** In residents of high altitude (Leadville, Colorado, elevation 10,150 feet), modest pulmonary hypertension renders the distribution of regional lung perfusion (A) as well as regional $\dot{V}A/\dot{Q}$ (B) more uniform than in sea level residents.[9]

more uniform lung function at rest is of any advantage in facilitating oxygen uptake. You could argue that exercise alone would make lung function more uniform, with no need to invoke pulmonary hypertension. To examine this possibility, Jim Will and I collaborated again, joined by Gerry Bisgard.[5] In our High Altitude Research Laboratory, we measured regional lung function with [133]xenon in Leadville residents, this time as they were performing mild exercise in the upright position. A significant upward redistribution of perfusion occurred making the ventilation-perfusion ratio more uniform. This redistribution did not occur in sea level residents performing comparable exercise, implying that the pulmonary hypertension at high altitude may indeed improve lung function. Sol Permutt would say, "I told you so."

The undisputed prime example of a high-altitude native is the llama of the Andes. If pulmonary hypertension is maladaptive, as some claim, then the llama would be expected to have no elevation of pulmonary arterial pressure at altitude, particularly because these animals have poorly muscularized pulmonary arteries. Natalio Banchero, Jim Will, and I obtained three llamas born at sea level and placed them in the Climax facility at 11,300 feet for 10 weeks. You guessed it; all three developed modest pulmonary hypertension. Mean pulmonary artery pressure increased from 14 to 23 mmHg, a response similar to that seen in man.[4]

If you have never been close to a young llama, you don't know what gentle, affectionate creatures they can be. When they are about one year old, they are delightful to work with. But young llamas grow up to be adult llamas. Ours became adults after our study at Climax was completed, and we returned them to the large animal facility in Denver. One day I was examining a calf that shared a corral with one of our llamas. While my back was turned on the llama, without provocation

he ran at me, reared on his hind legs, struck me in the back with his sternum (this is their normal mode of attack), and sent me sprawling on the ground. When I attempted to move, I felt a crunching pain in the side of my chest. I had a broken rib! So much for the gentle llama. Research certainly has its rewards, but it is not without its hazards!

## High Adventure in Peru

If cattle develop pulmonary hypertension at high altitude while sheep do not, what about humans? One of the earliest observations was made in 1932 by Alberto Hurtado.[27] A true pioneer in the study of human adaptation to high altitude, he established his now famous laboratory in the mining town of Morococha at 14,900 feet in the Peruvian Andes. On auscultation of the heart in Quechua Indians living in Morococha, he observed accentuation of the pulmonic second sound (P2), a recognized sign of pulmonary hypertension. However, not until the advent of cardiac catheterization in the mid-1940s could pulmonary arterial pressure be measured directly. Andres Rotta, an associate of Hurtado, first reported direct catheter evidence of moderate elevation of pulmonary arterial pressures at a symposium in 1949.[39] However, his pressure measurements in five Andean natives were not published until 1952, first in an obscure Argentinian journal[40] and then not again until 1956, in the *Journal of Applied Physiology*.[41] I believe this was the first documentation of hypoxic pulmonary hypertension in normal humans living at high altitude.

Obviously I had to meet Hurtado, particularly after our heroic experiences on Mt. Evans. So I wrote to him, and in 1961 Estelle and I flew to Lima, Peru. What an incredible experience! Hurtado proved to be an unpretentious man who invited us to his home for lunch with his family. He introduced us to Tulio Velasquez, Humberto Aste Salazar, Cesar and Baltazar Reynafarje, Andres Rotta, and Carlos Monge, Sr. and Jr., all authors of those landmark publications of the 1950s and earlier. Then we met the next generation of investigators, Dante Penaloza, Javier Arias Stella, Emilio Marticorena, and finally young medical students like Julio Cruz and Natalio Banchero. Penaloza and Arias Stella showed me their extensive new findings from the altiplano; humans do indeed develop pulmonary hypertension at 14,900 feet.[3,33] Altitude research was then at an all-time high in Peru (no pun intended!).

After visiting their laboratories in Lima, we were driven from sea level up over the 16,600-foot Ticlio Pass and on to Morococha for a tour of Hurtado's famous laboratory. I'll never forget that day. One minute I felt fine, the next everything went dark and I passed out cold. When I recovered, I was stretched out on a couch, breathing from an oxygen mask. I had experienced first hand the syncope that is now recognized as one manifestation of acute mountain sickness brought on by "going too high too fast." How embarrassing. Our tour continued on to Cerro de Pasco, another high mining town often used by the Peruvian investigators, then finally we went back down to Lima. Dante Penaloza invited me to speak to the *Sociedad Peruana de Cardiologia,* after which they presented me with a large certificate announcing that I was now a *Miembro Correspondiente* of that society. That certificate still hangs proudly on my wall at home, over 30 years later.

Although both Estelle and I spoke passable Spanish, through some misunderstanding our hosts got the idea we were having our wedding anniversary even though this was October, not July. As a surprise, on our last day we were taken to the country club for a lavish luncheon celebration. Those Peruvians really know how to entertain guests. Of course we couldn't let on they had the wrong date, so in 1961 we had two anniversaries. The second was especially memorable.

That first visit to Peru was informative, not only in terms of specific research projects, but also with regard to Hurtado's philosophy about research work in general. What I had observed was several generations of investigators working enthusiastically on various aspects of human adaptation to high altitude. Hurtado had made this possible by establishing a physical facility to conduct research in Morococha and then guiding his associates in obtaining research grants from the U.S. Air Force School of Aviation Medicine and later the U.S. National Institutes of Health. Thus, even though he personally was no longer in the laboratory, his efforts had facilitated others to continue in active research. Without Hurtado's efforts to create a research environment, much of the subsequent work by others probably never would have been carried out. I came to realize that I could perform a similar function back in Colorado and thereby further the research efforts of my associates as well as my own. That was a very important lesson.

## A Conference Among the Aspens

In the late 1950s, Roger Mitchell, Jack Durrance, and Giles Filley conceived the idea of holding annual international conferences devoted to various aspects of the lung. Through their efforts, the First Annual Conference on Research in Emphysema was held in Aspen, Colorado, in 1958. Today that series continues as the Tom Petty Aspen Lung Conference. Every conference requires a steering committee to organize things, and in 1961 the organizers selected a real novice to chair that committee; his name was Bob Grover. Imagine being handed the opportunity to put together a conference on my now favorite subject, the pulmonary circulation, and being able to invite anyone in the world. It was a fantastic opportunity for a young fellow like myself; I am still awestruck. Again, I say, the hand of fate moves in strange ways.

I plunged in with both feet, selecting investigators whom I believed were on the cutting edge of research on the lung circulation. Several again participated in this current conference: Kees Wagenvoort, Ewald Weibel, John Butler, Sol Permutt, Jack Reeves, and John West. I also brought in my new friends from Peru, Dante Penaloza and Javier Arias Stella, who presented their exciting work for the first time. And, to top it off, Andre Cournand performed the formidable task of summarizing the conference.[6] It was an outstanding success, and, for me, it marked the beginning of friendships with leaders in the field that I have continued to enjoy throughout my career.

## Finding "Gold" in Leadville

It's one thing to find pulmonary hypertension in people living at nearly 15,000 feet where the alveolar $PO_2$ is only 50 Torr, as Penaloza and his associates reported,[33] but would there be any significant elevation of pulmonary arterial pressure among people living at considerably lower altitudes in the Rocky Mountains? The place to look would be Leadville, Colorado, situated at 10,150 feet, where $PAO_2$ is 65 Torr. Undaunted by the local opinion that we wouldn't find anything, we contacted Dr. John Kehoe, the most active physician in Leadville, and found him receptive to our proposal. A clinical survey of the entire high school population of 508 teenagers was organized by Walt Weaver and conducted by our team of cardiologists. Sure enough, we found evidence of pulmonary hypertension through physical examination, electrocardiography, and chest x-ray.[35] We

had to document this by direct measurement.

They don't call Colorado "Ski Country USA" for nothing. The mountains get snow, lots of it, in the winter. And Leadville is in the mountains, so it too gets buried. Winters there are long. You hear Leadvillians say "last year, summer was on Thursday." In spite of this, we elected to perform our catheterizations in Leadville in February 1962. To get to Leadville from Denver, you must cross Loveland Pass. Today the Eisenhauer Tunnel bypasses the uppermost 1,000 feet, but back in 1962 you had no alternative but to climb over the 12,000-foot summit of the pass. In February in a snow storm, with an entire cath lab loaded in the back of your truck, that can get pretty hairy—and it did. But in two long weekends of intense work, Jack Vogel, Ray Rose, and I catheterized 28 individuals.[48] It may seem surprising, but the students agreed readily to heart catheterization, and without any remuneration. In fact, the kids teased one another by tapping an unsuspecting fellow on the shoulder any saying "you've just been selected for catheterization." Over subsequent years, we came to realize that residents of Leadville had a nagging concern that the high-altitude environment might somehow be injurious to their health. Therefore, when we arrived on the scene with an interest in their concerns, i.e., just what are the effects of living at high altitude, they were most cooperative and eager to help us find out.

Not only was pulmonary hypertension present in those young people (Fig. 9), but of a magnitude comparable to that found much higher in the Andes. We had Morococha right in our own backyard! We had struck scientific "gold." A whole vista of high-altitude research had suddenly stretched before us. Our catheterization studies had been conducted in St. Vincent's Hospital, run by the Sisters of Charity of Leavenworth, Kansas. We got to know Sister Mary Laboratory, Sister Mary

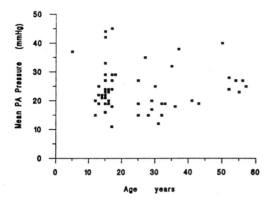

**Figure 9.** Individual variability in pulmonary hypertension observed at rest in 54 high-altitude residents catheterized in Leadville, Colorado, elevation 10,150 feet.

Kitchen, Sister Mary Administration, Sister Mary X-ray, and so on; they were a delightful bunch of women. This was a new hospital building for them, and they had not yet expanded to fill all their new space. Consequently, when we discussed with them the possibility of working over a number of years in more permanent facilities, they talked among themselves and ended up offering us a large basement room. Fantastic! We applied to NIH, obtained funds for fluoroscopic equipment, wall cabinets, sinks, and plumbing, and laboratory equipment. We had them installed, and by 1964 we had a fully equipped High Altitude Research Laboratory.

Not incidentally, the hospital and the community were justifiably proud to have such a facility in Leadville. Being a Catholic hospital, this new laboratory had to be blessed by the local bishop or cardinal or priest. It happened that on the day for the blessing ceremony, Jerry Dempsey and his crew from Madison were busy (Jerry was *always* busy) exercising their test subjects.[10] We had been told not to interrupt our schedule for the blessing. So this dignified figure appeared at the laboratory door, frocked and wearing a bishop's miter, only to be greeted by Jerry with this nearly naked, sweating, grinning, hirsute

subject named Schalub (not a Catholic). The unsuspecting priest looked shocked, mumbled his prayer, crossed himself, and beat a hasty retreat. We had been duly blessed.

Over the ensuing years, that High Altitude Research Laboratory provided facilities for an impressive series of projects, often conducted in collabortion with investigators from all over the country. As l anticipated, implementing Hurtado's philosophy of facilitating the research of others proved rewarding. The laboratory was, and still is, unique in that it is located in a modern community hospital with full medical services in a city with a resident population adapted to moderately high altitude. In a real sense, we put Leadville on the map, medically speaking.

Often our work in Leadville was conducted over the weekend. One Monday morning I received a phone call from the hospital's Business Office. It seems a concerned citizen had phoned the hospital to report seeing a car with state license plates parked on top of Loveland Pass on Sunday afternoon. Furthermore, the driver was accompanied by a *very attractive young woman.* Was this really official state business? The Business Office had checked the license number and found that the car had been checked out to me. What was the story? Well, yes, I was driving that car; yes, I did stop on the pass on the way back from Leadville; and, yes, I was accompanied by an attractive young woman—my wife! Estelle frequently participated in the research in Leadville, as everyone knew. The Business Office allowed they would contact the concerned citizen and assure him that what he had observed was indeed official state business. We've had many a good laugh over that episode.

## Was Darwin Correct?

Darwin's theory of evolution postulated that a process of natural selection operated through many generations, favoring those individuals who adapted well to environmental stress while culling out less well-adapted individuals. Survival of the fittest. When we discovered that at an altitude of 10,150 feet, pulmonary hypertension in the human population of Leadville was distinctly more severe than among natives of the Andes, we sought an explanation. Understandably, we invoked Darwin's theory of natural selection. Look, we said, people have been living at high altitude in the Andes for over 9,000 years, whereas Leadville was settled just over 100 years ago. Hence, the full spectrum of pulmonary vasoreactivity is still present in Leadville because not enough time has passed to weed out the hyperreactors. In contrast, natural selection operating through hundreds of generations in the Andes has resulted in a population of well-adapted hyporeactors. Sounds reasonable.

This argument presumes that pulmonary hypertension is maladaptive. Certainly if you are a cow that is true. Recall the steers we took to Mt. Evans. They displayed tremendous individual variability. After 8 weeks at high altitude, the mean pulmonary arterial pressure ranged from 50 mmHg to over 100 mmHg and full-blown brisket disease (Fig. 7). Had they not been removed from the hypoxic environment, the hyperreactive individuals would have died (through natural selection), leaving only the hyporeactors. In fact, this is the status of herds of cattle resident at 10,000 feet in South Park. Don Will and his associates found that among cattle native to this altitude, mean pulmonary arterial pressures averaged 38 mmHg.[55] whereas among the 10 steers we took to South Park in 1958, mean pressures after 6 months ranged from 41 to 109 mmHg (group mean of 63 mmHg).[52] Obviously natural selection does operate to minimize pulmonary hypertension, and because pulmonary vascular reactivity is a genetic trait, after only a few generations

you end up with an entire population of hyporeactive cattle. Survival of the fittest.

Nevertheless, adaptation has its limits, and given the fact that at 12,700 feet on Mt. Evans every steer had a mean pressure greater than 50 mmHg, you might think that, for cattle, extended survival would be impossible that high. Imagine our surprise when Estelle and I saw cattle grazing happily above 14,000 feet on the altiplano in Peru. It was incredible. I can't tell you what their pulmonary arterial pressures were, but when we showed photographs of them to our veterinary friends, they saw immediately they were all crossbreed "mongrels." The veterinarians then spoke of the concept of "hybrid vigor" and suggested that this, rather than generations of natural selection, was the clue to the survival of cattle at such extreme altitude. We had constructed our hypothesis based on our experience with purebred Hereford steers, by design lacking "hybrid vigor." Perhaps this had misled us.

Then we recalled our experience with the canine species. When Bob Johnson and I took purebred beagles to Leadville, they all developed mild pulmonary hypertension, 23 mmHg compared with 13 mmHg at sea level.[16] However, Alan Tucker reported no increase in pulmonary arterial pressure in mongrel dogs exposed to high altitude.[43] Was this difference analogous to that in cattle?

## Cultivating Research

Research cannot be conducted in a vacuum; it requires a nurturing environment. The original CVP Laboratory constructed in the early 1950s was intended to provide such an environment, and for several years it did. Within the CVP area was the cardiac catheterization laboratory directed by Gil Blount. The primary function of the cath lab was to provide hemodynamic and other information on patients being evaluated for possible cardiac surgery. A number of these patients had pulmonary hypertension, so the opportunity existed to explore their pulmonary vascular reactivity. For example, Jack Reeves and I demonstrated that a number of young children with ventricular septal defects had increased pulmonary vascular resistance, which could be reduced by the vasodilator tolazoline.[18]

Inevitably, as the cardiology service expanded, demands for diagnostic service from the cath lab increased. Consequently, less and less time and space remained for research. This competition for research facilities was relieved in 1965 with the opening of the newly constructed Colorado General Hospital and its updated diagnostic cath lab. I elected to remain in the original facility, now used exclusively for research, as director, while Jack Vogel was given responsibility for running the new diagnostic facility.

The newborn CVP Research Laboratory began modestly but grew steadily. Research funding was hand-to-mouth owing to several short-term individual grants. Fortunately, NIH recognized the need for a mechanism to stabilize and encourage small groups of investigators working on a common theme and established Program Project Grants (PPG). We competed successfully for one in 1972, and it has served as the economic foundation of the CVP Research Laboratory for the past 20 years.

Thanks to the PPG, a first-class research environment was established. Our permanent staff included Jack Reeves, Wiltz Wagner, John Weil, and later Ivan McMurtry, Lorna Moore, and Norbert Voelkel, with myself as director. We achieved a "critical mass," permitting the free exchange of ideas and criticism as well as mutual support for scientific problems. Young investigators considering careers in research were attracted to our laboratory, and with them came fresh ideas and great enthusiasm. It was wonderful, and privately I smiled, realizing that once again I had been successful in implementing Hurtado's philosophy of facilitating research opportunities for my colleagues.

## When High Flow Meets Mild Hypoxia

Jack Vogel and Peter Poole observed that patients with a congenital absence of one pulmonary artery seen in Denver often had pulmonary hypertension. However, a review of the literature indicated that pulmonary hypertension was rare in such patients seen elsewhere, i.e., living at lower altitudes.[34] The variable seemed to be Denver's altitude, even though the degree of atmospheric hypoxia is mild at 5,300 feet. This was 1961, the year after we had demonstrated the remarkable sensitivity of the bovine lung to hypoxia.

So Jack Vogel set out to create an animal model of the unilateral absent pulmonary artery syndrome by ligating the left pulmonary artery in calves soon after birth. The large animal facility I constructed with funds from the Colorado Heart Association, again to facilitate research, made such projects feasible. Sure enough, the calves developed rapid and severe pulmonary hypertension.[45] To examine the role of Denver's hypoxia, Jack shipped the hypertensive calves to Houston, Texas; the pulmonary hypertension promptly regressed. Next he reversed the sequence. Pulmonary arterial ligation performed in young calves at sea level resulted in only minimal elevation of the pulmonary arterial pressure. However, when those calves were shipped up to Denver, severe pulmonary hypertension developed rapidly[47] (Fig. 10). Keese and Noek Wagenvoort showed that medial hypertrophy developed in the pulmonary arteries of the overperfused right lung,[49] implying that the reversible pulmonary hypertension was due to vasoconstriction. The message was clear. The lung exposed to increased blood flow early in life has

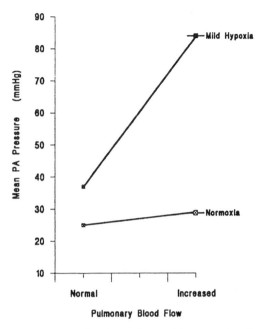

**Figure 10.** In bovine calves with normal pulmonary blood flow, only modest pulmonary hypertension results from the mild atmospheric hypoxia at 5,300 feet altitude in Denver, Colorado. Increasing pulmonary blood flow through the right lung by ligation of the left pulmonary artery (LPA) at sea level also produces only minimal pulmonary hypertension in the absence of hypoxia, i.e., normoxia. However, mild hypoxia combined with increased pulmonary blood flow act synergistically to produce severe pulmonary hypertension when LPA ligation is performed in Denver.[45,47]

enhanced pulmonary vascular reactivity to airway hypoxia. What a beautiful piece of research.

Vogel's definitive studies have many clinical implications. They help explain the observation that, among children with increased pulmonary blood flow secondary to left-to-right shunts through a ventricular septal defect or patent ductus arteriosus, the incidence of pulmonary hypertension is higher in Denver (and Mexico City) than at sea level.[46] Jack Reeves and I showed that this occurred because of pulmonary vasoconstriction, for the children responded to the pulmonary vasodilator tolazoline.[18] Further-

more, I have shown (but have never published my results) that in such patients, following surgical closure of the anatomical defect and restoration of normal pulmonary blood flow, pulmonary vascular hyperreactivity to acute hypoxia persists.

In another setting, Charles Houston observed a case of high altitude pulmonary edema in a patient with congenital absence of one pulmonary artery; he and Peter Hackett reported a series of such cases.[23] Some years earlier, Herb Hultgren and I had demonstrated that when otherwise normal men at sea level with a previous history of high altitude pulmonary edema were taken rapidly to Leadville, following exercise, they had abnormally elevated pulmonary arterial pressures, whereas they had no pulmonary hypertension at sea level[26] (Fig. 11). This implied

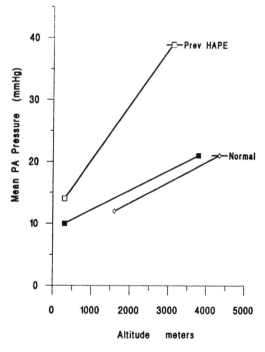

**Figure 11.** When normal men are exposed to high altitude for 24–48 hours, those with a past history of high altitude pulmonary edema (Prev HAPE) have an abnormally large increase in their pulmonary arterial pressure even though they are not clearly hyperreactive to acute hypoxia at sea level.[26]

that excessive hypoxic pulmonary vaso-constriction preceded the appearance of pulmonary edema. Hence, we believe that in Houston's patient we have seen again that the lung with chronically increased blood flow is extremely hyperreactive to the added stimulus of hypoxia, in a way analogous to Vogel's calves, although the calves did not develop high altitude pulmonary edema—but then no animal other than man appears to get high altitude pulmonary edema.

I have one further example of how pieces of the puzzle eventually fit together. Ivan McMurtry, studying isolated, blood-perfused rat lungs showed that the hypoxic pressor response could be prevented by the calcium channel-blocker verapamil.[30] Recently, Oswald Oeltz reported that another calcium channel blocker, nifedipine, is very effective in treating patients with high altitude pulmonary edema.[32] presumably by relieving hypoxic pulmonary vasoconstriction. Fascinating.

## A Most Remarkable Fellow

My phone rang one morning. It was my friend Paul Russell in the personnel department. Paul said to me, "Bob, I've just been talking with a most remarkable fellow. I think you would be interested in meeting him." Fine. Soon there was a knock at my office door, and in walked a callow youth who introduced himself as Wiltz Wagner. During the ensuing conversation I sensed what had excited Paul Russell; here was indeed an exceptional individual. True, he was a college dropout, but he wasn't the first young man who hadn't identified his direction. So I hired him as a technician and explained that he was going to learn a great deal about the lung circulation.

Wiltz developed rapidly. First he implemented the technique of microradiography to display the "pruning" of the pulmonary arterial tree that had occurred in our steers on Mt. Evans.[17] But he wanted to observe the pulmonary microcirculation in action, so I made it possible for Wiltz to develop the thoracic window technique to observe the blood vessels just beneath the surface of the living lung.[50]

Within a few years, Wiltz demonstrated his capacity for independent research, but such a career would be virtually impossible without academic credentials. Graduate school was the obvious route, but, recall, he had no bachelor's degree. To no one's surprise, the Graduate School of the University of Colorado would not even consider his application. However, there was an alternative, our strong association with members of the physiology department at Colorado State University. We discussed the situation, and they agreed to give Wiltz the opportunity to prove himself if I would act as his mentor. Wiltz disappointed no one and earned his Ph.D. in 1975. At last he was now qualified for research grants in his own name (Fig. 12). In addition, he was awarded a faculty position with me at the University of Colorado, although it soon became apparent that the academic opportunities for a Ph.D. in a clinical department were limited. To advance academically, Wiltz competed, successfully, for a faculty position at Indiana University. He is now a tenured full professor in physiology and holds an endowed chair in anesthesiology. Based on his research, Wiltz is an internationally recognized expert on the pulmonary microcirculation. All this from a simple phone call 30 years ago about a most remarkable fellow.

## Go West, Nobel Laureate!

Physiologists are taught to ask *"how"* but never *"why,"* because *"why"* implies purpose rather than mechanism, and that's teleology. Yet privately, teleology is our mistress. We do ask ourselves, what is

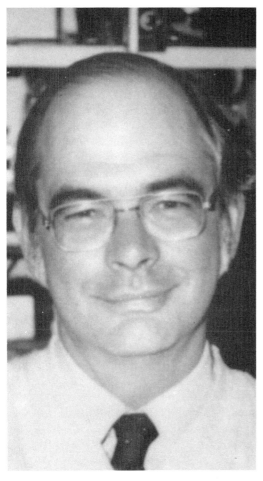

**Figure 12.** Wiltz W. Wagner, Jr.

the *purpose* of hypoxic pulmonary vasoconstriction? And we usually respond by saying that it serves to match local perfusion to regional ventilation throughout the lung, i.e. ventilation-perfusion balance, and thereby make gas exchange more efficient. Furthermore, if asked, most would say that notion originated with U.S. von Euler while he was working with Liljestrand back in 1946.[11] In 1982, Wiltz Wagner had the audacity to propose that we invite Professor von Euler to travel from Sweden to Denver to give us a lecture on his pioneering work on hypoxic vasoconstriction. The invitation was offered and, somewhat to my surprise, von Euler agreed to come, and he did.

In the world of science, U.S. von Euler is known for his discovery of the so-called slow reacting substance of anaphylaxis (SRSA), Substance P, the prostaglandins, and the neurotransmitter role of norepinephrine for which he received the Nobel Prize. Ironically, he never followed up on his 1946 report of the effects of airway hypoxia on the lung, and apparently it is only the pulmonary physiologists who remember that work. What is even more remarkable is that when von Euler arrived in Denver, he told us that never in his life had he ever delivered a lecture on that early work with hypoxia. Hence, his presentation in Denver was a "first" and it was wonderful.

There were problems to solve during his visit. For example, how do you entertain an elderly statesman of science, a distinguished Nobel Laureate, a visitor from a foreign land? Do you take him to the most elegant restaurant in town? Sometimes, but one special evening the answer was the Buckhorn, a turn-of-the-century eating place on the wrong side of the tracks in Denver's lower south side. There were four of us: von Euler, Wiltz Wagner, Ron Capen and myself. After several rounds of drinks, the conversation turned to the hunting trophies that adorn the walls of the Buckhorn: mule deer, elk, pronghorn antelope, black-bear – and jackalope. "I'm familiar with most of these, but what is a jackalope?" queried von Euler. We knew we had him going. Without cracking a smile Ron, the biologist, proceeded to explain that this was a rare cross between a jack rabbit and an antelope, and mating could occur only during the height of a severe electrical storm when the atmosphere was highly charged. The charged atmosphere at our table then exploded into laughter.

Before ordering dinner, appetizers were selected. Again von Euler was baffled. "What are Rocky Mountain oysters?" We insisted that he try them before we disclosed their non-aquatic source. It was fascinating to observe how our kind, gentle, distinguished guest warmed to being treated as just one of the boys, rather being held remotely on a pedestal. He enjoyed it immensely, and so did we.

The timing of von Euler's visit proved fortuitous, for he died within 6 months of returning to Sweden.

## Partnerships

If my career has been successful, it is because of the life-long partnership I shared with my wife Estelle. She was an active participant in all my endeavors, both scientific and otherwise. Together, we shared the labors, the anxieties, and the rewards of studying livestock on Mt. Evans,[36] of working with the wonderful residents of Leadville,[19] of testing Bolivian tin miners in Potosi, of exercising Quechua Indians in Cerro de Pasco, Peru,[15] of trekking to the base of Mt. Everest to learn more about acute mountain sickness,[24] and, yes, of touring the world exchanging ideas with other workers in the field of the pulmonary circulation. I conclude these

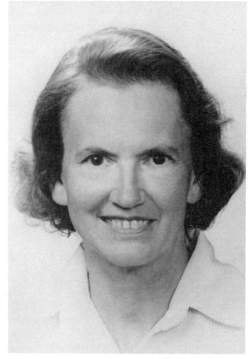

**Figure 13.** Estelle B. Grover.

reflections by dedicating them to my wonderful partner, Estelle (Fig. 13).

## References

1. Alexander, A. F., and R. Jensen. Gross cardiac changes in cattle with high mountain (brisket) disease and in experimental cattle maintained at high altitudes. *Am. J. Vet. Res.* 20: 680–689, 1959.
2. Alexander, A. F., D. H. Will, R. F. Grover and J. T. Reeves. Pulmonary hypertension and right ventricular hypertrophy in cattle at high altitude. *Am. J. Vet. Res.* 21: 199–204, 1960.
3. Arias-Stella, J., and M. Saldaña. The muscular pulmonary arteries in people living at high altitudes. *Med. Thorac.* 19: 484–493, 1962.
4. Banchero, N., R. F. Grover, and J. A. Will. High altitude-induced pulmonary arterial hypertension in the llama (*Lama glama*) *Am. J. Physiol.* 220: 422–427, 1971.
5. Bisgard, G. E., J. A. Will, I. B. Tyson, L. M. Dayton, R. R. Henderson, and R. F. Grover.

Distribution of regional lung function during mild exercise in residents of 3100 m. *Respir. Physiol.* 22: 369–379, 1974.
6. Cournand, A. Summary of conference. In: *Normal and Abnormal Pulmonary Circulation,* edited by R. F. Grover. Basel: Karger, 1963, p. 436–452.
7. Cournand, A., R. A. Bloomfield, and H. D. Lauson. Double lumen catheter for intravenous and intracardiac blood sampling and pressure recording. *Proc. Soc. Exp. Biol. Med.* 60: 73–75, 1945.
8. Dawson, A. Regional lung function during early acclimatization to 3,100 m altitude. *J. Appl. Physiol.* 33:218–223, 1972.
9. Dawson, A. and R. F. Grover. Regional lung function in natives and long-term residents at 33,100 m altitude. *J. Appl. Physiol.* 36: 294–298, 1974.
10. Dempsey, J. A., H. V. Forster, M. L. Birnbaum, W. G. Reddan, J. Thoden, R. F. Grover, and J. Rankin. Control of exercise hyperpnea under varying durations of ex-

posure to moderate hypoxia. *Respir. Physiol.* 16: 211–231, 1972.

11. Euler, U. S. von, and G. Liljestrand. Observations on the pulmonary arterial blood pressure in the cat. *Acta Physiol. Scand.* 12: 301–320, 1946.

12. Glover, G. H., and I. E. Newsom. Brisket disease (dropsy at high altitudes). *Colorado Agric. Exper. Sta. Bull.* 204, Jan. 1915.

13. Grover, R. F. *Biological Pressure Pulses: Their Registration and Interpretation* (Dissertation). Boulder: University of Colorado, 1951.

14. Grover, R. F. Chronic hypoxic pulmonary hypertension. In: *The Pulmonary Circulation: Normal and Abnormal,* edited by A. P. Fishman. Philadelphia: Univ. of Pennsylvania, 1990, p. 283–299.

15. Grover, R. F., J. Cruz, G. Jamieson, and E. B. Grover. Hypoxic ventilatory drive during exercise in man at 4300 m altitude. *J. Lab. Clin. Med.* 72: 879–880, 1968.

16. Grover, R. F., R. L. Johnson, Jr., R. G. McCullough, R. E. McCullough, S. E. Hofmeister, W. B. Campbell, and R. C. Reynolds. Pulmonary hypertension and pulmonary vascular reactivity in beagles at high altitude. *J. Appl. Physiol.* 65: 2632–2640, 1988.

17. Grover, R. F., and J. T. Reeves. Experimental induction of pulmonary hypertension in normal steers at high altitude. *Med. Thorac.* 19: 543–550, 1962.

18. Grover, R. F., J. T. Reeves, and S. G. Blount, Jr. Tolazoline hydrochloride (Priscoline): an effective pulmonary vasodilator. *Am Heart J.* 61: 5–15, 1961.

19. Grover, R. F., J. T. Reeves, E. B. Grover, and J. E. Leathers. Exercise performance of athletes at sea level and 3100 meters altitude. *Med. Thorac.* 23: 129–143, 1966.

20. Grover, R. F., J. T. Reeves, D. H. Will, and S. G. Blount, Jr. Pulmonary vasoconstriction in steers at high altitude. *J. Appl. Physiol.* 18: 567–574, 1963.

21. Grover, R. F., H. Swan II, and C. A. Maaske. Pressure changes in the pulmonary artery and aorta before and after ligation of the patent ductus arteriosus. *Fed. Proc.* 8: 63, 1949.

22. Grover, R. F., D. H. Will, J. T. Reeves, E. K. Weir, I. F. McMurtry, and A. F. Alexander. Genetic transmission of susceptibility to hypoxic pulmonary hypertension. *Prog. Resp. Res.* 9: 112–117, 1975.

23. Hackett, P. H., C. E. Creagh, R. F. Grover, B. Honigman, C. S. Houston, J. T. Reeves, A.

M. Sophocles, and M. vanHardenbroek. High-altitude pulmonary edema in persons without the right pulmonary artery. *N. Engl. J. Med.* 302: 1070–1086, 1980.

24. Hackett, P. H., D. Rennie, S. E. Hofmeister, R. F. Grover, E. B. Grover, and J. T. Reeves. Fluid retention and relative hypoventilation in acute mountain sickness. *Respiration* 43: 321–329, 1982.

25. Hanson, W. L., D. F. Boggs, S. E. Hofmeister, J. M. Kay, and W. W. Wagner, Jr. The pulmonary circulatory response of the coati mundi to high altitude. *FASEB J.* 2:724A, 1988.

26. Hultgren, H. N., R. F. Grover, and L. H. Hartley. Abnormal circulatory responses to high altitude in subjects with a previous history of high-altitude pulmonary edema. *Circulation* 44: 759–770, 1971.

27. Hurtado, A. Respiratory adaptation in the Indian natives of the Peruvian Andes. *Am J. Phys. Anthropol.* 17: 137, 1932.

28. Isbell, N. P., and E. Grover. The vaginal smear in office practice—the swab technique: an evaluation of 10,000 smears. *Am. J. Obstet. Gynecol.* 81: 784–791, 1961.

29. Isbell, N. P. and E. Grover. The vaginal smear in pregnant and nonpregnant women. *Acta Cytol.* 10: 87–88, 1966.

30. McMurtry, I. F., A. B. Davidson, J. T. Reeves, and R. F. Grover. Inhibition of hypoxic pulmonary vasoconstriction by calcium antagonists in isolated rat lungs. *Circ. Res.* 38: 99–104, 1976.

31. Newell, L. C. *A Course in Inorganic Chemistry for Colleges.* Boston: D. C. Heath, 1916.

32. Oelz, O., M. Ritter, R. Jenni, M. Maggiorini, U. Waber, P. Vock, and P. Bartsch. Nifedipine for high altitude pulmonary oedema. *Lancet* 2: 1241–1244, 1989.

33. Penaloza, D., F. Sime, N. Banchero, and R. Gamboa. Pulmonary hypertension in healthy man born and living at high altitude. *Med. Thorac.* 19: 449–460, 1962.

34. Pool, P. E., J. H. K. Vogel, and S. G. Blount, Jr. Congenital unilateral absence of a pulmonary artery: a review. The importance of flow in pulmonary hypertension. *Am J. Cardiol.* 10: 706–732, 1962.

35. Pryor, R., W. F. Weaver, and S. G. Blount, Jr. Electrocardio-graphic observations of 493 residents living at high altitude (10,150 feet). *Am. J. Cardiol.* 16: 494–499, 1965.

36. Reeves, J. T., E. B. Grover, and R. F. Grover. Pulmonary circulation and oxygen trans-

port in lambs at high altitude. *J. Appl. Physiol.* 18: 560–566, 1963.

37. Reeves, J. T., W. W. Wagner, Jr., I. F. McMurtry, and R. F. Grover. Physiological effects of high altitude on the pulmonary circulation. *Int. Rev. Physiol.* 20: 289–310, 1979.

38. Riley, R. L., E. J. M. Campbell, and R. H. Shepard. A bubble method for estimation of $P_{CO_2}$ and $P_{O_2}$ in whole blood. *J. Appl. Physiol.* 11: 245–248, 1957.

39. Rotta, A., A. Miranda, and R. Chavez. Heart catheterization at high altitudes. *Symposium Internacional de Biología de Altitud,* 1949.

40. Rotta, A., A. Canepa, T. Velasquez, A. Hurtado, H. Aste Salazar, and R. Chavez. Presión de la arteria pulmonar en el hombre que vive a 4,500 metros de altitud. *Rev. Argentina de Cardiologia* 19: 374, 1952.

41. Rotta, A., A. Canepa, A. Hurtado, T. Velasquez, and R. Chavez. Pulmonary circulation at sea level and at high altitudes. *J. Appl. Physiol.* 9: 328–332, 1956.

42. Ruiz, A. V., G. E. Bisgard, I. B. Tyson, R. F. Grover, and J. A. Will. Regional lung function in calves during acute and chronic pulmonary hypertension. *J. Appl. Physiol.* 37: 384–391, 1974.

43. Tucker, A., I. F. McMurtry, J. T. Reeves, A. F. Alexander, D. H. Will, and R. F. Grover. Lung vascular smooth muscle as a determinant of pulmonary hypertension at high altitude. *Am. J. Physiol.* 228: 762–767, 1975.

44. Tucker, C. E., J. A. Will, and R. F. Grover. Pulmonary hypertension in the goat at high altitude. *Physiologist* 12: 378, 1969.

45. Vogel, J. H. K., K. H. Averill, P. E. Pool, and S. G. Blount, Jr. Experimental pulmonary arterial hypertension in the newborn calf. *Circ. Res.* 13: 557–571, 1963.

46. Vogel, J. H. K., D. G. McNamara, and S. G. Blount, Jr. Role of hypoxia in determining pulmonary vascular resistance in infants with ventricular septal defects. *Am. J. Cardiol.* 20: 346–349, 1967.

47. Vogel, J. H. K., D. G. McNamara, G. Hallman, H. Rosenberg, G. Jamieson, and J. D. McCrady. Effects of mild chronic hypoxia on the pulmonary circulation in calves with reactive pulmonary hypertension. *Circ. Res.* 21: 661–669, 1967.

48. Vogel, J. H. K., W. F. Weaver, R. L. Rose, S. G. Blount, Jr., and R. F. Grover. Pulmonary hypertension on exertion in normal man living at 10,150 feet (Leadville, Colorado). *Med. Thorac.* 19: 461–477, 1962.

49. Wagenvoort, C. A., N. Wagenvoort, and J. H. K. Vogel. The pulmonary vasculature in cattle at an altitude of 1,600 metres with and without one-sided pulmonary arterial ligation. *J. Comp. Path.* 79: 517–523, 1969.

50. Wagner, W. W., Jr., and G. F. Filley. Microscopic observation of the lung *in vivo*. *Vasc. Dis.* 2: 229–241, 1965.

51. Weir, E. K., D. H. Will, A. F. Alexander, I. F. McMurtry, R. Looga, J. T. Reeves, and R. F. Grover. Vascular hypertrophy in cattle susceptible to hypoxic pulmonary hypertension. *J. Appl. Physiol.* 46: 517–521, 1979.

52. Will, D. H., A. F. Alexander, J. T. Reeves, and R. F. Grover. High altitude-induced pulmonary hypertension in normal cattle. *Circ. Res.* 10: 172–177, 1962.

53. Will, D. H., J. L. Hicks, C. S. Card, and A. F. Alexander. Inherited susceptibility of cattle to high-altitude pulmonary hypertension. *J. Appl. Physiol.* 38: 491–494, 1975.

54. Will, D. H., J. L. Hicks, C. S. Card, J. T. Reeves, and A. F. Alexander. Correlation of acute with chronic hypoxic pulmonary hypertension in cattle. *J. Appl. Physiol.* 38: 495–498, 1975.

55. Will, D. H., J. F. Horrell, J. T. Reeves, and A. F. Alexander. Influence of altitude and age on pulmonary arterial pressure in cattle. *Proc. Soc. Exper. Biol. Med.* 150: 564–567, 1975.

# 17

# Pressure, Flow, Stress, and Remodeling in the Pulmonary Vasculature

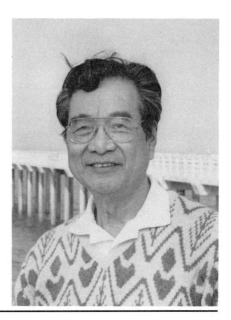

## Yuan-Cheng B. Fung, Ph.D.

*Professor Emeritus, Bioengineering and Applied Mechanics, University of California-San Diego, La Jolla, California*

## My Personal Experience

Personal experience has nothing to do with science but it has a lot to do with one's choice of topics and the approach one takes. To explain my approach I shall say a few words of my experience. I entered college in 1937 when Japanese militarists started the last big push to conquer China. I took my college entrance examination in Shanghai at the time Japanese troops landed in Shanghai. I chose to study airplane design because that seemed to be needed most by China to fight for its survival.

In wartime (1937–45) Chongqing, China had virtually no air defense. Our classes were usually held at the crack of dawn. Regularly, by 10:00 A.M. the Japanese air raid would arrive, and students and teachers would stay in the caves on the banks of Jialing River. One thing I saw most in those years around the caves was the clouds in the foggy sky of Chongqing. It was natural that my first publication was a small book on soaring and gliding in clouds.[7]

I entered the California Institute of Technology in 1946, obtained my Ph.D. in aeronautics and mathematics in 1948, and stayed on as a faculty member until 1966. My specialty was the mathematical theory of elasticity and nonstationary aerodynamics. The combined field is called *aero-*

From: Wagner WW, Jr, Weir EK (eds): *The Pulmonary Circulation and Gas Exchange.* ©1994, Futura Publishing Co Inc, Armonk, NY.

*elasticity.* It deals with the phenomenon of *flutter,* which is a dynamic instability of airplanes, supersonic aircraft, spacecraft, and birds when their flight speed exceeds their respective critical speed for flutter. It deals also with phenomena that occur when these flying objects encounter wind shear, gusts, clouds, clear air turbulences, or thunderstorms. It applies equally well to wind blowing on stationary structures. Indeed, the first paycheck I earned was for checking the safety of the design of the cantilever roof of the stadium of the University of Washington in Seattle against wind. I presented a systematic survey of the field in my book *An Introduction to the Theory of Aeroelasticity,* published in 1955.[8] My other papers were concerned with structures, vibrations, elastic waves, stochastic processes, protection of structures against nuclear bombs (the base-hardening problem). My endeavor to teach better led me to publish a book *Foundations of Solid Mechanics,* in 1965,[9] and *A First Course in Continuum Mechanics* in 1969, 1977, and 1993.[13] I was lucky to be recognized by my colleagues in engineering who elected me a fellow of the American Institute of Aeronautics and Astronautics in 1969, a fellow of the American Society of Mechanical Engineering in 1978, and a member of the National Academy of Engineering in 1979. Later I was even luckier and was elected a senior member of the Institute of Medicine of the National Academy of Sciences in 1990.

I began my self-study of physiology in 1957 because my mother had glaucoma, and out of concern and gratitude I periodically translated newly published articles on glaucoma into Chinese, which I sent to her and her surgeon in China. My sabbatical leave in Göttingen and Brussels in 1957–58 provided an excellent chance for me to read physiology papers. On returning to Caltech I joined Sidney Sobin, Wally Frasher, and Ben Zweifach in their studies of microcirculation. We wrote a few papers together.[10,11,35,51] In 1966 I resigned my professorship of aeronautics from Caltech and went to the University of California, San Diego, to devote myself full time to physiology and bioengineering.

How do you seduce a person comfortably established in one field to leave it and enter another field in which he is completely unknown? I suppose that there had to be a feeling that there was something in the new field for me to do. My first chance came when Ben Zweifach told me that capillary blood vessels are rigid. Looking at capillaries' ultrastructure, I could not believe this from my solid mechanics background. That led me to think about the contribution of surrounding gellike tissues that support the capillaries, and publish my first two papers in biology.[10,51] The same thought made me want to study the capillaries in the lung as a counterexample, because the pulmonary capillaries have virtually no surrounding tissue in the direction perpendicular to the interalveolar septa; hence, the distensibility of pulmonary capillaries must be very different from the systemic capillaries of the mesentery. The second chance came when Alan Burton and his students, Rand and Prothero, published their experiments on the deformation of red blood cells. I was a professional thin-walled shells man; I worked out a theory of red cell deformation and compared the theoretical results with experimental data to infer the bending and stretching rigidity of red cell membrane. This led to my third and fourth papers in biology.[11,46] Subsequently I made rubber models of red cells and studied the hemodynamics of red cell flow in capillaries.[59] Again I began to think of using the lung as a counterexample because Sid Sobin had shown me how different the pulmonary capillaries looked in comparison with the systemic capillaries. Then Wally Frasher introduced me to the determination of the mechanical properties of blood vessels.[58] I improved the experimental method and formulated a new theory to describe the mechanical properties of soft tissues.[14] So as soon as I spied the fringes of the new field, I knew how rich it was and was convinced that there would be plenty of things there for me to do.

Was something wrong with the old field that it repelled me? Not too much. At that time aerospace engineering still held sway. The government and military were pouring money into the field. The available financial, human, technological, and computational resources were almost infinite compared with individual initiatives. To me that suggested it was time to clear out.

Further, I did not need much imagination to see what contribution engineering can offer medicine. New instruments, devices, and prostheses are needed; new insight to physiology and pathology would be welcome. I was convinced that the science of biomechanics must be developed. The concerns of those in biomechanics—force, motion, flow, stress, strength, and remodeling—pervade the living world, yet the literature of biology has largely ignored these words. Hence I resolved to dedicate myself to the development of biomechanics.

## Cooperative Research with Sid Sobin and Mike Yen

Having Sidney Sobin and Michael Yen as close friends and collaborators is an extraordinary good luck for me. Sid was a prosperous cardiologist who accepted an NIH career professorship in 1965 to devote himself full time to physiology. Mike was my former graduate student and later my colleague at the University of California, San Diego. Our views on physiological research are similar. We would like to separate the work of searching for basic principles from that of solving boundary-value problems. We would like to identify the basic principles with as few ad hoc hypotheses as possible and base the boundary-value problems on the geometry and material properties of the real structure, i.e., geometry based on morphometry, material properties based on rigorous biorheological investigations. Then, for each clearly formulated boundary-value problem, we would like to solve the mathematical problem accurately so as to eliminate any inadvertent introduction of approximations, which are equivalent to additional ad hoc hypotheses. We thought this kind of approach would lead to greater understanding. Physicists, mathematicians, and engineering mechanicists call this kind of approach a *rational* approach. We would like to see if it works in physiology.

We chose to use the rational approach to study pulmonary circulation because in 1965 Sid had already made excellent progress in using the polymer casting method to study the morphology of pulmonary microvasculature. We saw that the pulmonary capillary blood vessels form a dense two-dimensional network in each alveolar wall. (See Figure 1, left panel, which is a photograph of the capillary network in a cat pulmonary interalveolar septum.) The capillary blood vessels occupy about 80% of the area in this plan view. Between the vessels are solid bits of tissue, which we call "posts."[35] The structure of pulmonary capillaries is so different from the systemic capillaries that we expect the hemodynamics to be different. We call the unique network a *capillary sheet*. We presented a theoretical study of pulmonary circulation at an ACEMB conference in November 1967[35] and at a FASEB meeting in April 1968.[36] Our first full theoretical paper was published in the *Journal of Applied Physiology* in 1969.[37] To complete the research proposed by this theory, we set up a program of study consisting of the following steps:

1. Measure the morphology of the vascular tree to understand the geometric structure.

2. Obtain basic data on the properties of matter involved in the system, including all of the gases, fluids, and tissues. Some mass transport data such as the diffusion constants, permeability, and solubility existed already. But rheological data on the apparent viscosity of the blood in small blood vessels and capillary network and on the mechanical properties of the pulmonary blood vessels of all generations were lacking and had to be measured.

3. Identify the applicable basic principles for the analysis. We decided to use as few ad hoc hypotheses as possible. We wanted to take the attitude of the reductionist to the extreme and allow only the following principles:
   • the conservation of mass,
   • the conservation of momentum,
   • the conservation of energy,

   and nothing else. For example, we know that waterfall phenomenon exists, as several authors before us have shown, but we are not going to make it a hypothesis. It should fall out as a result or conclusion of some specific boundary-value problem.

4. Formulate problems of pulmonary blood flow according to specific boundary conditions and appropriate geometric and material properties data. By "boundary conditions" is meant the external conditions applied to the lung, e.g., the pressure or flow at arterial inlet or venous outlet, the pleural pressure, any constraints imposed on the lung (e.g., a deformation due to a tumor, a movement of the diaphragm or chest wall), an external load applied on the lung (e.g., gravitation, inertial force due to acceleration or sports), and the mutual influence of blood vessels and airway. Each problem must have a special set of boundary conditions.

5. The basic equations and the boundary conditions together form a mathematical problem. In physics and engineering, these are called boundary-value problems. The next step is to solve the boundary-value problems of physiology.

6. Perform experiments and compare experimental results with theoretical predictions. If agreement is obtained, one gains confidence in the mathematical solution. If agreement is not obtained, one must reexamine the theory and experiment to identify the reasons for the disagreement. Inaccuracy of the material properties data, oversimplification of the mathematical analysis, neglect of extraneous factors in the experiment, mismatch of theory and experiment (e.g., dissimilar boundary conditions, wrong boundary values, etc.) are the usual culprits.

7. Finding genuine disagreement between theory and experiment provides opportunities for advancing scientific knowledge. Rectification often calls for major improvements in experimental control or accuracy and changes in theoretical concept or its mathematical description. One cannot rest until agreement is obtained.

8. The validated theory is then used to solve new problems and predict new events, which leads to new experiments, new comparisons between experiment and theory, new opportunities, and new understanding.

This program is straightforward, but it needed lots of work and documentation. It took us 12 years before we could close the first round of comparison between theory and experiment on the pressure-flow relationship of the whole lung[5-50,68-74,89-92,98-100]. But we had lots of fun on the way and found many pretty pebbles right and left. Furthermore, because a master plan exists, we know the value of every link in the chain, and the plan gives us greater patience in working out the details. A few highlights are given below.

## Anatomy and Morphometry

Much of the anatomy of the lung was well understood long before we began our work in mid-1960s. Data were incomplete, however, and a great deal of work was needed to fill the gaps. In mid-1960s, the data base was as follows: the branching pattern of human airway and arteries in the lung were known from the work of Drs. Weibel, Horsfield, Cumming, and their associates.[6,57,79] A lot of human clinical data existed but the majority of experimental physiological data was obtained from the dog, whose pulmonary arterial tree branching pattern is unknown. Elasticity data was known for only a few arterial segments of the rabbit and dog. The elasticity of the pulmonary capillary blood vessels was being measured by Sobin on the cat. We estimated that the measurement of the distensibility of pulmonary vessels of all generations would be a major effort. Because Sobin's work was progressing well, we chose the cat as our experimental animal.

The cat alveolar wall appears to be similar to that of man. The cat alveoli are almost twice as large as the dog alveoli and are closer to the human alveoli in size. Weibel had already idealized the capillary blood vessel network as made up of short circular cylindrical tubes arranged in a hexagonal pattern.[79] We looked at his picture and wondered how we could compute the pressure-flow relationship in such a network of tubes. Being schooled in fluid mechanics, we remembered the hypotheses under which Poiseuille's formula was derived. They are (1) the flow is laminar (i.e., not turbulent, no separation or secondary flow), (2) the tube is circular cylindrical in shape and is infinitely long, or, if it is of finite length, the velocity distribution at the entry and exit sections are parabolic over the radius, exactly as in

the long tube, and (3) the pressure distribution in any section perpendicular to the longitudinal axis is uniform. If these conditions are not met, Poiseuille's formula is not valid. That is why books on hydraulics are full of empirical formulas that are modifications of Poiseuille's formula: to take into account the finite length of the tube, the curvature of the tube axis, the existence of converging or diverging branches, and any special entry and exit conditions. There is no question that the individual tubes of the pulmonary capillary network do not satisfy the premise under which Poiseuille formula was derived. Modification is necessary, and trying to modify is in no sense disrespectful to Jean Poiseuille. Yet, strange it may seem, the resistance I encountered from the medical circle to our new theory came in large measure from our modification of Poiseuille formula.[54,68]

In deriving the pressure-flow relationship in pulmonary capillaries, we took advantage of the fact that the Reynold's number of capillary flow is very small (<0.001), so that the Navier–Stokes equation can be replaced by the Stokes equation. Even for the Stokes equation, we cannot handle the mathematical analysis of flow in the Weibel hexagonal-tube network.[79] We can manage the mathematics, however, to analyze a similar but different model of flow between parallel plates obstructed by round posts arranged in a periodic hexagonal pattern by means of the doubly periodic Weierstrass elliptic functions. In giving a name to this model we called it a *sheet-flow model*. J. S. Lee, Mike Yen, and I had little difficulty publishing the fluid mechanical analysis and its experimental verification in fluid mechanics and engineering journals.[12,15,19,44,45,60,76,83,84] Having obtained the basic solution, Sobin and I introduced further modifications to allow the sheet to be of finite size and to be distensible under positive transmural pressure and collapsible under negative transmural pressure.[38,39,72] In the meantime, we pursued morphometry of the alveolar sheet and compared our data with the data of other authors.[38,39,74] We believe that morphologically our model is as close to nature as Weibel's and is in some respects much better. In the first place, in the plane of the interalveolar septum the blood vessels of the real lung and our model have no corners, whereas Weibel's has. In the second place, with increased blood pressure the blood vessels of the real lung and of our model remain smooth, whereas the vessel walls of Weibel's model would have structural instability and buckle at the inner corners of tube junctions. With regard to the deformation of the capillary bed, when the blood pressure is varied, we can derive a theoretical relationship between the sheet thickness, transmural pressure, and tissue stress in the sheet model on the basis of the known geometrical and material properties.[38] This theoretical result fits our experimental results very well. On the other hand, if we used the tube network model, we would obtain some conclusions on the deformation pattern that contradict experimental results.

Knowing the capillary network in each interalveolar septum alone is useless to hemodynamics unless we know how the capillary networks are supplied and drained with blood. In other words, we would have to know the geometry of the arterioles that supply blood to the capillaries and the geometry of the venules that drain them. From photomicrographs such as those shown in Figure 1, we know that the capillary sheet of one interalveolar septum is connected to the neighboring sheets. In a sense the huge number of sheets of interalveolar septa form one big sheet. The arterial entry and venous drainage of each septum are rarely seen in alveolar micrographs, suggesting that they are very sparse relative to the capillaries.

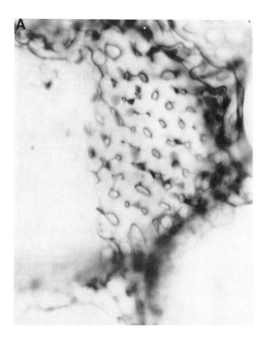 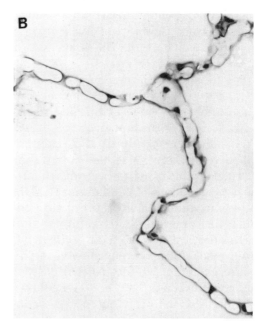

**Figure 1.** Two views of pulmonary alveolar wall (interalveolar septum) in a cat's lung. Left: Looking at the septum en face. Right: Cross section of a sheet. (Reproduced with permission from reference 37. Copyright 1969 American Physiological Society.)

Later we learned[92] that, on average, each arteriole supplies 24.5 alveoli and each venule drains 17.8 alveoli. This explains the experimental difficulty. To see the arterioles and venules along their length requires thick sections and low magnification. To identify the relationship of these vessels to the capillaries requires thin sections and high magnification.

A compromise method of identifying the capillary-arteriole-venule relationship is shown in Figure 2, which is a montage of micrographs representing a cross section of a cat lung.[69] On these micrographs every blood vessel larger than the capillaries was examined individually in the histological slide under an optical microscope to determine whether it is an artery (or arteriole) or a vein or (venule).[69] If a vessel was found to be arterial, then it was marked with a white dot. If it was venular, then it was marked with a bull's eye. The result shows a remarkable segregation of territories occupied by the arteries and veins. An artery is more likely to be surrounded by other arteries. A vein is more likely to be surrounded by other veins. An overlay of colored cellophane was used to cover areas in which there are only arteries. Looking at the colored cellophane against the background, we see a two-colored map. A geographic map of two colors can only represent islands and ocean. Hence our morphometric question becomes very simple: which are the islands? Arterial areas or venous areas? Which is the ocean? The montage gives the answer immediately: The arterial areas are the islands, the venous area is the ocean.[69]

How can we interpret this topological result in three-dimensional geometry? For this purpose, I can offer an analog. Imagine a tree, like a pine or a bonsai. The tree trunk branches and branches again and again. Each terminal branch occupies some volume of space. Suppose you find a specimen which is so shaped that when you pass a plane to cut the tree, the termi-

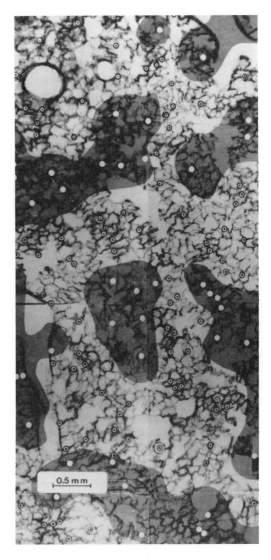

**Figure 2.** Only a two-colored geographic map can represent islands in an ocean. This is a lung map, representing a cross section of a cat lung, in which every arterial vessel is marked by a white dot and every venous vessel is marked by a bull's-eye. The domain of the pulmonary arteries are darker and the individual alveoli are seen. The arterial domains are like islands in a lung cross section. Such a map has many uses, e.g., it shows the relationship between microcirculation and respiration, it helps to locate the sites of "sluicing" or "waterfalls" in zone 2 condition, and explains the recruitment after capillary collapse in zone 2 condition. (Reproduced with permission from Sobin, Fung, Lindal, Tremer, and Clark, *Microvas Res* 19: 224, 1980.)

nal branch volumes are reasonably separated; that specimen's geometry is an analog of the geometry of the pulmonary artery. On the other hand, a garden variety analog of the pulmonary venous tree is hard to find. Perhaps a multitrunk banyan tree whose top covers a large area is a possible analog. In any case, the top branches of the venous tree must fill all the space left by the arterial tree within the envelope of the total volume.

Having clarified the topological relation between the pulmonary arterioles, venules, and capillaries, we can easily do some stereological measurements to obtain some needed morphometric data. Thus we obtain[69] that, for the cat lung, the average "diameter" of the arteriolar islands is $0.918 \pm 0.156$ (SD) mm, the average "width" of the venous zone is $1.158 \pm 0.410$ (SD) mm; the shortest path length between an arteriolar inlet into the capillary sheet to a venular outlet is $0.556 \pm 0.285$ (SD) mm. Furthermore, by counting the number of arteries, veins, and alveoli in several maps like that of Figure 2, Zhuong, Yen, Fung, and Sobin[92] obtained the ratios of arterioles, venules, and alveoli as mentioned earlier.

Turning to the relationship between pulmonary circulation and respiration, we need to know how the interalveolar septa are put together to form the alveoli and alveolar ducts and how the arterioles and venules are placed relative to the alveolar ducts. Hence I studied the models of the alveoli and alveolar ducts,[26] and the distribution of arterioles and venules relative to the alveolar ducts.[28,30]

Many people have made alveolar casts of wax, lead, vinyl, etc., to observe the geometry and structure of the alveoli and alveolar ducts. Miller[63] has reviewed earlier observations of historical importance, including his own contributions. More recently Hanson and Ampaya[55,56] presented a remarkably comprehensive set of data on the geometry of human alveoli and alveolar ducts. Oldmixon and

Hoppin[64] made sophisticated measurements. Mercer, Laco, and Crapo[62] used advanced computational techniques to make serial reconstruction of electron microscopic images to obtain data on alveolar geometry, surface area, etc. Ciurea and Gil,[5] Silage and Gil[67] made similar measurements of alveolar ducts. Budiansky et al.[3] have made theoretical calculations of alveolar elasticity on the basis of a pentagonal dodecahedron model. Wilson and Bachofen[81] have analyzed lung elasticity on the assumption that the structural elements of collagen and elastin are concentrated in the alveolar mouths, that the alveolar mouths lining the ducts can be represented by simple spirals, and that the alveolar walls contribute virtually nothing to lung tissue elasticity. But all this does not provide a clear three-dimensional mathematical description of the airway at the ducts-alveoli level.

I attempted to construct a mathematical model[26] with the following assumptions: (1) Alveolar ducts are formed by removing certain walls of the alveoli so that every alveolus can be ventilated to the atmosphere. (2) Before removal of walls to form ducts, all alveoli are equal and together fill the whole space of the lung. (3) Ducts are formed in a way that is efficient for gas exchange and structurally sound.

To begin constructing the duct model, we use a mathematical fact. There are only five known regular polyhedrons: the tetrahedron, the cube, the regular octahedron, the pentagonal dodecahedron, and a 20-faced icosahedron, of which each face is a triangle.[53,80] Of these, the pentagonal dodecahedron and the icosahedron are not space filling, and the tetrahedron and octahedron are space filling only if they are used in combination. Two nonregular polyhedra are known to be space filling: the rhombic dodecahedron and the 14-sided tetrakeidecahedron (14-hedron). The choice of space-filling polyhedron is thus limited to four. But because the interalveolar septa of the reconstructed alveoli given

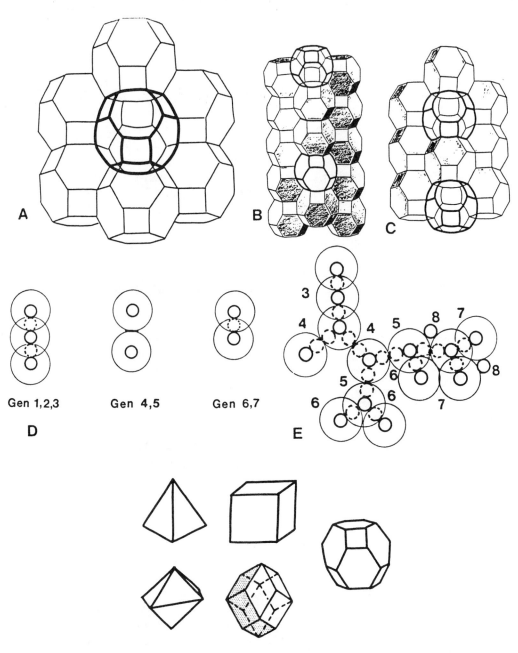

**Figure 3.** My model of pulmonary alveoli and alveolar ducts. At the bottom, five polyhedrons are shown. The three on the right-hand side are space filling. In (A), an order-2 14-hedron serves as my basic model. Fourteen 14-hedrons representing 14 alveoli are ventilated to a central duct, which is an empty 14-hedron. In (B), (C), the basic units are joined to form higher order structures. Fig. (D) shows 7 generations of ducts consisting of structures shown in (B), (A.A), and (C). Fig. (E) shows eight generations of alveolar ducts. (Reproduced with permission from reference 26. Copyright 1988 American Physiological Society.)

in references[5,55,56,62–64,67] do not appear to be all triangles or all squares or all parallelopipeds, we have to reject the 4-, 6-, and rhombic 12-hedrons as suitable models. Hence I choose the 14-hedron as the basic alveolar model,[26] Figure 3. Fourteen 14-hedrons surrounding a central 14-hedron form a unit called a second order 14-hedron. A second order 14-hedron with the walls of the central 14-hedron removed forms a basic unit of alveolar duct. The lung parenchyma is composed of second order and first order 14-hedrons. Successive second order 14-hedrons can be joined together to form longer alveolar ducts. My ducts model[26] is illustrated in Figure 3. The quantitative attributes derived from this model have been compared in detail with the data given by Hanson and Ampaya,[55,56] and I consider the validation successful.[26]

With this model and the data on pulmonary arterioles and venules, I deduced

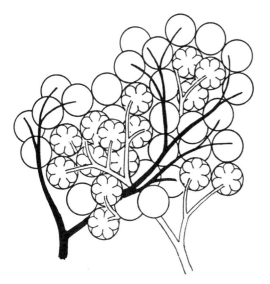

**Figure 4:** Conceptual illustration of how circulation and respiration systems are joined at the microvascular level. Arterioles are indicated by white. Venules are indicated by black. Alveoli are indicated by small circles. The basic units of duct, the order-2 14-hedra, are indicated by large circles. Alveoli in venular region are not shown. A similar drawing can be found in references 28 and 30.

the picture of the connection between the arterioles, venules, and capillaries, i.e., between the macrocirculation and microcirculation and between circulation and respiration, as illustrated in Figure 4.

In summary, I found the anatomical and morphometric study most rewarding. This study yielded a new model of the pulmonary capillary blood vessel network, laid the foundation for the sheet-flow theory, led to the basic concept of directional compliance of interalveolar septa: high in the direction perpendicular to the septal plane, low in the plane of the septa. We recognized for the first time the island-in-the-ocean type of arterial region distribution in an organ. We identified a mathematical model of the pulmonary alveolar ducts and alveoli. These results are new and fundamental, and we would not have studied them if they were not part of the information needed in the rational approach to pulmonary circulation. Yet they are basic to any boundary-value problems of pulmonary circulation. Hence, the rational approach is usually an economical one.

## Mechanical Properties of the Materials

A great deal was known about the properties of the gases and fluids in the lung and the mass transport characteristics across membranes. Least known in the 1960s were the mechanical properties of the pulmonary blood vessels. As I have explained earlier, due to the experimental work of Baez[1] on the capillaries in the mesentery, the capillary blood vessels were generally believed to be very rigid. Fung et al.[51] explained this rigidity in the mesentery on the basis of the tunnel-in-gel concept. Bouskla and Wiederhielm[2] showed that the capillaries in a bat's wing, in which the gel tissue surrounding the vessel is thin (about equal to the capillary diameter), are distensible. Now, in the pulmonary alveolar septa, capillaries are separated from the alveolar gas by a layer of tissue whose thickness is only on the order of 1μm (a small fraction of the capillary diameter), so the distensibility of the capillaries can be expected to be large. To document this expectation, Sobin and I worked out a theory of alveolar elasticity[38] and then set out to measure the change in the thickness of the pulmonary capillary sheet with the transmural pressure (i.e., the difference of blood pressure and alveolar gas pressure). We built a spherically rotatable microscopic stage to do it. The capillaries were perfused with a catalized liquid polymer. The static pressure was controlled while the flow was stopped before and during the solidification of the polymer. After solidification, histological slides were prepared and the thickness of the capillary vascular space was measured. We obtained the results shown in

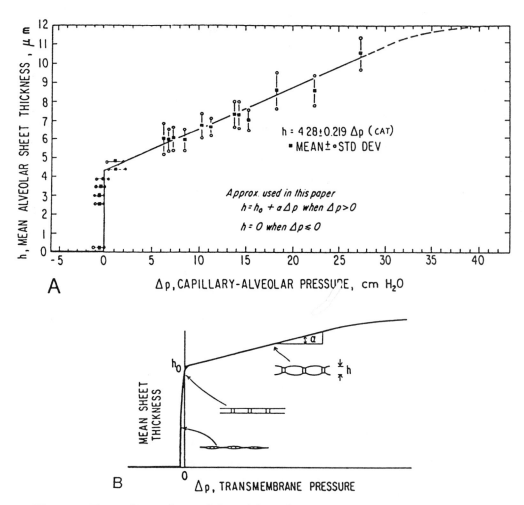

$$h = 4.28 \pm 0.219 \, \Delta p \ (\text{CAT})$$
■ MEAN ± • STD DEV

*Approx. used in this paper*
$$h = h_0 + a\Delta p \quad \text{when } \Delta p > 0$$
$$h = 0 \quad \text{when } \Delta p \leq 0$$

**Figure 5:** The nonlinear distensibility of the pulmonary capillary blood vessel is shown in the figure. The abscissa is the transmural pressure, $\Delta p$. the ordinate is the vascular sheet thickness, h. The distensibility curve starts at h = 0 for negative $\Delta p$, jumps up to $h_0$ at $\Delta p$ = 0, then follows a straight line at positive $\Delta p$ until $\Delta p$ = 3kPa (about 30 cm $H_2O$), and swings toward an upper limit at greater $\Delta p$. Theoretical deflection shapes are sketched. (Reproduced with permission from references 38 and 39. Copyright 1972 American Heart Association.)

Figure 5, which shows that when the transmural pressure is positive, the sheet is distensible. When the transmural pressure is negative, the sheet is collapsed.

Then Yen and I and our students[88,89] made morphometry of the branching patterns of the pulmonary blood vessels. We found that the arteries and veins are tree-like, whereas the capillaries are not. The fractal concept is applicable to arteries and veins, but not to capillaries. We then measured the pressure-diameter relationship of the small arteries and veins (with diameter less than 100 μm) by the silicone polymer cast method.[82,85] We measured also the pressure–diameter relationship of the larger vessels by x-ray angiography of isolated perfused lung.[82,85] Altogether we obtained the distensibility of the blood vessel of every generation.

The most important result we obtained in these studies, besides the nonlinear elastic behavior of the capillaries shown in Figure 5, was the observation that the pulmonary veins remain patent (not collapsed) when the difference of the local blood pressure minus the airway pressure turns negative in the physiological range.[43,82] This pressure difference is the net outward pressure acting on the blood vessel wall: when it is negative the vessel wall is compressed. For the vena cava or a vein without external tethering, the vessel wall becomes unstable when the critical "buckling" pressure is reached, and the vein will be collapsed if the critical pressure is exceeded. The critical "buckling" pressure of systemic veins is less than 1 cm of water. But the critical buckling pressure of the pulmonary vein is larger than 10 cm of water. This is because pulmonary veins are embedded in lung tissue, i.e., tethered by the parenchyma, which is composed of the alveolar walls—the interconnected interalveolar septa. In an inflated lung the interalveolar septa are stretched (in tension), and they give elastic support to the blood vessel wall. Figure 6 illustrates our experimental

results.[82] It refers to cat lung with pleural pressure equal to the values indicated in the figure (1 cm $H_2O$ is about 100 Pa). The airway pressure was zero (atmospheric). The blood pressure in pulmonary veins was varied, and the diameters of the veins were measured by x-ray angiography. The veins were perfused with a radio opaque material osmium tetraoxide, and the flow was stopped to make sure that the venous pressure was uniform everywhere. The horizontal axis of Figure 6 shows the value of blood pressure minus airway pressure. The vertical axis shows the ratio of the measured vessel diameter divided by its value when the pressure difference is 10 cm $H_2O$ at which the vessel cross section is circular. Thus, it is seen that the pressure–diameter curve is a straight line whose slope does not change as the blood and airway difference changes from positive to negative values.

Reference 43 presents photographic evidence of the patency of pulmonary veins under negative transmural pressure. Here we also provided the data from direct measurement of the diameter, length, and number of branches of the first three orders of the smallest pulmonary veins subjected to a wide range of negative transmural pressure.

This patency of pulmonary veins is of great importance to the understanding of pulmonary blood flow. In standing humans, part of the lung is above the level of the heart. The blood pressure in the left atrium is not far from the atmospheric value. For a pulmonary vein at a sufficient height above the left atrium, the hydrostatic pressure due to gravitational acceleration would decrease the blood pressure in the pulmonary vein to a value below the airway pressure. This is said to be in "zone 2."[65] If we do not know that the pulmonary veins can remain patent in this condition, we would worry about whether the veins in zone 2 would be collapsed. Now we know that they would not. We do know that the pulmonary capillaries will

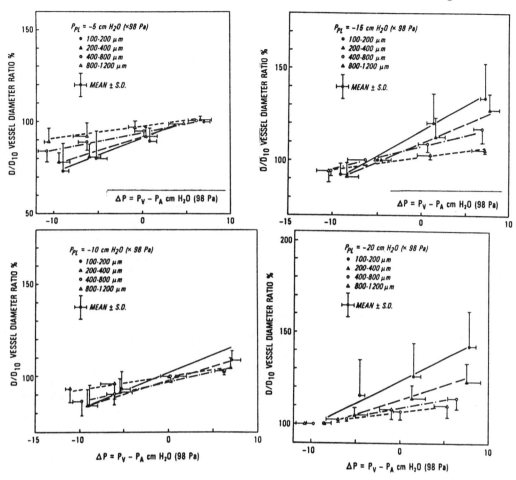

**Figure 6.** If waterfall or sluicing occurs in pulmonary circulation, the theoretical sites of action must be located at the ends of the capillaries where blood enters the venules. I reached this conclusion from the facts shown in this figure. Here the percentage change of diameter of pulmonary veins of the cat is plotted against the blood pressure, $p_V$. The airway pressure, $p_A$ is zero. The pleural pressure, $p_{PL}$, is listed in the figures. Note that the curves remain straight and they go through the point $p_V$ - $p_A$ = 0. The pulmonary veins do not collapse when the transmural pressure $p_V$ - $p_A$ turns negative, but the capillaries (see Figure 5). Blood pressure decreases downstream. Hence the first change for the blood vessels to collapse is at the ends of the capillaries. (Reproduced with permission from reference 82.)

collapse when the alveolar gas pressure exceeds the capillary blood pressure, such as at heights where the blood pressure is less than the airway gas pressure. For the blood flow analysis it is very important to know the exact sites where such collapse occurs. With the knowledge that the pulmonary veins do not collapse, our search for the collapsing sites is narrowed down to finding out where in the capillaries the

collapse will occur. The answer is pretty straightforward: due to viscous dissipation, blood pressure decreases downstream. Therefore the exit section where the capillary enters a venule is the place of the lowest blood pressure in the capillaries. That must be the site of first collapse in zone 2 condition.[38,39,41,43,48,50,91]

The sluicing of blood at a site of collapse of blood vessels leads to the "waterfall phenomenon" mentioned earlier. Observations and explanations of this phenomenon have been made by Permutt, Bromberger, Barnes, Bane, Riley, Zieler, and others.[65] The concept of waterfall is brilliant. A number of authors attributed the cause of waterfall to the action of vascular smooth muscle. Holding onto the idea that capillaries are rigid, they searched the sites of these waterfalls in arteries and veins. I considered the smooth muscle action as an extra hypothesis and proceeded to find out if it is possible to explain this phenomenon without the extra hypothesis. I recognize as an experimental fact that the capillaries will collapse under negative transmural pressure, whereas the pulmonary veins will not. A theoretical investigation on the stability of the capillaries[50] and the flow through the sluicing gates[48] led to the following conclusions for blood vessels in zone 2:

1. There is no waterfall in capillaries in the arterial "islands" of Figure 2.
2. All possible sites of waterfalls are located in the white "venous ocean" area of Figure 2.
3. A pulmonary capillary connected to a venule can be in one of the following three forms:
   a. completely collapsed (no flow),
   b. completely open: blood pressure in capillary remains larger than the alveolar gas pressure; there is no sluicing; while a rapid local pressure drop occurs after blood gets into a venule, or
   c. has a waterfall or a sluicing gate, and the pressure-flow relationship obeys the sluicing flow rule.
4. The number of capillaries in each of the three categories, a, b, c, named above depends on the size of the blood flow and the preconditioning (subjecting the lung to cyclic large flow) of the lung.

With these issues pinned down, a mathematical theory of zone 2 flow is then possible, leading to several simple, definitive formulas for the pressure-flow relationship of pulmonary blood flow.[29,30,48,86]

## Boundary-Value Problems

Once the geometry and material properties are known[14–16,29,31,82–85,93,94,98] we formulated many large and small problems by specifying various kinds of boundary conditions. We solved these problems and compared the theoretical results with experiments. The basic laws are the conservation of mass, momentum, and energy. Ad hoc hypotheses are avoided in deriving the basic equations.

The freedom of formulating small problems and testing the results along the way is the advantage of the rational approach we adopted. For example, our ultimate goal is to validate a theory leading to a computing program that can explain or test clinical conditions of patients. The system is the patient, the boundary conditions are the environment. This problem is too big to tackle all at once. Rushing ahead without proper preparation would not be productive. A more modest problem is determining the relationship between the pressures (arterial, venous, airway, pleural) and total flow in an isolated lung with nerves cut and environmental conditions maintained constant. The specified pressure and flows are the boundary values of the isolated lung. But the system is still very big. To further reduce the scope of the problem, we might ask: "When we keep on reducing the static pressure of the blood relative to the airway pressure, which blood vessel in the lung will be the first to collapse?" The system would be even smaller if the question were "For a pulmonary vein of order $n$ in an isolated lung subjected to specified values of airway and pleural pressures, what is the critical value of the static pressure of the blood that will cause the collapse of that vein?" The answer to the last question is dependent on the length of the vein, the conditions at the ends (details of bifurcation junction), and the interaction of the vein with the lung parenchyma attached to its outer wall. Further simplification can be obtained if one asked the same question of collapse of the capillary blood vessels in an interalveolar septum, because in that case no other tissue tethers the capillary sheet.

A big problem can often be broken down to a number of smaller problems. The lung is so big and complex that an infinite number of small problems can be formulated. I always turn a dozen or two such problems over in my mind, and every day I select one as my first priority. I train my students to do the same. I teach undergraduate courses in mechanics and biomechanics and ask students to formulate problems and solve them. Some students hate it, some love it. Many prefer to follow examples in the textbook to be assured of better grades. I try to get them to experience the pleasure of formulating problems for research or application.

Some little problems lead to nice little experiments. Some lead to nice little mathematics. My usual experience with theoretical problems is that at first the problems appears terribly difficult to solve. After tackling it for some time, I suddenly understand, and it becomes very simple, often too trivial to tell anybody. But I got lots of pleasure out of the experience anyway.

As I said at the outset, our objective is to obtain a validated theory that will enable us to compute the pressure, flow, stress, and strain in the whole lung, or anywhere in the lung, under specified boundary conditions. Our mathematical theory can be summarized quite succinctly, as I have done in reference 30, or, in greater detail as in references 23 and 29.

A brief summary may suffer a loss of clarity or precision. Hence I refer the readers to references 23, 29, and 30.

## Dynamic Remodeling of Pulmonary Blood Vessels

The stress-strain relationship of blood vessels mentioned above is an instantaneous relationship. Living tissues respond to stresses acting in them not only by an instantaneous deformation, but also by a slower process of remodeling their structures. I would like to show a picture of how fast the pulmonary blood vessels remodel themselves when the blood pressure is changed.

Liu and I[94,95] induced pulmonary hypertension in the rat by hypoxia. We used a commercial hypoxic chamber with a noncirculating gas mixture of 10% $O_2$, 90% $N_2$ at atmospheric pressure, 20°C, and 50% humidity. When a rat is placed in the chamber, its pulmonary blood pressure increases within minutes like a step function of time. Figure 7 shows a series of photographs of histological slides from four regions of the pulmonary artery of a normal rat and five hypertensive rats of the same initial age and body weight when put into the hypoxic chamber and kept there for different periods of hypoxia. The specimens were dissected and excised with the aid of a stereomicroscope, transferred into an aerated Krebs solution at room temperature (20 °C), fixed with 2.5% glutaraldehyde in phosphate buffer with pH 7.4 and osmotic pressure 310 mOsmol for 12 hours, postfixed with 2% Os $O_4$ for 2 hours, washed with distilled water, dehydrated, embedded in Medcast resin, cut into 1-μm sections, and stained with Toluidine Blue O. Marked swelling and thickening of intima were seen in the early period of exposure to hypoxia. Blebs appeared in intima in 2 hours and disappeared after 48 hours of exposure to hyp-

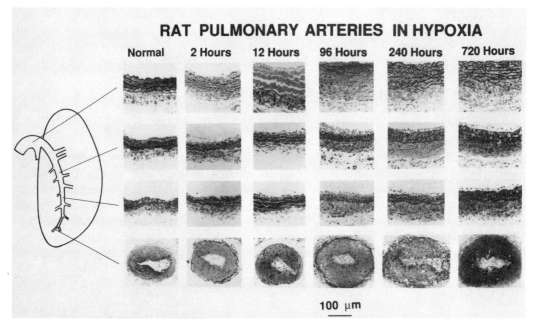

**Figure 7.** Photographs of histological slides from four regions of the main pulmonary artery of a normal rat and hypertensive rats with different periods of hypoxia. (Reproduced with permission from reference 34. Copyright 1991 American Physiological Society.)

oxia. The thickness of the medial layer increased slightly after 12 hours of exposure to hypoxia, more rapidly with a variable rate up to 240 hours, and then remained relatively stable in most regions of the vessel. The adventitia was thinner than the media in the normal group, changed little in the first 48 hours of exposure to hypoxia, but increased its thickness from 48 to 240 hours. It exceeded intimal-medial thickness by 96 hours. From 240 to 720 hours, the course of change of the thickness of both the endothelial-medial and adventitial layers ran parallel to each other. Thus the different layers of the vessel wall remodel at different rates.

Hypertension causes circumferential tensile stresses of variable magnitude in the blood vessel wall. Hence, one factor that can be correlated with the remodeling is the increased tensile stress. Other factors may be more directly responsible for

tissue growth and remodeling and may be changed because of stress changes, but our concern is with the stress.

To study the stress-growth relationship, we made use of another new observation. This is the finding that the zero-stress state of a blood vessel is not a tube but consists of segments of open-sectors whose opening angles vary along the length of the vessel. By cutting a vessel into short segments of rings and cutting the rings radially, they will open up into sectors. For the pulmonary artery, the opening angle of segments near the right ventricle can be as large as 360° or more. The variation of the opening angle along the pulmonary artery of a normal rat is shown in Figure 8. We can show that the opening angle correlates linearly with the thickness to radius ratio of the vessel wall if the vessel is straight. The opening angle is larger if the vessel is curved. When hypoxic hypertension is produced in the

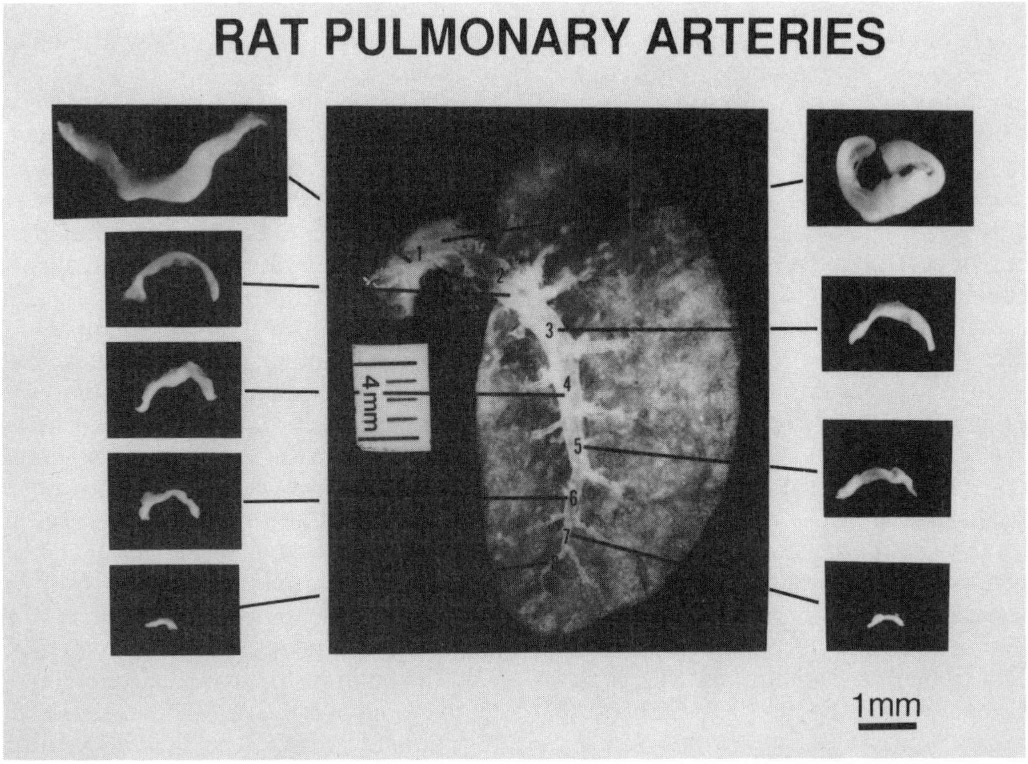

## RAT PULMONARY ARTERIES

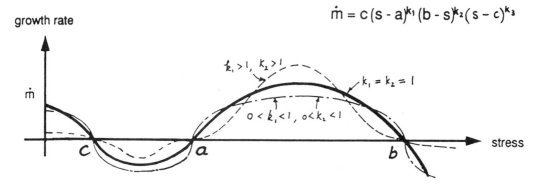

**Figure 8.** Photographs of the main pulmonary artery of a rat, and the zero-stress configuration of the artery at the locations indicated, with the endothelium facing downward. (Reproduced with permission from reference 34. Copyright 1991 American Physiological Society.)

rat, the opening angle at any given location changes with the length of time the animal suffered hypertension. Generally, at first the opening angle increases, then it decreases to values smaller than those of the control. This reflects the process of remodeling in the different layers of the blood vessel.[24,29,33,34,92–97]

Similar opening angle measurements and histological observations have been

$$\dot{m} = c\,(s - a)^{k_1}\,(b - s)^{k_2}\,(s - c)^{k_3}$$

**Figure 9.** The author's proposed stress-growth law. (Reproduced with permission from reference 29. Copyright 1991 Springer-Verlag.)

made on rat aorta in hypertension and hypotension, and diabetes.[33,95] These experiences lead me to speculate about the existence of a stress-growth law. I would like to present a possible form of such a law.[29] Referring to Figure 9, let the solid curve represent a relationship between the rate of growth of the mass of a material in the blood vessel (such as the smooth muscle, endothelial cells, collagen, elastin, or other substances) and the stress or strain acting in the material. The symbol $\dot{m}$ represents the rate of material growth. The symbol $s$ may represent a component of the stress or strain tensor, or a stress or strain invariant. Let $a$ represent a homeostatic value of $s$, at which the tissue can maintain a steady state. $\dot{m}$ is positive when $s$ exceeds $a$. $\dot{m}$ is negative when $s$ is less than $a$. The rate of growth $\dot{m}$, however, cannot increase indefinitely with increasing $s$. In orthopedics it is known that excessive $s$ causes resorption. Hence we assume that another homeostatic stress state $b$ exists beyond which resorption occurs. Similarly, the negative rate of $\dot{m}$ when $s < a$ cannot be unbounded. Suppose that resorption stops when $s = c$, where $c < a$; then $c$ is another homeostatic stress or strain. If the rate of growth $\dot{m}$ is a continuous function of $s$, and this function has zeros at a, b, c, and if the trend of change of $\dot{m}$ at a, b, c, is as discussed above, I propose the following simple relation.[29]

$$\dot{m} = C\,(s\text{-}a)^{k_1}\,(b\text{-}s)^{k_2}\,(s\text{-}c)^{k_3} \qquad (1)$$

in which a, b, c, C, $k_1$, $k_2$, $k_3$ are positive constants. This formula implies $\dot{m}$ to be positive when $s = 0$, as in cell culture in petrie dishes. The exponents $k_1$, $k_2$, $k_3$ determine how fast the growth rate changes when $s$ deviates from the homeostatic state. If $k_1 > 1$, the slope of the growth curve is zero at $s = a$, then small deviation has little influence. The slope of the growth curve is infinite at $a$ if $k_1 < 1$. $k_1 = 1$ signals a finite slope. I am using this

theoretical proposal as an experimental hypothesis.

In biomechanics of the bone, a relation between stress and growth is known as Wolff's law, which is over 100 years old.[29] Kummer[100] has posed Wolff's law in a manner similar to Eq. 1. Any formulation of growth-stress law for internal organs should refer to the literature on Wolff's law. There is also a huge literature on physical education, sports, sports medicine, and the science and art of surgery and rehabilitation, all concerned with stress and growth. thus a large stock of knowledge exists that has not, however, been distilled into mathematical form. In the new "tissue engineering" on the horizon, which aims to create tissue substitute with living cells to be used in surgery, the growth-stress law will play a decisive role.

The relationship of the topics of tissue remodeling and the growth-stress law to the study of pressure and flow in the lung is not far-fetched. Pressure and flow depend on the geometry and mechanical properties of the blood vessels, which are controlled by remodeling.

## Conclusion

I am a physiologist who entered the door by self-study, without formal training, because I found the subject more interesting than others and the people in the field nice. I made a plan to take a rational approach to studying pulmonary circulation, a plan that begins with morphometry, centers on the determination of the mechanical properties of materials involved, then follows a process of formulating boundary-value problems based on well accepted basic principles, solving the problems and testing the results experimentally in order to validate the analysis and gain confidence in the results, until it becomes possible to put all the blocks together to obtain the pressure-flow relationship of the whole organ. Then we compare the theoretical predictions with experimental results of the whole organ to validate the theory and seek to improve it. Once satisfactory agreement is obtained, then we can go to the next level of understanding and practical applications. Any success I have had I owe to my collaborators, Sid Sobin, Mike Yen, Shu Qian Liu, Herta Tremer, Feng Yuan Zhuang, and many others. In this chapter I present a few figures that represent some of the more interesting things picked up along the way. The explanations presented here are abridged and incomplete. For a more complete explanation, please see my books.[23,29,31] I would hope that I and my collaborators are remembered by the road we took and the vistas we opened. The odds and ends we picked up from the roadside are treasures for us. They gave us pleasure and enthusiasm; they illustrate the beauty of the road and the fertility of the land. But they are incidental. Only the road can give us direction.

# References

1. Baez, S., H. Lamport, and A. Baez. Pressure effects in living microscopic vessels. In: *Flow Properties of Blood and Other Biological Systems*, edited by Copley and Stainsky. London: Pergamon Press, 1960, p. 122–136.
2. Bouskela, E., and Wiederhielm, C. A. Microvascular myogenic reaction in the wing of the intact unanesthetized bat. *Am J. Physiol* 237: H59–H65, 1979.
3. Budiansky, B., and E. Kimmel. Elastic moduli of lungs. *J. Appl. Mech.* 109: 351–358, 1987.
4. Chuong, C. J., and Y. C. Fung. Residual stress in arteries. In: *Frontiers in Biomechanics*, (edited by G. W. Schmid-Schobein, S. L.-Y. Woo, and B. W. Zweifach. New York: Springer, 1986, p. 117–129.
5. Ciurea, D., and J. Gil. Morphometric study of human alveolar ducts based on serial sections. *J. Appl. Physiol.* 67: 2512–2521, 1989.
6. Cumming, G., R. Henderson, K. Horsfield, and S. S. Singhal. The functional morphology of the pulmonary circulation. In: *The Pulmonary Circulation and Interstitial Space.* edited by A. P. Fishman and H. H. Hecht. 1969, p. 327–340.
7. Fung, Y. C. *Gliding and Soaring in Clouds.* Chongking: Chinese Gliding Society, [In Chinese.] 1944.
8. Fung, Y. C. *An Introduction to the Theory of Aeroelasticity.* New York: John Wiley and Sons, 1955. Revised, Dover Publications, New York, 1969, and 1993.
9. Fung, Y. C. *Foundations of Solid Mechanics.* Englewood Cliffs, NJ: Prentice-Hall, 1965.
10. Fung, Y. C. Microscopic blood vessels in the mesentery. In: *Biomechanics,* edited by Y. C. Fung, New York: American Society of Mechanical Engineers, 25: 1966, p. 151–166.
11. Fung, Y. C. Theoretical considerations of the elasticity of red cells and small blood vessels. *Fed Proc* 25: 1761–1772, 1966.
12. Fung, Y. C. Blood flow in the capillary bed. *J. Biomech.* 2: 353–373, 1969.
13. Fung, Y. C. *A First Course in Continuum Mechanics.* 3rd ed. Englewood Cliffs, NJ: Prentice-Hall, 1993.
14. Fung, Y. C.: Stress-strain-history relations of soft tissues in simple elongation. In: *Biomechanics: Its Foundations and Objectives,* edited by Y. C. Fung, Englewood Cliffs, NJ: Prentice-Hall, 1971, Chap. 7, 181–208.
15. Fung Y. C. Theoretical pulmonary microvascular impedance. *Ann. Biomed. Eng.* 1: 221–245. 1972.
16. Fung, Y. C.: Biorheology of soft tissues. *Biorheology* 10: 139–155, 1973.
17. Fung, Y. C. Stochastic flow in capillary blood vessels. *Microvasc. Res.* 5: 34–49, 1973.
18. Fung, Y. C. Fluid in the interstitial space of the pulmonary alveolar sheet. *Microvasc. Res.* 7: 89–113, 1974.
19. Fung, Y. C. A theory of elasticity of the lung. *J. Appl Mech.* 41E: 8–14, March 1974.
20. Fung, Y. C. Does the surface tension make the lung inherently unstable? *Circ. Res.* 37: 497–502, 1975.
21. Fung, Y. C. 1975 Eugene M. Landis Award Lecture: Microcirculation as seen by a red cell. *Microvasc. Res.* 10: 246–264, 1975.
22. Fung, Y. C. Stress, deformation, and atelectasis of the lung. *Circ. Res.* 37: 481–496, 1975.

23. Fung, Y. C. *Biodynamics: Circulation.* New York: Springer, 1984.

24. Fung Y. C. What principle governs the stress distribution in living organs? In: *Biomechanics in China, Japan, and USA: Proceedings of an International Conference held in Wuhan, China, in May, 1983.* (edited by Y. C. Fung, E. Fukada, J. J. Wang), Beijing: Science, 1984, p. 1–13.

25. Fung, Y. C. Microrheology and constitutive equation of soft tissue. *Biorheology* 25: 261–270, 1988.

26. Fung, Y. C. A model of the lung structure and its validation. *J. Appl. Physiol.* 64: 2132–2141, 1988.

27. Fung, Y. C. Connecting incremental shear modulus and Poisson's ratio of lung tissue with morphology and rheology of microstructure. *Biorheology* 26: 279–289, 1989.

28. Fung, Y. C. Connection of micro- and macromechanics of the lung. In: *Microvascular Mechanics: Hemodynamics of Systemic and Pulmonary Microcirculation,* (edited by J. S. Lee and T. C. Skalak). New York: Springer, 1989, Chap. 13, p. 191–217.

29. Fung, Y. C. *Biomechanics: Motion, Flow, Stress, and Growth.* New York: Springer, 1990.

30. Fung, Y. C. Dynamics of blood flow and pressure-flow relationship. In: *The Lung: Scientific Foundations,* edited by R. G. Crystal and J. B. West. New York: Raven, 1991, Chap. 5.2.2.,p. 1121–1134.

31. Fung, Y. C. *Biomechanics: Mechanical Properties of Living Tissues.* New York, Springer Verlag, 1st ed. 1981 2nd ed. 1993.

32. Fung, Y. C., K. Fronek, and P. Patitucci. Pseudoelasticity of arteries and the choice of its mathematical expression. *Am. J. Physiol.* 237: H620–H631, 1979.

33. Fung, Y. C. and S. Q. Liu, Change of residual strains in arteries due to hypertrophy caused by aortic constriction. *Cir. Res.* 65: 1340–1349, 1989.

34. Fung, Y. C. and S. Q. Liu, Changes of zero-stress state of rat pulmonary arteries in hypoxic hypotension. *J. Appl. Physiol.* 70: 2455–2470, 1991.

35. Fung, Y. C., and S. S. Sobin. A sheet-flow concept of the pulmonary alveolar microcirculation: mophometry and theoretical results (Abstract). In: *Proceedings of the Conference on Annual Engineering in Medicine and Biology,* Vol. 9. Boston, MA, 1967, p. 97.

36. Fung, Y. C., and S. S. Sobin. Sheet-flow concept of pulmonary alveolar microcirculation: theory (Abstract). In: *Federation of the American Society for Experimental Biology,* 1968, p. 578.

37. Fung, Y. C., and S. S. Sobin. Theory of sheet flow in the lung alveoli. *J. Appl. Physiol.* 26: 472–488, 1969.

38. Fung, Y.C., and S. S. Sobin. Elasticity of the pulmonary alveolar sheet. *Circ. Res.* 30: 451–469, 1972.

39. Fung, Y. C., and S. S. Sobin. Pulmonary alveolar blood flow. *Circ. Res.,* 30: 470–490, 1972. Including an appendix by Y. C. Fung, R. T. Yen, and E. Mead, Model experiment on the stability of a collapsed Starling resistor in flow at low Reynolds number, p. 487–490.

40. Fung, Y. C., and S. S. Sobin. Mechanics of pulmonary circulation. In: *Cardiovascular Flow Dynamics and Measurements,* edited by N. H. C. Hwang and N. A. Norman, Baltimore: University Park Press, 1977, Chap. 17, p. 665–730.

41. Fung, Y. C., and S. S. Sobin. Pulmonary alveolar blood flow. In: *Bioengineering Aspects of Lung Biology,* edited by J. B. West, New York: Marcel Dekker, 1977, Chap. 4, p. 267–358.

42. Fung, Y. C., and S. S. Sobin. The retained elasticity of elastin under fixation agents. *J. Biomech. Eng.* 103: 121–122, 1981.

43. Fung, Y. C., S. S. Sobin, H. Tremer, R. T. Yen, and H. H. Ho. Patency and compliance of pulmonary veins when airway pressure exceeds blood pressure. *J. Appl. Physiol. 54 (Respirat. Environ. Exer. Physiol).* 1538–1549, 1983.

44. Fung, Y. C., and H. T. Tang, Solute distribution in the flow in a channel bounded by porous layers (a model of the lung). *J. Appl. Mech.* 41: 531–535 (*Trans. ASME,* Vol. 97, Ser. E), 1975.

45. Fung, Y. C., H. T. Tang. Longitudinal dispersion of tracer particles in the blood flowing in a pulmonary alveolar sheet. *J. Appl. Mech.* 42: 536–540 (*Tans. ASME,* Vol. 97, Ser. E), 1975.

46. Fung, Y. C., and P. Tong. Theory of the sphering of red blood cells. *Biophys. J.* 8: 175–198, 1968.

47. Fung, Y. C., P. Tong, and P. Patitucci. Stress and strain in the lung. American Society of Civil Engineers. *J. Eng. Mech. Div.* 104(EM1): 201–223, 1978.

48. Fung, Y. C., and R. T. Yen. A new theory of pulomonary blood flow in zone 2 condition. *J. Appl. Physiol.* 60: 1638–1650, 1986.

49. Fung, Y. C., R. T. Yen, Z. L. Tao, and S. O. Liu. A hypothesis on the mechanism of

trauma of lung tissue subjected to impact load. *J. Biomech. Eng.* 110: 50–56, 1988.

50. Fung, Y. C., and F. Y. Zhuang. An analysis of the sluicing gate in pulmonary blood flow. *J. Biomech. Eng.* 108: 175–182, 1986.

51. Fung, Y. C., B. W. Zweifach, and M. Intaglietta. Elastic environment of the capillary bed. *Circ. Res.* 19: 441–461, 1966.

52. Fung, Y. C., and S. Q. Liu. Strain distribution in small blood vessels with zero-stress state taken into consideration. *Am. J. Physiol., Heart and Circ.* 262: H544–H552, 1992.

53. Gasson, P. C. *Geometry of Spatial Forms.* New York: Wiley, 1983.

54. Gunteroth, W. G., D. L. Luchtel, and I Kawabari. Functional implications of the pulmonary microcirculation. *Chest,* 101: 1131–1134, 1992.

55. Hansen, J. E., and E. P. Ampaya. Human air space shapes, sizes, areas, and volumes. *J. Appl. Physiol.* 38: 990–995, 1975.

56. Hansen, J. E., E. P. Ampaya, G. H. Bryant, and J. J. Navin. The branching pattern of airways and air spaces of a single human terminal bronchiole. *J. Appl. Physiol.* 38: 983–989, 1975.

57. Horsfield, K., and G. Cumming. Morphology of the bronchial tree in man. *J. Appl. Physiol.* 24: 373–383, 1968.

58. Lee, J. S., W. G. Frasher, and Y. C. Fung. Comparison of the elasticity of an artery in vivo and in excision. *J. Appl. Physiol.* 25: 799–801, 1968.

59. Lee, J. S., and Y. C. Fung. Modeling experiments of a single red blood cell, moving in a capillary blood vessel. *Microvasc. Res.* 1: 221–243, 1969.

60. Lee, J. S., and Y. C. Fung, Stokes' flow around a circular cylindrical post, confined between two parallel plates. *J. Fluid Mech.* 37: 657–670, 1969.

61. Matsuda, M., Y. C. Fung, and S. S. Sobin. Collagen and elastin fibers in human pulmonary alveolar mouths and ducts. *J. Appl. Physiol.* 63: 1185–1194, 1987.

62. Mercer, R. R., and J. D. Crapo. Three-dimensional reconstruction of the rat acinus. *J. Appl. Physiol.* 63: 785–794, 1987.

63. Miller, W. S. *The Lung.* 2nd ed. Springfield, Il: Charles C. Thomas, 1947.

64. Oldmixon, E. H., J. P Butler, and F. G. Hoppin, Jr. Dihedral angles between alveolar septa. *J. Appl. Physiol.* 64: 299–307, 1988.

65. Permutt, S., B. Bromberger-Barnea, and H. N. Bane. Alveolar pressure, pulmonary venous pressure, and the vascular waterfall. *Med. Thorac.* 19: 239–260, 1962.

66. Rosenquist, T. H., S. Bernick, S. S. Sobin, Y. C. Fung. The structure of the pulmonary interalveolar microvascular sheet. *Microvasc. Res.* 5: 199–212, 1973.

67. Silage, D. A., and J. Gil. Morphometric measurement of local curvature of the alveolar ducts in lung mechanics. *J. Appl. Physiol.* 65: 1592–1597, 1988.

68. Sobin, S. S., and Y. C. Fung. Response to Guntheroth et al.'s challenge to the Sobin-Fung approach to the study of pulmonary microcirculation. *Chest,* 101: 1135–1143, 1992.

69. Sobin, S. S., Y. C. Fung, R. G. Lindal, H. M. Tremer, and L. Cleark. Topology of pulmonary arterioles, capillaries, and venules in the cat. *Microvasc. Res.* 19: 217–233, 1980.

70. Sobin, S. S., Y. C. Fung, and H. M. Tremer. The effect of incomplete fixation of elastin on the appearance of pulmonary alveoli. *J. Biomech. Eng.* 104: 68–71, 1982.

71. Sobin, S. S., Y. C. Fung, and H. M. Tremer. Collagen and elastin fibers in human pulmonary alveolar walls. *J. Appl. Physiol.* 64: 1659–1675, 1988.

72. Sobin, S. S., Y. C. Fung, H. M. Tremer, and T. H. Rosenquist. Elasticity of the pulmonary alveolar microvascular sheet in the cat. *Circ. Res.* 30: 440–450, 1972.

73. Sobin, S. S., R. G. Lindal, Y. C. Fung, H. M. Tremer. Elasticity of the smallest noncapillary pulmonary blood vessels in the cat. *Microvasc. Res.* 15: 57–68, 1978.

74. Sobin, S. S., H. M. Tremer, and Y. C. Fung. Morphometic basis of the sheet-flow concept of the pulmonary alveolar microcirculation in the cat. *Cir. Res.* 26: 397–414, 1970.

75. Tanaka, T. T. and Y. C. Fung, Elastic and inelastic properties of the canine aorta and their variation along the aortic tree. *J. Biomech.* 7: 357–370, 1974.

76. Tang, H. T., and Y. C. Fung. Fluid movement in a channel with permeable walls covered by porous media: a model of lung alveolar sheet. *J. Appl. Mech.* 42: 45–50 (*Trans. ASME,* Vol. 97, Ser. E), 1975.

77. Vawter, D. L., Y. C. Fung, and J. B. West. Elasticity of excised dog lung parenchyma. *J. Appl. Physiol.* 45: 261–269, 1978.

78. Wall, R. J., S. S. Sobin, M. Karspeck, R. G. Lindal, H. M. Tremer, and Y. C. Fung. Computer derived image compositing. *J. Appl. Physiol. (Respirat. Environ. Exer. Physiol.* 51(1): 84–89, 1981.

79. Weibel, E. R. *Morphometry of the Human Lung.* New York: Academic, 1963.

80. Weyl, H. *Symmetry.* Princeton, NJ: Princeton University Press, 1952.

81. Wilson, T. A., and H. Bachofen. A model for mechanical structure of the alveolar duct. *J. Appl. Physiol.* 52: 1064–1070, 1982.

82. Yen, R. T. and L. Foppiano. Elasticity of small pulmonary veins in the cat. *J. Biomech. Eng.* 103: 38–42, 1981.

83. Yen, R. T., and Y. C. Fung. Model experiments on apparent blood viscosity and hematocrit in pulmonary alveoli. *J. Appl. Physiol.* 35: 510–517, 1973.

84. Yen, R. T., and Y. C. Fung. Effect of velocity distribution on red cell distribution in capillary blood vessels. *Am. J. Physiol.* 235: H251–H257, 1978.

85. Yen, R. T., Y. C. Fung, and N. Bingham. Elasticity of small pulmonary arteries in the cat. *J. Biomech. Eng.* 102: 170–177, 1980.

86. Yen, R. T., Y. C. Fung, H. H. Ho, and G. Butterman. Speed of stress wave propagation in lung. *J. Appl. Physiol.* 61: 701–705, 1986.

87. Yen, R. T., Y. C. Fung, and S. O. Liu. Trauma of lung due to impact load. *J. Biomech.* 21: 745–753, 1988.

88. Yen, R. T., F. Y. Zhuang, Y. C. Fung, H. H. Ho, H. Tremer, and S. S. Sobin. Morphometry of cat's pulmonary arterial tree. *J. Biomech. Eng.* 106: 131–136, 1984.

89. Yen, R. T., F. Y. Zhuang, Y. C. Fung, H. H. Ho, H. Tremer, and S. S. Sobin. Morphometry of cat pulmonary venous tree. *J. Appl. Physiol.* 55: *Respirat. Environ. Exer. Physiol.* 236–242, 1983.

90. Zeng, Y. J., D. Yager, and Y. C. Fung. Measurement of the mechanical properties of the human lung tissue. *J. Biomech. Eng.* 109: 169–174, 1987.

91. Zhuang, F. Y., Y. C. Fung, and R. T. Yen. Analysis of blood flow in cat's lung with detailed anatomical and elasticity data. *J. Appl. Physiol.* 55: *(Respirat. Environ. Exer. Physiol.)* 1341–1348, 1983.

92. Zhuang, F. Y., M. R. T. Yen, Y. C. Fung, and S. S. Sobin. How many pulmonary alveoli are supplied by a single arteriole and drained by a single venule? *Microvasc. Res.* 29: 18–31, 1985.

93. Debes, J. C., and Fung, Y. C. Effect of temperature on the biaxial mechanics of excised parenchyma of the dog. *J. Appl. Physiol.* 73: 1171–1180, 1992.

94. Fung, Y. C., and Liu, S. Q. Elementary mechanics of the endothelium of blood vessels. *J. Biomechanical Engineering.* 115: 1–12, 1993.

95. Liu, S. Q., and Fung, Y. C. Influence of STZ-induced diabetes on zero-stress states of rat pulmonary and systemic arteries. *Diabetes.* 41: 136–146, 1992.

96. Liu, S. Q., and Fung, Y. C. Changes in the rheological properties of blood vessel tissue remodeling in the course of development of diabetes. *Biorheology.* 29: 443–457, 1992.

97. Liu, S. Q., and Fung, Y. C. Changes in the structure and mechanical properties of pulmonary arteries of rats exposed to cigarette smoke. *Am. Rev. Respir. Dis.* 148: 768–777, 1993.

98. Yager, D., Feldman, H., and Fung, Y. C. Microscopic vs. macroscopic deformation of the pulmonary alveolar duct. *J. Appl. Physiol.* 72(4): 1348–1354, 1992.

99. Yen, R. T., and Sobin S. S. Pulmonary blood flow in the cat: correlation between theory and experiment. In *Frontiers in Biomechanics* (ed. by G. W. Schmid-Schoenbein, S. L.-Y. Woo, and B. W. Zweifach, Springer-Verlag, New York, pp. 365–376, 1986.

100. Kummer, B. K. F. Biomechanics of bone: Mechanical properties, functional structure, functional adaptation. In *Biomechanics: Its Foundations and Objectives,* (ed. by Y. C. Fung, N. Perrone, M. Anliker), Englewood Cliffs, NJ, Prentice-Hall, pp. 237–269, 1972.

# 18

# The Exotic Gases, CO, $O_2$, and $CO_2$

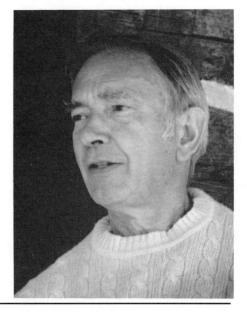

## Robert E. Forster II, MD

*Isaac Ott Professor Emeritus, University of Pennsylvania School of Medicine, Philadelphia, Pennsylvania*

This chapter is a personalized report of one path of my research on respiratory gas exchange with all the warts. It is part biographical, part review, part current, and part prognosticatory. In other words something old, something new, something borrowed, and something blue. I, by accepted standards, am old, as is my research. Some of it is new, I proclaim, but almost everything that is new is borrowed one way or another from my collaborators and students. As for my prognostications, they are blue sky.

After World War II the leaders of respiratory physiology were not only extremely able but also gentlemanly (as were the ladies) to each other and their juniors, which gave the whole field a feeling of community. I have been blessed with colleagues who have taught and stimulated me. I have mentioned only a few in this chapter, those whose collaboration was pertinent to the thread of rapid reaction kinetics.

This research in respiratory physiology has primarily involved exchanges and reaction/diffusion kinetics of CO, $O_2$ and $CO_2$ among blood, gas, and tissue. These familiar gases may perform in extraordinary fashions and have exotic aspects. I will say only a modest amount about older work on CO and very little about $O_2$, about which Professor Piiper says more elsewhere in this volume, but most about $CO_2$ kinetics, my current major interest.

This chapter affords me the opportunity to expound those profound principles of the conduct of physiological research,

From: Wagner WW, Jr, Weir EK (eds): *The Pulmonary Circulation and Gas Exchange.* ©1994, Futura Publishing Co Inc, Armonk, NY.

at least in the United States, which I have accumulated over a lifetime. I was reluctant to proffer these principles, as it seemed pompous and impertinent, but I have escaped this stigma because in the end I found that others had observed these principles before.[32] The first principle is

*Serendipity is the Dominant Strategy.*

This is a humbling and apparently unacceptable idea to administrators who try to plan research, committees of learned societies, principle investigators of NIH program projects, and would-be captains of the biomedical industry. If one knows enough about a problem to budget large expenditures of resources and time economically, both of course someone elses', the effort becomes one of development rather than research. The inability of our brightest and best to predict new research revelations has been frequently documented. A fine historical account of the converse, that discoveries of critical importance to biomedical science have not been foreseen nor have they resulted from administrative planning, is given in the articles by Julius Comroe and Robert Dripps in *Science*.[3–6] However, such is the seduction of large-scale research planning, that we repeat the errors of scientific history, although warned by Santayana that, "Those who cannot remember the past are condemned to fulfill it."[36] This is not to rule out the possibility of a stunning new and unexpected scientific finding uncovered by a committee; serendipity might even work through MBAs.

Principle I has a corollary in the dictum of Louis Pasteur,[31] "Dans les champs de l'observation le hasard ne favorise que les esprits préparés." Therefore, learning from the Boy Scouts and Sir Robert Baden-Powell, to do original science we should "Be prepared."

As a medical student I did some pedestrian research on the treatment of hypertension with SCN (thiocyanate), which had a efficacy approximating that of garlic, simply because a faculty member gave me a lab and encouragement. It did result in my first publication. As a house officer at the Peter Bent Brigham Hospital in Boston, I applied an ear oximeter, borrowed from Glenn Millikan, who had taught me in pharmacology, to cardiac patients with Samuel A. Levine, a superb clinical cardiologist. I measured, probably for the first time, human pulmonary arterial temperature during a catheterization with Lewis Dexter. All of these forays into research occurred because of individuals and serendipitous opportunities.

Through the efforts of George Thorn, I was assigned to the Quartermaster Corps Climatic Research Laboratory in Lawrence, Massachusetts, during World War II, which became the alma mater of other respiratory physiologists of more note. Our mission was to protect soldiers under a wide range of climatic conditions; one aspect of this mission was the physiology of temperature regulation. Under the guidance of Cuthbert Bazett and Richard L. Day, the New York pediatrician, my research resulted in my second publication, the first paper in the first issue of the *Journal of Applied Physiology,* which may contain the first experimental evidence for countercurrent exchange, the cooling of arterial blood in the hand by returning venous blood. I was the last author. I continued in this field at Harvard with Eugene Landis, but when I was offered a faculty position at the Graduate School of Medicine at the University of Pennsylvania by Robert Dripps and Julius Comroe, I accepted without a qualm because Julius had taught and inspired me at Penn and because the school offered more money (a figure that Landis thought was indecently high). I was fascinated by the physiology of temperature regulation and might happily have spent my life in it but changed my field to respiratory physiology because that was the focus of Julius Comroe's program (Fig. 1).

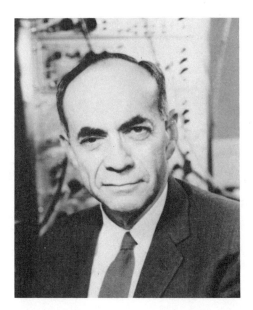

**Figure 1.** Julius Comroe, Jr., about 1956 in Philadelphia.

This brings me to the second principle:

*Inertia is a Powerful Force in Scientists.*

An investigator starts where he was taught and pushes on in small steps. He rarely makes a quantum jump into a new field but, stimulated by his observations, extends his horizon and may find in front of him, to his surprise, a new vista of discovery. If he does change fields, he is careful to do so under the umbrella of preceptors in his new area.

I was armed with experience in Experiment 26 of the medical school laboratory course in physiology at Harvard, long since gone by the board, as have so many. Run by John Pappenheimer and Baird Hastings, it taught students more about the alveolar air equation than they wanted to know and more than most chest physicians know today. Figure 2 is a charcoal drawing by John's son, Will, and suggests CO$_2$ and O$_2$ exchange among red blood cells, plasma, and alveolar gas, which became my forte.

It was humbling to my intellectualization of scientific research to realize in preparing this chapter that my work in respiratory physiology has been so dependent on the development of new apparatus for the measurement of rapid chemical reactions rather than as logical steps in the development of a master strategy to discover new physiology. The instruments were developed through small incremental innovations, the chronology of which is given in Table 1, borrowing from many and starting from what F. J. W. Roughton showed me in the early fifties.

## CO Research

I found on arriving back at Penn a small laboratory in the bowels of the Old Medical School Building, now called the John Morgan Building after an original prominence, in which was a breath analysis mass spectrometer and an infrared CO analyzer, which Julius Comroe and Seymour Kety had ordered before I came. With the help of Ward Fowler, David Bates,and Bernard van Lingen we followed the disappearance of CO from alveolar gas at different Po$_2$ (Fig. 3) using the new mass spectrometer to measure helium and O$_2$ and the infrared meter to measure CO.[15] This was certainly an early, maybe even the first, use of these instruments in physiology. Use of a mass spectrometer to measure respiratory gases had been reported in an abstract by Fred Hitchcock.

The raw data in Figure 3 shows that increasing alveolar Po$_2$ decreases the rate of CO disappearance in seconds. Only a drop in the rate of the chemical reaction of CO with intracellular hemoglobin, resulting from the competitive reaction of O$_2$, can occur this rapidly. Therefore this also means that the velocity of gas uptake by red cells in the alveolar capillaries can be rate limiting, a new concept at the time. To interpret the results quantitatively, we needed measurements of the rate of CO

**Table 1.**
Chronology of Rapid Reaction Instruments

| Continuous-Flow Rapid-Mixing Apparatus | Stop-Flow Rapid-Mixing Apparatus |
|---|---|
| *Reversion spectroscope*  1957 <br> then soon <br> *Split beam, two color*  1957 <br>  CO + Hb; $O_2$ + Hb in RBC | |
| *$PO_2$ electrode* <br>  $O_2$ + Hb: top of curve  1959 | |
| | *Split beam; two color.* |
|  Rate of Bohr shift  1963 | |
| | $HbO_2$ + dithionite in RBC 1965 |
| *$PCO_2$ electrode* <br>  $CO_2$ uptake by RBC  1965 | |
| | $O_2$ + Hb in RBC  1966 |
|  $CO_2$ + Hb solution  1968 <br>  Root Shift, eel Hb  1969 | |
| *pH electrode* <br>  $NH_3$ uptake by RBC  1972 | *pH electrode* <br>  OH-permeability of RBC  1971 |
| *Split beam; two-color: pH dye* <br>  Quantitative CA  1990 <br>  activity: solution | <br>  Quantitative CA  1990 <br>  activity: solution |
| *$^{18}O$ Exchange between $CO_2/HCO^-_3$ and HOH* <br>  RBC CA and $P_{HCO_3-}$  1977 <br>  Mitochondrial CA  1980 <br>  Quantitative CA  1990 <br>  activity: cells & solution | *$^{13}C$ NMR* <br>  RBC $CO_2/HCO^-_3$ exch.  1984 |

uptake by human red cells at 37°C, so I wrote F. J. W. Roughton at Cambridge to see if he had such data. He did not but came to Philadelphia to obtain the measurements (Fig. 4), bringing with him a continuous-flow gas pressure driven rapid-mixing apparatus, having managed to avoid U.S. Customs with the help of the Air Transport Command of the U.S. Air Force. The mixing apparatus is shown in Figure 5. Its principle was developed by Hartridge and Roughton[19] and is in its simplest form a tee-tube in which a solution of CO and a suspension of red cells at a given $PO_2$ are driven in each side arm and the turbulent reacting mixture flows out the central shaft at a rate about 0.2 cm/ms, so that by observing the HbCO/ $HbO_2$ at progressive distances down the tube, the course of the reaction can be followed. The beauty of this apparatus is

that the analytical apparatus, or observer, can have as slow a response time as convenient, limited only by the volume of reactant available.

Roughton brought with him a reversion-spectroscope, an ingenious optical instrument built by Hamilton Hartridge (who had learned fluid mixing from work on airplane carburetors in World War I) that reverses and superimposes the two absorption bands of HbCO or $HbO_2$ in the green (540 to 568 µm). As [HbCO] increases, the peak of $HbO_2$ at 576 µm moved toward that of HbCO at 578 µm and this movement can be quantitated by superimposing the two bands. It was a subjective instrument requiring experience and rapport to use, so that only Roughton operated it, turning reactant flows on and off with hemostats while peering into the spectroscope. On one historic occasion he

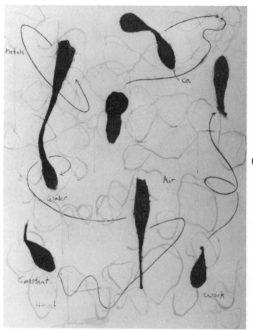

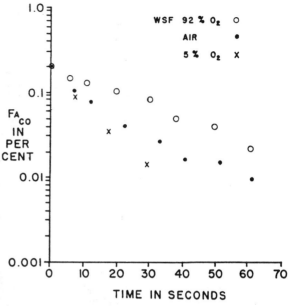

**Figure 2.** Objective Participants. Gouache, pastel, and charcoal on paper by Will Pappenheimer, 1989. Dimensions 52 in by 41 in. Reproduced by permission of the artist.

**Figure 3.** The effect of altering the $O_2$ and $CO_2$ tensions in inspired gas on the rate of disappearance of CO from the alveolar gas. $FA_{CO}$ is alveolar CO concentration in % atmosphere. (Subject: Ward S. Fowler).

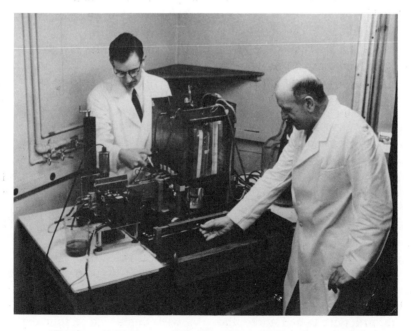

**Figure 4.** R. E. Forster II (left) and F. J. W. Roughton (right).

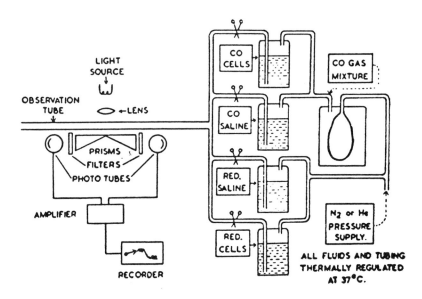

**Figure 5.** Cartoon of the pressure drive continuous-flow rapid-mixing apparatus, HARMDYF (Hartridge, Roughton, Millikan, Daziel, and Forster [last]). The rubber-bag-in-box was needed to transmit gas driving pressure equally to all four reactant bottles (1L) while preventing the admixture of CO with the unliganded cells suspension and CO free solution. The storage bottles are within a temperature-regulated bath, and the mixing chamber and observation tube are within a temperature regulated aluminum block. *CO cells* is a suspension of red cells containing enough CO to produce 100% HbCO, while *Red. cells* is a suspension containing no CO or $O_2$. *CO saline* and *Red. saline* are physiological saline containing dissolved CO at a predetermined partial pressure or no dissolved CO, respectively. The bottles were submerged in a temperature-controlled water bath, and the observation tube was water jacketed at the same temperature (generally 37°C). Hemostats on the rubber tubing were used to control the flow of the liquid reactants.

groped for a hemostat but instead seized a pair of scissors, severed the rubber tubing, and rapidly disposed of two bottles of reactants that had taken half a day to prepare. At this point, Bill Briscoe and I decided an automatically recording photoelectric instrument was needed and developed the split-beam two-color analyzer shown in Figure 5 using a prism purloined from Britton Chance[16]. By measuring the changes in the difference of absorption by the cell suspension at two colors, most of the artifacts produced by light scattering were eliminated. Using this apparatus Roughton, Briscoe, Ferdinand Kreuzer, and I measured the rate of uptake of CO by human red blood cells ($\theta$) at 37°C with increasing $PO_2$ and, with Leon Cander, the diffusing capacity ($D_L$) at different alveolar

$PO_2$[17] Summing the resistances to gas CO transport in the alveolar capillary, which are the reciprocals of the conductances or diffusing capacity, we obtained the convenient relationship.[35]

$$1/D_L = 1/D_M + 1/\theta V_C, \qquad (1)$$

where $D_L$ is the diffusing capacity of the whole lung and $D_M$ is the diffusing capacity of the alveolar membrane alone, both in ml CO/min/mmHg; $\theta$ is in ml CO/min/mmHg/ml normal blood; and $V_C$ is the volume of the capillaries in ml.

These measurements of $D_L$ and $\theta$ as a function of $PO_2$ plus the theoretical interpretation permitting calculation of $D_M$ and $V_C$ were contained in four papers[16,17,34,35] in the *Journal of Applied Physiology* in

1957 by Roughton and myself; the senior authorship was divided equally but arbitrarily. This demonstrates a minor principle concerning the order of authorship designated the "Gilbert and Sullivan rule," Things are never what they seem; skim milk masquerades as cream. The papers in which I was senior author were primarily the work of Roughton, and vice versa. I believe this is still the only method to measure pulmonary capillary blood volume.

The next improvement was the introduction of a fine platinum teflon-covered P$_{O_2}$ electrode into the reacting stream to measure the disappearance of [O$_2$] with time when a suspension of deoxygenated red cells was mixed with an O$_2$ solution.[42] This was the first use of an electrode in a rapid reaction apparatus and had the potential theoretical artifact that the inevitable stagnant layer on the teflon surface would be delayed in comparison to the average in the stream cross section so that the measured P$_{O_2}$ would be correspondingly later in time. Fortunately this did not turn out to be an important error, so we were encouraged to use other electrodes later, such as pH and P$_{CO_2}$. The response time of the electrodes was measured in seconds to tens of seconds, so large volumes of reactants were consumed to obtain a measurement, and the development of more rapidly responding electrodes became a high priority. In this P$_{O_2}$ electrode reaction apparatus we also used for the first time in our experiments motor-driven pistons to deliver the reactants (Glenn Millikan had done the same at Cambridge in the 1940s).

The reason for using a P$_{O_2}$ electrode rather than continuing to use photospectroscopy was heightened sensitivity, since a mmHg P$_{O_2}$, which is easily measured, represents a very small Δ[HbO$_2$]. With this apparatus, we (Bishop, Staub and I) measured the rate of O$_2$ uptake by red cells starting at a high HbO$_2$ saturation. The apparatus also provided an entree into red cell CO$_2$ kinetics because we could measure the displacement of O$_2$ by CO$_2$ in the Bohr shift.[9]

The next advance in kinetic apparatus was the application of the stopped-flow rapid mixing apparatus developed by Quentin Gibson, to the exchanges of red cells (an example is given in Figure 6). In this instrument the two reactants are impelled by pistons into a mixing chamber; the mixture flows into a third syringe whose plunger hits a stop, causing all flow to cease in a millisecond. In 1954 Roughton and I talked with Gibson in his home in Sheffield about the possibility of using the apparatus for cells but worried about stagnant layers of fluid developing around the cells immediately after the flow was stopped, slowing the reaction measurements. Sirs and Roughton[41] at Colloid Science in Cambridge built a stopped-flow spectrophotometric apparatus, a copy of which Lawson, Holland, and I used to measure the rate of egress of O$_2$ from red blood cells by mixing an oxygenated cell suspension with a solution containing dithionite, which reduces the O$_2$.[26] Because the dithionite will penetrate to the surface of the cells, we hypothesized that any stagnant layer effect would be minimal. Holland and I[21] measured the rate of O$_2$ uptake by human red cells and concluded the values we obtained were not significantly different from those obtained with a continuous-flow instrument. With this agreement we were confident that the stopped-flow apparatus could be used on cell suspensions. There were reports that the stagnant layer around the cells did retard the reactions[2] but the conditions were extreme and we still thought the artifact was negligible. More recently, however, we (Krawiec, Gottliebsen, Fish and Lin, unpublished) compared stopped-flow and continuous-flow photocolorimetric measurements of θ$_{O_2}$ and found the stopped-flow values were about half those from continuous-flow measurements. Not all investigators agree with us, however.

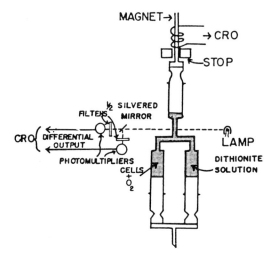

**Figure 6.** Diagram of a stop-flow rapid-mixing apparatus set up to measure the rate of deoxygenation of human red cells. The two lower syringes are pushed upward, and reacting mixture flows until the third, or upper, syringe hits the stop, halting flow in less than a millisecond. The white light beam passes through the reacting mixture, is split, and each half passes through a 559 mμ or 573 mμ interference filter and onto two separate photomultiplier tubes, the difference of whose output is amplified and fed into a cathode ray tube. By taking the difference of the two transmitted colors, most of the changes in output resulting from light scattering are eliminated. The output is essentially linear with [HbO₂]. The movement of the magnet through the coil produces a signal, also fed into the oscilloscope (CRO) which is proportional to volume flow rate.

Masaji Mochizuki from Sapporo came to Philadelphia to help me in the early 1960s, and we measured the facilitated flux of CO through a thin layer of hemoglobin solution absorbed on to a millipore membrane, stimulated by analogous studies of Pete Scholander.[29] In this form of transport, CO reacts to form HbCO on one surface, and this liganded form diffuses to the other surface where the CO dissociates, contributing to the total diffusion of CO. We demonstrated that the facilitated flux rate was limited by the velocity of the dissociation of HbCO so that this flux could be used to measure the reaction velocities of CO and Hb. Ian Longmuir,

Woo, and I applied this to the facilitated diffusion of $CO_2$.[27] Unfortunately, because [H⁺] as well as [$CO_2$] and [$HCO_3^-$] vary, it is impossible to obtain an analytic solution, so the method was of limited usefulness until Donaldson and Quinn[13] modified the experiment to measure the exchange of isotopically labeled $CO_2$ at chemical equilibrium in which [H⁺] is constant, thereby permitting a useful analytic solution.

## $CO_2$ Research

Roughton and colleagues had tried to estimate the physiological rate of the carbonic anhydrase catalyzed hydration of $CO_2$ in red cells by measuring the rate at increasing concentrations of hemolysate and extrapolating to the normal intracellular concentrations. They could not measure the reaction at carbonic anhydrase concentrations greater than one-third of the normal intracellular value; the reaction was too fast for the mixing time of their apparatus. We saw the possibility of using a $P_{CO_2}$ electrode in a continuous-flow instrument to measure $CO_2$ uptake by human red cells. While the concentrations of carbonic anhydrase and hemoglobin were physiological in each red cell, the suspension was dilute (1/20), so the rate of change of $P_{CO_2}$ in the reacting mixture was easily measured. Typical results are shown in Figure 7. The initial rate of $CO_2$ uptake, calculated from the initial slope of the $P_{CO_2}$ curve, was, however, only 60% of the value predicted by extrapolation from in vitro measurements on hemolysate. We concluded that the reaction was most likely impeded by the accumulation of end products, particularly H⁺. This finding demonstrates that one cannot measure correctly the rate of $CO_2/HCO_3^-$ reactions inside an intact lipid membrane, which is impermeable to H⁺ by any method involving a net formation or consumption of $CO_2$.

Figure 7 also shows the effect of a sulfonamide carbonic anhydrase inhib-

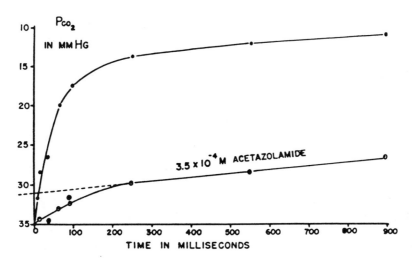

**Figure 7.** Decrease in $P_{CO_2}$ at 37°C with time after mixing a 1:10 suspension of normal human blood in physiological buffer at $P_{CO_2}$ of 2 Torr, $[HCO_3^-]$ of 25.8 mM, and pH 8.66 with a physiological saline solution containing a $P_{CO_2}$ of 71 Torr, $[HCO_3^-]$ of 29.4 mM, and pH 7.25 (upper curve). In the lower curve, the cell suspension contained in addition 350 μM acetazolamide, 20,000 times Ki. The dashed line represents the extrapolated uncatalyzed reaction (modified from 18).

itor, sufficient in concentration to fully eliminate the enzyme activity. The remaining uncatalyzed rate should be linear on the graph; the initial upward convexity is produced by the formation of hemoglobin carbamate. This stimulated us to go on later and measure the kinetics of the $CO_2$ reaction with hemoglobin,[18] and this in turn brought Research Principle III to my attention. About 1979 a distinguished American scientist complimented me on this paper saying it provided the first experimental results that convinced him that hemoglobin carbamate really existed. This was in spite of the fact that Meldrum and Roughton had published data on this topic in 1933 and the results had been in physiological and some biochemical text books for decades. I assume from this conversation that many scientists had not accepted their conclusions but did not make the public aware of their skepticism.

The third research principle is

### Don't Forget the Silent Majority

The egalitarian and permissive mores of the American scientific community dic-

tate that one does not disagree in public with another scientist's conclusions with the same strength as one's private convictions. However, these convictions will still surface in Study Sections and at Site Visits.

The next modification of the stopped-flow apparatus was to introduce an electrode, a glass pH electrode, into the reacting mixture to follow rapid changes in $[H^+]$. We were not optimistic that the instrument would work because in the first place pH electrodes are notoriously slow in their response.[40] Part of this lag we thought resulted from their high electrical resistance, which we hoped could be overcome by modern high impedance DC amplifiers. Second, we were concerned that the inevitable stagnant layer on the electrode surface would increase on cessation of flow and magnify the artifact. We were pleased to find that, in the stop-flow apparatus with the reactant mixture directed as a jet against the glass tip, the response time was as little as 0.005 seconds. We concluded that the slow response of the ordinary laboratory glass pH electrode was in large part due to a failure to change the fluid on the glass surface fast enough with any test solution. The stopped-flow apparatus does this more successfully. We—Chow, Lin, and myself (unpublished)—found that the response time decreased with increasing buffer concentration in the test solution. We surmised that the buffer facilitates the transport of H+ to the active surface.

We used the stopped-flow pH apparatus to measure the effective permeability of the red cell membrane to OH-[7] and to $HCO_3^-/Cl^-$ exchange.[1] In considering the classic diagram of red cell gas and ion exchanges in the capillary beds of Roughton,[33] we suddenly realized that the necessary cyclic changes of [H+] in the plasma could not be produced by the movements of $HCO_3^-$ and Cl- across the cell walls but were produced by the hydration of $CO_2$ and dehydration of $HCO_3^-$ in the plasma. Some years later I found that Roughton had pointed this out in his 1935 review.[33] Since there was no carbonic anhydrase in the plasma, these reactions were necessarily slow, could not be completed in the capillary transit time, and might never be complete as the blood cells

cycled through lung and peripheral capillary beds. There the matter should have rested if at least three groups of investigators[8,14,24] had not looked for the predicted disequilibrium between plasma [$CO_2$] and [H+][$HCO_3^-$]. They could only find this in the presence of carbonic anhydrase inhibitors, demonstrating the presence of carbonic anhydrase available to the capillary plasma. There is a large amount of carbonic anhydrase in the lung, among which are several different isozymes (Fig. 8), including a carbonic anhydrase IV isozyme type, which is generally found in membranes and could be on the capillary endothelium.

Clearly we needed a method of measuring carbonic anhydrase activity or, rather, the velocity of $CO_2/HCO_3^-$ reactions uninhibited by end products. In 1977 Nobutomo Itada and I applied the $^{18}O$ exchange method of Mills and Urey[22,28] to this purpose. The principle is illustrated in Figure 9. When $^{18}O$ labeled $HCO_3^-$ is added to water, labeled $CO_2$ is produced and reaches almost complete isotopic equilibrium with $H^{18}O^{16}O_2^-$. The $^{18}O$ exchanges with $^{16}O$ in water more slowly and is enormously diluted so that

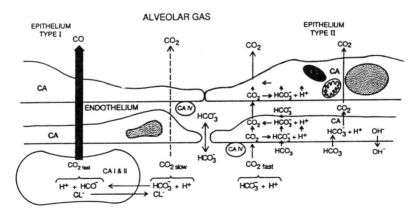

**Figure 8.** Cartoon of lung showing location of possible functions of its carbonic anhydrase isozymes. The leftmost broad arrow represents the major flux of $CO_2$ transported by blood. The dashed arrow indicates the flux of $CO_2$ arising from uncatalyzed dehydration of $HCO_3^-$ in plasma. The third set of arrows indicate the flux of $CO_2$ that may be facilitated by carbonic anhdyrase in the endothelium and in the epithelium. The last arrows on the right indicate the possible production of $CO_2$ from $HCO_3^-$ exchanged with plasma.

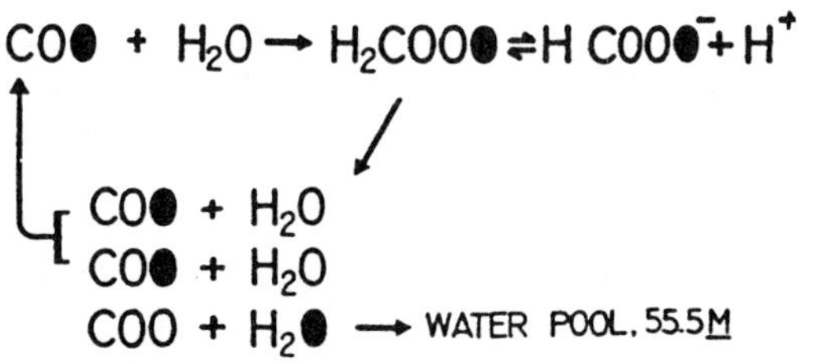

$$CO\bullet + H_2O \rightarrow H_2COO\bullet \rightleftharpoons H\,COO\bullet^- + H^+$$

$$\begin{array}{l} CO\bullet + H_2O \\ CO\bullet + H_2O \\ CO + H_2\bullet \rightarrow WATER\ POOL,\ 55.5\underline{M} \end{array}$$

**Figure 9.** Cartoon of the exchange of $^{18}O$, solid O's, in CO$_2$ and HCO$_3^-$ with those of H$_2$O. The oxygens in HCO$_3^-$ are symmetrical, so when the molecule is dehydrated, the probability of an $^{18}O$ forming labeled H$_2$O is 1/3, while the probability of its forming labeled CO$_2$ is 2/3.

$C^{18}O^{16}O$ essentially disappears, and at an exponential rate that can be measured conveniently in a mass spectrometer. From this rate, the unidirectional velocity constants can be calculated. Experimental results on red cells and hemolysate are shown in Figure 10. Hemolysate accelerates the disappearance, and the effect of carbonic anhydrase can be quantified. The results with an intact red cell suspension showed a "step," or first a rapid and then a second slower exponential disappearance, a double exponential process. This occurs because CO$_2$ can diffuse easily into the cell where the $^{18}O$ exchange with water occurs 17,000 times faster than out-

side, and $[C^{18}O^{16}O]$ drops because the extracellular labeled $[HCO_3^-]$ carbonic anhydrase which is 21 times the $[CO_2]$ and thus 95% of the $^{18}O$ in the solution in the absence of carbonic anhydrase, cannot dehydrate to form $C^{18}O^{16}O$ fast enough. This also means that the intracellular labeled $HCO_3^-$, which is in nearly complete isotopic equilibrium with $C^{18}O^{16}O$, is much less than extracellular $HC^{18}O^{16}O_3^-$. This transmembrane gradient causes the flux of labeled $HC^{18}O^{16}O_3^-$ into the cell providing a measure of membrane permeability to $HCO_3^-$ as well as the activity of carbonic anhydrase in the cell. Silverman and colleagues independently developed a similar method, and, on the basis of their finding that carbonic anhydrase was not inhibited in intact cells to the same extent as in solution, concluded that red cell membrane resistance to CO$_2$ diffusion was rate limiting.[38,39] We believe our disagreement can be explained by the relative impermeability of the red cell membrane to the sulfonamides used.

The advantages of the method are:

1. It is carried out at chemical equilibrium so $[H^+]$ is constant.

2. It can measure carbonic anhydrase activity inside a membrane, which other methods cannot.

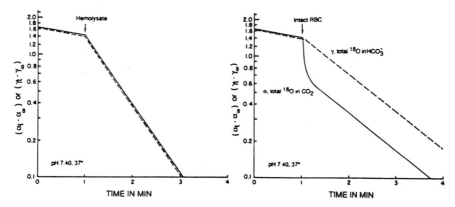

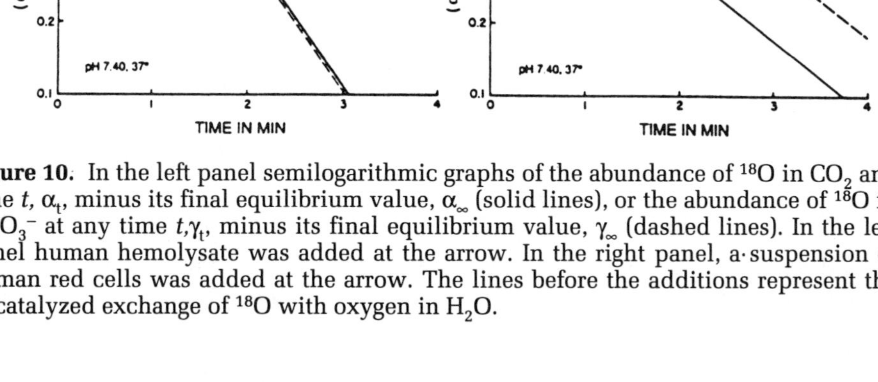

**Figure 10.** In the left panel semilogarithmic graphs of the abundance of $^{18}O$ in CO$_2$ any time $t$, $\alpha_t$, minus its final equilibrium value, $\alpha_\infty$ (solid lines), or the abundance of $^{18}O$ in HCO$_3^-$ at any time $t$,$\gamma_t$, minus its final equilibrium value, $\gamma_\infty$ (dashed lines). In the left panel human hemolysate was added at the arrow. In the right panel, a·suspension of human red cells was added at the arrow. The lines before the additions represent the uncatalyzed exchange of $^{18}O$ with oxygen in H$_2$O.

3. It can measure $HCO_3^-$ self-exchange across the cell membrane.

4. It can be modified to give the most sensitive method for carbonic anhydrase activity.

At the same time the method has disadvantages; it requires expensive equipment and is slower than some other techniques.

Using the $^{18}O$ exchange method we found the same carbonic anhydrase activity, 17,000 times the uncatalyzed rate at 37°C in intact and lysed human red cells.[23] This answers the original question of Roughton as to whether the enzyme activity of carbonic anhydrase in the highly concentrated milieu of red blood cells is the same as in a dilute solution. The answer is yes; the intracellular activity is proportional to the concentration of enzyme and can be extrapolated from values in dilute solutions.

$^{18}O$ exchange between $CO_2$ and water can also be used to measure carbonic anhydrase activity in a test tissue exposed to labeled $CO_2$ in a gas phase. This modification was used by Shoko Nioka to determine the average carbonic anhydrase activity in an isolated perfused guinea pig lung rebreathing a physilogical $CO_2/O_2$ mixture containing $^{18}O$ labeled $CO_2$.[30] The $CO_2$ equilibrates with the $HCO_3^-$ buffer system in the pulmonary parenchymal tissue in several seconds. The rate of $^{18}O$ loss from the labeled $CO_2$ in the alveolus gas to the pool of unlabeled oxygen in the tissue water is slower but can be used to measure carbonic anhydrase activity in the parenchymal fluid. By adding sulfonamide inhibitors of different membrane permeability to the lung perfusate, she was able to show that almost all of the carbonic anhydrase was present within the cells of the lung and not on the endothelium of the capillaries.[30] This agreed with the results of Henry et al,[20] who homogenized rat lung and measured the carbonic anhydrase activity in the different cellular and subcellular fractions.

One other technique that can measure the velocity of the reversible reactions of $CO_2$ and $HCO_3^-$ is nuclear magnetic resonance (NMR) with $^{13}C$ labeled $CO_2$. The broadening of the nuclear magnetic resonance peak indicates quantitatively the speed of interchange of the labeled atoms between $CO_2$ and $HCO_3^-$.[37] However this measurement must be done deep inside a strong magnet and is impractical for many purposes.

In 1980 we embarked in a new and exciting direction, the result again of serendipity in the laboratory. Leena Mela was investigating the effects of hypoxia on mitochondrial function. The mass spectrometer and reaction chamber/inlet system was available, so Susanna Dodgson and Bayard Storey measured the carbonic anhydrase activity of these subcellular particles, finding there was considerable activity in liver mitochondria (Fig. 9).[10] The "step" in the record of the intact mitochondria shows that there is carbonic anhydrase activity inside the inner membrane and that $HCO_3^-$ is less permeable than $CO_2$. The mitochondrial carbonic anhydrase turned out to be a new isozyme, now designated carbonic anhydrase V.

There had been prior suggestions in the literature that liver mitochondria contained carbonic anhydrase, but there also were strong denials. We submitted the manuscript to an English biochemical journal, which rejected it rapidly because they said everyone already knew there was carbonic anhydrase in mitochondria so why publish old information. We then submitted it to an American biochemical journal, which criticized it because of published evidence that carbonic anhydrase was not present in liver mitochondria. This brings me to my fourth principle:

*Scientists Don't Really Like New Ideas . . .
Except Their Own.*

This sounds harsh, and I almost deleted it, but then found I am not the first nor the most distinguished to point this out. "A new scientific truth does not triumph by convincing its opponents and making them see the light, but rather because its opponents eventually die and a new generation grows up that is familiar with it"—a statement of Max Planck.[32]

It is an accepted fact in the mitochondrial field that the inner mitochondrial membrane is impermeable to HCO$_3^-$. While Figure 11 demonstrates that the liver mitochondrion is less permeable to HCO$_3^-$ self-exchange than CO$_2$, it is still permeable to the anion, albeit 1/10 as permeable as human red cell membrane.[10] In spite of this low permeability, because a mitochondrion has about 1/200th the volume of a red cell, labeled HCO$_3^-$ should equilibrate between a mitochondrion and its ambient in a fraction of a second.

The most fascinating question concerning carbonic anhydrase V is its function. Our hypothesis was and continued to be that carbonic anhydrase V is present in liver mitochondria to produce HCO$_3^-$ from CO$_2$ fast enough to provide substrate for one or more of the syntheses that require this anion.[12] In this context it is important to note that while the decarboxylation reactions of the mitochondrion produce CO$_2$, not HCO$_3^-$, it is the latter that is required to react with ATP and NH$_3$ to form carbamoyl phosphate in the urea cycle, to react with pyruvate to form oxaloacetate in gluconeogenesis, and to react with acetyl CoA to form malonyl CoA in fatty acid synthesis (Fig. 12).[11,25]

A major weakness in our hypothesis, at least for me, is that the uncatalyzed hydration of CO$_2$ should be rapid enough to provide the necessary HCO$_3^-$ from CO$_2$ without the acceleration of carbonic anhydrase and that, while carbonic anhydrase inhibitors reduce the rate of urea formation, they do not reduce it as much as expected.

Thus my interest in respiratory CO$_2$ exchanges has led me from the respiratory dead space to studying CO$_2$ handling by

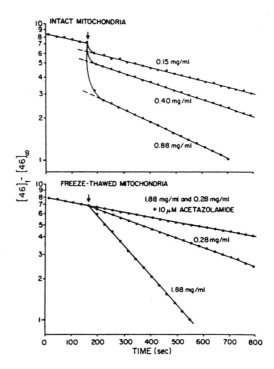

**Figure 11.** Semilogarithmic graphs of mass 46 peak height-mass 46 peak height at final equilibrium against time. Dry NaHCO$_3$ 2% enriched with $^{18}$O was added to a solution of 300 mosM mannitol-sucrose at 25°C pH 7.4 to give a 25 mM solution. In upper panel, guinea pig liver mitochondria were added at the arrow to give the mgm protein/ml indicated on the curves. In lower panel freeze-thawed guinea pig mitochondria were introduced at the arrow to give the concentration of mitochondrial protein indicated. In curve 1, 10 µM acetazolamide was added to the initial solution before the freeze-thawed mitochondria were added in the same concentrations as in curves 2 and 3.

mitochondria, where we are now finding that either CO$_2$ is channeled among enzymes without being free to exchange with the ubiquitous CO$_2$/HCO$_3^-$ or there are gradients for CO$_2$/HCO$_3^-$ within a single mitochondrion.

**Acknowledgement:** I wish to recognize all my friends and colleagues who are not mentioned in this chapter. This chapter was not planned as a complete survey of my research and collaborators, but it is restricted to development of measurements of the rapid reactions of these exotic gases with tissue and red blood cells. I have resisted straying, which means

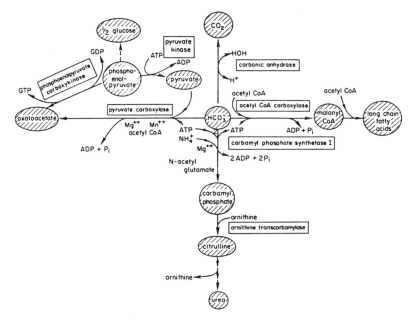

**Figure 12.** Pathways of synthesis of urea, glucose, and fatty acid that involve intrahepatocytic $HCO_3^-$ (reference 11, reproduced with permission).

that other areas of my interests and many fellow workers and instructors may not be mentioned. Among the neglected research topics are temperature regulation; gas exchange in lungs, gills, and placentae; pulmonary function testing; pulmonary circulation; CO metabolism; and red cell permeability.

# References

1. Chow, E. I., E. D. Crandall, and R. E. Forster. Kinetics of bicarbonate-chloride exchange across the human red blood cell membrane. *J. Gen. Physiol.* 68: 633–652, 1976.
2. Coin, J. T., and J. S. Olson. The rate of oxygen uptake by human red blood cells. *J. Biol. Chem.* 254: 1178–1190, 1979.
3. Comroe, Julius H., Jr., and R. D. Dripps. Ben Franklin and open heart surgery. *Circ. Res.* 35: 661–669, 1974.
4. Comroe, J. H., Jr., and R. D. Dripps. Scientific basis for the support of biomedical science. *Science* 192: 105–111, 1976.
5. Comroe, J. H., Jr. Retrospectroscope: Insights into Medical Discovery. Menlo Park, CA: Von Gehr, 1977.
6. Comroe, J. H., Jr. *Exploring the Heart: Discoveries in Heart Disease and High Blood Pressure.* New York, Norton: 1983.
7. Crandall, E. D., R. A. Klocke, and R. E. Forster. Hydroxyl ion movements across the human erythrocyte membrane. *J. Gen. Physiol.* 57: 664–683, 1971.
8. Crandall, E. D., and J. E. O'Brasky. Direct evidence for participation of rat lung carbonic anhydrase in $CO_2$ reactions. *J. Clin. Invest.* 62: 618–622, 1978.
9. Craw, M. R., H. P. Constantine, J. A. Morello, and R. E. Forster. Rate of the Bohr shift in human red cell suspensions. *J. Appl. Physiol.* 18: 317–324, 1963.
10. Dodgson, S. J., R. E. Forster II, B. T. Storey, and L. Mela. Mitochondrial carbonic anhydrase. *Proc. Nat. Acad. Sci. USA* 77: 5562–5566, 1980.
11. Dodgson, S. J., R. E. Forster II, and B. T. Storey. The role of carbonic anhydrase in hepatocyte metabolism. In: *Biology and Chemistry of the Carbonic Anhydrases,* edited by R. E. Tashian and D. Hewett-Emmett. *Ann. N. Y. Acad. Sci* 429: 516–524, 1984.
12. Dodgson, S. J., and R. E. Forster II. Carbonic anhydrase: inhibition results in decreased urea production by hepatocytes *J. Appl. Physiol.* 60: 646–652, 1986.
13. Donaldson, T. L., and J. A. Quinn. Kinetic constants determined from membrane transport measurements: carbonic anhydrase activity at high concentrations. *Proc.*

*Nat. Acad. Sci. USA* 71: 4995–4999, 1974.

14. Effros, R. M., R. S. Y. Chang, and P. Silverman. Acceleration of plasma bicarbonate conversion to carbon dioxide by pulmonary carbonic anhydrase. *Science* 199: 427–429, 1978.

15. Forster, R. E., W. S. Fowler, D. V. Bates, and B. Van Lingen. The absorption of carbon monoxide by the lungs during breatholding. *J. Clin. Invest.* 33: 1135–1145, 1954.

16. Forster, R. E., F. J. W. Roughton, F. Kreuzer, and W. A. Briscoe. Photocolorimetric determination of rate of uptake of CO and O₂ by reduced human red cell suspension at 37 C. *J. Appl. Physiol.* 11: 260–268, 1957.

17. Forster, R. E., F. J. W. Roughton, L. Cander, W. A. Briscoe, and F. Kreuzer. Apparent pulmonary diffusing capacity for CO at varying alveolar O₂ tensions. *J. Appl. Physiol.* 11: 277–289, 1957.

18. Forster, R. E., H. P. Constantine, M. R. Craw, H. H. Rotman, and R. A. Klocke. Reaction of CO₂ with human hemoglobin solution. *J. Biol. Chem.* 243: 3317–3326, 1968.

19. Hartridge, H., and F. J. W. Roughton. A method of measuring the velocity of very rapid chemical reactions. *Proc. Roy. Soc. Ser.* 104: 376–394, 1923.

20. Henry, R. P., S. J. Dodgson, R. E. Forster, and B. T. Storey. Rat lung carbonic anhydrase: activity, localization, and isozymes. *J. Appl. Physiol.* 60: 638–645, 1986.

21. Holland, R. A. B., and R. E. Forster. The effect of size of red cells on the kinetics of their oxygen exchange. *J. Gen. Physiol.* 49: 727–742, 1966.

22. Itada, N., and R. E. Forster. Carbonic anhydrase activity in intact red blood cells measured with ¹⁸O exchange. *J. Biol. Chem.* 252: 3881–3890, 1977.

23. Itada, N., L. Pfeiffer, and R. E. Forster. Intracellular enzyme activity. In: *Frontiers of Biological Engergetics.* New York, Academic, 1978, p. 715–724.

24. Klocke, R. A. Catalysis of CO₂ reaction by lung carbonic anhydrase. *J. Appl. Physiol.* 44: 882–888, 1978.

25. Lane, M. D. Comparison of enzymatic carboxylation mechanisms. In: *CO₂: Chemical. Biochemical and Physiological Aspects,* edited by R. E. Forster, J. T. Edsall, A. B. Otis, and F. J. W. Roughton. Washington, DC: National Aeronautics and Space Administration, 1968, p. 195–206.

26. Lawson, W. H., Jr., R. A. B. Holland, and R. E. Forster. Effect of temperature on deoxygenation rate of human red cells. *J. Appl. Physiol.* 20: 912–918, 1965.

27. Longmuir, I. S., R. E. Forster, and C. Woo. Diffusion of carbon dioxide through thin layers of solution. *Nature* 209: 393–394, 1966.

28. Mills, G. A., and H. C. Urey. The kinetics of isotopic exchange between carbon dioxide, bicarbonate ion and water. *J. Am. Chem. Soc.* 62: 1019–1026, 1940.

29. Mochizuki, M., and R. E. Forster. Diffusion of carbon monoxide through thin layers of hemoglobin solution. *Science* 138: 897–898, 1962.

30. Nioka, S., R. P. Henry, and R. E. Forster. Total CA activity in isolated perfused guinea pig lung by ¹⁸O-exchange method. *J. Appl. Physiol.* 65: 2236–2244, 1988.

31. Pasteur L. Inaugural speech as dean and professor of the Faculté de Sciences at Lille, September, 1854. In: *Life of Pasteur,* R. Vallery-Radot. New York: Doubleday, 1920, p. 74ff.

32. Rescher, N. The ethical dimension of scientific research. In: *Introductory Readings in the Philosophy of Science,* edited by E. D. Klemke, R. Hollinger, and A. D. Kline. Buffalo, NY: Prometheus Books, 1980. p. 238–253.

33. Roughton, F. J. W. Recent work on CO₂ transport by blood. *Physiol. Rev.* 15:241–296, 1935.

34. Roughton, F. J. W., R. E. Forster, and L. Cander. Rate at which carbon monoxide replaces oxygen from combination with human hemoglobin in solution and in the red cell. *J. Appl. Physiol.* 11: 269–276, 1957.

35. Roughton, F. J. W., and R. E. Forster. Relative importance of diffusion and chemical reaction rates in determining rate of exchange of gases in the human lung, with special reference to true diffusing capacity of pulmonary membrane and volume of blood in the lung capillaries. *J. Appl. Physiol.* 11: 290–302, 1957.

36. Santayana, G. In: *Life of Reason,* vol. 1, chap. 12. Flux and constancy in human nature. New York: Macmillan, 1981.

37. Shporer, M., R. E. Forster, and M. M. Civan. Kinetics of CO₂ exchange in human erythrocytes analyzed by ¹³C-NMR. *Am. J. Physiol.* (*Cell Physiol.*) 246: C231–234, 1984.

38. Silverman, D. N. A new approach to measuring the rate of rapid bicarbonate ex-

change across membranes. *Mol. Pharmacol.* 10: 820–836, 1974.

39. Silverman, D. N., C. Tu, and G. C. Wynns. Depletion of $^{18}O$ from $C^{18}O_2$ in erythrocyte suspensions: the permeability of the erythrocyte membrane to $CO_2$ *J. Biol. Chem.* 25: 4428–4435, 1976.

40. Sirs, J. A. Electrometric stopped flow measurements of rapid reactions in solution. *Trans. Faraday Soc.* 54: 207–212, 1958.

41. Sirs, J. A., and F. J. W. Roughton. Stopped-flow measurements of CO and $O_2$ by hemoglobin in sheep erythrocytes. *J. Appl. Physiol.* 18: 158–165, 1963.

42. Staub, N. C., J. M. Bishop, and R. E. Forster. Velocity of $O_2$ uptake by human red blood cells. *J. Appl. Physiol.* 16: 511–516, 1961.

# 19

# A Physician-Scientist's Tale

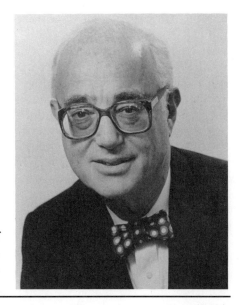

## Alfred P. Fishman, M.D.

*William Maul Measey Professor of Medicine, University of Pennsylvania Hospital, Philadelphia, Pennsylvania*

*. . . at the Tabard as I lay*
*Redy to wenden on my pilgrymage*
*To Canterbury with ful devout corage,*
*At nyght was come into that hostelrye*
*Well nyne and twenty in a compaignye,*
*On sondry folk, by aventure yfalle*
*In felaweshipe, and pilgrims weren they alle.*
    *—Chaucer, The Canterbury Tales[12]*

Supper was over and we were just lounging. A hearty meal had capped a day of exciting scientific sessions. But what to do next? The meeting place was out in the country, far beyond city lights. It was too early for bed, too dark for a stroll, and there was no particular place to go. Each person at the table took a turn at stoking the conversation. We were running out of topics and spontaneity.

Suddenly, the animated voice of the host, who was seated at our table: each person would tell the tale of how he or she got started in research. What were the circumstances? The motivation? How easy the first passage? The lessons?

New life at our table. The two seated closest to the host told their tales. The following was my story.

As my medical residency was drawing to a close, I was summoned to the chairman's office. As a rule, this sort of invitation presaged either an admonition, a fresh assignment, or, uncommonly, a reprimand. The chief, Dr. Snapper, was a professor of the old school, a Hollander by birth and Germanic by training. He was well known internationally for his studies of metabolic bone disease and was highly regarded for his clinical skills.

Dr. Snapper was in a congenial mood. His friend in Holland, Dr. Wilhelm Kolff, had invented an artificial kidney. This kidney had been tried in a few instances of

From: Wagner WW, Jr, Weir EK (eds): *The Pulmonary Circulation and Gas Exchange.* ©1994, Futura Publishing Co Inc, Armonk, NY.

uremia and seemed to hold promise as a last resort in acute renal failure. Dr. Kolff had offered to send one of his machines to our hospital for testing. Dr. Snapper thought that I was the ideal person to take on this assignment because I was on the verge of completing my medical residency and about to begin one year of pathology. What would be more natural than having the former chief medical resident responsible for the medical management of patients in acute renal failure, use the artificial kidney when medical management proved ineffective, and do the autopsy in his role as resident in pathology if things did not turn out well?

The apparatus arrived a few weeks after our meeting (Fig. 1). In essence, it consisted of a large, unwieldy bathtub on which was mounted a rotating drum. The dialysis membrane was sausage casing that was wound around the drum in a continuous spiral; at each end the casing was connected to a special rotating joint that enabled the casing to remain untangled while the drum continued to revolve. The sausage casing was obtained from a meat-packing house in Chicago and had to be thoroughly rinsed before use. Gallons and gallons of bath fluid had to be prepared fresh for each patient in accord with the individual's uremic state and electrolyte imbalance. By the time the apparatus arrived, Dr. Snapper had put together a team of two urologists and one cardiac fellow to assist me in the placement of arterial and venous catheters and to participate in the round-the-clock monitoring of the patient during dialysis.

No member of the team had any formal training in science, and none had previously engaged in this type of invasive human experimentation.

Unbelievably, the apparatus did work. Lives were saved. In the course of managing patients who were expected to be candidates for the artificial kidney, we also learned a great deal about the management of acute renal insufficiency. In-

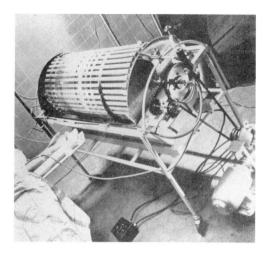

**Figure 1.** The Kolff artificial kidney. (Reproduced from Fig. 2 ref. 4.)

deed, by the time I had finished my year in pathology, we had established the efficacy of the artificial kidney, written several papers about both the management of acute renal insufficiency and the application of the artificial kidney, and *Life* magazine had featured our research in one of its issues.[4] We also received visitors from other institutions. Among them were physicians from the Peter Bent Brigham Hospital, who, impressed with our results, returned home to build a better model, which, in turn set the stage for modern renal dialysis.

This heady experience with the artificial kidney also had a sobering aspect. My understanding of research on the kidney and in hemodynamics was sorely inadequate. To remedy this deficiency, I obtained a research fellowship from the American Heart Association. I was to spend 6 months in Homer Smith's laboratory at New York University, and 6 months in the Cournand–Richards laboratory at Bellevue Hospital (Fig. 2). Little did I expect that this year would lead to a 5-year term as an established investigator of the American Heart Association. But that is another story. Here I will deal with only the 6 months in the Cournand–

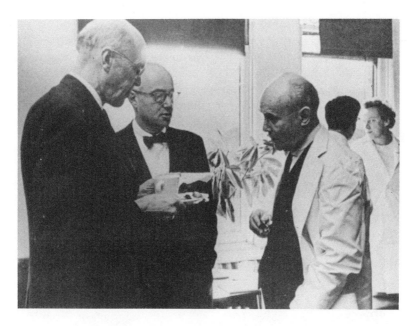

**Figure 2.** A. Cournand (right), A. P. Fishman (center), and D. W. Richards (left) at a small laboratory party after being awarded the Nobel Prize. (Reproduced from Fig. 7, ref. 9.)

Richards laboratory, which played a critical role in shaping my lifelong career in research.

My first encounter with Cournand did not auger well. I showed up at Bellevue Hospital well before the appointed hour. To escape the crowds milling aimlessly in the lobby, I took the stairs to the first floor where the Cournand-Richards laboratory was presumably housed. The stairs emptied onto a long corridor with windows on one side and closed heavy doors on the other. No one was in sight. I walked down the corridor looking for an open door. Finally I found two in a row: the first was clearly a secretarial office, but no one was there. I moved on to the next open door. Success. There, in the far corner, was Dr. Cournand himself. I recognized him immediately, even though I had only seen him once before, from afar, in a large lecture hall. He sat on the edge of his chair at a large desk in the far corner near the window, totally immersed in the papers on his desktop and completely unaware of

my presence in his doorway. I still remember the room. Everything about it was gray—even the light that filtered in through the unwashed window. His desk faced one wall; behind his back were tall green-gray files crowned with heaps of books and papers in calculated disarray. Even now I think of his office as a prison cell without bars.

Instinct told me that I could not have arrived at a worse time. However, my reflexes were too slow. Before I could retreat, Cournand sensed my presence and turned quickly to face me. (I learned later that his practice was to leave his office door open in case some procedure or test in one of the adjacent rooms called for his immediate attention.) Half out of his chair, looking directly at me, he challenged, "What do you want? Where's Ruth?"

"My name is Fishman."

No response. Arrested in midair, he stared at me, clearly upset at being disturbed.

I continued lamely, "I am from the

American Heart Association. I am scheduled to work with you during the coming year."

No response.

By now, he was standing. A pause. "You must be mistaken. I am not expecting any trainees. You probably want Stan Bradley." (I had never met Dr. Bradley, but I knew of his research on the liver at the Columbia-Presbyterian Medical Center—at the opposite end of New York City.)

It was a standoff. He was ready to turn back to his writing. I had no choice but to leave. Suddenly a new actor appeared on stage. A young, attractive woman stood behind me, in the way of my retreat.

She spoke past me, over my shoulder, directly to Cournand. "He is right. You and Dr. Richards did accept him. The letter is on my desk. I have set up a desk for him in my office."

Cournand did not turn a hair. He simply shrugged, sank back into his chair, and went back to his writing. It was Ruth who beckoned me to follow her to her office next door. This was to be my headquarters in the months ahead.

For weeks thereafter, Cournand was civil but disinterested. Left to my own devices, I explored the laboratory and met the members of the two teams: one was devoted primarily to cardiac catherterization and heart failure; the other to gas exchange. Each team was run by distinguished investigators, but each team had all the hands it needed. I was welcome to watch, to ask questions, to learn techniques, and occasionally to lend a hand. But I was clearly an observer. In my spare time I attended conferences and made ward rounds with J. Burns Amberson and Julia Jones. Every now and then I visited with Dickinson Richards. But, I did not belong.

Tired of reading and bored with the aimless mastering of analytic techniques and recording machines, I turned to the old data books in the blood gas laboratory. All samples of blood and gas were done in duplicate on separate machines—and redone immediately if any inconsistency was found. The books were carefully guarded by Mrs. Lester. Every now and then, in the course of a cardiac catheterization, Cournand would dash in, study the results, and order repeats if there were any question about any of the data. It was in these old data books that I found the roots of my future research on the pulmonary circulation.

Before proceeding, let me remind the reader of the state of understanding of the pulmonary circulation in the 1950s. In 1946, von Euler and Liljestrand had published their seminal paper on the effects of the respiratory gases on the pulmonary circulation of the open-chest cat. They showed that acute hypoxia (and hypercapnia) raised pulmonary arterial pressure.[1] They measured neither cardiac output nor pH. However, they reasoned with powerful insight that acute hypoxia was a potent pulmonary vasoconstrictor and that it was a mechanism by which local alveolar hypoxia would automatically adjust local blood flow to local ventilation.

A word is also in order about the state of determination of cardiac output at that time. Estimates of the cardiac output in humans were both indirect and inaccurate. The Fick principle had been published long ago in the brief proceedings of the Würzburg Physikalische-Medizinische Gesellschaft for July 9, 1870.[6] The communication went as follows:

> *Herr Fick has a contribution on the measurement of the amount of blood ejected by the ventricle of the heart with each systole, a quantity the knowledge of which is certainly of great importance.—It is surprising that no one has arrived at the following procedure by which this important value is available by direct de-*

termination, at least in animals. One measures how much oxygen an animal absorbs from the air in a given time, and how much $CO_2$ it gives off. One takes during this time a sample of arterial and a sample of venous blood; in both samples oxygen content and $CO_2$ content are measured. The difference of oxygen content gives the amount of oxygen each cubic centimeter of blood takes up in its passage through the lungs; and as one knows how much total oxygen has been taken up in given time, one can calculate how many cubic centimeters of blood have passed through the lungs in this time, or if one divides by the number of heartbeats during this time, how many cubic centimeters of blood are ejected with each beat.

Since for the demonstration of this method two gas pumps are needed, your reporter unfortunately is not in a position to communicate experimental data.

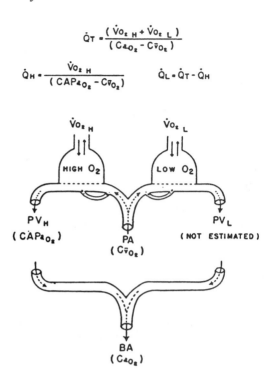

**Figure 3.** The blood flow through each lung in man during unilateral hypoxia. (Reproduced from Fig. 1 ref. 5.)

Having enunciated the concept, Fick undertook no experimental proof. Stating the principle was an end in itself. Eighteen years after his short communication, Grehant and Quinquaud applied the principle to the determination of cardiac output in dogs, followed in a few years by a more detailed study of the cardiac output in the horse. The arteriovenous oxygen difference in humans was not yet known.[6] Indeed, not until the late 1930s did Cournand and Richards resort to right-heart catheterization for the sake of obtaining samples of mixed venous blood for the determination of the cardiac output in humans (Fig. 3).[9] When I came into the Cournand-Richards laboratory, the Fick principle was in the air.

Having developed the technique of right-heart catheterization for physiologic studies in intact, unanesthetized human subjects, it was natural for the Cournand-Richards laboratory to extend the observations of von Euler and Liljestrand on open-chest cats by adding determinations of cardiac output. Motley et al. reproduced the pressor effect in normal human volunteers by administering an inspired mixture containing 10% oxygen and nitrogen.[10] The test gas was administered for 10 minutes before blood and gas samples were drawn for the determination of the cardiac output by the Fick principle. Their paper, based on five human subjects, was published in the *American Journal of Physiology*. One reviewer, Dr. Wallace Fenn, while recommending publication, expressed surprise in his cover letter at the finding that cardiac output decreased during acute hypoxia. To him, this decrease made no sense physiologically.

On reviewing the results of these experiments in Mrs. Lester's data books, I was impressed by the tendency of the values for the respiratory exchange ratios to be lower during hypoxia than during ambient air breathing. My attention was drawn to the respiratory exchange ratios, because recent research from Fenn's own laboratory had pointed out that when low oxygen mixtures were inspired, it might take a long while to reach a steady state of respiration and circulation.[11] Failure to achieve a steady state would be reflected in a low value for the respiratory exchange ratio, leading in turn to a low value for oxygen uptake (the numerator of the Fick equation). If one recalculated the data of Motley et al. assuming that oxygen uptake during hypoxia remained unchanged rather than decreased, cardiac output turned out to be either normal or increased, as Fenn had anticipated.

I showed my calculations to Cournand. He was annoyed. He recalculated the data. He ran back and forth between his office and the blood gas laboratory, checking numbers. Finally, he was convinced. I was told to present the results at *the* Saturday morning conference. This was the test. At the conference, all agreed that although the paper by Motley et al. had confirmed the pulmonary pressor effect of acute hypoxia, the values for cardiac output seemed to have been unduly low because of a lack of a "steady state." The 10 min exposure to 10% $O_2$ had simply been too brief for oxygen uptake, measured at the mouth, to reflect accurately the oxygen uptake by blood coursing through the lungs and by systemic tissues and organs. A new set of experiments were to be undertaken with milder degrees of acute hypoxia and, if necessary, using the respiratory exchange ratios as a guide for longer periods of equilibration.[5]

These observations on the effects of acute hypoxia marked the beginning of my acceptance as an active player in the laboratory. Moreover, Cournand and Richards

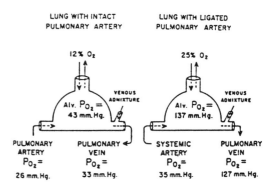

**Figure 4.** The "effective" pulmonary collateral blood flow in man. (Reproduced from Fig. 1, ref. 7.)

became interested in having me acquire additional training in hemodynamics and respiratory physiology. In the laboratory they encouraged my interplay with Aaron Himmelstein, a thoracic surgeon, who was extraordinarily adept at cardiac catheterization and bronchospirometry. In time, the association with Himmelstein and with Fritts was to lead to further applications of the Fick principle, including the measurement of blood flow through each lung separately during acute hypoxia,[7] the determination (Fig. 4) of pulmonary collateral blood flow in humans,[3] and to a succession of attempts to unravel the mechanisms responsible for the hypoxic pressor effect.[2]

Tales of this sort generally have a moral. Chaucer's pilgrims often concluded their narratives with timeless lessons, such as "success often occurs in the face of adversity," "the universe is directed so that everything happens for the best," or "what must be should not only be tolerated, but also celebrated."[8] One can add others: "one person's oversight can begin another person's career" or "mistakes occur in the best of laboratories." Perhaps all of these morals apply to my story. But the reader will be in a better position to draw the proper lesson when the other tales in this book have been told.

## References

1. Euler U. S. von, and G. Liljestrand. Observations on the pulmonary arterial blood pressure in the cat. *Acta Physiol. Scandinav.* 12: 301–320, 1946.
2. Fishman, A. P. Hypoxia on the pulmonary circulation: how and where it acts. *Circ. Res.* 38SS: 221–231, 1976.
3. Fishman A. P., A. Himmelstein, H. W. Fritts, Jr. and A. Cournand. Blood flow through each lung in man during unilateral hypoxia. *J. Clin. Invest.* 34: 637–646, 1955.
4. Fishman, A. P., I. G. Kroop, H. E. Leiter, and A. Hyman. Experiences with the Kolff artificial kidney. *Am. J. Med.* 7: 15–34, 1949.
5. Fishman, A. P., J. McClement, A. Himmelstein, and A. Cournand. Effects of acute anoxia on the circulation and respiration in patients with chronic pulmonary disease studied during the "steady state". *J. Clin. Invest.* 31: 770–781, 1952.
6. Fishman, A. P., and D. W. Richards. *Circulation of the Blood.* Men and Ideas. Bethesda, MD: American Physiological Society, 1982, p. 96, 97.
7. Fishman, A. P., G. M. Turino, M. Brandfonbrenner, and A. Himmelstein. The "effective" pulmonary collateral blood flow in man. *J. Clin. Invest.* 37: 1071–1086, 1958.
8. Hussey, S. S. *Chaucer: An Introduction.* 2nd ed., London: Methuen, 1981, p. 245.
9. Malm, J. R. New York: a bellwether for thoracic surgery. *J. Thorac. and Cardiovasc. Surg.* 92: 169–180, 1986.
10. Motley H. L., A. Cournand, L. Werkö, A. Himmelstein, and D. Dresdale. The influence of short periods of induced acute anoxia upon pulmonary artery pressures in man. *Am. J. Physiol.* 150: 315–324, 1947.
11. Rahn, H. and A. B. Otis. Man's respiratory responses during and after acclimatization to high altitude. *Am. J. Physiol.* 157: 445–462, 1949.
12. Robinson, F. N. (Ed). The Works of Geoffrey Chaucer. Boston: Houghton Mifflin Co, 1957, p. 17.

# 20

# Reflections on the Waterfalls in the Chest

## John Butler, M.D.

*Professor of Medicine, Division of Pulmonary and Critical Care Medicine, University of Washington, Seattle, Washington*

My story begins long, long ago and far, far away, in a place called Birmingham in England. I had been chief resident at the university hospital, the Queen Elizabeth Hospital. Most English hospitals are named after queens or saints. The advantage of naming a hospital after a queen is that you can get her to open it and visit it occasionally—which increases its visibility and encourages donations. This is difficult with saints. The Queen Elizabeth Hospital was the teaching hospital for the University of Birmingham. After being subjected to a period of character formation as chief resident there, one was expected to join the Medical Professorial Unit. There was only one professor of medicine in those days: Professor, now Sir, Melville Arnott (Fig. 1). Actually the professorial unit was run by a triumvirate

(Fig. 2). This picture is true; only the faces have been changed to protect the innocent. One of the seated members of the triumvirate was Peter Harris, who was senior lecturer in the Department of Medicine and is a contributor to this book. He is seated on the right, but has shaved and changed his clothes since that time.

When I followed the traditional path to the unit, Sir Melville thrust a paper labeled "The mechanics of breathing in man" by Otis, Fenn, and Rahn,[15] into my hands and said, "You'd better do some research, Butler." Because I had been in the army, I was good at swallowing things, and, after reading in this paper about measuring esophageal pressure changes as reflections of intrapleural pressure changes, I was not surprised to find I could easily swallow esophageal balloons. Otis

From: Wagner WW, Jr, Weir EK (eds): *The Pulmonary Circulation and Gas Exchange.* ©1994, Futura Publishing Co Inc, Armonk, NY.

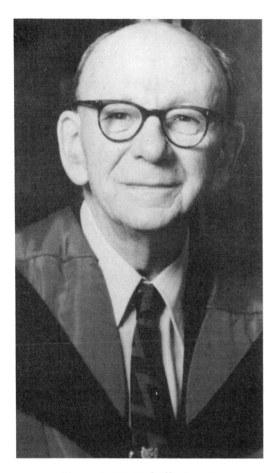

**Figure 1.** Sir Melville Arnott.

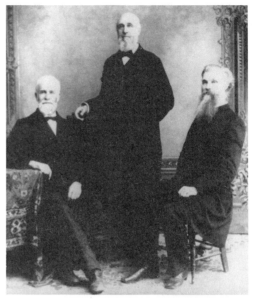

**Figure 2.** The professor, first assistant (left), and senior lecturer (right).

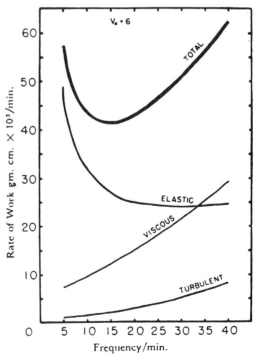

**Figure 3.** Relation of the rate of the mechanical work done on the lung to the breathing frequency. Minimal work is at a rate between 10 and 15 breaths/min.

and his colleagues had used the esophageal balloon to measure the work of breathing and had found that the normal breathing rate was that at which the work was least (Fig. 3). So I decided to measure the work of breathing at different end-expiratory volumes throughout the vital capacity to see if it changed and at what chest volume it was least (Fig. 4).

I found that the volume at which the work was least was the end-expiratory volume or functional reduced capacity at which each subject normally breathed (Fig. 5). This was pleasing to me because it fulfilled my preconceptions. I wrote up the studies and, in the discussion, waxed rather too lyrical about the Wisdom of the Respiratory Apparatus and the evidence

Pressure Volume Loops at Different Lung Volumes

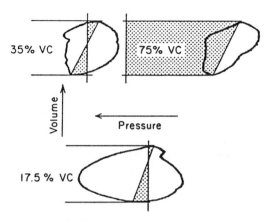

**Figure 4.** Esophageal pressure-lung volume loops at different lung volumes (%VC). Total work on the lung is made up of elastic work (dotted) and frictional work (enclosed in loop). Breathing at 15 breaths/min with 0.5 L tidal volume. The zero pressure (vertical line) was not corrected for the small chest wall effect over this volume.

of Purpose in Nature shown by the selection of both the rate and the volume at which the work of breathing was least. I showed the manuscript to Sir Melville, who was also the editor of *Clinical Science,* the journal in which I hoped to get the work published. He was unperturbed until he came to the discussion. After reading that he clutched his head and looked at me over his spectacles.

"I must tell you that *Clinical Science* does not like teleology, Butler."

I crept out of his sanctum with my unhappy masterpiece and went to look up "teleology" (Fig. 6). It occurred to me then, and it has occurred to me several times since, that it is no more disgraceful to look for a purpose in physiology than it is to look for an adaptation by evolution in nature. The latter is Darwinism and is now widely accepted. Why not the former? I have encountered this prejudice throughout my research efforts, as I shall show you. Others, such as Lynne Reid, have been similarly perplexed.

Because Sir Melville was the editor, my paper was published after I had excised the offending parts of the discussion.[5] Flushed with success, I cast around for a "Big Problem" to solve. At this stage of knowledge of the mechanics of the chest, the Big Problem was obviously the lack of knowledge about its normal pressure-volume relationships (Fig. 7). The Relaxation Pressure curve, as carried out by Rahn and his colleagues, depended on complete muscle relaxation after inhalation or exhalation to different volumes; they themselves had pointed out that such complete relaxation was impossible.[17] My brainstorm was to ensure complete relaxation by measuring these pressures and volumes in normal subjects whose mus-

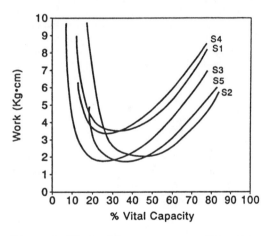

**Figure 5.** Work of lung movement (Fig. 4) in relation to lung volume at end exhalation. $S_1$ to $S_5$ = 5 normal subjects.

# TELEOLOGY

• "Evidence of Purpose in Nature"

(Oxford English Dictionary)

**Figure 6:** Teleology.

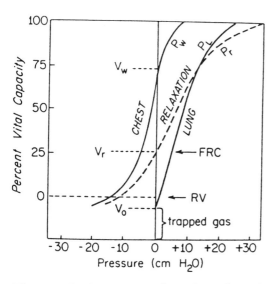

**Figure 7.** Static pressure volume (compliance) relations of the thorax. The relaxation pressure (Pr) is made up of the lung ($P_L$) and chest wall ($P_W$) pressure at each volume. Vr is the relaxation volume when the system is in balance. The lung exerts no pressure at $V_O$, the chest wall at $V_W$. FRC = functional residual capacity; RV = residual volume (Rahn, Otis, Chadwick, and Fenn.[15])

cles had been paralyzed with a relaxant. I could do this because I had become friendly with the surgeons and the anesthesiologists while I was chief medical resident.

Of course, the idea of obtaining a true value of the elastic properties of the lungs and chest wall by inducing paralysis proved to be extremely naive. Instead of the more compliant chest that I expected, the relaxation pressure curve in the paralyzed patient showed a loss of volume below that during voluntary apnea and a compliance that was only about half that obtained in the same patient during voluntary relaxation.

At this time, the Professorial Unit was visited by a friend of Sir Melville's, a famous researcher in physiology from America, Julius Comroe, Jr. (Fig. 8). Although I had no inkling at the time, J. C., Jr., was to change my life. I showed him my work, and he told me of work that he

had recently carried out with an anesthesiologist called Nims.[14] They had done exactly the same study as I had and found the same loss of volume and increase in rigidity. It was, of course, devastating to find that what I had imagined to be a most important contribution had already been contributed. This was the first of a series of Great Discoveries I was to make, only to find that they had already been discovered long before.

Nims and Comroe had attributed the increased rigidity in their anesthetized, paralyzed patients to a failure of the normal inspiratory muscle tone in the chest wall. On the other hand, it seemed to me, because I had used my favorite research instrument, the esophageal balloon, that it was the lungs rather than the chest wall that had changed. With trepidation I told J. C., Jr. (a la Jesus Christ, Jr.) about this. He pointed out that esophageal pressures were erroneous in the supine patient but, because my control measurements had been made in the same position, reassured me that there might be something in what I had found. Could I come over to Philadelphia to work in his lab and so arrive at the truth?

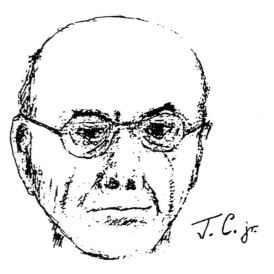

**Figure 8.** Julius Comroe, Jr. This and the sketch in Fig. 12 were made during his lectures, when the author should have been paying attention.

In those days it was not so difficult to get research grants (Fig. 9). I got a Rockefeller Traveling Fellowship. This success stunned my colleagues in the Professorial Unit. On arriving in Philadelphia, I found that Julius Comroe had fled to the west coast to become director of the Cardiovascular Research Institute in San Francisco. At his Graduate School of Medicine in Philadelphia I was, however, lucky enough to work with Arthur DuBois. Arthur was undoubtedly the person who gave the greatest help to my research career. With him and Colin Caro I studied another technique, suggested by Colin, for chronically reducing the functional residual capacity to a similar or greater extent than that consequent to muscle paralysis. This was strapping the chest and abdomen. Within a few minutes, the lung compliance invariably fell, sometimes to less than half normal, depending on the degree of constriction that was tolerated. Only Arthur could breathe with his lungs voluntarily held at a volume low enough to cause this compliance change without the aid of strapping. The low compliance, which persisted as long as the lungs were held in an expiratory position, reverted to normal immediately after a deep breath (Fig. 10). Normally the expiratory position is associated at first with a more positive intrapleural pressure and with narrower airways and blood vessels than those at the functional residual capacity. It seemed to us that this adaptation of the lungs by "shrinking" at low volumes was useful in maintaining the normal low intrapleural pressure and thus the

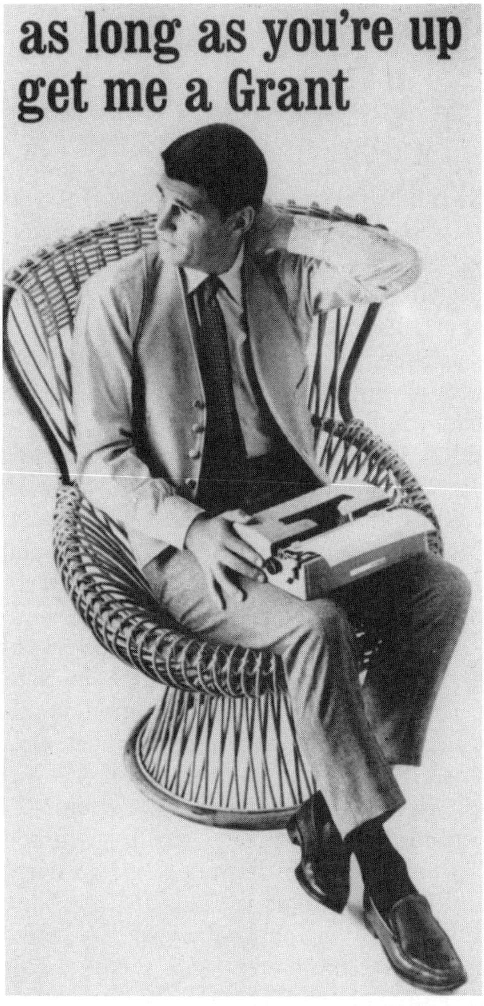

## as long as you're up get me a Grant

**Figure 9.** Availability of research fellowships in the 1950s, thought to be one of the first advertisements of NIH.

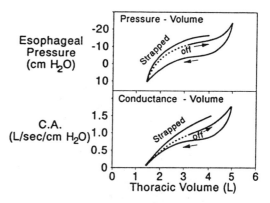

**Figure 10.** *Top:* Quasi-static pressure-volume relations of the lung (lung compliance slopes) with chest strapped and during first breath to total lung capacity after removal of strapping ("off" arrows). Note low compliance abolished by lung inflation. *Bottom:* Quasi-static conductance-volume relations under same conditions. Note increased conductance at each volume in the low compliance state.

normal airway caliber, airway resistance, and gradient for venous return (Fig. 11). Colin Caro and I wrote this up, aiming for the stars, that is, for the *Journal of Clinical Investigation.* After many months it bounced back rejected in part because two referees had found that the amount of teleology in the discussion section "did not befit good scientific work."

We removed the offending passages, modified other parts as requested, and it became acceptable.[7] I returned to England after this exciting glimpse of American research and, thanks to Sir Melville, obtained a job as first assistant in the Professorial Unit in Manchester. Julius Comroe (Fig. 12) wrote to me while I was there, asking me whether I would join him in San Francisco to exploit his body plethysmograph, about which I had learned so much from Arthur DuBois. This was an unexpected windfall, and as in many other stages of my career, I knew exactly what to do. I wrote and accepted his proposal. Later after I had thought about it a little, I wrote back that I regretted having to decline the position. I then thought about it for a month or two more and sent

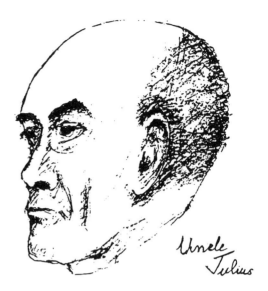

*Unele
Julius*

**Figure 12.** Julius Comroe, Jr.

him a telegram saying that I would accept the position if the job were still open. It was. And so I moved to America.

After the windfall began the quest for waterfalls. I had learned the nitrous oxide technique for measuring instantaneous pulmonary capillary blood flow using the body plethysmograph while I was with Arthur DuBois in Philadelphia (Fig. 13). After the plethysmograph began to work in San Francisco, I pursued the idea that the maintenance of a low intrapleural pressure was important for regulating venous return. I had to assume that the pulmonary capillary flow reflected the rate of venous flow into the chest, since the right atrium, right ventricle, and pulmonary circulation in the normal person act as a conduit through the lungs to the left atrium. Together with Paul Vermeire, I studied the pulmonary capillary blood flow in a series of normal subjects when they changed their intrapleural pressure (reflected by esophageal pressure) during respiratory maneuvers and breath holds with open glottis (Fig. 14).[21] We found that the pulmonary capillary blood flow and the venous return increased at the beginning of a slow inhalation but then failed to

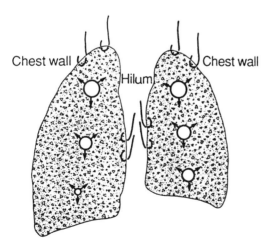

**Figure 11.** Usefulness of increased recoil pressures in unexpanded regions of lung in keeping airways and blood vessels patent. *Left:* Normal lung. *Right:* Restricted lung. Hooks represent suspension of lung from chest wall and hilum.

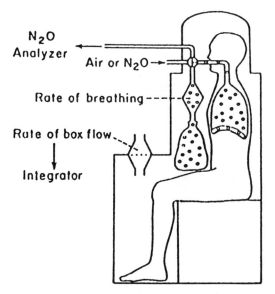

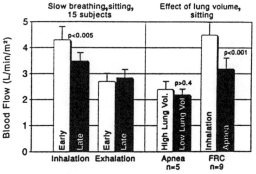

assumed to partially collapse to form a waterfall at their distal ends when the alveolar pressure compressing them rose above the left atrial pressure within them. To me the waterfall concept has always been wonderfully evocative of the beauty of flow (Fig. 16). The rate at which water

**Figure 13.** Nitrous oxide ($N_2O$) technique for measuring instantaneous pulmonary capillary blood flow in man. The subject in a closed box (plethysmograph) takes a breath of air containing a very soluble gas ($N_2O$) from a bag in the box. The $N_2O$ is absorbed (disappears) into the pulmonary capillary blood as it pulses into the gas exchanging regions. This causes air to flow in through the flowmeter in the wall. The rate of this flow is proportional to pulmonary blood flow, which can be calculated from the alveolar $N_2O$ concentration and solubility. The airflow trace after a breath of air must be subtracted from the $N_2O$ tracing so that non-$N_2O$ events can be excluded.

**Figure 14.** Blood flow into the lungs ($N_2O$ method), assumed to reflect systemic venous return. *Right:* Flow was higher in early inhalation to vital capacity than later, in spite of more negative intrapleural pressures later. There was no further change during slow exhalation. *Left:* Pleural pressure and lung volume during prolonged (10 to 15 s) apnea with the glottis open had no effect on blood flow. Blood flow was higher when functional residual capacity (FRC) was reached early, during inhalation, than when functional residual capacity was held during prolonged apnea.

rise further in spite of a continued fall in intrapleural pressure. During exhalation venous return was lower but unchanging. We stressed the system even more by slowly inhaling through a high resistance (Fig. 15). In spite of quite negative intrapleural pressures, pulmonary capillary blood flow did not increase. This was extraordinary because we had thought that the more negative the intrapleural pressures, the greater the increase in systemic venous return.

A few years previously Permutt and his colleagues in the U.S.[16] and Bannister and Torrance in the U.K.[1] had described the alveolar "waterfall" or "sluice" effect. The delicate alveolar microvessels were

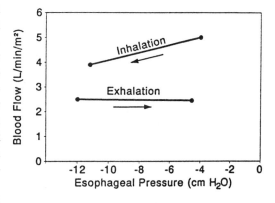

**Figure 15.** Pulmonary capillary blood flow, reflecting systemic venous return at the same negative esophageal pressures during inhalation and the start of exhalation. More negative pressures did not increase blood flow.

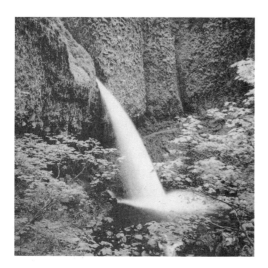

**Figure 16.** Waterfall.

falls over a cliff is not influenced by how far it falls. Only when the base of the falls is brought up above the level of the top of the cliff is the rate of flow diminished.[10] To strengthen the analogy, the falling water can be thought of as enclosed in a flexible sheath with blood flow in a very thin elastic walled vessel. In reality, the flow need not plunge to a lower hydrostatic level. It is sufficient if the downstream pressure of a vessel, inclined in any direction, falls below the value at which the transmural pressure causes its walls to buckle inward (Fig. 17).[10,11] This pressure and its locus are influenced by the rate of upstream inflow in relation to the downstream pressure; no more can be pulled through than is put in. The segment may be long if the collapsing transmural pressure continues downstream. Or it may be short if the transmural pressure is restored, as happens, for instance, where the veins enter the negative pressure domain in the chest. The compliance of a tube changes dramatically as the transmural pressure distorts the cross-sectional area of its lumen. Entering the partially collapsed segment it is high; upstream (fully distended) and in the partially collapsed segment (fully distorted) it is low. Com-

plete stoppage of flow is prevented by the rigidity of the partially collapsed segment and the abrupt rise in transmural pressure that would occur as intravascular pressure upstream of a complete obstruction rose to input pressure. There is instability ("flitter") when a flow-limiting segment forms, which may be audible as a venous hum.

After deep cogitation we surmised that there must be a flow-limiting or "waterfall" effect in the systemic veins as they enter the chest such that increasingly negative intrapleural pressure would not affect the rate of venous return. For several days, I was happy that we had finally made the Great Discovery. But then Paul found that the work of G. A. Brecher, which had been published 16 years previously,[3] and then that of J. P. Holt, published 11 years before that.[11] Both described flow limitation due to partial venous collapse where the veins enter the thorax. Brecher had applied increasingly negative pressures acutely to the downstream end of the vena cava and had shown that, after the pressure had reached $-15$ cm $H_2O$, further decreases did not affect the rate of flow (Fig. 18). He showed

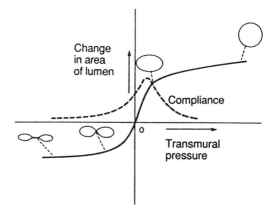

**Figure 17.** Venous caliber in relation to transmural pressure. The dramatic change in luminal area when transmural pressure is zero in this schematic causes the waterfall effect. Venous compliance (dotted) is highest at slightly positive transmural pressures (Hoffman and Spaan.[10])

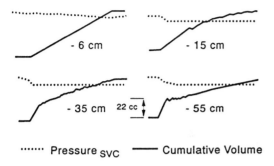

······· Pressure $_{SVC}$ ——— Cumulative Volume

**Figure 18.** Negative pressures applied to the downstream end of the superior vena cava (SVC) detached from the right atrium. At −6 cm the cumulative volume extracted increases rapidly during the depleting phase as the veins collapse. At −15 cm and more negative pressures the rates of outflow become the same, limited by the venous collapse (Brecher, Mixter, and Share.[2])

that when the pressure falls there is first an increase of flow as the veins empty and partially collapse. This "depleting" phase is followed after 2 or 3 seconds (faster with more negative pressures) by a flow-limitation phase when the partial collapse of the veins prevents any further rise in flow rate. The reader can demonstrate this waterfall effect in the systemic veins by holding his wrist at a level below the chest and observing the distended veins on the back of the hand. Inspiratory efforts against a closed glottis (Mueller maneuver) do not alter their distension, showing that the veins are still emptying into the thorax at the same rate as they are filling on the back of the hand, in spite of very negative intrapleural pressures. However, if the upstream pressure is increased by raising the wrist above the level of the axilla, the veins collapse as blood flow into the thorax increases.

Very negative intrathoracic pressures are necessary during inhalation in severe lower airway obstruction such as asthma but are counterbalanced by very positive pressures during exhalation. Very negative intrathoracic pressures are present with upper airway obstruction during in-halation (snoring, adenoids, etc.), but these are not negated by high exhalation pressures. Were such pressures to cause a torrential inflow of systemic venous blood, the vessels in the chest and the pulmonary vasculature would overdistend and pulmonary edema could ensue. Indeed pulmonary edema has been described in such patients since the diphtheria days.[22] Happily the systemic venous waterfall usually prevents such dramatic displacements of blood during sustained inspiratory efforts.

We pointed out this potentially important physiological role in the discussion section of the paper we sent to *Circulation Research*. Julius Comroe was the new editor of the journal. We got the reviews back in record time; J. C., Jr. regretted that the paper was "unacceptable in its present form" and suggested that we heed the suggestion of one of the referees that we omit our speculations about the "wisdom of the body" in pulmonary edema prevention. We did so but slipped in a little gas exchange teleology because we thought this would be too much for cardiologists to cavil about in a rereview— and indeed it was.[21]

After getting out of my depth in systemic waterfalls, I decided to continue the search downstream in the friendly flows of the pulmonary circulation.

The measurement of pulmonary venous pressure by passing catheters retrogradely up the pulmonary veins had proved an unrewarding technique. If the catheter is pushed to the wedged position, pulmonary arterial pressure is registered. As the catheter is unwedged and pulled toward the larger veins, the pressure falls, depending on how much the catheter blocks the flow. However, Caro and McDonald have shown that pressures can be measured without obstructing flow if thin catheters with a bell-shaped distension on one end and a point on the other are passed retrogradely out through the lung surface so that the bell-shaped end wedges in a bifurcation of the vascular system (Fig. 19).[6] We used this method to measure the pressures in the veins of the excised lung. Using several such catheters, we obtained upstream venous pressures in both small and large intrapulmonary veins. These were unaffected during constant flow when the downstream pressures in the left atrium or in the pulmonary veins in the intrapleural space were reduced below about 7 $cmH_2O$, even to very low pressures.[20] We were able to find the site in the vein—the waterfall or partially collapsed segment—at which there was a sudden fall from upstream venous pressure to the low left atrial pressure. This was just before the veins passed out of the lungs (Fig. 20). When the lung surface was resected back 1 or 2 cm, the abrupt pressure change again occurred inside the new surface. We showed subsequently that we could make similar measurements in the living, open-chested animal and that the results were identical.[19] We were reasonably certain that this discovery of a pulmo-

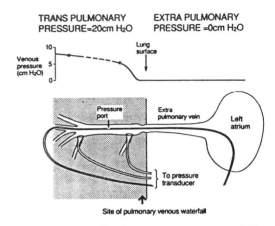

**Figure 20.** Site of pulmonary venous waterfall. Flared catheters were wedged in small and large intrapulmonary veins. A fine catheter with a single side hole pressure port was withdrawn through the lung from the left atrium. Pressure increased suddenly as the port was pulled just within the surface of the lung.

nary venous waterfall would finally make us famous. However, it turned out that Duomarco and his colleagues had shown the pulmonary venous waterfall effect some fifteen years before.[8] He had even drawn an elegant diagram of the venous narrowing and of the pressure relationships that must exist between the perivenous pressure within the lungs and that outside the lungs in the intrapleural space (Fig. 21). Another Great Discovery that wasn't!

The position of this waterfall, just within the lungs, remains a puzzle. Although not as low as that around the arteries, the pressure around the veins within the lung has been measured and shown to be similar to that in the intrapleural space.[12] Indeed Fung and his colleagues concluded that extra alveolar vessels in the lung "do not collapse" when subjected to alveolar pressures considerably higher than intravascular pressures.[9] They used the term *collapse,* however, to signify a complete closure of a vessel, assessed using an elegant silicone elastomer cast technique. Part of the explanation for the position of the venous waterfall can likely be

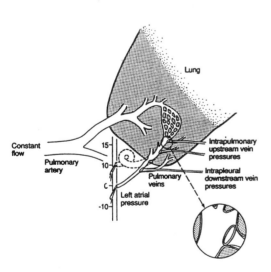

**Figure 19.** Excised lung perfused at constant rate while varying the downstream pulmonary venous (left atrial) pressure. Intrapulmonary and extrapulmonary pressures in main veins were measured via venous tributaries using catheters that did not obstruct the lumen of the main veins.

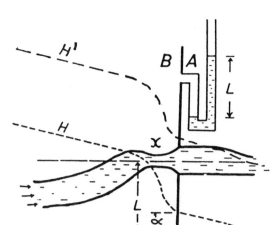

**Figure 21.** Diagram of physical factors involved in pulmonary venous hemodynamics. X is the site of collapse. A is the low pressure domain (atmospheric or intrapleural), whereas B is the high pressure domain (intrapulmonary). H′ relates intravenous to extrapulmonary pressure at the level of the vein, H to intrapulmonary pressure around the vein. L is the hydrostatic level of the surrounding pressure necessary to deform and collapse the vein when its intravascular distending pressure is $\alpha$. $\alpha$ is set by the rate of flow and the frictional resistance upstream of the vein. (From Duomarco, Rimini, and Giambruno.[7])

found in the work of Younes and others.[4] They have shown that, in a system of collapsible tubes, the intravascular pressure fall toward their downstream ends is compounded by the narrowing it causes. This leads to a further rise in resistance. Also, the compliance of individual veins increases as they get bigger downstream; they have a poor intrinsic resistance to buckling and are less well tethered than are the arteries in the bronchovascular bundles. Presumably they partially collapse and a flow-limiting waterfall segment forms where they are particularly poorly supported just before they exit from the lungs. Although the intravascular pressure at the waterfall is hardly influenced by alveolar pressures up to 15 $cmH_2O$ and the corresponding lung volume changes, it rises when these increase further.[19] Thus near its edge the lung

seems to be compressing rather than expanding the veins.

Another piece of this puzzle was put in place some years later by Grant Lee. Using dogs, he and his colleagues showed that the veins lying between the lung and the left atrium in the intrapleural space are easily distensible and, when distended, contain a volume that can be as large as the left ventricular stroke volume.[18] Lee the cardiologist was interested in the damping of the flow pulse from the right ventricle by this distensible reservoir formed by the pulmonary veins. My interest in it, as a respiratory physiologist, was that it must also be a reservoir capable of holding the increase in flow from the partially collapsing intrapulmonary veins at the start of inspiration. This flow increment would otherwise distend the left atrium before the protective pulmonary venous waterfall formed to limit venous outflow from the lungs. Were it not for this waterfall effect, every time a person yawned, there would be an immediate and dramatic increase in cardiac output as pulmonary venous return to the left atrium rose in proportion to the fall in intrapleural pressure. Such a rise in output would be particularly inappropriate for the bored reader.

This paper went to the *Journal of Applied Physiology.* It was reviewed by two of my friends and finally accepted with these teleological warts untreated.[19]

Are there, then, three waterfalls affecting blood flow in the chest (Fig. 22)? To my knowledge the alveolar waterfall has never been seen or shown by direct pressure measurements, as has the pulmonary venous waterfall.[8,19,20] The many elegant studies of its formation have relied on raising pulmonary venous or left atrial pressure, downstream of both waterfalls, and showing an effect on upstream flow or pressure when the waterfall pressure was exceeded. So either, or both, could have caused the changes. However a micropuncture study of the pressures in 50 μm venules showed no further fall as down-

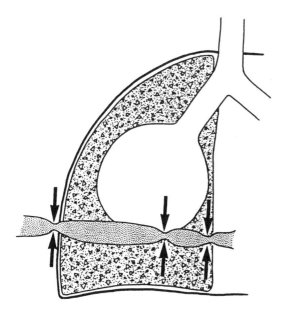

**Figure 22.** The three waterfalls along the systemic vein-pulmonary vessel channel. The systemic veins collapse before entering the intrapleural space, the alveolar vessels at the downstream end of the alveolar pressure domain, and the pulmonary veins collapse before entering the intrapleural space.

heart. But the pulmonary venous waterfall serves the same purpose. Must one postulate that there is an alveolar waterfall because pericapillary pressures in the alveoli should be so much higher than perivenous pressures in the extra-alveolar compartment? We now know that surface tension lowers pericapillary pressures, particularly around corner vessels, and that interstitial pressures measured in the extra-alveolar compartment depend on the circumstances and the location. Thus the vascular effect of the alveolar to extra alveolar interstitial pressure difference could have been over emphasized. This remains a fascinating field of study.

The natural waterfall does not have an opaque, plain vascular encasement. Thus, it can be seen to be beautiful. I think that one might be excused, however, for arguing that the waterfalls in the circulation are there for a beautiful physiological purpose. This is arrant teleology and unworthy of a scientist (Fig. 23). But this time I am not worried, for I know that my manuscript must be accepted.

stream venous pressure was lowered below 7 cmH$_2$O (alveolar pressure)[2] consistent with an effect downstream of the alveolar vessels.

The effect of the alveolar waterfall is to prevent more blood flowing through zone 2 of the lungs, when left atrial pressure falls, unless there is an augmented inflow (pulmonary arterial) pressure from a more vigorous right heart. In other words, although acute differences can still occur, it ensures the long-term matching of the stroke volumes of the right and left

Teleology is like a mistress;
a person one cannot do without,
but with whom one dare not be
seen in public

**Claude Bernard**

**Figure 23.** From the French father of physiology.

---

### References

1. Bannister, J., and R. W. Torrence. The effects of the tracheal pressure upon flow: pressure relations in the vascular bed of isolated lungs. *Q. J. Exp. Physiol.* 45: 352–367, 1960.
2. Bhattacharya, J., S. Nanjo, and N. C. Staub. *Ann. NY Acad. of Sci.* 384: 107–114, 1982.
3. Brecher, G. A., G. Mixter, and L. Share. Dynamics of venous collapse in superior vena cava system. *Am. J. Physiol.* 171: 194–203, 1952.
4. Bshouty, Z., and M. Younes. Distensibility and pressure flow relationship of the pulmonary circulation. II. Multibranched

model. *J. Appl. Physiol.* 68: 1514–1527, 1990.

5. Butler, J., and W. M. Arnott. The work of pulmonary ventilation at different respiratory levels. *Clin. Sci.* 14: 703–710, 1955.

6. Caro, C. G., and D. A. McDonald. The relation of pulsatile pressure and flow in the pulmonary vascular bed. *J. Physiol. (London)* 157: 426–453, 1961.

7. Caro, C. G., J. Butler, and A. B. Dubois. Some effect of restriction of chest cage expansion on pulmonary function in man: an experimental study. *J. Clin. Invest.* 4: 573–583, 1960.

8. Duomarco, J. L., R. Rimini, and C. E. Giambruno. The collapse of the pulmonary veins. *Acta Physiol. Latinoam.* 7: 8–17, 1957.

9. Fung Y-C, S. S. Sobin, H. Tremer, M. R. T. Yen, and H. H. Ho. Patency and compliance of pulmonary veins when airway pressure exceeds blood pressure. *J. Appl. Physiol.* 54: 1538–1549, 1983.

10. Hoffman, J. I. E., and J. A. E. Spaan. Pressure-flow relations in coronary circulation. *Physiol. Revs.* 70: 331–390, 1990.

11. Holt, J. P. The collapse factor in the measurement of venous pressure. *Am. J. Physiol.* 134: 292–299, 1941.

12. Lai Fook, S. J. Perivascular interstitial fluid pressure measured by micropipettes in isolated dog lung. *J. Appl. Physiol.* 52: 9–15, 1982.

13. Little, R. C. Volume-pressure relationships of the pulmonary-left heart vascular segments. *Circ. Res.* 8: 594–598, 1960.

14. Nims, R. G., S. Y. Bothelo, O. Nissel, and J. H. Comroe, Jr. Pressure volume measurements upon the lungs and thorax (Abstract). *Fed. Proc.* 7: 113–114, 1952.

15. Otis, A. B., W. O. Fenn, and H. Rahn. The mechanics of breathing in man. *J. Appl. Physiol.* 2: 592–607, 1950.

16. Permutt, S., B. Bromberger-Barnea, and H. N. Bane. Alveolar pressure, pulmonary venous pressure and the vascular waterfall. *Med. Thorac.* 19: 239–260, 1962.

17. Rahn, H., A. B. Otis, L. E. Chadwick, and W. O. Fenn. The pressure volume diagram of the thorax and lung. *Am. J. Physiol.* 146: 171–178, 1946.

18. Rajagopalan, B., C. D. Bertam, T. Stallard, and G. Lee. Blood flow in pulmonary veins. III. Simultaneous measurements of their dimensions, intravascular pressure, and flow. *Cardiovasc. Res.* 134: 684–692, 1979.

19. Smith, H. C., and J. Butler. Pulmonary venous waterfall and perivenous pressure in the living dog. *J. Appl Physiol.* 38: 304–308, 1975.

20. Takahashi, S., and J. Butler. A vascular waterfall in extra alveolar vessels of the excised dog lung. *J. Appl. Physiol.* 26: 578–584, 1969.

21. Vermeire, P., and J. Butler. Effect of respiration on pulmonary capillary blood flow in man. *Circ. Res.* 22: 299–308, 1968.

22. Willms, D., and D. Shure. Pulmonary edema due to upper airway obstruction in adults. *Chest* 94: 1090–1092, 1988.

# Acute and Chronic Lack of Oxygen:
## Consequences for the Lung and Carotid Body; A Journey with *Bacillus investigationis,* the Curiosity Bug

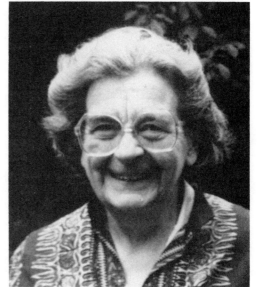

## Gwenda R. Barer, M.D.

*Royal Hallamshire Hospital, Department of Medicine, Sheffield, England*

*For there are indeed many who openly confess that the greatest part of those things which we do know is the least of the things which we know not.*

(William Harvey, 1628)

A life-long infection with the curiosity bug has been a great asset to me. It has been the driving force for a research life, has overcome disappointments and frustrations, sustained interest, and also overwhelmed those destructive impulses—the pursuit of fortune and distinction.

I was lucky to have studied physiology in Ernest Starling's laboratory. It was an exciting place. Starling had died early, but we learned his tradition of controlled artificial circuits for circulatory studies from Charles Lovatt Evans. A. V. Hill ran a biophysics laboratory that attracted brilliant people from all over the world. Wallace Fenn was one of them; Hill had won the Nobel Prize with Otto Meyerhof for studies on muscle heat production and metabolism (Fig. 1A). He taught us to do everything ourselves and make our own apparatus when we could. Bernard Katz, a future Nobel laureate, had just escaped from Nazi Germany; he worked late into the night looking at end-plate potentials with early cathode ray tubes. Tom Lewis of ECG fame taught simple bedside "clinical science." Contact with these great men

From: Wagner WW, Jr, Weir EK (eds): *The Pulmonary Circulation and Gas Exchange.* ©1994, Futura Publishing Co Inc, Armonk, NY.

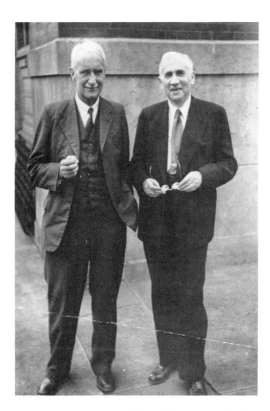

**Figure 1A.** A.V. Hill and Otto Meyerhof.

aroused our enthusiasm and set standards for a lifetime.

It is more than 360 years since Harvey demonstrated that the whole cardiac output flows through the lungs, though he knew nothing of their function and would never see a capillary.[24] His deductions from observations were fantastic. In my student days (1935–42) there was still great ignorance about the pulmonary circulation, and after the Second World War scientists still argued as to whether a membrane separated the alveolar capillaries from air.[41] In 1946 von Euler and Liljestrand cannulated the pulmonary artery directly in cats and showed that pressure rose during ventilation with low $O_2$ or high $CO_2$ mixtures.[21] Their great contribution was to suggest that these gases caused vasoconstriction in the lung as opposed to causing a dilator effect, as they did in other organs. Von Euler and Liljestrand's

conclusion was speculation because they could not measure cardiac output; if cardiac output had risen with these stimuli, the result would have been the same. One must be right for the right reason and have supporting evidence, yet speculation is a great stimulus to research. It was soon shown that the Scandinavians had been correct; in controlled isolated perfused lung preparations hypoxia and hypercapnia both caused vasoconstriction.[18] This phenomenon, not yet explained, has been studied from that day to this.

My husband was offered a university post while racing across Europe with the tanks in the final stages of World War II. Thus we arrived in postwar Oxford, and I soon got a job in the Nuffield Institute for Medical Research. This period in Britain has been called a "golden age." There was no difficulty in funding research; science was valued. In the Nuffield Institute, Geoffrey Dawes and his team were studying the fetal circulation (Fig. 1B). Geoffrey had been named director of the institute before he turned thirty. Under him this laboratory became a centre to which physiologists, pediatricians, and obstetricians came from all over the world; clinical

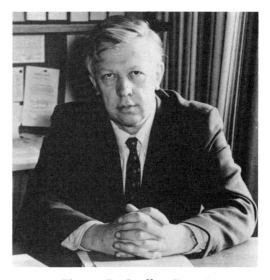

**Figure 1B.** Geoffrey Dawes.

problems were considered side by side with basic physiology.

After the Second World War right heart catheterization made possible direct measurement of pulmonary arterial pressure in humans. Clinicians measured pulmonary vascular resistance as the ratio of pulmonary artery pressure to cardiac output or that of pulmonary artery-wedge pressure to cardiac output. However, the important work of Alan Burton taught us that this ratio is an unreliable guide to haemodynamic changes. One needs to measure the relation between pressure and flow over a wide range; if the line is curved or forms an intercept on the pressure axis, the ratio will vary passively due to simple geometry. If there is a true vasomotor or mechanical change, then the whole line will shift.[39]

We began to study pulmonary haemodynamics in the anaesthetized open-chest cat.* We inserted a tall column into the left pulmonary artery (Burton's method)[39] and allowed it to fill with blood and then empty through the lung. From the pressure at the base of the column and the cross sectional area of the tube, we could calculate blood flow. Figure 2 shows some results; the line moved from A to B in a parallel fashion when we raised tracheal pressure.[12] The young Dr. Grant Lee remarked perceptively that the shift "looked like an obstruction in the vascular bed." In a nearby laboratory Banister and Torrance were perfusing isolated cat lungs. They showed that, when tracheal pressure was raised above left atrial pressure, flow was unaffected by left atrial pressure until it exceeded tracheal pressure. In this circumstance tracheal pressure became the downstream pressure for flow, which now depended on pulmonary artery pressure-tracheal or alveolar pressure and not pulmonary artery-left atrial pressure. They introduced the idea of sluice flow.[2] Per-

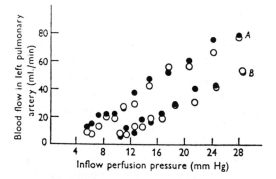

**Figure 2.** Parallel shift of pressure/flow line in the lung with raised tracheal pressure. Pressure/flow lines measured in left pulmonary artery of anaesthetized open-chest cat. A tall column was inserted into the artery, allowed to fill with blood and then empty through the lung; pressure was recorded at the base of the column. Flow was calculated first from the rate of change of pressure and cross-sectional area of the tube (solid circles) and second from a volume recorder attached to the top of the tube (open circles). Between A and B tracheal pressure was raised. (Reproduced with permission from reference 12.)

mutt and Riley in Baltimore were also showing that the driving pressure for blood flow through the lung was not always pulmonary artery-left atrial pressure. They showed that small collapsible vessels with muscle tone could act like the resistors used by Starling in his heart-lung preparation.[40] Starling's resistors consisted of a collapsible rubber tube inside a glass tube. The space between the tubes could be raised to any "surrounding pressure," and this formed the outlet or downstream pressure; the inner tube fluttered open and shut with flow. The great contribution of the Baltimore group was to show that small muscular vessels could behave like Starling resistors and that tone in their walls could act as the surrounding pressure, if it was effectively greater than left atrial pressure. They called this "waterfall flow" and showed that it corresponded

---

*All experiments on living animals were conducted under full anesthesia.

with Burton's "critical closing pressure."[15,35]

Waterfall or sluice flow is a useful explanation but not necessarily the sole explanation for events in the pulmonary circulation. In an artificial circuit, the pressure-flow line can be shown to change its slope or resistance if the tubing is narrowed with a screw clip but to shift in a parallel manner, as in Figure 2, if the surrounding pressure in a Starling resistor is raised.

## Changes in Pulmonary Vascular Resistance in Collapsed Lung

Geoffrey Dawes's team was showing that blood flow through the fetal lung varied tremendously when the ewe was ventilated with high $CO_2$ or low $O_2$ mixtures. He suggested that it would be interesting to compare the adult collapsed lung with the fetal unexpanded lung. We needed a reliable instrument to measure blood flow, and our physicist, Derek Wyatt, designed an electromagnetic flow meter that has played a crucial role in our research and has never been equaled or surpassed by commercial instruments.[52] We inserted this flow meter into a loop in the left pulmonary artery of cats. The two lungs were separately ventilated, the left with $O_2$. When the left tube was occluded, the gases were rapidly absorbed and the lung became solid like liver in about one minute. The rapidity of collapse dismayed visiting pediatricians, for they were still using high $O_2$ mixtures for babies. Figure 3 shows that the blood flow to the collapsing lung fell rapidly when ventilation ceased.[4] Pressure-flow lines were obtained by progressively occluding first the right and then the left pulmonary artery; they moved to and fro with collapse and reexpansion (Fig. 3, right). We tried to estab-

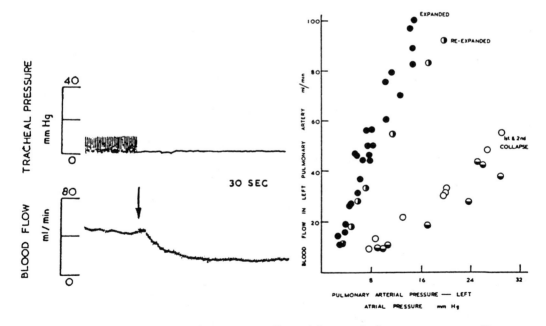

**Figure 3.** Reduction in blood flow in a collapsed lung and changes in pressure/flow lines. Left: Blood flow in the left pulmonary artery of an anaesthetized cat, measured with an electromagnetic flow meter, falls rapidly when ventilation to the left lung ceases. Right: Pressure/flow line measured by progressive occlusion of first the left and then right pulmonary artery shifts when the lung is collapsed, returns on reexpansion, and shifts again on recollapse. (Compiled from reference 4).

lish the cause of flow reduction. Was it due to gas tensions in the unchanged venous blood flowing through the lung, to mechanical changes, or to release of vasoactive substances?

## Hypoxia and Lung Vessels

There was intense interest at the time in hypoxic pulmonary vasoconstriction. It had been demonstrated to be a local mechanism in isolated perfused cat lungs under controlled conditions.[18] We began to study the phenomenon in anaesthetized cats in vivo. The left lung was supplied with blood by a connection to the left carotid artery, in which flow and pressure were measured. An adjustable clip re-

duced the pressure to pulmonary arterial levels and enabled us to keep blood flow constant. Thus, if left atrial pressure remained constant (and it did), rises in pressure in the loop meant that vasoconstriction was taking place in the lung. Ventilation of the cat with 10% $O_2$ caused sustained and reproducible increases in pulmonary arterial pressure, which still took place after removal of the adrenal glands[4] (Fig. 4, top). Vasoconstriction caused by hypoxia is surprising, because lack of $O_2$ is usually associated with negative effects. We set out to see whether vasoconstriction was caused by release of a transmitter, which in turn would cause vascular smooth muscle to contract. We found that several "α catecholamine in-

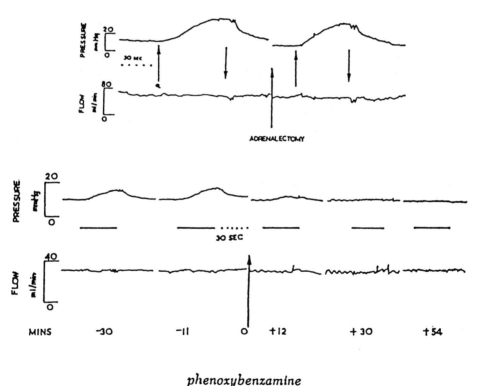

*phenoxybenzamine*

**Figure 4:** Hypoxic Vasoconstriction: Effect of α Catecholamine "Blockade" Anaesthetized cats. Left pulmonary artery supplied from left carotid artery; pressure reduced to pulmonary levels, and blood flow, measured with an electromagnetic flow meter, kept constant. Above: On ventilating cat with 10% $O_2$ between arrows, pulmonary arterial pressure rose, also after adrenalectomy. Below: Pressure rises during hypoxia, during bars, but this effect is slowly lost after 10 mg/kg phenoxybenzamine. (Compiled from reference 4.)

hibitors'' (the terminology used at that time) abolished hypoxic vasoconstriction (phenoxybenzamine in Fig. 3, bottom). Also, $\alpha$ inhibitors decreased and $\beta$ inhibitors increased pulmonary vascular resistance; we were excited and thought we had found the transmitter. Yet we had trouble with the paper on this work, which we had submitted to an eminent journal. It was returned with rude remarks. We were rescued, however, by a timely visit from Dr. A. P. Fishman, whose fine literary talent helped make it acceptable.

Unfortunately, soon after the paper was published, our hypothesis was shattered by two papers from Anton Hauge in Norway. They seemed to show conclusively that histamine was the transmitter in the rat.[25,26] However, testing his hypothesis we found that the antihistamine (H1) inhibitor he had used in rats did not abolish hypoxic vasoconstriction in either cats or dogs.[31] Indeed, given to rats *during* hypoxia, histamine caused dilatation.[44] We then found that the $\alpha$ catecholamine inhibitors, so promising in cats, were ineffective in dogs and rats. So we had both been wrong. We became friends and learned the limitations of pharmacological "blockade." Differences can be instructive! Another lesson was that species differ profoundly. Over the 45 years since this phenomenon was discovered many transmitters have been proposed, but all so far have been discarded. Yet the pharmacological inhibitors used have been relatively specific in that they abolished hypoxic but not other forms of pulmonary vasoconstriction. There is surely some clue here.

## Hypoxia and the Lung in Health, Disease, and at High Altitude

In the 1960s I continued work on hypoxia in the Department of Medicine in Sheffield. Charles Stuart-Harris, head of the department, was studying chronic bronchitis and emphysema in that formerly very polluted city (Fig. 5). I still thought of this disease as smoker's cough, but Stuart-Harris was showing the lethal nature of this terrible smokers'-pollution disease. It was valuable to compare physiological mechanisms in the lung with disordered function in disease. I owed my opportunity to Stuart-Harris's vision that one should study patients and fundamental mechanisms side by side. Many of his patients were extremely hypoxic, so much so that one marveled at their survival; one patient walked into the laboratory, and his arterial $PO_2$ was measured as 28 mmHg, close to estimated value on the summit of Everest. A further widening of my horizons came when a mountaineering colleague, John Clegg, arrived with a hypobaric chamber in which we started to keep rats and mice. We began to consider hypoxia of the lung in many contexts, its role in the healthy fetus and in the adult and its effects on mountaineers and high-altitude dwellers and in our laboratory animals. We looked for similarities and differences. Why, for example, do the pa-

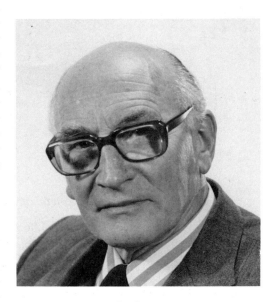

**Figure 5.** Charles Stuart-Harris.

tients with hypoxic lung disease, aptly named "blue bloaters," die, whereas dwellers at very high altitudes are capable of sustaining heavy exercise? What is the cause of the mountain sickness so common among climbers? Our laboratory animals were subjected to conditions that mimicked these states.

## Role of Blood-Gas Tensions in Unventilated Lung and Response Curves of Lung Vessels to Hypoxia and Hypercapnia

We tried to find out whether hypoxia caused blood flow changes in collapsed lungs. In cats we measured blood flow in a loop in the left pulmonary artery, which had a connection to the left carotid artery. On occlusion of the left bronchus during normal perfusion with venous blood, the flow to this lung fell rapidly as before. When we switched to arterial blood at the same pressure, the control flow rate was almost restored, and it fell again on returning to the venous supply.[10] (Fig. 6, top). Pressure-flow lines shifted during collapse, as in Figure 3, but returned nearly or wholly to the control position during continued collapse with arterial blood perfusion (Fig. 6, bottom). Thus some property of venous blood rather than a mechanical effect caused flow to fall; the low $PO_2$ in venous blood was a likely candidate.

We set out to determine the quantitative relationship between blood flow and blood-gas tensions. We devised circuits in which the left lower lobe of lung was autoperfused under controlled conditions and separately ventilated with different gas mixtures. In dogs and cats we put a loop into the vein, draining this lobe in which we could measure flow and pressure and sample blood for gas tensions.[11] When we ventilated this test lobe with decreasing $O_2$ concentrations or increas-

ing $CO_2$ concentrations, each step led to a fall in blood flow (Fig. 7), but there was little or no change in pulmonary arterial pressure or left atrial pressure. From measurements of blood-gas tensions in the effluent blood we were able to plot the relationship between blood flow % control and both $PO_2$ and $PCO_2$. Hypoxia led to an S-shaped curve. There was a slow fall in flow above normal oxygen tensions followed by a steeper fall within the physiological range. The arteriovenous difference in $PO_2$ caused a mean 47% fall in flow in cats, rather less in dogs; this reduction would be expected in unventilated areas of lung. There was a curvilinear relationship between flow and $PCO_2$, but the arteriovenous difference was associated with only a 6% fall in flow. Thus one would expect hypoxia to be the most important factor in ventilation-perfusion matching. It was of much interest to us that the flow-$PO_2$ curve resembled in shape and $PO_2$ range the curve relating $PO_2$ to ventilation and also the relation between $PO_2$ and impulse traffic in the carotid nerve. A similar sensor might detect $PO_2$ in these two organs, as once suggested by Torrance.[48]

We had problems with this paper as well. A referee for one eminent journal asked, "Why did you try two species?" Such miseries have to be borne. Another important journal took the paper at once. Figure 8 shows similar curves measured during hypoxia in ferret lungs in vivo.[47] On the left are flow-$PO_2$ lines, and on the right are lines relating pulmonary arterial pressure to $PO_2$ in a second preparation; the lobe was perfused with blood drawn from the right atrium at a constant flow rate. These curves show the expected changes in pressure if the whole lung becomes hypoxic, as in an hypoxic environment at high altitude or when insufficient oxygen enters the body because of lung disease. The curves on the left, like those in Figure 7 for the cat, show how local hypoxia may divert blood away from hy-

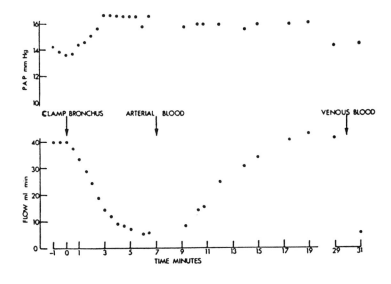

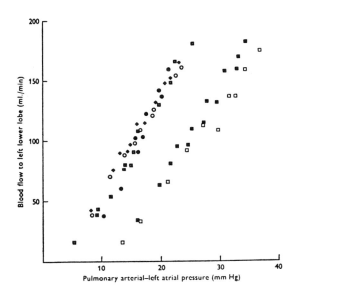

**Figure 6.** Effect of collapse of a lung perfused with arterial or venous blood: Above: Anaesthetized cat. Measurements of blood flow and pulmonary arterial pressure in a loop in the left pulmonary artery. A connection to a carotid artery permits perfusion with arterial blood. Blood flow falls on bronchial occlusion, while the lobe receives its normal pulmonary arterial supply (venous blood). A switch to carotid arterial blood at the same pressure restores flow, while a return to venous blood again reduces flow. Below: Anaesthetized dog. Pressure/flow lines measured during ventilation or collapse during perfusion with arterial or venous blood as in cat, above. Ventilated, arterial (○), venous (◆), Collapsed, venous (■), arterial (●), venous (□). Reexpanded, venous (❑).

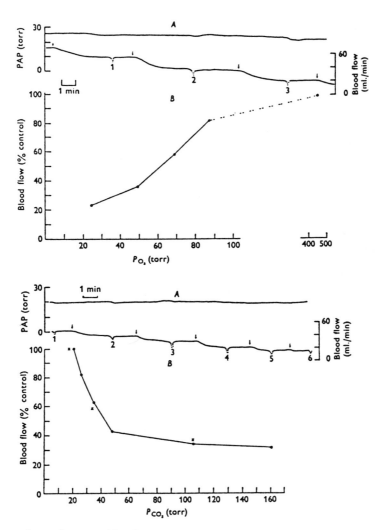

**Figure 7.** Relation between blood–gas tensions and local blood flow. Anaesthetized cats. Blood flow and gas tensions were measured in a loop in the left lower lobe pulmonary vein: pulmonary arterial pressure was measured in the main pulmonary artery. Above: A, test lobe ventilated with increasingly hypoxic gas mixtures (at arrows); flow fell at each change. B. $PO_2$ in effluent blood, measured at 1, 2, 3, etc., is plotted against blood flow, % control. Below: A, test lobe ventilated with progressively higher concentrations of $CO_2$ in air (at arrows); B, $PCO_2$ is plotted against flow, % control. (Reproduced with permission from reference 11.)

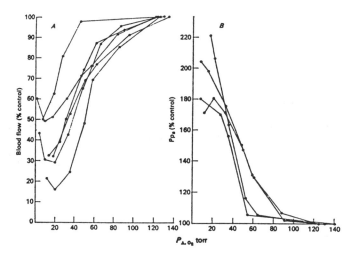

**Figure 8.** Local hypoxia causes flow diversion; general hypoxia raises pulmonary artery pressure: ferrets. A: 6 ferrets. Blood flow % control related to alveolar $PO_2$ (measured by mass spectrometry), circuit as in Figure 6; flow is diverted to better ventilated lung in local hypoxia. B: 4 ferrets. Venous blood from right atrium is pumped at constant flow to left lower lobe pulmonary artery. Lobe ventilated with decreasing $O_2$ concentrations. Pressure rises with each change in $PO_2$ as in generalized hypoxia in the lung. (Reproduced with permission from Barer et al. *J. Physiol* 281: 40–41P, 1978.)

poxic regions of lung. For both sets of curves the $PO_2$ for half the maximal effect is about 45 mmHg.

We compared the stimulus-response curves to hypoxia and hypercapnia with the changes seen in collapsed lungs (Fig. 9). If lungs were ventilated with oxygen briefly before collapse, we noticed in both cats and dogs that the reduction in flow after bronchial occlusion took place in two phases.[11] In phase 1, $PO_2$ remained high as there was a store of oxygen, whereas $PCO_2$ rose and pH fell; phase 2 coincided with a fall in $O_2$ tension. We measured gas tensions in the two phases and compared that reduction in flow at these times with the reductions caused by hypoxia or hypercapnia of similar degree in the same lobe. The lower part of Figure 7 shows that the flow changes in phase 1 of collapse fitted well with changes caused by hypercapnia, whereas on the right a good correlation is shown between the reductions in flow in phase 2 of collapse and those due to hypoxia. It is probable, therefore, that the effect of collapse

under these experimental conditions is due to the combined effects of hypoxia and hypercapnia.

Is this mechanism important in adult humans? At first thought, the very low $PaO_2$ seen in patients with hypoxic lung disease suggests that it is not. However, the damage to their lungs is so widespread that a shutdown of all affected areas would not be possible; the whole cardiac output must pass through the lung. Marshall and Marshall were later to show in dogs that hypoxic diversion of flow becomes less effective the larger the area that is made hypoxic; it is replaced by a rise in pressure, as we saw in Figure 8, right.[36] Also, in these patients bronchoconstrictor drugs that are also vasodilators (aminophylline, isoprenaline) sometimes reduce arterial $PO_2$; this could be due to an increase in blood flow through poorly ventilated areas of lung. Yet the view is held by some that hypoxic vasoconstriction in adults is only a vestige of an important fetal mechanism; in the fetus it diverts blood flow away from the non-

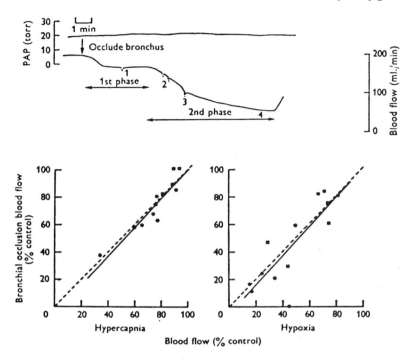

**Figure 9.** Correlation of flow changes in unventilated lung with flow changes caused by hypoxia and hypercapnia. Above: Flow changes in cat during collapse of left lower lobe after brief preventilation with 100% $O_2$, pulmonary venous loop preparation. Blood flow falls in 2 phases. In phase 1, $PO_2$ remains high but $PCO_2$ rises, whereas in phase 2 $PO_2$ falls. Below: Correlation in cats (●) and dogs (■) left, of flow changes in phase 1 with flow changes caused by hypercapnia of similar degree in same lobe and right; correlation of flow changes in phase 2 with those of similar degree of hypoxia. Solid lines = regression lines, dashed lines = lines of identity. (Compiled from reference 11.)

ventilated lung through the ductus arteriosus and towards the umbilical artery. Yet diversion of blood flow from hypoxic lung regions has been clearly shown in humans,[19] and in certain postures changes in ventilation-perfusion measurements during hyperoxia suggest redistribution of flow.[1] In humans generalized hypoxia certainly leads to a rise in pulmonary arterial pressure. In hypoxic sleep apnoea, pressure also rises. In our experiments the changes in blood flow with gas tensions were of the same order as those found in fetal lambs. So there is probably some redistribution of flow in favour of better ventilated regions, although calculations have shown that the gain of the mechanism is not great.[23] Without evidence I am predisposed to think that when we doze in

lectures, some lung units may close and their blood flow diminish, to open again when we yawn.

## Chronic Effects of Hypoxia on the Pulmonary Circulation

In the 1970s we began to study the effects of prolonged exposure to hypoxia in rats and mice. We hoped to throw light on changes in patients and highlanders and perhaps to find means of preventing or reversing them. We used either a hypobaric chamber at half an atmosphere or a normobaric chamber at 10% or 12% $O_2$; $CO_2$ levels were kept normal. We detected no difference between results with the two chambers. We looked first to see whether the arteries had become more muscular. There seemed to be a change in wall thickness in very small vessels, but we could not pinpoint it in routine sections. After more than a year of effort, a pathology technician suggested an elastic stain might be helpful. We used one and immediately saw that the small pulmonary arterioles, which are normally thin-walled with little or no muscle and only one elastic lamina, had developed a second internal elastic lamina bounding a new muscular coat.[32] Later measurements with the lung perfused with contrast medium at known pressures showed that the lumen was narrowed 10–14%, a change with profound haemodynamic consequences.[22] We sent a slide to Professor Donald Heath, who replied that the changes closely resembled those he had found in his bronchitic patients. This was the first of many fruitful exchanges. The crucial observation was that there was peripheral extension of new muscle to tiny vessels beside alveolar ducts and among alveoli. The proportion of these "thick-walled peripheral vessels" increased several fold in chronically hypoxic rats and mice. Also the right ventricle became hypertrophied, the packed cell volume increased, and pulmonary arterial pressure rose.[32]

Pulmonary arterial pressure was measured with a special catheter designed by Dr. Jan Herget, visiting us from Prague; it could be introduced into the pulmonary artery of anaesthetized rats.[27] The mean value in normal rats was 16 mmHg, whereas in rats exposed for several weeks to 10% $O_2$ it was 36 mmHg when they were breathing air. Thus the rise was not due to hypoxic vasoconstriction but to structural changes and to the increased blood viscosity caused by polycythaemia. After 6 weeks recovery in air, the mean pressure was still 27 mmHg, but it was back to normal after 20 weeks in air. These pressures corresponded with the vascular changes. The muscularization appeared fully developed after 10 days hypoxia but was still raised after 6 weeks in air; after 20 weeks recovery we could still detect some residual abnormalities in these vessels.[29] So there was rapid remodeling but slow resolution, which has implications for disease states and recovery. Yet the right ventricular hypertrophy and polycythaemia resolved more quickly. It seems that different growth factors and stimuli cause different changes. This is an area of great current interest and importance. During the events and illnesses of life our bodies are subject to changes of which we are quite unaware.

Some diverse observations on these rats may bear fruit in the future. Growth changes observed during hypoxic exposure might be relevant to hypoxic episodes during growth in humans. The lung and chest grew abnormally fast relative to body size, for skeletal growth and weight increase were retarded. In young animals, lung size did not return to "normal" after recovery in air.[32] Then, with possible relevance to clotting problems at high altitude, platelet volume was increased, a change associated in other circumstances with increased platelet activity. Also the megakaryocytes in bone marrow from which platelets are derived showed an increase in polyploidy.[8] We also found that the endocrine cells in the conducting airway and alveolar walls contained more calcitonin-gene-related peptide than normal.[45] We have no idea what this could mean; indeed we have no notion of the function of these endocrine cells.

Haemodynamic consequences of hypoxic exposure were demonstrated by measurement of pressure-flow relations in isolated blood-perfused rat lungs; left atrial pressure was zero.[20,16] Figure 9 shows mean lines for groups of rats measured during air ventilation (look only at lines CS and CHS; the other lines are described below). Note that by this time we plotted the lines correctly, with flow as the independent variable on the abscissa!

Compared with control rats, line CS, the line for chronically hypoxic rats, CHS, is steeper and has a larger projected intercept on the pressure axis. We attribute the intercept to activity of the small, newly muscularized vessels in a state of tone, which now forms the downstream pressure for flow. The increased slope, which is a measure of resistance in larger vessels as opposed to resistor properties of small collapsible vessels, could have several causes. We found arterial compliance reduced; the vessels were stiffer, which could be due to deposition of new connective tissue in the walls of larger vessels. Alternatively the volume of the vascular bed could be smaller. Pressure in the rat and human pulmonary circulations is similar, although the flow in the latter is at least 100 times greater. However, vascular volume measured with [125]-I-labeled serum albumin was similar to normal rats; this is an expression of the relatively large lung size in these rats. In these tests, both groups of lungs were perfused with normal blood of normal haematocrit; in chronic hypoxia there was polycythaemia, which made a substantial contribution to vascular resistance, as we found when we varied the haematocrit artificially.[8]

Like others, we tried to find drugs that would prevent or reverse the high pressure and structural changes of chronic hypoxia. We had some success with α methyl dopa, which, given daily during exposure, attenuated pulmonary hypertension, right ventricular hypertrophy, and muscularization of arterioles.[28] The basis of this effect is obscure. More exciting was a drug brought to us by Professor Yingnian Cai from Beijing. It was ligustrazine, synthesized principle of an ancient Chinese herbal remedy grown in peasants' gardens and used for more than 2,000 years for "heart disease." It proved to be a potent pulmonary vasodilator. When given daily during hypoxic exposure, it attenuated the right ventricular

hypertrophy, pulmonary hypertension, and vascular changes.[16] Figure 10 shows the results. There were four groups of rats: controls treated with saline (CS), controls treated with ligustrazine (CL), chronically hypoxic rats treated with saline (CHS), and chronically hypoxic rats treated with ligustrazine (CHL). The saline-treated

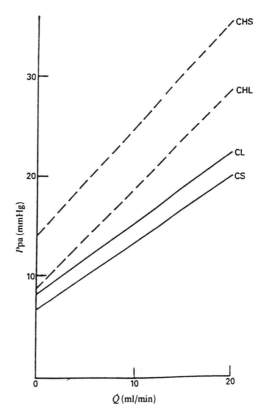

**Figure 10.** Altered pressure/flow lines in chronically hypoxic rat lungs: the effect of ligustrazine. Mean pressure/flow lines from four groups of rats measured in isolated blood-perfused lungs. (1) CS 5 control rat lungs, treatment with 0.9% saline (placebo); (2) CL 5 control rats treated with ligustrazine; (3) CHS 11 rats exposed to 10% $O_2$ for 2 weeks treated with saline; (4) CHL 11 rats similarly exposed treated with ligustrazine. Note steeper lines and higher intercept on pressure axis in CHS compared with CS rats. Ligustrazine has no effect in control rats, but in chronically hypoxic rats the intercept is normal, the slope unaltered. (Reproduced with permission from reference 16.)

lines have already been described; they are similar to those always found in normal and hypoxia-exposed rats. The controls treated with the drug had an unchanged line, but the chronically hypoxic treated rats had a line whose slope was unchanged but whose intercept had returned to control values. Thus only one feature of the remodeled vascular bed was altered, and we expected that this would prove to be the muscularization of arterioles. Indeed our count of thick-walled peripheral vessels in the ligustrazine-treated chronically hypoxic rats was significantly less than that in the saline-treated group. This very interesting finding requires further confirmation. The unchanged slope suggests that changes in larger vessels, perhaps stiffening due to connective tissue proliferation, was undiminished.

## Reactivity of the Pulmonary Circulation in Chronically Hypoxic Rats

We looked to see whether the chronically hypoxic rat pulmonary circulation had abnormal responses to natural stimuli and drugs. In the perfused lung of normal rats, almost no tone can be demonstrated, as in the normal human lung—that is, vasodilator drugs have little or no effect unless there is preconstriction. In the chronically hypoxic rat, as in human hypertensive pulmonary disease, there is resting "tone," and dilatation is easily shown. We perfused the lungs with blood and defined reactivity as the rise or fall in pulmonary arterial pressure at constant flow. This is a superficial definition, but it describes the change the right heart experiences during systole. Responses to vasoconstrictor substances (angiotensin I and II, PGF2α), dilator substances (isoprenaline, adenosine) and substances with mixed effects (bradykinin, ATP, histamine, arachidonic acid, platelet-activating factor) were enhanced.[5,20,42] Increased muscularity, increased tone, and narrowed lumen could account for most of these changes. However, there were peculiar changes in hypoxic vasoconstriction. We found in young rats of our strain an increased response to hypoxia over a wide range of oxygen tensions, as in Figure 11.[20] However, the group in Denver and Dr. Kentera in Belgrade found exactly the opposite. Responses to hypoxia were attenuated, despite more muscular vessels.[37,34] Once again differences stimulated further research, and it became clear that enhancement or attenuation depended on the age and strain of rat and on the length of hypoxic exposure. An exaggerated response was always found after a few days' recovery and a diminished response after only 36–48 hours of hypoxic exposure. It seems that there is a balance between the effects of increased muscle and metabolic changes.[14] Metabolic changes could be due to changed activity of the endothelium adjacent to the new muscle, to special properties of the new muscle, or to altered numbers or expression of receptors. Reactivity changes could have important consequences during development of pulmonary vascular disease.

## Oedema of Hypoxic Exposure

We tried hard to reproduce the forms of oedema associated with hypoxia. Mountaineers and high-altitude residents are sometimes afflicted by pulmonary oedema that can be fatal. Patients with hypoxic lung disease frequently develop systemic oedema. Our rats exposed to 10 or even 8% $O_2$ did not develop oedema, nor, when we measured fluid and sodium balance, could we detect retention of either. However, when we tried to mimic the circumstances in which mountaineers and highlanders get pulmonary oedema, we had partial success.[43] Highlanders who spend some time at sea level and then

**Pulmonary vessels in chronic hypoxia**

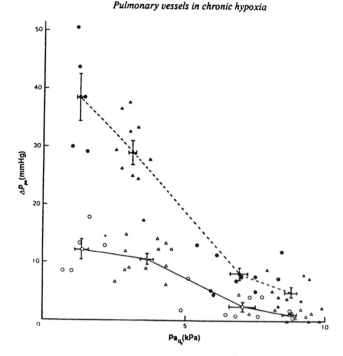

**Figure 11.** Changed reactivity to hypoxia in chronically hypoxic rats. Relation between effluent blood $PO_2$ and pulmonary arterial pressure in control (open symbols, solid line) and chronically hypoxic rats (closed symbols dashed line) in isolated blood-perfused lungs during ventilation with increasing hypoxia; four $O_2$ mixtures, represented by different symbols, were used. Points represent mean pulmonary arterial pressure and mean $PO_2 \pm$ SEM for each level of hypoxia. (Reproduced with permission from reference 20.)

return home are prone to pulmonary oedema. We kept rats for several weeks in hypoxia, allowed them to recover in air for a few days, and then returned them to the hypoxic environment. They developed oedema of the alveolar wall but not florid oedema in alveolar spaces. Mountaineers are susceptible to oedema when they first ascend to high altitude. So we placed unadapted rats in severe hypoxic surroundings for a few hours and found that the endothelium of alveolar capillaries became detached and formed bullae that obstructed the capillaries. Professor Heath's group had also made this observation.

We never succeeded in causing systemic oedema but made observations that might provide a clue for future research.

The prevailing view has been that the systemic oedema of chronic hypoxic lung disease is due to right heart failure secondary to pulmonary hypertension. Yet the cardiac output remains normal until near death, and the hypertension is mild. The Sheffield group found in the 1950s that these patients had an unexplained reduction in renal plasma flow.[46] An alternative hypothesis emerged that fluid and sodium retention could be due to disturbance of mechanisms that control water and sodium balance. Honig had shown in cats that hypoxia caused a diuresis and natriuresis, which was due to a carotid body reflex; the efferent limb of the reflex seemed to involve release of a hormone.[30] He also deduced from the literature that in severe hypoxia there is, by contrast, water and sodium retention. Karim et al. have shown this in dogs and think it also due to a carotid body reflex, which in this case causes a reduction in renal blood flow through sympathetic nervous activity.[33]

In the 1970s we had been introduced to the extraordinary drug almitrine, which has the unique property of mimicking the positive actions of hypoxia both at the carotid body, where it causes reflex stimulation of respiration, and in the pulmonary circulation, where it causes vasoconstriction (though this action is more complex). Honig had shown that almitrine also caused natriuresis in cats. In our group P. Bardsley extended these observations and showed that almitrine causes a reflex diuresis and natriuresis abolished by section of the carotid nerve in rats. Because the effect is seen in rats with only one transplanted and therefore denervated kidney,[3] the effect must be attributed to a hormone. Could it be, in severe hypoxic disease, that the natriuretic reflex is overwhelmed by the one in which there is reflex neural reduction in renal blood flow?

## The Carotid Body in Hypoxia: Structure and Function

The carotid body and the pulmonary vessels are the only sites known where hypoxia causes a positive change, an increase in ventilation and vasoconstriction. Both tissues are derived from branchial arches, and several functional links between them have been detected whose importance remains obscure.

In those humans with hypoxic lung disease or who live at high altitude, the carotid body is abnormally large. We found similar enlargement in rats exposed either to hypobaric or normobaric hypoxia. Initially we did this work with Donald Heath's group.[6] Figure 12 shows gross enlargement in a chronically hypoxic rat. The blood vessels are greatly dilated. Using morphometric techniques derived from the work of Ewald Weibel, we found other important changes. The number of Type I and endothelial cells and the amount of connective tissue increased; angiogenesis occurred. The harmonic mean distance between the capillaries and glomus tissue, a measure of diffusion distance, was reduced.[17]

While I was reporting this work at a symposium on the carotid body, someone shouted out, "You are wrong. Type 1 cells are neurons; they can't divide." I am glad to say that we identified cell division in Type 1 cells after 1–4 days hypoxia by arresting mitosis in metaphase with vincristine, as shown in Figure 9.[13] The cells are identified by their dense-cored vesicles, which contain dopamine. We do not know what these growth changes mean, but they suggest that the carotid body is a labile organ. Its size was reduced but not normal after 4 weeks in air.

A characteristic of long-term residents at high altitude is that they have a blunted ventilatory response to hypoxia. Figure 13 shows that our rats, immediately after removal from the hypoxic chamber, also had a response curve to hypoxia that was lower than that of the controls.[6,49] Moreover, the relationship between almitrine dose and ventilation was also lower.[49] We were excited about this, as it seemed to reproduce the high-altitude state. Disappointingly, the hypoxic response returned to normal after a few days in air,[6] so we do not know if the reduced response is the beginning of "blunting." We did, however, observe that dopamine, an inhibitor of carotid body stimulation by hypoxia, was present in increased quantities in the carotid bodies of these rats. When we gave normal and chronically hypoxic rats a dopamine 2 inhibitor, domperidone, ventilation increased in both groups. The increase was greater in the chronically hypoxic group. The difference between chronically hypoxic and control rats was wiped out, and response curves to

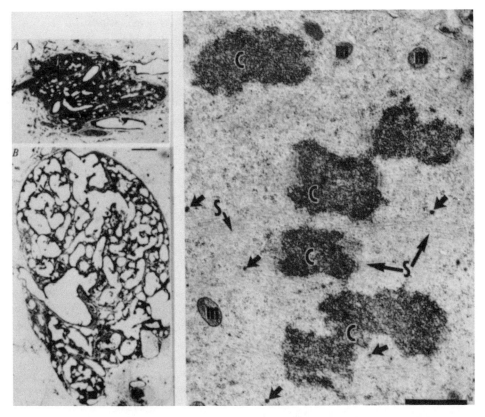

**Figure 12.** The rat carotid body in chronic hypoxia. Left: A, light photomicrograph of normal rat carotid body. B, section of carotid body from rat exposed to 10% $O_2$ for 4 weeks (Note enlargement and dilatation of capillaries). Right: Electron micrograph of Type I cell from carotid body of rat exposed 2 days to 10% $O_2$, identified by dense-cored vesicles (small arrows). Chromosomes are lined up on spindle fibres (s). Mitosis arrested in metaphase by vincristine. (Compiled from references 13 and 17.)

both hypoxia and almitrine were superimposed. Several explanations have been advanced for the blunted ventilatory response to hypoxia at high altitude; a local dopaminergic mechanism is yet another.

## Site of Hypoxic and Almitrine Vasoconstriction in Normal and Chronically Hypoxic Rats

In the 1980s we examined the effect on hypoxic vasoconstriction of inflating the lung to high alveolar pressures. One must admit that the motive for conducting

experiments is often evident in retrospect when, at the time, one was just following one's nose. Looking back I believe we thought that, when alveolar pressure exceeds left atrial pressure, any vasomotor effects detected would be occurring in upstream vessels. We measured pressure-flow lines in isolated perfused rat lungs during lung inflation to an alveolar pressure of 5 and then 15 mmHg while the left atrial pressure was $\leq 0.50$ Figure 14 shows mean lines for groups of normal rats on the left and chronically hypoxic rats on the right. The solid lines, measured during normoxia, shift about 10 mmHg in a parallel fashion when the alveolar pressure is

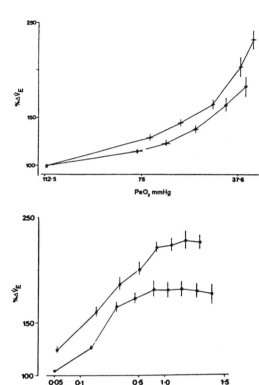

**Figure 13.** Attenuated Ventilatory Responses to hypoxia and almitrine in chronically hypoxic rats. Ventilation measured under anaesthesia immediately after removal of rats from hypoxic chamber (exposure 2–5 weeks at 10% $O_2$) and in control rats of comparable age. Initial ventilation was similar in the two groups; % increase in $\dot{V}_E$ with the stimulus is plotted. For each experiment the control rats showed greater increases in ventilation (upper lines). Above: relation between $PO_2$ during progressive nonisocapnic hypoxia and increase in ventilation in 8 control and 10 chronically hypoxic rats. Below: relation between almitrine dose (cumulative doses during continuous infusion) and increase in ventilation in the same groups of rats, breathing air, $CO_2$ not controlled. (Modified from reference 49.)

hypoxic rats some muscular action must be causing the higher intercepts. During hypoxic vasoconstriction, dashed lines, the lines at the lower alveolar pressure, become steeper, with a higher intercept in both groups of rats attributable to muscle action. At the high inflation pressure of 15 mmHg, the two groups respond very differently. In controls the line shifts by much less than 10, whereas in chronically hypoxics it shifts by greater than 10 mmHg.

Virtually identical results were found during almitrine vasoconstriction. A possible explanation is illustrated in a diagram that we owe to a most helpful correspondence with Dr. Richard Riley. It shows that, in a normal rat, hypoxia or almitrine may cause constriction in small, collapsible vessels upstream from alveoli to form Starling resistors and become the downstream pressure. A rise in alveolar pressure is not transmitted to pulmonary arterial pressure until it is high enough to open up the Starling resistor and become once more the downstream pressure. Note that the intercept has come back to about 15 mmHg in the control group. However, in the chronically hypoxic rat, the new smooth muscle extends down to tiny precapillary vessels, which are surrounded by alveoli. During vasoconstriction these vessels form Starling resistors and create the downstream pressure. The high alveolar pressure sums with the muscular activity in these vessels and in some way enhances it; this pressure is fully transmitted to pulmonary arterial pressure. This explanation fits the facts and implies that in chronic hypoxia the main site of hypoxic and almitrine vasoconstriction has moved peripherally to the newly muscularized arterioles. However, some anomalies remained, which are evident in our paper.[50] The implications of this change for pulmonary function cannot be imagined at present. In hypoxic lung disease and also in chronically hypoxic rats,[9] the lung is held at a higher volume than normal so that

raised from 5 to 10 mmHg, although the chronically hypoxic rats have steeper slopes and higher intercepts. Note that in the controls the intercepts are very close to alveolar pressure, which therefore forms the downstream pressure. In chronically

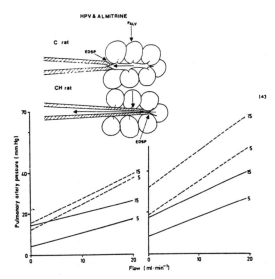

**Figure 14.** Changed effect of hypoxia during lung inflation in chronically hypoxic rats. Mean pressure/flow lines from 9 control (left) and 11 chronically hypoxic rats (right) during inflation of the lungs to 5 and 15 mmHg alveolar pressure in normoxia (solid lines) and hypoxia (broken lines). Note big difference in effect of high pressure inflation during hypoxia in the two rat groups. Diagram, top left, shows a possible explanation that depends on the peripheral extension of new arteriolar muscle into the alveolar region of lung in chronically hypoxic rats. EDSP = effective downstream pressure caused by development of "Starling resistors" during vasoconstriction; see text. (Modified from reference 50.)

these observations might have importance.

### Implications of Endothelial Damage for the Pulmonary Circulation: Endothelial Control Mechanisms

Damage to the endothelium and intimal coat is a central feature of much hypertensive pulmonary vascular disease. Thus our aims at the time of writing were to cause endothelial damage in the lung and to determine the role of endothelial-derived factors in controlling the pulmonary circulation. In the systemic circulation Moncada and colleagues have shown that the endothelial-derived relaxant factor, nitric oxide, is continuously released and attenuates pressure.[38] Is it responsible for the low vascular tone of the normal pulmonary circulation? Some years back it was suggested that this low tone might be actively maintained.[51] Our results so far suggest that continuous release of nitric oxide cannot be the cause. Synthesis of nitric oxide from L-arginine in endothelial cells can be inhibited by L-arginine analogues. Two such analogues had trivial effects on pulmonary arterial pressure in normal rat lungs ventilated with air but raised pressure substantially in lungs of chronically hypoxic rats.[7] Perhaps some change in the chronically hypoxic hypertensive rat lung stimulates release of nitric oxide, which then attenuates pressure through a negative feedback. If endothelium is damaged in pulmonary vascular disease, could the loss of this restraining effect of nitric oxide be responsible for the precipitate rises in pressure sometimes encountered? In severe pulmonary vascular disease, dilator therapy may be required, for example, in preparation for lung transplantation. We may need dilator drugs that are endothelial independent. Our Chinese herbal remedy proved to be endothelial independent!

### Vale!

As the journey nears its end one should take stock. Luck, help, the patience of great teachers, and constant support of a life partner have made a research life possible. Above all it has been fun, but has anything substantial been achieved? Individually very little, but with the efforts of fine colleagues and good friends the world over, we have made progress. We have not solved hypoxic vasoconstriction in the past 45 years, but we no longer think that alveolar capillaries are in direct contact with air. Looking back, what was better and what was worse 40 years ago? Apparatus is now more complex and difficult to maintain and design oneself. Statistics, which then took weeks to calculate, now take minutes, but the maxim remains true that in biology if an effect is "genuine" statistics are unnecessary. Free exchange of ideas, so crucial to science and medicine, was once taken for granted. I believe it must now be defended. It retreats a little before severe competition for grants and jobs; equipment is much more expensive, and it is tempting to keep one's ideas secret to be "first." Then in Britain there is ALF. The Animal Liberation Front attracts criminals prepared to kill humans, steal animals, and "liberate" them in midwinter, only to be destroyed by predators. But it also attracts civilized people who teach us to consider animal suffering as we do our own. In every experiment human and animal rights must be balanced.

The curiosity bug will never be satisfied, and our ignorance remains very great.

**Acknowledgments:** I thank Professor Geoffrey Dawes and Professor Sir Charles Stuart-Harris for their help and support, which have made this journey possible. Among my many splendid colleagues, I specially thank Derek Wyatt, Alan Ryder, Peter Howard, John Clegg, Christine Brown, Graham Tate, Celia Emery, Enid Leach, Jan Herget, Andrew Suggett, Denise Bee, and Richard Wach. I have drawn heavily on work they have done, as well as work we have done together. Finally, to Robert Barer and our family, I owe everything.

# References

1. Arborelius, M., V. Granquist, B. Lilja, and C. W. Zanner. Regional lung function and central haemodynamics in the right lateral body position during hypoxia and hyperoxia. *Respiration* 31: 193–200, 1974.
2. Banister, J., and R. W. Torrance. The effects of tracheal pressure on pressure-flow relations in the vascular bed of isolated lungs. *Q. J. Exp. Physiol.* 45: 352–367, 1960.
3. Bardsley, P. A., B. J. Johnson, A. G. Stewart, and G. R. Barer. Natriuresis secondary to carotid body stimulation with almitrine bismesylate in the rat: the effect on kidney function and the response to renal denervation and deficiency of antidiuretic hormone. *Biomed. Biochim. Acta.* 50: 175–182, 1991.
4. Barer, G. R. Reactivity of the vessels of collapsed and ventilated lungs to drugs and hypoxia. *Circ. Res.* 18: 366–378, 1966.
5. Barer, G. R., Y. Cai, P. C. Russell, and C. J. Emery. Reactivity and site of vasomotion in pulmonary vessels of chronically hypoxic rats; relation to structural changes. *Amer. Rev. Respir. Dis.* 140: 1483–1485, 1989.
6. Barer, G. R., C. Edwards, and A. I. Jolly. Changes in the carotid body and the ventilatory response to hypoxia in the chronically hypoxic rat. *Clin. Sci.* 50: 311–313, 1976.
7. Barer, G. R., C. Emery, A. Stewart, D. Bee, and P. Howard. Endothelial control of the pulmonary circulation in normal and chronically hypoxic rats. *J. Physiol.* 463: 1–16, 1993.
8. Barer, G. R., C. J. Emery, D. Bee, and R. A. Wach. Mechanisms of pulmonary hypertension: an overview. In: *The Pulmonary Circulation in Health and Disease,* edited by J. A. Will, C. A. Dawson, E. K. Weir, and C. K. Buckner. Orlando, FL: 1 Academic, p. 409–422.
9. Barer, G. R., J. Herget, P. J. M. Sloan, and A. J. Suggett. The effect of acute and chronic hypoxia on thoracic gas volume in anaesthetized rats. *J. Physiol.* 277: 177–192, 1978.
10. Barer, G. R., P. Howard, J. R. McCurrie, and J. W. Shaw. Changes in the pulmonary circulation after bronchial occlusion in anaesthetized dogs and cats. *Circ. Res.* 25: 747–764, 1969.
11. Barer, G. R., P. Howard, and J. W. Shaw. Stimulus-response curves for the pulmonary vascular bed to hypoxia and hypercapnia. *J. Physiol.* 211: 139–155, 1970.
12. Barer, G. R., and E. Nusser. Pulmonary blood flow in the cat: the effect of positive pressure respiration. *J. Physiol.* 138: 103–118, 1957.
13. Bee, D., D. J. Pallot, and G. R. Barer. Division of Type 1 and endothelial cells in the hypoxic rat carotid body. *Acta Anatomica* 126: 226–229, 1986.
14. Bee, D., and R. A. Wach. Hypoxic pulmonary vasoconstriction in chronically hypoxic rats. *Respir. Physiol.* 56: 91–103, 1984.

15. Burton, A. C. On the physical equilibrium of small blood vessels. *Amer. J. Physiol.* 164: 319–329, 1951.

16. Cai, Y. N., and G. R. Barer. Effect of ligustrazine on pulmonary vascular changes induced by chronic hypoxia in the rat. *Clin. Sci.* 77: 515–520, 1989.

17. Dhillon, D. P., G. R. Barer, and M. Walsh. The enlarged carotid body of the chronically hypoxic and hypercapnic rat: a morphometric analysis. *Q. J. Exp. Physiol.* 69: 301–317, 1984.

18. Duke, H. N. Pulmonary vasomotor responses of isolated perfused cat lungs to anoxia and hypercapnia. *Q. J. Exper. Physiol.* 36: 75–88, 1951.

19. Durand, J., M. Leroy Ladurie, B. Ranson-Bitker. Effects of hypoxia and hypercapnia on the repartition of pulmonary blood flow in supine subjects. *Prog. Resp. Res.* 5 (*Pul. Circ.*): 156–165, 1970.

20. Emery, C. J., D. Bee, and G. R. Barer. Mechanical properties and reactivity of vessels in isolated perfused lungs of chronically hypoxic rats. *Clin. Sci.* 61: 569–580, 1981.

21. Euler, U. S. von, and G. Liljestrand. Observations on the pulmonary arterial blood pressure in the cat. *Acta. Physiol. Scand.* 12: 301–320, 1946.

22. Finlay, M., G. R. Barer, and A. J. Suggett. Quantitative changes in rat pulmonary vasculature in chronic hypoxia: relation to haemodynamic changes. *Q. J. Exp. Physiol.* 71: 151–163, 1986.

23. Grant, B. J. B., E. E. Davies, H. A. Jones, and J. M. B. Hughes. Local regulation of pulmonary blood flow and ventilation-perfusion ratios in the coatimundi. *J. Appl. Physiol.* 40: 216–228, 1976.

24. Harvey, W. *An Anatomical Disputation Concerning the Movement of the Heart and Lung in Living Creatures,* [1628], translated by Gweneth Whitteridge. Oxford: Blackwell, 1976.

25. Hauge, A. Role of histamine in hypoxic pulmonary hypertension in the rat 1: blockage or potentiation of endogenous amines kinins and ATP. *Circ. Res.* 22: 371–383, 1968.

26. Hauge, A., and K. L. Melmon. Role of histamine in hypoxic pulmonary hypertension in the rat 11: depletion of histamine, serotonin and catecholamines. *Circ. Res.* 22: 385–392, 1968.

27. Herget, J., and F. Palecek. Pulmonary arterial blood pressure in closed chest rats: changes after catecholamines, histamine and serotonin. *Arch. Internat. de Phar-*

*mocdynamie et de Therapie* 198: 107–117, 1972.

28. Herget, J., and A. J. Suggett. Effect of α methyl dopa on the pulmonary vascular changes induced by chronic hypoxia in the rat. *Clin. Sci.* 53: 397–400, 1977.

29. Herget, J., A. J. Suggett, E. Leach, and G. R. Barer. Resolution of pulmonary hypertension and other features induced by chronic hypoxia in rats during complete and intermittent normoxia. *Thorax* 33: 468–473, 1978.

30. Honig, A. Role of arterial chemoreceptors in the reflex control of renal function and body fluid volumes in acute arterial hypoxia. In: *Physiology of Arterial Chemoreceptors,* edited by H. Acker and R. O'Regan. Amsterdam: Elsevier, 1983, p. 395–429.

31. Howard, P., G. R. Barer, B. Thompson, P. M. Warren, C. J. Abbott, and I. P. F. Mungall. Factors causing and reversing vasoconstriction in unventilated lung. *Respir. Physiol.* 24: 325–345, 1975.

32. Hunter, C., G. R. Barer, J. W. Shaw, and E. J. Clegg. Growth of the heart and lungs in hypoxic rodents: a model of human hypoxic disease. *Clin. Sci. Molec. Med.* 46: 375–391, 1974.

33. Karim, F., S. M. Poucher, and R. A. Summerhill. The effects of stimulating carotid chemoreceptors on renal haemodynamics and function in dogs. *J. Physiol.* 392: 451–462, 1987.

34. Kentera, D., D. Susic, and V. Kanjuh. Experimental evidence that hypoxic pulmonary hypertension can be altered by drugs. *Progr. Respir. Res.* 30: 26–30, 1985.

35. Lopez-Muniz, R., N. L. Stephens, B. Bromberga-Barnea, S. Permutt, and R. L. Riley. Critical closing pressure of pulmonary vessels analyzed in terms of a Starling resistor model. *J. Appl. Physiol.* 24: 625–635, 1968.

36. Marshall, B. E., C. Marshall, J. Benumof, and L. J. Saidman. Hypoxic pulmonary hypertension in dogs: effect of segment size and oxygen tension. *J. Appl. Physiol.* 51: 1543–1551, 1981.

37. McMurtry, I. F., M. D. Petrun, and J. T. Reeves. Lungs from chronically hypoxic rats have decreased pressor response to acute hypoxia. *Amer. J. Physiol.* 235: H104–H109, 1978.

38. Moncada, S., R. M. J. Palmer, and E. A. Higgs. Nitric oxide: physiology, pathophysiology, and pharmacology. *Pharmacol. Rev.* 43: 109–142, 1991.

39. Nichol, J., F. Girling, W. Jerrard, E. B. Claxton, and A. C. Burton. Fundamental instability of the small blood vessels and critical closing pressure in vascular beds. *Amer. J. Physiol.* 164: 330–344, 1951.

40. Permutt, S., and R. L. Riley. Hemodynamics of collapsible vessels with tone: the vascular waterfall. *J. Appl. Physiol.* 18: 924–932, 1963.

41. Policard, A. Le poumon. 2nd ed. Paris: Masson, 1955, p. 56.

42. Russell, P. C., C. J. Emery, Y. N. Cai, G. R. Barer, and P. Howard. Enhanced reactivity to bradykinin, angtiotensin 1 and the effect of captopril in the pulmonary vasculature of chronically hypoxic rats. *Eur. Respir. J.* 3: 779–785, 1990.

43. Scott, K. W. M., G. R. Barer, E. Leach, and I. P. F. Mungall. Pulmonary ultrastructural changes in hypoxic rats. *J. Path.* 126: 27–33, 1978.

44. Shaw, J. W. Pulmonary vasodilator and vasoconstrictor actions of histamine. *J. Physiol.* 215: 34–35P, 1971.

45. Springall, D. R., G. Collina, G. Barer, A. J. Suggett, D. Bee, and J. M. Polak. Increased intracellular levels of calcitonin-gene-related peptide-like immunoreactivity in pulmonary endocrine cells of hypoxic rats. *J. Path.* 155: 259–267, 1988.

46. Stuart-Harris, C. H., J. McKinnon, J. D. S. Hammond, and W. D. Smith. The renal circulation in chronic pulmonary disease and heart failure. *Q. J. Med.* 25: 389–405, 1956.

47. Suggett, A. J., F. H. Mohammed, G. R. Barer, C. Twelves, and D. Bee. Quantitative significance of hypoxic vasoconstriction in the ferret lung. *Respir. Physiol.* 46: 89–104, 1981.

48. Torrance, R. W. The idea of a chemoreceptor. In: *Pulmonary Circulation and Interstitial Space,* edited by A. P. Fishman and H. H. Hecht. Chicago: University of Chicago Press, 1969, p. 223–237.

49. Wach, R. A., D. Bee, and G. R. Barer. Dopamine and the ventilatory effects of hypoxia and almitrine in chronically hypoxic rats. *J. Appl. Physiol.* 67: 186–192, 1989.

50. Wach, R. A., C. J. Emery, D. Bee, and G. R. Barer. Effect of alveolar pressure on pulmonary artery pressure in chronically hypoxic rats. *Cardiovasc. Res.* 21: 140–150, 1987.

51. Weir, E. K. Does normoxic vasodilation rather than hypoxic vasoconstriction account for the pulmonary pressor response to hypoxia? *Lancet* 1: 476–477, 1978.

52. Wyatt, D. G. A 50 c/s cannulated electromagnetic flowmeter. *Electron. Engng.* 33: 650–655, 1961.